Parkinson's Disease for Dummies®

Michele Tagliati, MD
Gary N. Guten, MD, MA
Jo Horne, MA

16pt

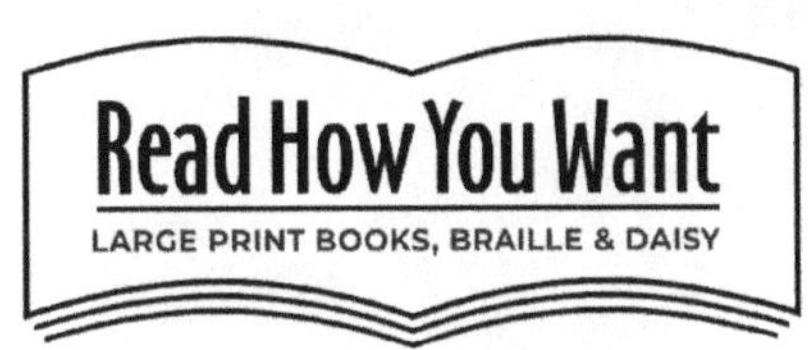

Copyright Page from the Original Book

Parkinson's Disease For Dummies®

Published by
Wiley Publishing, Inc.
111 River St.
Hoboken, NJ 07030-5774
www.wiley.com

Published by Wiley Publishing, Inc., Indianapolis, Indiana
Published simultaneously in Canada

For general information on our other products and services, please contact our Customer Care Department within the U.S. at 800-762-2974, outside the U.S. at 317-572-3993, or fax 317-572-4002.

For technical support, please visit www.wiley.com/techsupport.

Wiley also publishes its books in a variety of electronic formats. Some content that appears in print may not be available in electronic books.

Library of Congress Control Number: 2006939494

ISBN: 978-0-470-07395-7

Manufactured in the United States of America

10 9 8 7 6 5 4 3 2 1

1O/QZ/QR/QX/IN

TABLE OF CONTENTS

Foreword by Deborah W. Brooks

President and CEO of The Michael J. Fox Foundation for Parkinson's Research

About the Authors

Michele Tagliati, MD, is a movement disorders specialist with extensive experience in the diagnosis and treatment of Parkinson's disease. As Director of the Parkinson's Disease Center at Mount Sinai Medical Center in New York, he follows hundreds of patients at several stages of disease progression. He dedicates his professional life to caring for PD patients and developing research protocols that will ultimately improve their condition. In particular, Dr. Tagliati is a leader in the field of deep brain stimulation for PD and dystonia. He currently serves as teaching faculty at the annual courses given on DBS programming at the American Academy of Neurology and the International Movement Disorders Society. He has published over 40 peer-reviewed articles and 20 book chapters. A medical graduate and neurologist specialist from the University of Rome in Italy, he moved to New York in 1991 with a PD research scholarship. After completing a second neurology residency at Mount Sinai Medical Center, Dr. Tagliati served as a faculty member at Albert Einstein College of Medicine and then moved back to Mount Sinai to become Division Chief of Movement Disorders. He is currently Associate Professor of Neurology at Mount Sinai School of Medicine and a diplomate of the American Board of Psychiatry and Neurology.

Gary N. Guten, MD, MA, is qualified to contribute to this book for three reasons: He's a sports medicine orthopedic surgeon, author, and Parkinson's patient. As an orthopedic surgeon, he specializes in sports medicine, exercise, and nutrition. He was the founder of Sports Medicine and Orthopedic Center in Milwaukee, Wisconsin. The center now has eight doctors. As an author, he has published six books on sports medicine and 27 medical journal publications—14 are on the Web site of the National Library of Medicine accessible at www.pubmed.co m. As a Parkinson's patient, his insight and understanding of Parkinson's disease comes from the fact that he developed

PD in 1995. He had to stop doing surgery—but continues to actively do office practice and consultations. Gary received his medical degree from the University of Wisconsin, and as a lifelong learner received a Master of Arts degree in 2005 in Bioethics from the Medical College of Wisconsin. His master's thesis subject was *Placebo Surgery* with a critical analysis of stem cell surgery for PD.

Jo Horne, MA. Many factors came together to lead Jo to this project. After receiving her master's degree in communications from the University of Cincinnati, she spent the early years of her career as a college lecturer. Later as she began an eight-year journey as the long-distance caregiver for her parents, she became aware of the need for a comprehensive guide for caregivers. Over the next several years she wrote three such guides, all published by AARP. At the same time, she left teaching to work with her husband as he and others pioneered the concept of adult day care in the state of Wisconsin. She was also a fellow of the Midwest Geriatric Education

Center's initial class and was tapped to deliver the keynote address at the national meeting of the Association of University Professionals in Health Administration for her work in developing curriculum on professional/patient interactions in long-term care. Her work as a communications manager in the dual corporate worlds of long-term care insurance and later the pharmaceutical industry further prepared her to research and write on the effects of Parkinson's on patients and their care partners. Finally when her sister was diagnosed with PD, Jo found herself up close and personal with the impact PD can have. Her unique combination of personal and professional experience has made her a popular speaker and workshop leader as well as a guest expert for national television and radio talk shows.

Dedication

Michele Tagliati, MD—In memory of my father, Silvano Tagliati, who suffered with great dignity from Parkinson's disease, and my beloved wife, Tracy, who greatly inspired my life as a man and a doctor.

Gary N. Guten, MD, MA—This book is dedicated to the lasting memory of my neurologist, Dr. Steven Park, who died in 2006 from a tragic accident. Not only was he a Parkinson's disease maven, but he was my medical mentor, respected colleague, and golfing buddy.

Jo Horne, MA—Every book is for Larry, whose belief in me has never wavered. This one is also especially for Patsy Horne DeBord—my sister and friend—whose fight with PD brought our family closer in spite of the years and miles separating us. It is also for my siblings, Betsy and Earle, and in-laws, Tom and Carole, who took on the demanding role of care partner for Patsy without hesitation and—learning on the job—performed it with love.

Authors' Acknowledgments

Michele Tagliati, MD—I would like to thank Jo, whose enlightened spirit envisioned and inspired this book, and all my patients, who teach me a great deal about their disease every day. In addition, I would like to thank the Department of Neurology at Mount Sinai Medical Center and the Bachmann-Strauss Dystonia & Parkinson Foundation for their continuous support.

Gary N. Guten, MD, MA—One person stands out as being responsible for my insight, knowledge, and fight against Parkinson's disease. That person is my piano teacher—Rita Shur. She has taught me to play the piano (or write)—not with my fingers—but with my heart and my head.

Jo Horne, MA—Without the unique expertise and indefatigable dedication of Michele and Gary, this project would still be on the drawing board. I am indebted to both of them for their insights and humor as we made this journey. I am also deeply indebted to my agent Natasha Kern and everyone on the project team at Wiley Publishing. But as Willie Loman said in the Arthur Miller play *Death of a Salesman,* "Attention must (also) be paid" to the dozens of PWP, their care partners, and healthcare professionals who contributed to the work just by showing me what it means to live with PD. Finally I am profoundly indebted to those fearless and tireless warriors at the foundations and organizations who daily wage the battle to find a cure. My deepest wish is that they make this book obsolete in a very short time.

Publisher's Acknowledgments

We're proud of this book; please send us your comments through our Dummies online registration form located at www.dummies.com/register/.

Some of the people who helped bring this book to market include the following:

Acquisitions, Editorial, and Media Development

Senior Project Editor: Alissa Schwipps

Acquisitions Editor: Michael Lewis

Copy Editor: Pam Ruble

Technical Editor: Ramón Luis Rodríguez, MD

Senior Editorial Manager: Jennifer Ehrlich

Editorial Assistants: Erin Calligan, Joe Niesen, David Lutton

Cover Photo: © Stockbyte

Cartoons: Rich Tennant (www.the5thwave.com)

Composition Services

Project Coordinator: Jennifer Theriot

Layout and Graphics: Lavonne Cook, Denny Hager, Stephanie D. Jumper, Barry Offringa, Alicia B. South, Erin Zeltner

Special Art: Kathryn Born, Medical Illustrator

Anniversary Logo Design: Richard Pacifico

Proofreaders: Jessica Kramer, Techbooks

Indexer: Techbooks

***

Publishing and Editorial for Consumer Dummies

Diane Graves Steele, Vice President and Publisher, Consumer Dummies

Joyce Pepple, Acquisitions Director, Consumer Dummies

Kristin A. Cocks, Product Development Director, Consumer Dummies

Michael Spring, Vice President and Publisher, Travel

Kelly Regan, Editorial Director, Travel

Publishing for Technology Dummies

Andy Cummings, Vice President and Publisher, Dummies Technology/General User

Composition Services

Gerry Fahey, Vice President of Production Services

Debbie Stailey, Director of Composition Services

Foreword

A diagnosis of Parkinson's disease is a life-altering event. There is no one way to deal with it. Everyone has a unique set of circumstances, and every patient experiences Parkinson's differently. That's why one book on PD can never be all things to all people. Whether you are living with the disease or are a caregiver or friend to someone who is, you will come to rely on a wide variety of high-quality books, manuals, Web sites, resources and tools. You may be surprised by the voracity of your appetite for newer, better, and just plain more information about PD. And since Parkinson's is—for now, at least—a disease that stays with you for life, your information needs may evolve and change over time.

This book represents something incredibly important: a place to start. We commend its emphasis on tenets that we at The Michael J. Fox Foundation strive to incorporate into our work: an action orientation, a problem-solving mentality, and the distillation of a great deal of complicated information into clear, logical next steps.

Most importantly, the Foundation shares with the authors of this book a commitment to keep patients front and center in every decision we make. As the largest funder of Parkinson's research outside the federal government, we actively partner with scientists to innovate new funding mechanisms that can maximize the quality, quantity and pace of PD research. With a comprehensive view of the field and proactive management of the grants in our portfolio, we are ideally positioned to bridge the gap between basic research and the clinic. For years scientists have asserted that with sufficient research funding, a cure for Parkinson's is within reach. We are working urgently to prove them right.

I am continually inspired by the patients I meet who are endeavoring to live their lives beyond the potentially limiting effects of this disease, defining themselves by their achievements, not their struggle with PD. But no one who knows Parkinson's would suggest that a positive outlook is achievable all the time. Do everything you can to put the odds on your side: Find doctors you trust and can build relationships with; eat well and exercise as much as possible; appreciate and invest in your family and friendships; investigate ways to reduce stress and practice what works for you.

And know that work is continuing aggressively to make this disease, finally, a thing of the past.

Debi Brooks

President and CEO, The Michael J. Fox Foundation for Parkinson's Research

Introduction

If the very idea of a Parkinson's disease diagnosis scares the bejeebers out of you, take a deep breath and pay attention. Although Parkinson's is a chronic and progressive condition with no cure (yet), the strides made in just the last decade to control and manage symptoms are impressive and hopeful. Also the number of national organizations (not to mention big-name celebrities) that are placing the spotlight squarely on the need for a cure is unparalleled.

And we're here to help: An experienced neurologist and lecturer on the treatment of Parkinson's disease (PD); another physician—not a neurologist but rather one who has been living with his own PD (and finding new and innovative ways to maintain control over his life) for over a decade; and a writer of books on aging and giving care whose oldest sister has PD. Together we give you the facts you need, resources you can rely on, and tips on how best to structure your life so that—to paraphrase the popular slogan—you have PD, but it doesn't have you.

This book is your guide to understanding and living with PD. While you—the person with Parkinson's (PWP) are the primary audience—feel free to share *Parkinson's Disease For Dummies* with family, friends, and especially that person who will most likely make this journey with you—your care partner.

We—the doctor-athlete who's fought PD for over ten years, the writer who's seen dozens of people triumph over their PD, and the neurologist who's not in the business of giving up—wish you the strength to persevere, the will to keep fighting for a cure, and the physical and emotional stamina for a long, productive life.

About This Book

At first glance the idea of a *For Dummies* guide to Parkinson's disease may seem ludicrous or even downright insulting. But those of you who have used these guides understand that the dummies reference indicates a guide that presents its topic in simple, straightforward terms. Although PD doesn't have a cure, it can be well managed for years before a person faces its more challenging aspects. And that's what this guide is about—practical ways you can control and manage the symptoms of your Parkinson's so you can get on with your life!

Now, this is not some sugar-coated Pollyanna guide to living with PD. It's a realistic look at what you're facing. It provides solid information and resources to help you and your family come to terms with PD as a factor in all your lives. It offers proven techniques and tips to help you prepare for the future without projecting the worst. And most of all, it reminds you that living a full and satisfying life—in spite of PD—is definitely possible, even probable.

We designed each chapter of *Parkinson's Disease For Dummies* to be self-contained so that you don't have to read the book sequentially or read the first parts to understand any later chapters. You can dip in and out wherever you please and concentrate only on what you need. The table of contents and the index can help guide your search.

Conventions Used in This Book

The following conventions are used throughout the text to make the info consistent and easy to understand:

- New terms appear in *italic* and are closely followed by an easy-to-understand definition. We also clearly define the terms in the handy glossary at the back of the book.
- **Bold** is used to highlight the action parts of numbered steps.

This guide has a few special conventions that are widely accepted by Parkinson's researchers and advocates as well as by people with PD and their families:

- Parkinson's disease is often abbreviated *PD.*
- A person diagnosed and living with PD is often referred to as *PWP,* or person (or persons) with Parkinson's.

- Because PWP are fully capable of making decisions and planning their care for many years following diagnosis, we refer to their primary care-givers as *care partners.* There may come a day when you need more hands-on care and assistance. Should that day come, that's when your *care partner* takes on the additional role of *caregiver.*
- Although we hope your family and close friends will read many portions of this guide, some sections are do-not-miss for these folks. Several chapters have a section titled "A Word for the PD Care Partner" at the end. Be sure to share these sections with the person (or persons) most likely to be your support and eventual caregiver.

Foolish Assumptions

In putting together this guide to living with PD, the three of us have assumed the following about you:

- That you have (or suspect you have) PD yourself or are close to someone who does.

- That you want reliable information about PD, and you're looking for proven ways (techniques and resources) to treat and manage its symptoms.
- That you intend to take a proactive role in facing this challenge and not simply (blindly!) do everything the first healthcare provider you see tells you to do.
- That you're open to lifestyle adjustments and complementary or alternative techniques that are proven to manage symptoms and prolong functions.
- That you realize PD is not just a physical condition that affects only you; it has elements that impact you—and everyone who cares about you—physically, mentally, and emotionally. You all need to be proactive in preparing for and meeting those challenges head-on.

How This Book Is Organized

All *For Dummies* books are divided into parts and chapters. The goal is for you to easily move from one part or chapter to another without having to read a gazillion pages of information that aren't essential at the moment. Clever, right? The following sections describe each part.

Part I: Understanding PD

The chapters in this part explain what PD is and isn't. Chapter 1 gives an overview: statistics and background information plus the differences between primary PD and other conditions that can look like it. Chapter 2 gets into the potential causes—genetic and environmental—that researchers study to find new treatments and even a cure. You also find out who's at risk for getting PD. In Chapter 3 we take a closer look at the four major symptoms and signs that distinguish Parkinson's from related conditions. The chapter concludes with the stages of the disease and why these stages have no clear markers.

Part II: Making PD Part—But Not All—of Your Life

These chapters walk you through those initial steps following your suspicions of PD. We begin with guidance on getting an accurate diagnosis, finding a specialist, and understanding the tests and techniques that confirm your diagnosis. We explain how to connect with other health experts—therapists, counselors, and such—who will play a vital role in managing your PD. In addition, you need to focus on sharing the news with people around you. Chapter 7 gives you tips on how, when, and who to tell. The final chapter in this part addresses the special needs of people with young onset PD (before age 50).

Part III: Crafting a Treatment Plan Just for You

This is your guide to the current options for treating PD and managing symptoms over the long term. We look at prescription medicines, the possibility of surgery, and proven complementary or alternative therapies that are viable assets. The largest chapter is on diet and exercise, and that's intentional. We include a program of exercises specifically designed to enhance flexibility and build muscle strength. We also insist that you show this program to your physician and physical therapist before trying it on your own! Because PD is a neurological condition (affecting the brain), we include a separate chapter on depression and anxiety, which can be treatable symptoms of the condition itself. Wrapping up this part is a chapter on clinical trials. We discuss how to find such trials as well as the pros and cons of being a participant.

Part IV: Living Well with PD

Because living with PD for many years—even decades—is not only possible but also likely, this part discusses special areas of your life (people, work, and independence) that may need fine-tuning. We explain how people often react differently to a person who now has a chronic and progressive condition and how it's up to you to maintain normalcy with your family, friends, and co-workers. We also address PD and the workplace: the issues you face when you can work as well as the options you have when you can't work. Finally we cover ways to maintain independence and control over your life despite changes in your mobility and mental prowess.

Part V: Coping with Advanced PD

As with any progressive condition, you'll eventually delegate responsibilities and rely on other people to keep you mobile, mentally alert, and emotionally upbeat. This part of the book is as important for your primary care partner as it is for you, so both of you need to read it. We cover important decisions and planning processes that you should address early on, and we discuss the onset of later-stage symptoms that can be incapacitating. We also address the gradual shift of your partner's role from care partner to caregiver, based on ground rules the two of you make. Early discussions on housing, finances, and legal issues are also covered in this part.

Part VI: The Part of Tens

Every *For Dummies* book includes a section of lists, that is, key information that readers can use right away. In *Parkinson's Disease For Dummies,* those lists include ten ways to manage difficult feelings (anger, guilt, sadness, and such), ten ways you (the PWP) can care for your care partner, and—possibly the most important list—ten ways you and your care partner can become active in the fight for a cure.

Part VII: Appendixes

Appendix A contains a glossary of Parkinson's-related terms to use as reference. Appendix B summarizes the many PD resources we mention through-out this guide: organizations, care partner resources, support groups, and assistive devices for making life with PD easier.

Icons Used in This Book

To make this book easier to read and simpler to use, we include icons that help you find (and fathom) key information. Here's what they look like and highlight:

This icon flags essential information that cautions and protects you against potential pitfalls and problems. Do *not* skip over these paragraphs.

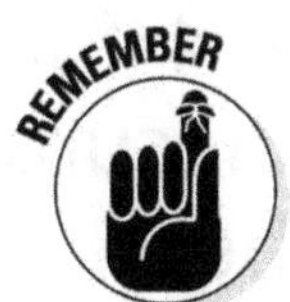

This icon signals essential information that's important enough to bear repeating. It's information you should keep in mind.

This icon identifies information that may save you time, offer a resource, or show you an easier way of doing some task or activity.

Where to Go from Here

Where you open this book—Chapter 1, Chapter 18, or somewhere in between—depends on where you are in your journey through Parkinson's. If you suspect PD is the cause behind some troubling symptoms, you may want to start with Chapter 4 for tips on the best way to get an accurate diagnosis. If you've already been diagnosed, then Part III, where we discuss treatment options, may be your first stop.

The point is that this is a *guide,* a roadmap to help you on the path to living with PD. We offer information and resources that you can trust—tools that help you adapt to life with PD without making it your whole life. In the long run, however, it's your resolve to face each day with renewed strength and energy that will see you through. And it's your example that will set the stage for those people who intend to partner with you in the fight.

Part I

Understanding PD

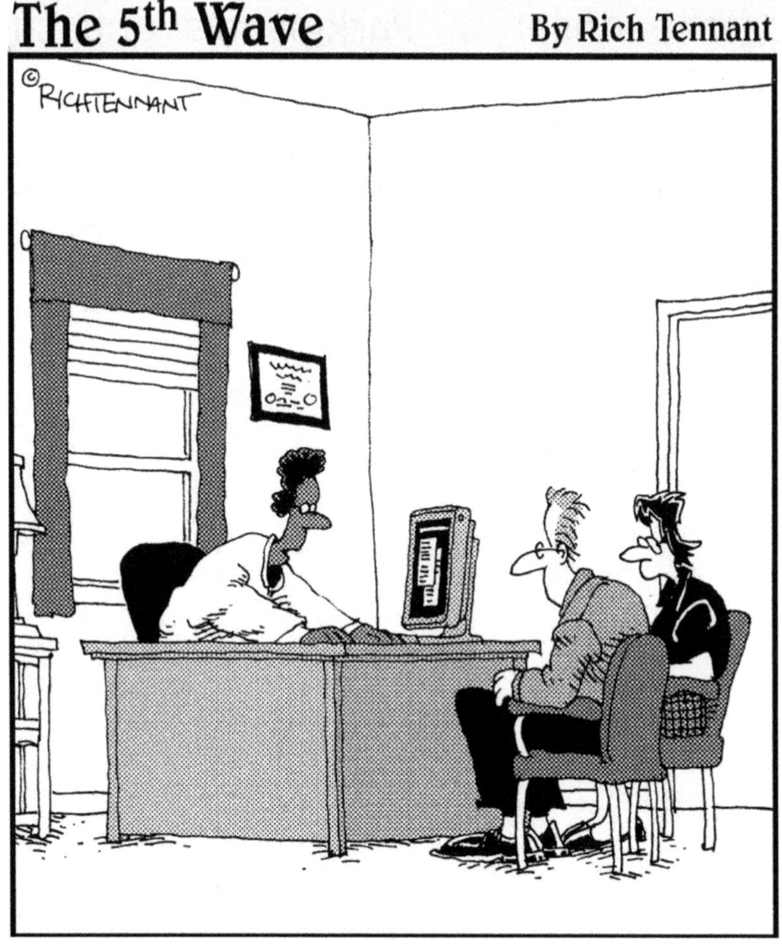

"As explained, Parkinson's disease is a depletion of dopamine in the brain. But before you fill up that space with a lot of negative thoughts, let's discuss your treatment options."

In this part...

You discover what Parkinson's disease is and how it differs from related forms of parkinsonism. We identify the current theories on causes for the onset of Parkinson's and the risk factors that may play a part for some people. Finally you get a good idea of what symptoms to watch for and what signs doctors look for to diagnose and stage this condition.

Chapter 1

Parkinson's Disease: The Big Picture

In This Chapter

- Setting the stage: What Parkinson's disease is—and isn't
- Making a plan to establish your care
- Maximizing your care options
- Living (and loving) your life
- Getting from here to there: Your present and future with PD

The National Center for Health Statistics (a division of the Centers for Disease Control) reports that approximately 1 percent of all Americans over the age of 65 receive a diagnosis of Parkinson's disease (PD). Sixty thousand new cases are diagnosed every year. But you didn't pick up this book because you're interested in mass numbers. You opened it because you're only interested in one number—yours or someone you love. You opened it because you've noticed some symptoms that made you think *Parkinson's,* or you just got a confirmed diagnosis and you're wondering what's next.

What's next is for you to go into action mode—understand the facts (rather than listen to the myths) about PD—what causes it, how it's treated, and, of huge importance to anyone diagnosed with PD, how to live with it. (Notice we said *live,* not just *exist.*) In this chapter, you find the big picture of the rest of the book and (more to the point) where to find the information that you need right now.

Defining Parkinson's—A Movement Disorder

Parkinson's disease is a disease in a group of conditions called *movement disorders*—disorders that result from a loss of the brain's control on voluntary movements. Dopamine (a neurotransmitter in the brain) relays signals from the substantia nigra to those brain regions (putamen, caudate, and globus pallidus—collectively named the *basal ganglia*—in the *striatum*) that control movement, balance, and coordination (see Figure 1-1). In the brain of people with Parkinson's (PWP), cells that produce this essential substance die earlier than normal.

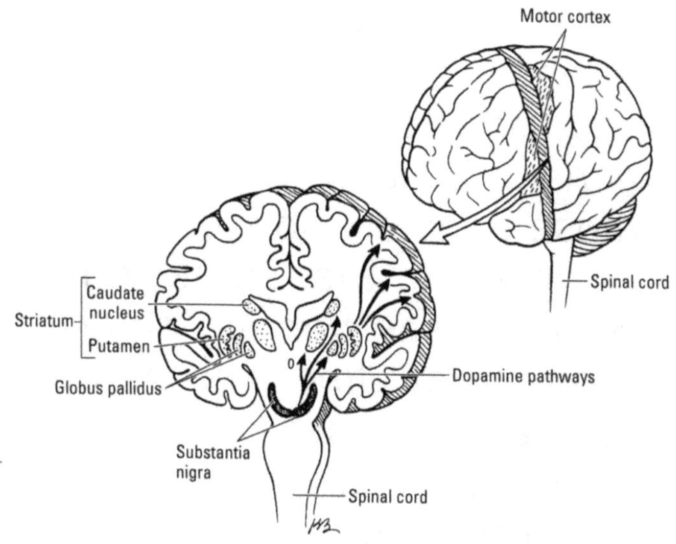

Figure 1-1: The dopamine pathway.

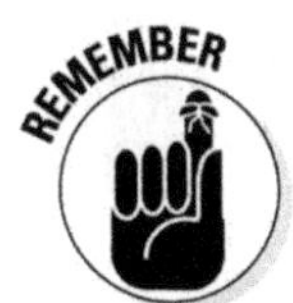

Although a whole group of conditions are known as *parkinsonism,* the one that most people know is called *idiopathic PD,* a Greek word that means arising spontaneously from an unknown cause. As the term suggests, the jury is still out as to the underlying cause (though theories do exist).

Go into a room filled with 50 people with Parkinson's (PWP) and ask how they first suspected they had PD. You're likely to hear 50 different stories. Take ten of those people who were diagnosed at approximately the same time and you're likely to see varying signs of PD progression—from almost no progression to more rapid onset of symptoms. Similarly, you're likely to experience a variety of attitudes and outlooks from the individuals dealing with their PD.

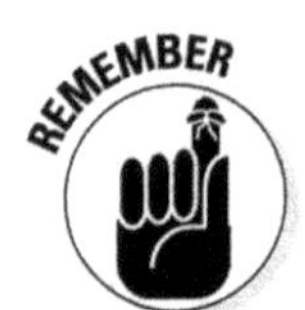

When you're diagnosed with PD, you set out on a unique journey—one where your outlook, lifestyle changes, and medical treatment can be key directional maneuvers along the way. In truth, this disease is one that you can live with, surrender to, or fight with everything you've got. The road veers and curves differently for each person. Some people may choose one path for managing symptoms, and some people choose another. Sometimes the disease itself sets the course. The bottom line? No clear roadmaps are available. But one fact is certain: Understanding the chronic and progressive nature of PD can take you a long way toward effectively managing your symptoms and living a full life.

Accepting the chronic progressive factors

Chronic and progressive can be scary words when you're talking about your health. But keep the words in perspective. Any number of chronic conditions occur with age—arthritis, high blood pressure, and cholesterol management to name three. So, take a realistic look at the terms, accept them for what they are (and aren't), and move on.

Chronic—it's part of you now

In medical terms, illnesses are either *acute* (develop quickly and usually go away with treatment or time) or *chronic* (develop over time, may be managed with treatment, but have no cure at this time). In short, a chronic illness like PD (or arthritis or high blood pressure) is now part of you—a fact that can help or hinder you in the fight.

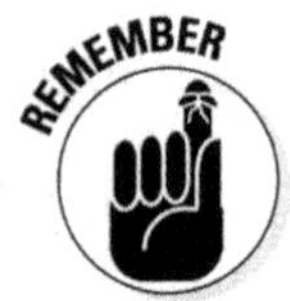

If you refuse to accept that PD is a fact of life for you, then you're wasting precious time and energy in denial. But, if you accept that most people get challenges in life and PD is yours, then you're ahead of the game. Facing PD is no different than facing any situation that changed the way you thought your life would be.

Progressive—it will get more challenging

Progressive, advancing, worsening—more scary stuff. Here's some good news: For millions of PWP, the progression takes years, even decades. Many PWP live relatively normal life spans following their diagnosis. However, two factors are essential for successfully containing PD's progressive effects: your attitude and your willingness to attend to lifestyle and medical therapy.

Throughout this book we address both factors in multiple ways, but for now, remember:

- **Your attitude**—refusing to allow this diagnosis to color every part of your routine and life—is a huge factor in coping with the management of new symptoms through the years.
- **Your willingness to take lifestyle changes seriously** and get involved in the fight to find a cure can make all the difference between you managing the disease or the disease managing you.

To figure out how you're going to live with PD—if you have it—you first need to understand the basics: what it is (and is not), how you get it, what to look for, and how it progresses.

Distinguishing between Parkinson's disease and related conditions

Several neurological conditions may appear to be *idiopathic* (without known cause) PD at first, but they eventually trace back to known causes, progress differently, and respond differently to therapy. (Chapter 3 has more on this.) These other conditions include the following:

- **Essential tremor** (ET) is perhaps the most common type of tremor, affecting as many as five million Americans. ET differs from the tremor in idiopathic PD in several ways: ET occurs when the hand is active (as in eating, grasping, writing, and such). It may also occur in the face, voice, and arms. The renowned actress, Katherine

Hepburn, had ET, not PD. Differentiating ET from PD is very important because each condition responds to completely different sets of medications.

- **Parkinson-plus syndromes** may initially have the same symptoms as PD. But these syndromes also cause early and severe problems with balance, blood pressure, vision, and cognition and usually have a much faster progression compared to PD.
- **Secondary parkinsonism** can result from head trauma or from damage to the brain due to multiple small strokes (*atherosclerotic* or *vascular parkinsonism*). Both forms can be ruled out through scans (CTs or MRIs) that produce images of the brain (see Chapter 4).
- **Pseudoparkinsonism** can appear to be PD when in fact the person has another condition (such as depression) that can mimic the inexpressive face of PWP.
- **Drug- or toxin-induced parkinsonism** can occur from taking antipsychotic medications

(drug-induced) or from exposure to toxins such as carbon monoxide and manganese dust (toxin-induced). Drug-induced symptoms are usually (but not always) reversible; toxin-induced symptoms usually aren't.

The subtleties of diagnosing idiopathic PD may lead your family doctor to send you to a *neurologist,* a specialist in the treatment of neurological conditions. If that happens, don't panic. Getting the correct diagnosis, discussed in Chapter 4, is the first step toward figuring out what comes next for you.

Debunking some commonly held myths about PD

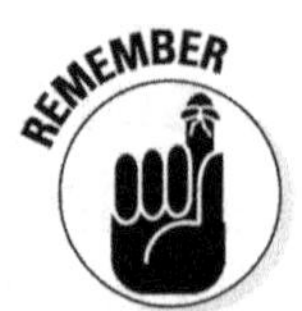

It's to your advantage to get a grasp on some of the more commonly held myths about PD—what it is and what it isn't.

- PD is not:
    - Contagious
    - Curable (at this writing, but research is hopefully getting closer!)
    - Normal for older people—or impossible for younger people
    - A reason to make immediate life-changing decisions (like assuming you won't be able to work or that you need to move)
    - Bound to get you if you live long enough
- PD is:
    - Chronic (when you have it, you have it—like arthritis or diabetes)
    - Slowly progressive (over time—often years) even with treatment
    - Manageable (often for years) with proper treatment and key lifestyle changes
    - Life-changing for you, your family, and friends (Whether that's good or bad is up to you and how you decide to face it.)

In many ways these debunkers are the key messages we want you to take away from this book. If you have PD, you have an enormous challenge before you, but tens of thousands of people successfully face it every day. You can get through this—and we're here to show you how.

Recognizing symptoms that raise questions

First things first: Do you have PD? Although researchers may not yet have a clear idea of the cause(s) for PD (see Chapter 3), they have established that idiopathic PD starts on only one side of the body and includes one or more of these four key symptoms:

- Tremor at rest (trembling in the hands, arms, feet, legs, or face when that body part isn't engaged in activity)
- Rigidity (stiffness in the limbs and trunk)
- Akinesia or bradykinesia (lack of movement or slowness of movement)
- Postural instability (impaired balance or coordination of movement)

Notice how the first letters of the symptoms spell out the handy acronym

TRAP to help you remember (like you need to be reminded!). You'll have times when the symptoms of PD make you feel trapped inside your body. In this book, we work hard to show you a number of ways to fight back and maintain control of your life in spite of the *TRAP.*

Chapter 3 discusses symptoms (what you report to the doctor) and signs (what the doctor observes) in more detail.

Seeking the Care You Need

Perhaps more than any other chronic condition, managing PD is a team effort. You're going to be working with an entire front line of healthcare professionals (doctors, therapists, and the like) as well as non-professionals like your family and friends and other PWP that you'll meet along the way.

From medical professionals

At least two doctors are likely to be intricately involved: your primary care physician and a neurologist. In addition, you'll possibly connect with several other healthcare professionals along the way: your pharmacist; physical, occupational, and speech therapists; counselors and advisors to help manage any depression, anxiety, diet changes, and exercise regimens; advisors to help manage financial, legal, housing, and other major decisions that'll affect you and your family over the long term. Chapter 6 offers more information about this group.

From loved ones

You'll also have a personal care team: your spouse or significant other; your children (and possibly grandchildren); your close friends and (if you're diagnosed with young onset Parkinson's—YOPD) your parents and siblings. Benchwarmers who may surprise you with their willingness to help out include neighbors, co-workers, members of groups you belong to, and others. In Chapters 7 and 16 we talk more about how to break the news and get these folks involved. Chapter 8 covers questions and situations specific to YOPD.

As your PD progresses

One of the toughest truths you'll face as your PD progresses is that you have to rely on other people's help to some degree. Years may pass before this becomes a factor, but you and your loved ones need to plan for it. In Chapter 18 we discuss the symptoms that can crop up as your PD progresses. Every case of PD is different though; symptoms that occur in another person may never be a problem for you. Knowledge is good, but assuming that you'll have to endure every symptom in this book is just wrong on so many levels.

The more positive approach is to *prepare* without *projecting.* For example, will you have swallowing difficulties? Maybe, but you can have a speech therapist as a part your care team, as we talk about in Chapter 6. She's there on the bench, ready to get in the game if you need help. Will your spouse or significant other have to dress you, feed you, bathe you? Chances are good that he'll need to assist you in these basic daily activities in the advanced stages of your PD. We cover that step in Chapter 19.

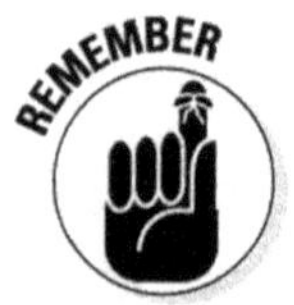

Reaching decisions about advanced PD questions before they occur (such as identifying a caregiver and having a family meeting to plan an extended network of support) is just smart planning. (That's in Chapter 19 too).

Treating Parkinson's—Previewing Your Options

After you've educated yourself with facts (not myths or hearsay) and drafted your care team(s), it's time to get down to the serious business of treating your PD and managing symptoms as they appear. In this book we cover the options—in fact, a growing number of options—for treating and managing your PD symptoms. In addition to medications (Chapter 9) and—in some advanced cases—surgery (Chapter 10), you can find relief in complementary treatments (such as physical and occupation therapies) and alternative treatments (such as yoga or acupuncture). See Chapter 11 for more about all of these.

In the beginning your doctor may want you to postpone a prescription-medication regimen in favor of trying some lifestyle changes—for example, diet and exercise (see Chapter 12) and counseling for your PD-related anxiety and depression (Chapter 13). With today's bright spotlight on research for a cure, you may even want to participate in one of the many clinical trials for new treatments (Chapter 14).

As new symptoms appear (usually years after your initial diagnosis), you'll want to check out Chapter 18 to understand the difference between symptoms that can be PD-related and symptoms that can be related to the aging process or another condition entirely(such as high blood pressure).

Starting the Course, Staying the Course

Not surprisingly, for many people and their families, the diagnosis of PD comes as a shock. *Progressive* and *incurable* are likely to be the words that register in these early hours. But as the news begins to sink in, you have choices to make. The following sections provide advice.

Dealing with the here and now

As Debi Brooks, President and CEO of the Michael J. Fox Foundation, notes in the foreword to this book, if you're going to truly have a life with PD, you need to do three things: develop an attitude of action, form a problem-solving mentality, and possess the ability to take a great deal of information coming at you from all directions and distill it into clear, logical next steps.

Here are some tips to get you on the road:

- Stay in the here and now—not the distant future. PD is a condition you can successfully manage, perhaps for many years, before you must rely on other people.

- Work with your healthcare team to focus on *your* PD and how you can most effectively manage those symptoms.
- Do *not* compare your situation, symptoms, or ability to manage to other PWP. This is not a contest and you are not those persons.
- Get organized. What are your questions? Write them down. Who are the best medical professionals to treat your PD? If finding that doctor means traveling to another community, at least consider it. This is your life, after all.
- Maintain some sense of control over your destiny by educating yourself. Use only reputable sources such as those we list throughout this guide and in Appendix B.
- Use the lingo. Everyone else will—your doctors, the people in your support group, the authors of the articles you read. We define terms as we go, but Appendix A is a glossary for your convenience.
- Be a team player by:
    - Taking the time to prepare for doctor appointments with questions

and information about your current symptoms.

• Taking charge of your own health by making changes to your diet and exercise routine as needed—and sticking with it.

• Understanding that, although you have every right to maintain independence and autonomy over your decisions, you also have a responsibility to care for the people who will care for and eventually speak for you.

• Encouraging innovation in your health team, your family and friends, and yourself. (For example, if you used to love playing jazz saxophone but your tremor makes that impossible, does that mean you have to give up loving jazz?)

• Celebrating even the smallest victory and allowing yourself a decent interval to mourn the greater losses.

• Remembering that your PD is not all about you. Other people are affected, some of them in major, life-changing ways.

- Advocating for new and more effective treatments and a cure. (You can't be more effective than when you're speaking out for those 60,000 PWP who are being diagnosed each year.)
- Learn as much as you can, lean on the support of other PWP who have been there (done that), laugh with other people and at yourself, love in return those people who offer love in their support and care, and LIVE with the single determination that you won't be reduced to a PD-only identification ("That's Jack Wilson—he's really an amazing person!").

Working, playing, and having a life

Okay, the medical experts are in place, you're on a regimen customized to manage your symptoms. What's next? How about getting a life—at least getting back to some semblance of the one you had before the diagnosis?

Part IV of this guide is all about living with PD: keeping up with the relationships that are so vital to you as an individual (Chapter 15), maintaining a job (even continuing to build a career if that's important for you; see Chapter 16), and getting out and about—you know, living (Chapter 17).

Making plans for your future

Any diagnosis of a chronic and progressive condition—no matter how slowly it progresses—is a wakeup call for attending to those financial and legal matters everyone needs to address. For you, that time is now. You and your family need to get together with an experienced team of financial and legal consultants and take steps to protect you and your loved ones in the event that you become incapacitated.

If at some point you can no longer speak for yourself or make the complex decisions in managing finances, your care partner must know your choices and have the power to act on your behalf. This advice is just common sense whether a person has PD or not. Chapter 20 offers guidelines and tips that can save you and your family a lot of stress and worry in the future on these matters.

If your current housing become an issue later on (for example bedrooms and the only bath are on the second floor), Chapter 21 takes a look at the growing range of options, including adapting your current residence so you can stay there.

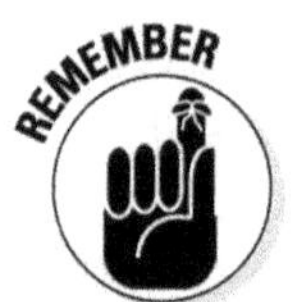

In the course of our individual careers and our collaboration on this book, the three of us have seen case after case of people living full and satisfying lives in spite of PD. We understand that it isn't always easy, but we have seen the incredible results when PWP succeed in living beyond their disease.

Although no single resource can provide all the answers, we believe that in these pages you can find the information you need to make the best decisions for living your life with PD.

Chapter 2

Considering Possible Causes and Risk Factors

In This Chapter

- Understanding theories behind the possible causes of Parkinson's disease
- Determining risk factors
- Assessing your at-risk quotient

Although James Parkinson described the disease nearly two centuries ago and research has been ongoing ever since, the underlying cause—the factor that sets Parkinson's disease (PD) in motion—is still unknown. A number of theories are under discussion and research, any one of which may lead to the breakthrough in managing symptoms or even curing the disease. The medical community has also made progress in assessing risk factors—some more common than others. In this chapter we cover these potential causes and risk factors so you can better understand them as the hunt for a cure continues.

Considering Theories on Causes

The underlying event behind the onset of PD is a loss of neurons (nerve cells) in the *substantia nigra* region of the brain. These neurons normally produce *dopamine,* a neurotransmitter that helps the brain communicate with other parts of the body, telling them to perform common movements (such as walking, handling objects, and maintaining balance) almost automatically.

PD is a little like diabetes because in both diseases

- You lose a vital chemical (insulin in diabetes; dopamine in PD).
- The chemicals are essential to the body's ability to function properly.
- The chemicals can be replaced.

Of course, the diseases are more complex than that, but you get the idea. As we age, all of us lose dopamine-producing neurons, which results in the slower, more measured movements. But the decline of dopamine in people with Parkinson's (PWP) is not normal.

Why PD targets the substantia nigra at the stem of the brain remains a mystery. But the damage results in abnormal protein deposits that can disrupt the normal function of the cells in that area. These protein clumps are called *Lewy bodies,* named for Freiderich H. Lewy, the German physician who discovered and documented them in 1908. The presence of Lewy bodies within the substantia nigra is associated with a depletion of the brain's normal supply of dopamine. For this reason, their presence is one of the pathological hallmarks of PD (although Lewy bodies are present in other disorders).

In reality, Lewy bodies have been found in other parts of the brain affected by PD, which suggests that the problem may be more widespread. This more extensive pathology may explain the occurrence of non-motor and levodopa-unresponsive symptoms (see Chapter 9). Nevertheless, researchers still don't know whether Lewy bodies cause the damage to the nerve cells or are a by-product of damage caused by another factor.

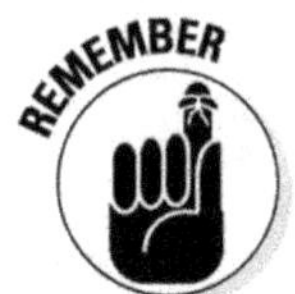

Theories on causes abound—family history, environment, occupation, and so on. Today's researchers generally agree, however, that the onset of PD is a *multi-factorial* process; that is, several conditions are at play in the onset of PD rather than one specific and single cause. But the true causes behind the onset of PD in one person and not another—in one family member and not another—are unknown.

Much of the research today focuses on environmental and genetic factors that may contribute to the onset of PD. This section takes a look at those environmental conditions and then considers genetic issues and other factors that scientists have identified as potential causes.

Taking a close look at environmental factors

According to the National Institute of Environmental Health Sciences, PD is the second most prevalent neurodegenerative disorder behind Alzheimer's disease. Of the three primary risk factors for PD (age, genetics, and environmental exposures), a line of research that began in the 1980s shows an increasing association between environmental factors and PD. The following sections explore the variety of environmental exposures that may play a role in triggering PD.

Free radicals—the internal battle

Free radicals are unstable molecules that lack one electron. In their quest to replace that missing link, they rub against other molecules, seeking a connection that will stabilize them.

Even when the free radical doesn't make a connection, it keeps digging, damaging other molecules in the cell in a process known as *oxidation* or *oxidative stress.* Normally your body has enough antioxidants to stabilize the free radical and repair the damage, but if it doesn't, then those damaged cells die.

Key players in controlling oxidative stress are the *mitochondria* (the part of the cell outside the nucleus that converts nutrients into energy) because they're a potential source of free radicals. In addition, several of the toxins associated with PD seem to damage specifically the mitochondria. Researchers believe a connection may exist between oxidative stress and the death of cells in the substantia nigra, which causes PD symptoms. This theory is one of the main reasons that some doctors recommend a diet rich in antioxidants. (See Chapter 12 for more on diets for PWP.)

Location, location, location

For the overwhelming number of PD patients who get Parkinson's, certain environmental factors seem to put the person at higher risk for getting the disease. Consider that family members share not only a genetic history but also an environmental history—at least for a portion of their lives. They live in the same house, drink the same water, eat the same food from the same sources, have exposure to the same chemical compounds, and so on. Therefore, researchers are studying geographic environmental factors as a possible link to the onset of PD. These factors include living in a rural area and using well water for drinking, cooking, and such.

Exposure to toxins

Toxins that people inhale or ingest can damage the body in many ways, including cell function interference. Research shows that excessive exposure to specific environmental or industrial toxic chemicals such as pesticides and herbicides can increase the risk of developing PD. For example, the damage by the pesticide *rotenone* is directed at the *mitochondria* (the power plant of our brain cells) and can critically reduce the energy produced by the cell until the cell dies. (See the "Free radicals—the internal battle" sidebar for more on this topic.)

In some cases environmental toxicity and genetic factors may operate in tandem. Scientists have discovered that the gene CYP2D6, when functioning normally, produces an enzyme that breaks down the toxicity of pesticides.

But in some people the gene is less effective, leaving those people more sensitive to the toxicity of pesticides. More studies are needed to verify whether there may be a correlation between genetic predisposition to pesticide toxicity and PD.

Links to viral problems

Although PD is not contagious, a viral factor may be associated with its cause. This hypothesis is mainly based on the occurrence of *post-encephalitic parkinsonism* after the influenza pandemic of 1918. More Americans died from this flu in a single year than from the all the wars from World War I through the Vietnam War.

To complicate matters, many patients developed the so-called *sleeping sickness (encephalitis lethargica),* characterized by the progression from severe headache to drowsiness to possible coma and death. Patients who survived the encephalitis (brain infection) often developed symptoms of parkinsonism, including bradykinesia, rigidity, hypomimia, postural instability, and eye movement abnormalities *(oculogyric crises).* The memoir *Awakenings* by Oliver Sacks (Vintage) and the 1990 movie by the same title starring Robin Williams and Robert de Niro provide an insightful and accurate representation of this disease.

In reality, the relationship of a virus (such as influenza) and the brain degenerative lesions causing parkinsonism has not been proven. Furthermore, the pathology described in the brain of patients with post-encephalitic parkinsonism is very different from PD and actually bears more of a resemblance to Alzheimer's disease. So the possible viral link with parkinsonism remains elusive.

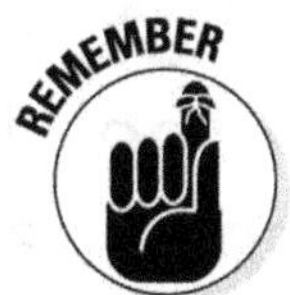

Although these environmental factors and cellular interactions appear to significantly contribute to the onset of PD, the Parkinson's Disease Foundation notes "no conclusive evidence that any single environmental factor, alone, can be considered a cause of the disease." (Go to the foundation's Web site at www.pdf.org /aboutPD/ and click on *Causes* for more information on this topic.)

Looking at possible genetic factors

Every human being plays host to a gazillion genes in their DNA molecules. Genes determine everything from the color of your eyes to the possibility of developing a certain disease or condition. Note the use of the word *possibility.* Because you carry genes in double copies, if one of your genes has the propensity for a condition, the other copy may offset that vulnerability.

According to the National Human Genome Research Institute, evidence now shows a genetic factor in the development of PD. People with a close relative (parent or sibling) who has PD are slightly more likely to contract Parkinson's than someone who has no family history of the disease. But, according to the Mayo Clinic, the link is a small one—less than 5 percent—and more common when the onset occurs before age 30, which is also very rare. (For more information on early onset PD, check out Chapter 8.)

So why waste time and money studying genes? Oddly enough, the very fact that PD is one of the most typical nongenetic diseases makes the genetic study of PD patients interesting. In other words, if PD is typically not inherited, then what else is going on?

In the last decade, scientists have identified multiple genes with definite links to the onset of PD in families where PD is present in multiple generations. An abnormality in one such gene, *Parkin,* may be a predictor of the onset of Parkinson's at a young age (before age 50). Because Parkinson's is present and progressing for several years before any symptoms become obvious, a gene predictor can mean earlier diagnosis and earlier intervention.

Another recent discovery shows that a *mutation* (change) in the protein-producing gene *alpha-synuclein* may change the gene's amino acid composition and thereby contribute to the development of *clumps* (separate cells bonding together) in dopamine neurons, eventually damaging or destroying the dopamine-producing neuron. Interestingly, alpha-synuclein is part of the Lewy bodies, the hallmark protein deposit in dopamine cells affected by Parkinson's disease. If researchers can find a way to break up those clumps and get rid of the excess proteins, then they may have found a way to slow or even stop the progression of PD. (See the section "Occupational causes" later in this chapter for more about clumping.)

Keep in mind that less than 5 percent of PWP appear to have inherited it; at this writing, any genetic factor seems limited to a relatively small number of families. However, the study of genes enhances the ability to understand which molecules a scientist may target for treatment. If you have a family history of PD or are interested in more information on genetic research, visit www.ninds.nih.gov/disorders/parkinsons_disease.

Checking out other possible causes

If it's not family history and it's not the environment, what caused your PD? Unfortunately, that's a difficult question to answer at this stage. And any time a chronic illness has no definitive cause, theories will fly. At the moment, PD has its fair share of such theories. The following sections describe instances where the jury is still out regarding a link with the onset of PD.

Latent effects of war

Links between PD and Agent Orange (an herbicide used during the Vietnam War) and chemical weapons during the Gulf War continue to be relevant questions for PD researchers. For example, in 2003 the Salk Institute identified a gene (called neuropathy target estrase or NTE). In studies with mice, scientists found that when NTE genes are exposed to organophosphate chemicals (such as those used in the Gulf War), the gene's normal activity was inhibited and even changed. While this discovery has certainly opened new doors (not to mention raised new questions), the evidence is far from conclusive. Remember that age is a consideration in the onset of PD and Vietnam vets are reaching the age that onset of PD is more common simply because of their generation. Whether exposure to Agent Orange may also be a contributing factor is still not clear. The good news is that the Veterans Administration (VA) is conducting ongoing research. If you're a veteran of either war, you can find out more information by contacting the U.S.

Department of Veterans Affairs online at www.va.gov.

Overmedication and drug use

Certain drugs taken to excess or over a long period of time may produce the symptoms of PD. Some of the conditions and their drugs include

- Schizophrenia, major depression, or agitation in older people: haloperidol (Haldol) and chloropromazine (Thorazine)
- Control of nausea: metoclopramide (Reglan) and prochlorperazine (Compazine)

Side effects of such medicines usually subside after the medicine is out of the body's system. ***Note:*** Symptoms brought on by drug use commonly occur on both sides of your body at the same time, unlike primary PD. The question remains whether a drug reaction of this nature is a predictor for PD.

Illicit drug use may also be a factor. In one case, a group of young people brewed up what they thought was a hallucinogenic drug called *meperidine* and mistakenly produced a heroin-like drug. When injected, this drug, which contained the toxin 1-methyl-4-phenyl-1,2,3,6-tetrahydropyridine (MPTP), headed straight for the substantia nigra, destroying dopamine cells in its path and leaving the youngsters with signs of advanced PD. The tragedy has led to more research on the possibility of a connection between illicit drug use and the onset of PD.

Occupational causes

Many people have theorized that Muhammad Ali's PD was brought on by his years in the boxing ring. "Too many times getting hit in the head," they assert. Indeed some studies suggest an association between head trauma and the development of PD. Possibly Ali's years in the ring brought the underlying presence of his PD to light.

Another class of work associated with onset of PD is the welding profession. At this writing, an absolute connection doesn't exist between prolonged exposure to metallic fumes or dust and the onset of PD-like symptoms. Nevertheless, researchers continue to explore the possibility of a link because studies show that exposure to heavy metals and pesticides—each already linked to a possible cause for onset of PD—can accelerate the clumping of certain protein cells called *alpha-synuclein.* (See the earlier section "Looking at possible genetic factors" for more on this gene.)

Sounds like sci-fi, but a word about neuroprotectors

The brain has two types of cells: *neurons* (nerve cells) and *glia* (cells that respond to injury and regulate the chemical composition surrounding them, among other tasks). Although glia cells are far more prevalent, the neuron cells do the heavy lifting when it comes to brain work. According to the National Institute of Neurological

Disorders and Stroke, the three classes of neurons are:

- Sensory neurons to carry information from the senses (eyes, ears, and such) to the brain
- Motor neurons to carry messages from the central nervous system (comprised of the brain, spinal cord, and network of nerves running through the body) to the body's muscles and glands
- Interneurons that communicate only within their immediate location

Within each category, hundreds of neuron types operate with the very specific messaging abilities that make each person unique. But the neurons affected by PD control the body's ability to move. When those neurons die in large enough numbers, the brain's ability to signal the body to move is compromised.

Researchers are working hard to understand the death of these neurons and to develop treatments and therapies that can protect them. One potential value of stem cell research is that neural stem cells may reproduce the variety of neurons in the brain. Scientists could then figure out how to maneuver these new neurons to become

- A protector of healthy neurons (preventing or at least slowing further damage or loss)
- A replacement for damaged or dead neurons

In addition, ongoing research considers whether certain therapies—such as certain drugs, vitamin supplements, and rigorous exercise therapy—may act as a protector and slow the loss of these vital neurons. For more information on the role of neuroprotection in the battle against PD, check out Chapters 11 and 12.

Oddly enough, in more than one occupational study, teachers and healthcare workers showed a higher incidence of PD—as much as two to three times higher than other professions. Researchers are puzzled because the commonality in the two professions seems to be exposure to infection, even though PD is clearly not a contagious disease.

Weighing Your Risk Factors

Your suspicion that you have PD (or an actual diagnosis from your doctor) can raise all sorts of questions starting with, "How did this happen to me?" It's perfectly normal to look back and consider the risk factors that were present (although unknown at the time) as you also look forward to protecting your children and others around you from those same risks.

Start with what is known for sure:

- PD is not contagious—you can't get it from or give it to another person.
- Most cases (at least three-fourths) show up after age 60, and incidence increases every decade after that.
- Head trauma (a serious fall or accident involving injury to the head) can be a risk factor for PD.
- Men are more likely to get PD than women.

Your particular risk factors (or family members' risks if you suspect you have PD) are the life and lifestyle details that can increase the chances of developing PD. They may be *multi-factorial.* (You may be at risk from more than one source or situation).

Considering your age and gender

The one concrete risk factor for developing PD is age. Most people develop symptoms in middle age, but the risk for developing PD increases simply because dopamine production declines with age. The average age for onset is 60, and risk increases until around age 75. Some research has shown a significant decrease in the number of people who develop PD after age 75.

At least three studies have confirmed that men are more likely to develop PD than women—in some studies twice as likely. One theory suggests that the production of estrogen may protect women. At the 2006 meeting of the American Academy of Neurology, a research team from the Mayo Clinic presented evidence that points to a possible link between risk for contracting

PD and three genes that control the production of estrogen. Simply put, if the presence of estrogen reduces the risk, a decrease in estrogen increases a woman's risk factor for getting PD. However, more studies are needed to confirm a protective role for estrogen in PD.

Taking a look at ethnicity

Studies have shown that non-white populations, such as African Americans and Asian Americans, have a lower risk of developing primary Parkinson's disease but may be more vulnerable to other forms of parkinsonism such as essential tremor and multiple system atrophy (see Chapter 1). However, whether this difference is tied to an economic and class-based imbalance in the delivery of medical care—especially specialized medical care, like seeing a neurologist—has not been fully considered.

Regarding other risk possibilities

Although they aren't definitive causes, some factors we discuss in this chapter may contribute to your risk for developing PD. In a world where pesticides and herbicides have so many uses, it's hard to avoid exposure to chemicals that put you at risk for all sorts of health problems including PD. Similarly, in an eat-on-the-run fast-food society, people may be denying their body's needs for key vitamins and nutrients. And what about the dangers of such evils as smoking and caffeine? Can these all be factors that put people at greater risk for getting PD?

Overexposure to herbicides and pesticides

Your everyday exposure to chemical toxins can range from the chemicals to control weeds on your lawn to the unseen sprays that coat and polish fresh produce from overseas. Because prolonged or consistent exposure to such toxins is a possible cause of PD (check out "Taking a close look at environmental factors" early in this chapter for more on toxins), take the following precautions:

- Wash all fresh produce thoroughly—even those items like melons or citrus where you normally discard the skin.
- Limit your exposure to the use of toxins such as pesticides and insecticides.
- Use all chemical materials in open areas and wear a protective mask.

If your job requires you to work with chemical compounds such as those in industrial pesticides and herbicides, talk to your employer about precautions to protect you and other employees from exposure and contamination.

Factoring in your weight

Face it: Being overweight sets you up for all kinds of health risks. A 2002 study showed that carrying excess weight during your middle and later years can put you at greater risk for PD. A report in the May, 2003 issue of *Psychology Today* magazine shows an increased rate of PD linked to dietary fat and sugar intake. Although the association between weight gain and PD hasn't been proven, the benefits of a diet rich in antioxidants and a regular program of exercise can't hurt. (In some cases, these benefits have prolonged the time before PD symptoms needed to be treated with medication (see Chapter 12).

Reduced levels of B6, B12, and folate

B6, B12, and folate are essential nutrients for maintaining many of the body's functions. Researchers are beginning to explore whether reduced levels of these nutrients may be a factor in PD. Although studies are in preliminary stages to verify any role the nutrients may play in the management of PD, consider asking your doctor about increasing or supplementing your intake of nutrients.

Regardless of the research and the nutrients' potential for managing your PD, people over age 50 are at increased risk for deficiencies of these three essential nutrients. A diet rich in these nutrients and a supplement (if your doctor advises) may be helpful. However, these need to be carefully monitored by your doctor. Too much B6, for example, can cause additional neuropathic problems such as a profound inability to feel your legs.

Check with your doctor before taking any vitamin or herbal supplement. Claims for these products often lack solid research. The overuse of such products may do more harm than good.

Smoking and caffeine

Get this: As many as 50 published studies over two decades have shown that smoking cigarettes reduces the risk of Parkinson's in people who have smoked steadily most of their adult lives. Caffeine also appears to offer some protection.

But these factors are not a guarantee (as Michael J. Fox noted in an NBC *Dateline* interview in 2006). And the negative effects of these factors (such as lung cancer from smoking) that can greatly shorten your stay on this planet are way too grim to think a two-pack-a-day habit may be worth the risk.

Changing Don't Know to Know

The more researchers tackle the problems of PD, the more complex the challenges become. This section takes a quick look at the unknowns of PD and offers ways that PWP and the general public can help PD research move forward.

The need-to-know info

Questions for PD researchers abound, but one of the greatest challenges is simply getting a good handle on the accurate numbers and extent of PD. For example

- Scientists really don't know how common Parkinson's is.
- They don't know whether the numbers are changing over time or

simply reflecting longevity and an aging population.

- They don't know whether geographic cluster patterns exist (places in the United States where PD is unusually prevalent or absent).

The Muhammad Ali Foundation has established a voluntary registry where patients may record their PD diagnosis and information. (Register at www.alicenter.org.) However, because this information is random and voluntary, it has limited practicality.

At this writing, PD has no national registry where doctors can report the diagnosis of PD in the United States. (California is the only state where doctors must report cases of Parkinson's.) A mandatory national registry for the diagnosis of PD would be an enormous step forward (a global registry would be even better!) and one of the best ways to help researchers gather the knowledge and data they need. This registry may seem an invasion of your privacy, but information that allows researchers to track patterns is the best way to gain vital knowledge that leads to new treatments and a cure.

The attitude that busts research barriers

At the 2006 World Parkinson's Congress in Washington, D.C., Joan Samuelson (founder of the Parkinson's Action Network) said that when first diagnosed, she believed her job was to be a *patient patient.* That attitude quickly changed as Joan understood more about the known and unknowns of PD. Today her motto is that patients need to be *in the room*—the PD patient community needs to take a vocal and proactive role in helping research move forward.

You may not be ready to take on this larger fight, but keep it in the back of your mind as you use this book. ***Note:*** In many ways you've taken a key first step—you're educating yourself about Parkinson's and what a diagnosis may mean for you and your loved ones. But getting involved with the greater Parkinson's community at a local, state, and national level is one of the most empowering steps you can take to live a full and productive life in spite of PD. (And when you are ready to get more involved, see Chapter 14 for more information on clinical trials and Chapter 24 for ideas on advocacy roles.)

Chapter 3

Sizing Up Symptoms, Signs, and Stages

In This Chapter

- Getting the terms straight
- Taking stock of your symptoms
- Prioritizing: Primary and secondary signs
- Categorizing the progression of PD
- Keeping the care partner in the loop

Whenever you have a concern about your health, you've usually taken note of certain troubling (and unexplained) symptoms. Perhaps you seem more clumsy than usual or your joints seem unusually stiff and rigid. If these symptoms are troubling enough, you're likely to make an appointment with your primary care physician (PCP) to have them checked out. After you describe your symptoms, your doctor conducts a clinical exam looking for signs that may explain your symptoms.

In this chapter, we describe the *symptoms* that can signal Parkinson's disease (PD) as well as the *signs* your doctor looks or to reach a diagnosis. Although many chronic, progressive conditions move through defined stages, this chapter stresses how progression in PD is unique for each patient.

Familiarizing Yourself with the Lingo

In the medical world, a *symptom* is

- What you feel or perceive before you see the doctor.
- The reason you ultimately decide to make an appointment.
- The details (vague or specific) you give when the doctor or nurse asks why you've come in.

For example, you may say that you're more tired than usual or moving more slowly because you lack energy. Or perhaps you're depressed or experiencing dizziness or shaking.

In contrast, medical *signs* are what your doctor observes during the examination. The best doctors use their senses in addition to the data from the usual medical imaging techniques and screening tools (see Chapter 4 for more about these instruments). For example, a doctor's touch may sense tightened muscles, or his eyes may observe a fine tremor when your hand's at rest, or he may note a compromised balance or slight shuffle when you walk. His ears may detect softer speech, a searching for words, or unusual sounds in your lungs or intestines.

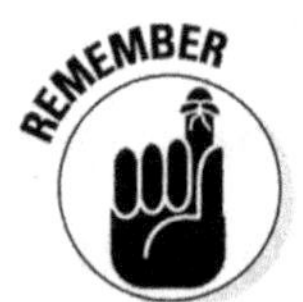

Simply put, symptoms make up your subjective report of your experiences, and signs contribute to your doctor's objective basis for a diagnosis.

Disease *staging* divides a chronic and progressive illness into levels that usually correspond to the advancement of symptoms and disease. Generally, stages have the following labels:

- *Early stage:* The disease is manageable with little outside assistance.
- *Moderate stage:* The patient needs more assistance and lifestyle changes.
- *Advanced stage:* The disease has advanced to the point that can be difficult to manage; the patient may face the end of life.

The following sections take a closer look at symptoms (what you tell your doctor), signs (what your doctor observes and discovers via tests and examination), and staging (where you are in the progression if you do have PD).

Symptoms—What You Look for

Let's cut to the chase. You suspect that you or someone you love may have PD or you wouldn't be flipping through this book and you definitely wouldn't have turned to this chapter.

Ask yourself what's behind those suspicions.

- **A slight shakiness in the hands?** Does it occur in only one hand? If the shaking occurs while the hand is at rest, does it stop when that hand picks up a cup of coffee, a pen, or a tennis racket? If the shakiness is in both hands and doesn't stop when the person grasps something, then PD probably isn't the cause (but get it checked out anyway).
- **A general slowing down of movement?** Does it take longer to walk from one place to another or to get in and out of the car? Has there been an increase in stumbling, clumsiness, or loss of balance? Do you (or does the person) feel tired, stiff, or just not *yourself?*
- **A significant change in energy level or outlook?** Everyone experiences days when they're tired or weaker than usual. And everyone has the blues from time to time. But if you've been feeling unusually weak, fatigued, depressed, or anxious for longer than two weeks,

those symptoms need attention—even when you have a plausible cause (such as an unusually busy week at work or the death of a loved one).

- **Gastrointestinal problems (like constipation) or psychological problems (like increased nervousness or anxiety)?** In some cases, patients show none of the usual symptoms, so don't stop with the more traditional PD symptoms.

These are the symptoms—the feelings, aches, and pains that have made you think something's not right. It may be PD or it may not. Either way, you owe it to yourself to get your doctor's assessment.

Signs—What Your Doctor Looks for

When you see your doctor, she'll listen as you describe your symptoms and then conduct an examination to determine what those symptoms indicate. As you talk about your symptoms, your doctor begins a *differential diagnosis* if your symptoms indicate several possibilities. For example, if your symptoms are in keeping with PD, your doctor also looks for signs that indicate PD. But any doctor worth her salt doesn't offer a firm diagnosis before she's seen the results of several tests and a specialist has confirmed her suspicions.

In addition to four primary signs of PD (which may or may not be evident when you first go to the doctor), your doctor considers several secondary signs and symptoms. And because PD is a neurological condition, it doesn't just affect your physical movement; it can also trigger non-motor or cognitive signs and symptoms. We discuss all of these signs and symptoms in the following sections.

Four primary signs

Although the actual causes and risk factors for getting PD are still mysterious (see Chapter 2 for more on these factors), the primary signs that signal the presence of PD are very clear. You may have noticed one or more of these signs but then dismissed it as something slight, easily explained, or due to an entirely different condition.

Several resources use the acronym *TRAP* to illustrate the four primary signs of PD. And, because PD seems to trap your body with your brain's compromised ability to communicate, the acronym makes the top four symptoms easy to remember.

T=Tremor at rest (uncontrolled shaking)

PD was originally called *shaking palsy* because the *resting tremor* (it goes away as soon as the hand is engaged) rarely occurs in other illnesses. Characteristically, the resting tremor begins in one hand and moves to the other hand years later in the disease. The tremor may extend to the leg or foot on the same side and sometimes to the lips and jaw—or you may have no tremor at all. Tremor in the head and neck, however, is less common in primary Parkinson's disease.

Variations of the resting tremor include:

- Postural tremor (obvious when arms are extended to hold a position or posture)
- Action tremor (present when certain tasks, such as holding, are performed)
- Internal tremor (the patient feels the tremor but can't show it, almost as if it's coming from inside)

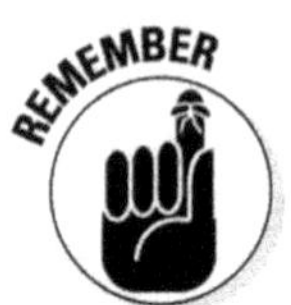

While tremor is the most obvious symptom of PD, it doesn't have to be present for diagnosis.

R=Rigidity (stiff muscles)

Rigidity is probably the most ignored and easy-to-explain-as- something-else sign. In plain English, *rigidity* means *stiffness.* (Who doesn't experience stiffness in joints and limbs that makes movement more difficult as they age?) If your doctor observes rigidity (without other signs of PD), he may first suspect arthritis and prescribe an anti-inflammatory medication. But, if medicine doesn't relieve the stiffness, you need to let your doctor know.

A=Akinesia (absence or slowness of movement)

Especially early on, people with PD (PWP) may experience slight *bradykinesia* (unusually slow movement). Much later in the progression, that slowed movement may become *akinesia* (no movement).

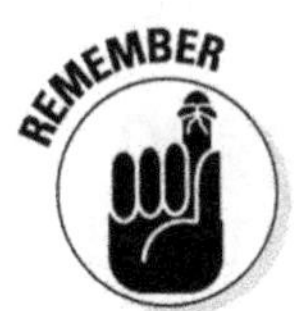

Get to know these terms because, if indeed you or a loved one has PD, you'll hear these words again and again. *Kinesia* means *movement* in the sense of knowing what you want your body to do. So *akinesia* and *bradykinesia* indicate problems initiating or continuing an action. For example, to walk across the room, you stand up and your brain tells your foot to step out—but with bradykinesia, your body doesn't move right away.

The problem can extend well beyond simply walking from here to there. Bradykinesia can also affect

- Facial expression because it slows blinking eye movement and the ability to smile. Read more about this *facial mask* in the next section, "Secondary signs and symptoms."
- Fine motor movements, such as the ability to manage buttons or cut food because the fingers lack the necessary speed and coordination to perform these detailed actions. In addition, fingers may curl or stiffen because of rigidity.
- The ability to easily turn over in bed because of lack of coordination between the various parts of the body that need to move in sequence; again muscle stiffness and rigidity may further complicate

this normally routine task. (See discussion of secondary signs and symptoms later in this chapter.)

P=Postural instability (impaired balance)

In a healthy person, the natural movement is to alternately swing the arms and step forward with assurance. For PWP, however, the swing slowly decreases; in time the person moves with small, uncertain, shuffling steps. (PWP may adapt by propelling themselves forward with several quick, short steps.) Other PWP experience episodes of *freezing* (their feet feel glued to the floor).

Problems with balance (resulting in falls that can cause major injuries, hospitalization, and escalation of symptoms) are usually not a factor until later stages in PD. In time, PWP may lose the ability to gauge the necessary action to regain balance and prevent a fall. They may grasp at doorways or other stationary objects in an effort to prevent the loss of balance. Unfortunately, these maneuvers can make PWP appear to be under the influence of alcohol or other substances.

Secondary signs and symptoms

Many of the following indicators—although not essential to a PD diagnosis—are observable early on and can contribute to the diagnosis of PD. During your appointment, tell your physician anything that is troublesome regarding these secondary symptoms. They're part of your symptomatic history that helps your doctors see the total picture of your condition.

Facial mask

The mask (lack of facial expression) is a common sign of PD, and it can lead people to assume that you're not listening or not understanding the conversation. The difference may simply be a change in your facial expression due to decreased animation or emotion. Maybe someone has said, "You don't smile as often," and you're thinking, "I'm smiling just as often as before!" Likewise, people may accuse you of staring, but the real problem is that the number of eye-blinks has decreased.

Slowed or slurred speech

You (or other folks) may notice that your voice is softer or fades away after a strong start. Your doctor may further note that your voice lacks normal variations of tone and emotion or that you sound hoarse but report nothing to explain that hoarseness. In some cases you may have trouble saying a word clearly; you slur it instead of enunciating.

As PD advances, other speech issues (such as stuttering or speaking very rapidly) can appear; swallowing difficulties may develop later in the disease. (See Chapter 18 for more info about advanced symptoms of PD.)

Small, cramped handwriting

Handwriting that once was free-flowing and smooth may appear increasingly cramped and jerky. This *micrographia* typically appears as letters that become progressively smaller (for example: *Parkinson*) and closer together.

Constipation and urinary incontinence

Most people (even some doctors) associate constipation with aging. But PD can also slow the bowels (as it does the rest of the body), so mention any unusual changes in bowel habits or routine to your doctor.

By the same token, *urinary frequency* (having to urinate often) and *urinary urgency* (NOW!) are common sideshows in the aging process. Although these problems may be signs of a totally unrelated condition, they are not uncommon in PD. Definitely bring these symptoms to your doctor's attention.

Increased sweating or oily skin

A sensitivity to heat and cold and excessively oily (or dry) skin are other signs that may indicate PD.

Non-motor signs and symptoms

Although the *TRAP* signs (check out the earlier section, "Four primary signs") are often enough evidence to raise the possibility of PD, non-motor factors may be present before those primary signs appear. Your doctor may ask questions to discover underlying symptoms that you've been ignoring or simply discounting.

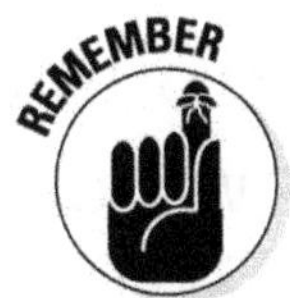

It is vital that you keep an open mind and answer your doctor's questions as honestly and fully as possible. Any one of the following symptoms or a combination of them may indicate a condition other than PD. Don't jump to conclusions or try to self-diagnose. Trust your doctor on this!

Anxiety or depression

Anxiety and depression are such an integral part of PD that they get their own chapter (Chapter 13) in this book. For now, remember that these feelings may be some of the earliest symptoms of PD. Anxiety episodes can range from a mild, underlying feeling of uneasiness to a full-blown panic attack. Depression may disguise itself as a general lack of interest in normal activities, or it may be severe enough for you or your family to consider counseling or medication.

Executive dysfunction and cognitive abnormalities

Do you have trouble balancing your checkbook, following directions, or making decisions? In medical terms, these symptoms are examples of *executive dysfunction.* Another term, *cue-dependent function,* is also part of the non-motor symptom package, and it means you need a reminder of some sort. For example, you may need an alarm that tells you to take your medicine or attend a meeting. Or you have labels on cabinets and drawers to remind you of their contents. Of course, many people use these reminders, especially when their lives are jammed with multiple responsibilities and a calendar brimming with appointments and commitments. But if you notice an escalation in the need for such reminders, mention it to your doctor.

In addition as many as half of all PWP experience problems with memory, thought processing, and word finding. These symptoms are usually more pronounced in later stages (see Chapter 18).

Dizziness or lightheadedness

In some cases dizziness or lightheadedness is due to a drop in blood pressure when you stand up, especially in warm weather or over-heated rooms. Although dizziness can be a factor in a number of conditions, don't ignore mentioning it to your doctor if it's one of your symptoms.

Sleep disturbances

PWP usually have no trouble getting to sleep. The more common problems are staying asleep, napping throughout the day, and moving restlessly when asleep. In some cases, the PWP has intense dreams that add to the restlessness and disturbance of normal sleep.

Sexual dysfunction

As with many medical conditions, PD can adversely affect sexual desire and performance. The underlying causes may or may not be related to PD; however, if the problem is part of your PD, it may be relieved with proper medication and treatment.

Visual hallucinations

Visual hallucinations (seeing people or objects that really aren't present) can be a side effect of many medications. In the case of antiparkinsonian meds, hallucinations are usually benign. ***Note:*** If a patient reports hallucinations before the PD diagnosis and before she begins taking PD meds, the doctor will look for other medications or causes that may be at the root of the problem.

Stages—Understanding the Unique Path PD Can Take

The key to living with any chronic, progressive illness is taking responsibility to maintain your life beyond that condition. We discuss this in much greater depth throughout the book. For now, the significant question is: If this is PD and it does progress, then how fast and to what extent?

Some *chronic* (long-lasting) and *progressive* (advancing or worsening) diseases have clear-cut divisions between *stages* (obvious and even predictable changes in the patient's condition). However, PD isn't one of those—it affects each patient differently. In rare cases, PD can progress rapidly; the person quickly becomes dependent on others for assistance with basic daily activities. However, for most PWP the progression takes years. With proper treatment and management of new symptoms, PWP can live independently for quite some time before they need close care.

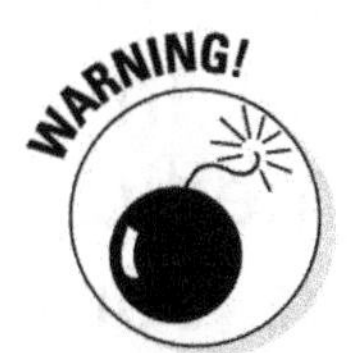

Don't let yourself or others try to project the future. *Prepare*—plan for what may happen—yes. *Project*—assume it will happen on a certain timetable—no. Projecting only adds to your anxiety and may actually prevent you from taking some measures that prolong the time between stages.

In spite of PD's lack of clearly defined and timed steps, your doctor may describe your condition in terms of stages. This breakdown is common practice in the medical profession because it permits doctors to use a common and accepted language when making notes about your condition. If you need to change doctors midstream, the new physician's ability to understand the previous doctor's notes can save you valuable time and enhance the new doctor's ability to address your needs.

Although your PD takes a path unique to you and in response to your lifestyle and medical choices, the disease does have some broad outlines of progression. For a fuller discussion of PD rating scales that determine its various stages, turn to Chapter 4.

Early stage PD: When life can be fairly normal

You may have experienced (and ignored) certain warning signals from PD for several years before you went to your doctor. Maybe you were constantly tired or had a vague, don't-feel-good sensation. As your general movement slowed, maybe you dismissed it as *getting older* or *lack of energy today.*

Then you began to notice some troubling (not to mention, annoying!) symptoms: stiffness that was different from the not-as-young-as- I-used-to-be version, shakiness, dizziness, or mood changes. You know the list.

If you have tremor, you may have barely noticed it at first, or maybe you dismissed it as a spasm. It may have appeared in one finger, so you noticed it only when you were performing a certain task, like tying your shoe or buttoning a jacket.

In *early* stage PD, the following conditions may occur:

- Symptoms are mild and often easily explained.
- Symptoms are annoying when they occur, but they don't significantly interfere with normal activity.
- Symptoms occur on only one side of the body.
- Tremor is present in one limb—usually the hand—and is most noticeable when the hand is at rest.
- Other people may comment on changes related to appearance, posture, energy, and facial expression.

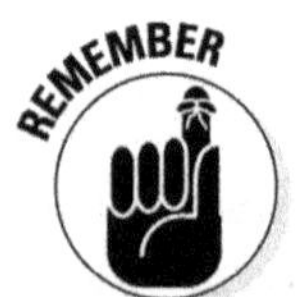

In the early stages of PD, you can manage for some time with no pharmacological intervention. In other words, you don't need pills to control the symptoms.

Moderate stage PD: When you need to accept help

The defining signal of progression in PD is symptoms on both sides of the body. However, even at this stage, the diagnosis of PD has been missed in some cases simply because the symptoms (rigidity, gait change, tremor) were taken as normal signs of aging.

Other factors that may signal the *moderate* stage include the following:

- Your posture becomes stooped; your head is more often bent forward with your chin toward the chest.
- Movement of all body parts is significantly slower. When you walk, you often experience *freezing* (your feet feel glued to the floor); your hand tremor may now affect your entire arm, making activities such as shaving or brushing your teeth more difficult.
- Cognitive and executive function (see "Non-motor signs and symptoms" earlier in this chapter) is more impaired. Short-term memory, putting thoughts into

words, balancing a checkbook, and making decisions are all more challenging.

- *Late-moderate* denotes increasing need for anti-dopaminergic medications. Problems with balance and risks of falls (which may result in injuries that require hospitalization) can actually speed the onset of late stage PD. (See Chapter 17.)
- PWP must rely on medicines as well as assistance from other people to pursue many of the activities they took for granted before PD. Examples of these activities are driving, getting in and out of a chair or bed, and going to the bathroom.

As symptoms progress, the challenging task for you and your doctors will be to manage your symptoms (see Chapter 9).

After you begin taking them, antiparkinsonian medicines can be amazingly effective. But they also have some serious and unsettling side effects. (For more about PD meds and their side effects, check out the discussion in Chapter 9.) Balancing the dosages and timing is a constant challenge that becomes more difficult as you move from the moderate to the late stage. The good news is that new medicines become available every year, medicines that—ideally—can be more effective without the frustrating side effects.

Late stage PD: When planning keeps you in control

When a PWP reaches the point of serious disability (that is, unable to lead a normal, independent life without major assistance), the medical community describes the stage as *late* or *advanced.* At this stage even the medications that were working so well in the earlier stages start creating problems and complications, and unless the PWP is a candidate for deep brain stimulation surgery (see Chapter 10), he may face unprecedented challenges. This is the stage (for most patients, it's years after the initial diagnosis) when all your planning and preparing (that we preach about throughout this book) pays off for you and your family. In spite of advancing frailty, you are still in control. You have made the decisions necessary to see you through this time, and your family understands and accepts your wishes. You can probably guess the signs:

- Walking is possible only with a walker and for short distances, if at all.
- The entire body is stiff and rigid; balance is significantly compromised.
- The PWP can no longer manage without considerable assistance.
- Cognitive impairments worsen; physical limitations increase.
- The benefits of medication wear off earlier between each dose.

- The PWP is usually confined to bed and requires round-the-clock care (most advanced stage).

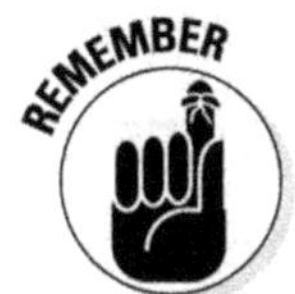

The length of each stage is unique to each PWP. With lifestyle and medical therapies and even with certain interventions along the way, PWP can maintain the early-stage status quo for several years.

A Few Words for You and Your Care Partner

If you're living with someone that you suspect has PD, encourage that person to seek a definitive diagnosis. The symptoms may or may not be PD. Many symptoms associated with PD are also factors in illnesses and conditions that are treatable and curable. Neither you nor the other person should jump to conclusions, but you shouldn't ignore the warning signs either.

If the diagnosis is PD, then your first job is to understand that this person you love can continue to live an independent and self-reliant life for some time, even many years.

If you're the person's care partner:

- Don't assume you need to be Super-Caregiver. Resist the urge to go into full-on nurturing mode; encourage independence and self-reliance.
- Understand that adding PD to your already busy life can lead to problems if you aren't proactive and don't take the necessary steps to integrate your new role into the rest of your life.
- Be aware that a decline in the PWP's self-reliance and confidence may be a sign of depression—a common symptom of PD.

If you're the PWP:

- Maintain your independence and refuse to permit PD to rob you of the normal roles you've always played in all your relationships.
- Understand that depression is perfectly normal when you first hear that you have PD; however it is not

normal for such depression to be pro-longed to the point that it actually escalates the progression of your PD and your need for hands-on care.

For each of you, the second task is to realize (and accept) that all the medicines and physician advice in the world can't be effective unless the PWP follows treatment recommendations, including changes in lifestyle. Self-management (the ability to take responsibility through changes in attitude and behavior) is the key to living with chronic illness of any type—and vital for living with PD. If you're the partner, consider what changes you can make in your own routines and habits that support and encourage the PWP to fight this disease.

The following tips may help both of you cope in these early stages:

- Find out everything you can—from reliable and respected sources—about PD. (See Appendix B for many of the best resources.)
- Ask questions. Chapters 4 and 5 deal specifically with the diagnosis

and the steps immediately following it.

- Take an active role in partnering with the PWP and medical professionals to consider treatment options and manage symptoms (See Chapter 6 for teaming up with the pros and Chapters 9, 10, and 11 for more about treatment options.)
- Maintain emotional balance as you each cope with your fears and anxieties about the meaning of this diagnosis for you and other people close to the PWP. (Chapter 7 offers ideas on dealing with other people. Chapters 15 and 19 address relationship questions you may be asking.)
- Remind each other of times when the PWP faced a difficult situation and didn't just cope, but triumphed in handling it.
- Whether you're the PWP or the care partner, don't wait to get help for obvious anxiety and depression. (Chapter 13 covers this piece of PD in more detail.)

If the diagnosis is PD, don't panic. You and the PWP are now members of a unique, extraordinarily proactive, well-organized community. If you open yourself to that community, you'll be richer for the friends you make, the information you exchange, and the comfort you share.

Part II

Making PD Part—But Not All—of Your Life

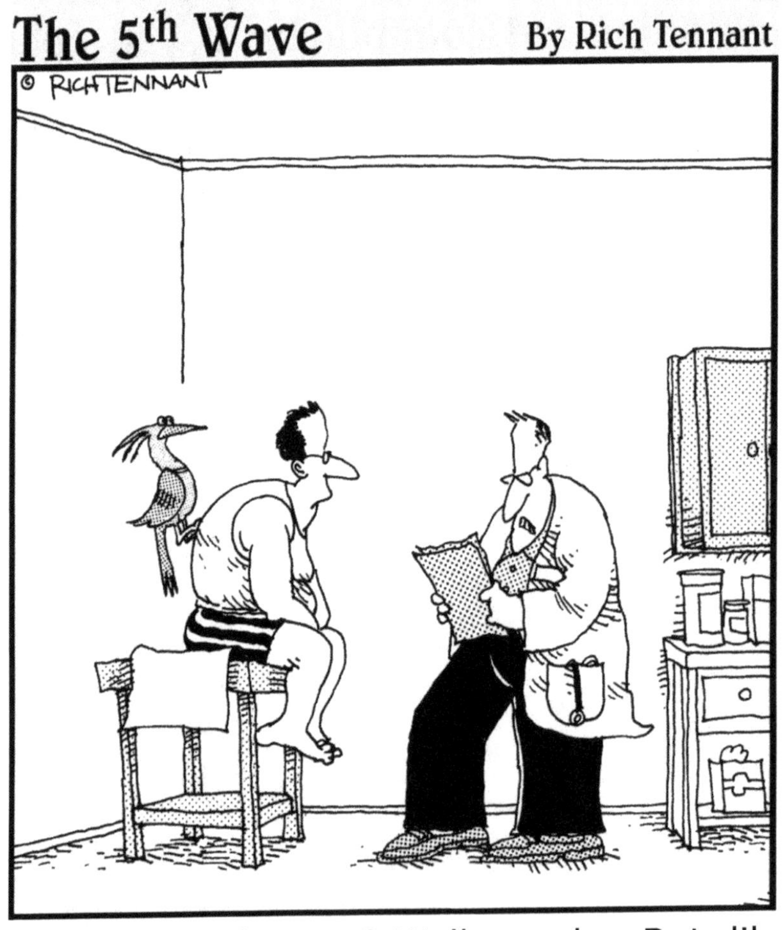

"Parkinson's disease? Well, maybe. But, like that pain in your shoulder, it could be a lot of things."

In this part...

We explore the intricacies of making an accurate diagnosis and why you should see a specialist—a neurologist—to develop a plan for treating your PD and managing your symptoms. You get the basics on how to assemble the healthcare support team you're going to need and the best way (and time) to let other people know of your diagnosis. This part includes a special chapter filled with information for people under age 50 who have young onset Parkinson's disease (YOPD).

Chapter 4

Getting an Accurate Diagnosis

In This Chapter

- Prepping for your primary care doctor
- Partnering with a neurologist
- Understanding the diagnosis process
- Looking for a second opinion

Okay, perhaps you've checked out Chapters 2 and 3 to see the causes and risk factors of Parkinson's disease (PD) as well as its signs and symptoms. And maybe the more you read, the more you worried that you (or someone you care for) may actually have it. Before you freak out, get to a doctor and find out for sure. Your imagination about PD and its consequences is far worse than living with it. In reality, many people with PD live relatively normal and fully active lives for many years after diagnosis. It's your call, but you can set this book aside right now and go bury your head in the sand, or you can take a measured, proactive approach to checking out those symptoms.

Ah, you're still here—great! (Okay, so the book's a little sandy. No problem.) The first step is to get an accurate diagnosis of your symptoms, starting with an accurate list of your current symptoms and medical history. Follow that with a visit to your primary care physician (PCP), who may recommend that you see a specialist. No doubt, you'll be prodded and tested, but you'll finally have a diagnosis. Last step? You want to get that diagnosis confirmed. Ready? Here we go.

Bringing Up the Subject with Your Doctor

This isn't going to be the usual appointment with your doctor. You're not going for an annual check-up or some routine test. You're making this appointment because you have symptoms that you can't explain and that don't seem to be going away. And you're making this appointment because you're concerned something is seriously wrong. An appointment for these reasons needs careful planning all along the way, from scheduling the appointment to gathering information to preparing questions you want to ask. All of this needs to happen *before* the appointment.

Scheduling an appointment

When you call your doctor's office to schedule the appointment, ask to speak to the doctor's nurse or assistant. Tell that person why you're scheduling the appointment. (Yes, go ahead and say it, "I'm concerned that I may have Parkinson's disease.") Then add that you want an appointment when the doctor will have more time—especially if your suspicions are correct. Also ask the nurse what information you should bring with you. When you do make the appointment (usually through the office manager or receptionist), only you can weigh the possible wait (perhaps several weeks until the doctor has this extra time) against the earliest available appointment. ***Note:*** If you choose the latter, consider booking that later appointment as well in case you want to follow up in more detail with the doctor. In either case, ask to be on the call list. In the event of a cancellation, you can then get to see the doctor sooner.

Preparing for your initial exam

Before seeing your PCP, plan to take the following steps to make that first meeting as productive as possible.

Gathering your medical records

First, be sure that your PCP has copies of all medical records. For example, if you've been seeing a cardiologist, your PCP needs copies of any lab work or stress test results as well as that doctor's notes on observations and treatment.

As soon as you schedule the appointment with your PCP, ask the office staff of any specialist you're seeing to fax copies of recent lab results to your PCP's office. Preparing and transferring such information can take time. So, if time is short, call the clinic where the tests were done or the doctor who ordered the tests and ask for a copy of the results. Then you can pick up these reports and take them with you to your appointment.

Prioritizing your symptoms

Next, make a list of your symptoms and prioritize them. For example, maybe the following is your list of symptoms:

- Anxious and not my usual upbeat self
- Shaky—especially in my right hand
- Unusually fatigued—no get-up-and-go
- Not sleeping well

If you suspect PD because you've noticed a slight tremor, you may want to move the second bullet (shaky) to the top of your list.

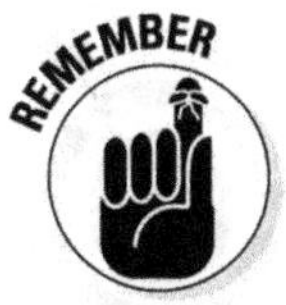

Keep in mind that the doctor's staff may interview you first. When the nurse asks you why you came in, the first words out of your mouth get her attention. So, if you say, "I haven't been sleeping that well," rather than "Over the last few weeks I've noticed a slight shakiness in my right hand," the nurse writes that your primary issue is *sleep disturbance.* And that statement can take matters in a whole different direction, wasting precious time.

Your doctor refers to the first symptom as your *chief complaint.* When she follows up on your answer with some form of "What makes you suspect Parkinson's?" then you can offer the rest of the symptoms on your list.

For heaven's sake, if you suspect PD, don't be afraid to introduce it into the conversation right away. Life—and doctor's appointments—are too short to beat around the bush!

Compiling your medical history

Writing down your personal medical history helps you prepare for the many questions along the way to your diagnosis. Preparing your history in advance also gives you time to think carefully about the specifics instead of trying to remember details on the spot.

If you've seen a doctor recently, you know that the questions are usually the same—no matter how many times you give the information. First, one or two members of the staff gather your information, and then the nurse or physician assistant (PA) may ask the same questions. But, with a trusty print-out of your history, you can provide a clean copy for their file and still have a copy in-hand (you made two copies, right?) to prompt you on dates and details. This step saves everyone precious time during the appointment and spares you the frustration of recalling every detail for every question.

Don't let this multiple quizzing frustrate you. There's a method to the madness of three different people asking you the same question—usually some form of "Why have you come to see the doctor?" They know that the second or third time a patient answers that question, he may provide additional information without even realizing it.

Many doctors send a questionnaire to help patients gather essential information about themselves and their medical histories. Even if you don't receive such a document, be prepared for your doctor's questions by writing down the following information and taking it with you to your initial exam:

- Patient's legal (full) name and maiden name
- Date of birth
- Birthplace
- Parents' names with dates and causes of death
- Current prescribed (Rx) medications, dosing routine, and purpose (example: diazide, 10mg 1 x day for hypertension); list each Rx separately
- Current over-the-counter (OTC) medications taken regularly, including vitamins, supplements, and such (example: calcium+D, 600 mg 2 x day); list each separately
- Any medications (Rx or OTC) taken over the past year but not currently taken
- Known allergies or adverse reactions to medications or common medical equipment (example: latex gloves)
- Other physicians seen regularly (example: allergist,

cardiologist)—name, address, telephone

- Current health problems and dates of onset
- Dates and circumstances of past illnesses or medical events (example: fractured rib, heart attack, accident)
- Dates and reasons for hospitalizations
- Dates and reasons for surgeries
- Recent changes in physical health
- Recent changes in mental or emotional health
- Current situations that may contribute to health changes (consider family, work, and other factors)

Stepping through your initial exam

Okay, you have everything in order and today's the appointment. Take some-one with you. If you think you have PD (and it turns out that your doctor agrees), you'll need that extra set of ears to hear what you're bound to miss after you hear that you may have a chronic and progressive condition. Most likely, this will be your care partner if the diagnosis turns out to be PD. The role of this person is to take notes and listen during the appointment and then help you digest and decipher that discussion after the appointment.

Much of what happens at the doctor's office is already familiar to you: the wait (complete with dog-eared selections of last year's magazines); the weigh-in, blood pressure and updating of your medical history; the second wait (this time in the exam room). Use this time to go over the information and questions you've prepared. The doctor's going to ask why you think you have PD, and you need to be prepared to offer specifics (your symptoms, when and how often they occur, when they began, what seems to relieve them, and so on). If you've made a list, you're ready and can just review it.

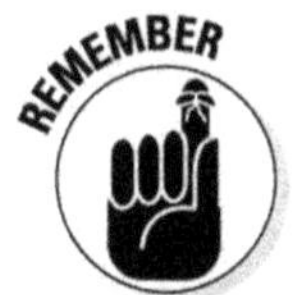

The doctor may be giving you extra time for your appointment, but that's not the same as endless time. You need to use the time you have wisely by coming to the appointment as well prepared as possible. For more tips on knowing what to expect from a diagnostic appointment and getting the most from that appointment, see "Working with Your Neurologist to Determine Whether This Is PD" section later in this chapter.

Leaving with the answers you need

You'll probably have a gazillion questions by the end of the initial appointment, and you're just as likely not to be able to think of a single one. So once again, be prepared. Prepare a list of questions in advance and use that list. You may even want to hand a copy to your doctor.

If you've brought another person with you to listen and take notes, this is the time she may want to speak up and ask questions also. You can use the following sets of questions as a guide during the appointment. But feel free to add your own.

If the diagnosis seems pretty clear from the start

Although your PCP may believe the diagnosis is clear, he most likely will deliver the news as *possibly* or *likely* Parkinson's and recommend you see a neurologist (a specialist in disorders of the central nervous system). Your PCP may talk in lingo that's unfamiliar to you (*parkinsonism, bradykinesia, postural instability,* and such). Don't be afraid to ask for a clear, layperson's explanation by asking the following questions:

- What is the diagnosis—in plain English?
- What is the prognosis (how quickly will the condition progress)?
- How will the diagnosis be confirmed?
- Does this diagnosis require me to see a specialist?
- Can you recommend a specialist and help set an appointment for me?
- In the meantime, what should I do?

If the doctor orders tests

Even if your doctor believes the diagnosis is fairly clear, she may want to rule out other possibilities. For example, some of the medications you've been taking may be interacting in a way that produces a slight shaking (tremor) in your hand. Or, maybe your primary symptom seems to be depression and apathy; the doctor may want to refer you to a psychologist for evaluation. If she recommends these or other tests, ask the following questions:

- What are the tests and why are you ordering them?
- What is the procedure for each test?
- How quickly will you have the results?
- What will be the next steps after you have the test results?

If the PCP recommends treatment

Especially if you live in a small community or rural area, your PCP may be the only name in town for treating a wide variety of complex conditions. Even if you live in a larger community that has several specialists including neurologists, your doctor may be aware that your economic situation and lack of adequate insurance may keep you from seeking these services. In any case, if your PCP does not recommend seeking a specialist as a next step but does recommend a plan of treatment, ask the following questions:

- What is the treatment?
- Why are you choosing this treatment option?
- What are the risks or possible down sides of taking these medicines or

following the recommended therapies?

- What is the cost and will this be covered by my insurance?
- What are the benefits?
- How quickly should the treatment work?
- How will you monitor and follow up on the treatment plan?
- What are the alternatives to this treatment plan?

If It Looks Like PD ... Connecting with a Neurologist

The initial suspicions of you and your PCP will likely lead to an appointment with a neurologist who can administer further tests to confirm the diagnosis. (If your PCP has already diagnosed PD, then your neurologist helps manage your care.) The following sections suggest how to find a specialist in your area and how to know whether you'll make a good team.

Locating an experienced and qualified neurologist

If possible, look for a neurologist who specializes in movement disorders (like Parkinson's). If you're very fortunate, you live in or near a community that has a Morris K. Udall Parkinson's Disease Research Center of Excellence program. These programs—often in a medical university or institution—are involved in clinical research specifically for the benefit of PD patients. (See the "Morris K. Udall Parkinson's Disease Research Centers of Excellence" sidebar for more information.)

This section suggests resources for finding a neurologist who can help you deal with your PD—now and down the road.

Surfing the Web

The Internet can be a huge help to locate a doctor. Several sites locate physicians by specialty as well as by location, and the sites provide important information about a doctor's training, expertise, possible ethical or treatment violations, and so on. Try an online search with the phrase *neurologists finding.*

You can also get information by checking with the local or regional chapter of a national PD organization. (See the next section and Appendix B for the national organization's info.) Ask whether your area has a local PD support group. If it does, ask for the name and contact information of the group's facilitator. When you call the facilitator, ask whether any members of the group have been treated by neurologists that you're considering. If possible, contact those patients (preferably including patients who have changed doctors) and ask about their experiences with those doctors.

Checking with the local chapter of PD groups

The following organizations have chapters and support groups in communities across the country. You can call them to get names of neurologists in your area.

- National Parkinson's Foundation (NPF): 800-327-4545
- American Parkinson's Disease Association (APDA): 800-223-2732
- Parkinson's Action Network (PAN): 800-850-4726

If you live in a small community, you may have to connect with the group in a larger community nearby (or even at the state level), but the information from these experienced groups is invaluable as you look for a neurologist that's right for you.

Asking your family doctor

Your PCP may be an internist or, if you live in a small community or rural area with limited access to medical care, he may be a general practitioner. For some women, an Obstetrician/Gynecologist (OB/GYN) is their PCP. Whatever your doctor's focus, he's probably aware of local leading doctors in various specialties.

A key question to ask your PCP is: Which specialist do you recommend for working in tandem with you (the PCP) and me to manage my overall health and PD? This question is important for many reasons, but mainly because it is enormously important that your neurologist be consulted before any other doctor prescribes medications or treatment that may adversely affect your PD medication routine or worsen your symptoms.

When your town has no neurologists

Speaking of small communities, what are your options if the closest neurologist is some distance away? First, consider that you're not going to see this specialist weekly or even monthly after the diagnosis is confirmed and you begin routine treatment. Second, assuming the neurologist and your PCP are willing to work together, you have the emergency backup of your PCP if you need immediate attention.

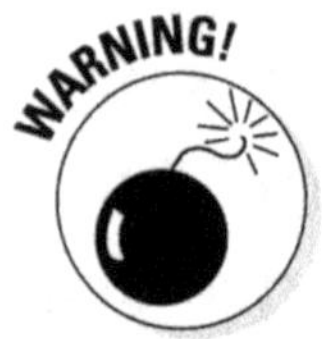

Don't be tempted to just let your PCP manage your PD for the sake of convenience. At the very least, you want to have your neurologist reevaluate your treatment and status two to four times a year depending on how much change you experience between visits. If you have questions between appointments, try the phone and e-mail. But, taking a day every two to three months to see the neurologist—the specialist in treating your PD—is time well spent. You're worth every minute of it!

Evaluating your neurologist

First things first. You can't expect a neurologist to cure you because a cure for PD doesn't exist—yet. But you can and should expect a professional partnership. You and your neurologist (as well as other team members that we introduce in Chapter 6) will work together to manage your PD symptoms and maintain your physical, mental, and emotional health to the highest possible levels during the years ahead.

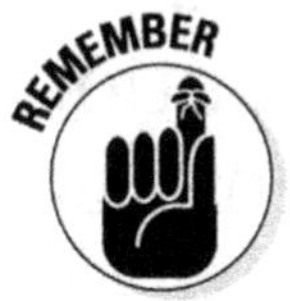

You're looking for a specialist who seems curious about *your* Parkinson's:

- How it's affecting you now
- How you can manage those symptoms best
- How to postpone onset of new or worsening symptoms for as long as possible

Morris K. Udall Parkinson's Disease Research Centers of Excellence

Morris K. Udall served in the United States Congress for 30 years and was well-respected by colleagues on both sides of the aisle. He also lived with Parkinson's disease from his diagnosis in 1979 until his death in 1998, serving in the House of Representatives until 1991. In 1997, Congress passed the Morris K. Udall Parkinson's Disease Research Act, and President Clinton signed it into law in 1998. This legislation contributed to the establishment of 12 Parkinson's research centers funded by the National Institute of Neurological Disorders and Stroke (NINDS), a division of the National Institutes of Health (NIH). As a result, the legislation cast a national spotlight on the need for collaborative, coordinated research efforts for new treatments and a cure for PD.

The 12 centers are:

- Brigham and Women's Hospital, Boston, MA
- Columbia University, New York, NY
- Duke University, Durham, NC
- Harvard University (McLean Hospital), Belmont, MA
- Johns Hopkins University, Baltimore, MD

- Massachusetts General Hospital (Massachusetts Institute of Technology), Boston, MA
- Mayo Clinic, Jacksonville, FL
- Northwestern University, Evanston, IL
- University of California Los Angeles (UCLA), Los Angeles, CA
- University of Kentucky Medical Center, Lexington, KY
- University of Virginia, Charlottesville, VA
- University of Pittsburgh, Pittsburgh, PA

The 1997 legislation was a good start, but more work is needed. In 2005, Congressman Lane Evans of Illinois, who also has PD, introduced H.R. 3550, a bill to amend and further the work of the original legislation. The new bill would require NIH to hold a conference to review the progress of the work at these Centers for Excellence every two years and produce a strategic plan (including a budget, expected results, actual spending, and actual results) and a report to Congress. H.R. 3550 was

> referred to a subcommittee in August of 2005. As of this writing, that was the last action on the bill. The Parkinson's Action Network (PAN) maintains a watch on this bill and other legislation critical to the fight. The Web site is www.parkinsonsaction.org.

Along with expertise, you're looking for a certain quality of empathy—a chemistry between the two of you. (See more discussion on this relationship in the next section.) You don't want a godlike figure that makes decisions *for* you rather than *with* you. After all, who has to live with this PD? Not the neurologist.

Preparing for that first visit

Use the following checklist as you prepare for meeting the neurologist:

- When you make the appointment, ask for the first or last appointment of the day. This choice should assure additional time for questions.
- Make sure your PCP has sent copies of your records to the neurologist's

office. Assuming that it was your PCP who referred you to the specialist, you may think that the records are transferred automatically. Guess again. You need to stay on top of this transfer and follow up with both offices to make sure the transfer actually takes place.

- Take a copy of your personal medical history and the results of any recent lab work with you. (Refer back to the section "Preparing for your initial exam" earlier in this chapter for more about the history.)
- Be sure to update that history to include your medications with the strength and dosage routine (or pack up the actual meds in a plastic bag—seriously!). Also list any vitamins, supplements, or other OTC meds you take on a regular basis.
- A few days prior to the appointment, call the office to confirm the appointment and ask whether they've received your records. If they haven't, follow up with your PCP. You may need to

pick up copies of the records and take them with you to the appointment.

- Arrive half an hour before your scheduled appointment so you can complete their paperwork without cutting into your time with the doctor.

Interviewing the good doctor

Everyone wants the best neurologist out there. But, because of PD's chronic and progressive nature, you also need a neurologist who's a good fit for you and your care partner. Start with the basic nuts and bolts. The following list contains the most essential factors you need consider:

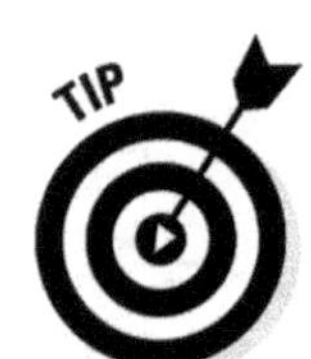

- Of course the neurologist has a medical degree, but is he *board-certified* (has he completed and passed nationally recognized exams to test his expertise)? If he has special training in *movement disorders* (PD is one), count yourself ahead of the game.

- What professional organizations and societies does he belong to?
- How many people with Parkinson's (PWP) are currently under his care?
- How long has the doctor been treating PWP? (If the good doctor is a good *older* doctor, how long does he anticipate practicing?) If the doctor is relatively young, check background and experience. Has this person worked with more experienced PD specialists?
- Who are the partners in his practice, and what are their backgrounds? No partners? Where does he send patients when he's unavailable?
- What days and hours does he see patients? (If the doctor is well known and sought after but has really limited office hours, that situation may send up a red flag for getting appointments when you need them.)

• Are the office hours and location convenient for you? If not, is that a deal breaker for you? Keep in mind that in the early stages of your PD (see Chapter 3) you'll probably see your neurologist infrequently, perhaps every six to eight weeks. If the distance and schedule still seem inconvenient, you can look elsewhere, but please try not to sacrifice experience and skill for convenience.

• If the doctor orders lab work, does his office provide the service? If not, is the office part of a hospital-physician complex where labs are easily available? If the answer is "No" to both questions, you'll most likely go to your area hospital or walk-in clinic for the lab work.

• What's the cost of an office visit?

• If you need to consult with him by phone, does he charge you for it?

• Does he accept your insurance? If you're on Medicare, does he *accept assignment* (charge only what Medicare assigns as the cost)? See Chapter 20 for more help on those sticky insurance questions.

Reviewing your first impressions

Okay, the neurologist passes your basic tests. Now for the tough part: How well will the two of you work together? First impressions can say a great deal, so pay attention to details like the following:

- Does the doctor seem rushed or distracted when she meets you?
- Does she listen and ask questions that draw out additional information, or does she cut you off making pronouncements rather than recommendations?
- What is her treatment philosophy on PD? Medication right away? Medication only after symptoms start to interfere with life routines? What about the use of new or proven surgical procedures?

The right answer, of course, includes a reminder that all patients progress differently and under varying circumstances, so the treatment regimen varies person to person.

• What is the doctor's philosophy about partnering with the patient (and eventually, when your care partner becomes your advocate and spokesperson, with the care partner)?

• Is there chemistry (we're not talking magic here, just good vibes)? Do you feel an intangible connection—where you can rely on this doctor's partnership to explore ways to manage symptoms and maintain functionality as long as possible?

Moving forward if it's a good fit

Finally, if this doctor seems a good fit, you have just a few more questions to ask him:

- How does the doctor prefer that you prepare for an appointment? For example, does he want you to e-mail questions or concerns in advance, or can you bring written questions to the appointment? Can you bring a tape recorder to tape the conversation so you can listen to it again?

- What is his preferred way of communicating with you between appointments: by phone or e-mail; through his nurse or physician assistant? (If you're to contact the nurse or physician assistant, be sure you meet this person and get direct contact information.)
- What hospital does the doctor use for treating patients?

And what if, after all of this, the doctor just isn't for you? No chemistry. Of course, you can move on and start the whole process with another doctor. On the other hand, if this doctor is considered the best in your area, perhaps you should give the relationship a chance. After all, the two of you are relative strangers. How well did you click with other professionals in your life on the first appointment? Keep in mind that this is first and foremost a professional relationship; you will rely on this expert to plot the course you'll navigate through the challenges of PD. This doctor may not be especially interested in seeing pictures of your first grandchild, but if the treatment plan he puts together clearly focuses on your individual journey through PD and helps you enjoy that grandchild for years to come, do you really need anything more?

Working with Your Neurologist to Determine Whether This Is PD

Neurologists use a variety of methods to make a definitive diagnosis of PD:

- The physical examination
- An assessment of your function through mental and performance testing
- Sophisticated imaging equipment that permits a look inside your brain

Despite all these methods, your doctor may still need to rule out other explanations for your symptoms before she's prepared to state, without question, that you have PD.

This section takes you through the usual steps of that first visit.

Navigating the clinical exam

No single diagnostic test (like doctors have for measuring blood pressure or cholesterol levels) can confirm a clinical diagnosis of Parkinson's disease. So your neurologist's skill of observation and his experience in diagnosing and treating PWP is key. Your initial appointment will probably include the following three levels of examination:

History taking

The first level of examination is a discussion of your complete medical history. The printed copy you provide (see "Compiling your medical history" earlier in this chapter for help with this step) can help, but you'll probably hear some questions two or three times in this first appointment. Be a *patient* patient (pun intended). A good neurologist asks these questions not only to review your symptoms but also to rule out less-typical types of parkinsonism or other neurological conditions, which sometimes entail radically different management. (See "Parkinsonism, But Not PD" later in this chapter.)

Physical exam

After recording your medical history, the doctor performs a physical examination that may include such standards as:

- Measuring your blood pressure (while you're lying down and then again standing up)
- Checking your pulses, heartbeat, lungs, and abdomen

The point of such routine observations is to make sure your symptoms aren't due to problems in other parts of your body.

Neurological exam

The final level is the neurological examination, which is largely a process of observation. The neurologist tests your coordination and balance while observing you walk, stand, sit, turn, extend your arms and hands, and so on.

This exam may also include any of the following tasks:

- Opening and closing your fists or tapping your fingers several times
- Touching the doctor's finger and then your nose with your index finger (it looks silly but can give the neurologist a wealth of information)
- Recovering your balance after the doctor pulls you gently from behind your shoulders as you stand with your eyes open or closed
- Answering several simple questions from the doctor to test your attention and memory
- Drawing a figure on a piece of paper and then duplicating it

Don't be surprised by the apparent simplicity of these questions and tests; they are all part of a standardized exam!

After the neurologist has completed the initial interview, the physical exam and neurological observations, he (or an assistant) may use standard screening tools to further confirm the diagnosis or the stage or severity of your PD. This next section covers those tools.

Establishing the severity and staging the progression of your PD

Your neurologist may use a variety of tools for establishing your PD's progression through the various stages or levels. (See Chapter 3 for more about these stages.) The rating scales in the next section are useful in setting a benchmark for the doctor. Neuroimaging tools are also helpful in tracking progression and ruling out other possibilities for symptoms you may experience.

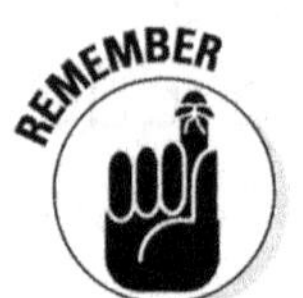

Rating scales and neuroimaging tests are tools available to your doctor to assist in establishing the progression of your PDC. They aren't used in confirming the diagnosis.

Rating scales

In any major disorder like PD, neurologists may use standardized rating scales to measure symptoms and stage the disease. (For a refresher on *staging,* flip over to Chapter 3.) These instruments are helpful in determining how advanced your symptoms are and how best to address them. The scales also form the basis for a more extensive medical history if a patient needs to change doctors in the future. In addition, clinical researchers frequently use these scales to monitor the effects of new and experimental therapies on patients. (See Chapter 14, where we discuss the trials more completely.)

- **Hoehn and Yahr Rating Scale:** This diagnostic tool stages the level of a person's PD by using broad measures of disability. This scale was originally devised by Melvin Yahr and Margaret Hoehn following a detailed study of the natural progression of PD in the late

1960s. They observed five general stages in PD, ranging from Stage 1 (unilateral disease, limited to one side of the body) to Stage 5 (wheelchair bound or bedridden unless aided). However, as we mention often in this book, PD doesn't progress in neat, little, predictable stages. Therefore, the more complex (and more informative) Unified Parkinson Disease Rating Scale (see the next section) usually accompanies and complements this tool.

- **Unified Parkinson Disease Rating Scale (UPDRS):** The UPDRS focuses on several facets of PD's disability, such as its effects on daily activities, motor skills, and mental capacity (including behavior and mood). It consists of a painless interview and a focused neurological exam, with a score for each item from 0 (normal) to 4 (severe). Therefore, the higher the UPDRS score, the greater the disability from PD.

The UPDRS—when administered correctly—is "an exquisitely sensitive test for detecting early PD," according to a Parkinson's Disease Foundation article. It may be the best tool for the neurologist to assess symptom levels and design treatment plans. The UPDRS is currently under revision by the Movement Disorders Society and will be soon updated to better reflect the multifaceted reality of PD disability.

- **Schwab and England Activities of Daily Living:** This tool rates a person's ability to perform the normal routine activities of daily living using a percentage rating. The patient usually rates himself with the help of set definitions presented by the doctor.

For example, people who consider themselves to be completely independent and functional qualify for a 100 percent rating. They can perform all activities without difficulty. In contrast, a person who takes three to four times the normal time to perform a task (such as dressing) has a 70 percent independence rating. And a person who can manage only a few chores from time to time (and always with great effort) has a 30 percent rating.

Neuroimaging

A thorough neurological exam and the proper administration of the UPDRS is usually enough to diagnose a new case of PD. However, neuroimaging techniques now permit neurologists to pinpoint the diagnosis of PD and follow its progression by observing the affected nerve cells.

Two recently developed imaging techniques, positron-emission tomography and single photon emission computed tomography, can confirm the diagnosis of PD and distinguish PD from other Parkinson-like disorders. (See "Parkinsonism, But Not PD" later in this chapter for more discussion on other disorders.) Both scans use low levels of radioactive materials and pose little, if any, risk for the patient. I describe both of these scans in the following:

- The *positron-emission tomography* (PET) scan uses a radioactive form of *levodopa* (the drug that enhances dopamine production in the brain), which is injected intravenously into the patient, to highlight the loss of normal *dopamine* cells (the neurons primarily affected by PD) in the brain. As dopamine cells uptake levodopa, a reduced signal from labeled (radioactive) levodopa is usually found in PD.

- The *single photon emission computed tomography* (SPECT) scan is another imaging technique able to measure metabolic and physiological functions of specific areas of the brain. When using radioactive markers able to link to dopamine cells, SPECT scans can measure the progressive loss of these neurons caused by PD.

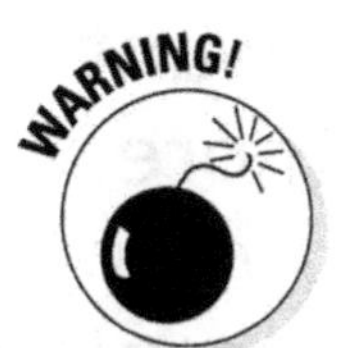

A couple of factors limit the use of neuroimaging: cost and availability. At this writing, some insurance companies consider such scans experimental and as a result, don't cover any of the costs. In addition, the equipment and expertise for performing and interpreting the scans aren't widely available.

Ruling out the red herrings: What else can it be?

What else looks like PD? That answer may depend on your presenting symptoms (the information you tell the doctor) or on other facts that the doctor gathers through interviewing and examining you.

For example:

- If you don't present with any of the *TRAP* symptoms (check out Chapter 3 for a quick review of these) but you talk about a loss of energy, the doctor may want to explore that symptom more. After further questioning, your doctor may see that depression plays a role in your loss of energy. If so, is the depression associated with PD, or is it related to some other life-changing event, such as the death of a loved one or the loss of a job?
- Even if a hand tremor was your reason for seeing a neurologist, is the tremor confined to one hand or both? Does it stop after the hand

is engaged in activity, or does the tremor continue?

Don't try to second-guess your symptoms. Is it PD? Maybe. Is it something else—something easier to treat and cure? Possibly. Either way, you need to know. Why postpone treating a curable condition simply because you think it may be more serious? And if it does turn out to be PD, then you want to get a jump on managing symptoms as early as possible—when you have the greatest opportunity to maintain independence and flexibility.

Parkinsonism, But Not PD

If it walks like a duck and quacks like a duck, it's a duck, right? So if it looks like PD and acts likes PD, then it's PD, right? Not always.

The same symptoms that indicate PD can also indicate other conditions, thus *parkinsonism* is a generic term referring to slowness and mobility problems that look like PD. Parkinsonism is a feature in several conditions that have different (and perhaps known) causes, but those conditions don't progress like PD. As a result, years may go by before the differences between PD and the other disorder are apparent; the PD diagnosis may then be reversed.

Taking antiparkinsonian medications (such as levodopa) may be the first indicator that parkinsonism isn't actually PD. By definition, PD promptly responds to this medication, which improves its symptoms in a consistent way, at least for a few years. But, in parkinsonism, improvement is often erratic or nonexistent from the beginning. In fact, your neurologist will always closely monitor your response to treatment in order to rule out the possibility that your condition is a disorder other than PD.

Two categories of non-PD disorders are:

- **Parkinson's Plus syndromes:** This group of neurodegenerative disorders has parkinsonian features, such as *bradykinesia* (slowness), *rigidity* (stiffness), *tremor* (shaking), and *gait disturbances* (balance). See Chapter 3 for more about these PD symptoms. However, they are also associated with other complex neurological symptoms that reflect problems in brain areas other than the *dopaminergic system* (the network of neurons able to make and release the neurotransmitter *dopamine*). These conditions progress more rapidly than PD and don't respond as well (or at all) to antiparkinsonian medications. The most common Parkinson's Plus syndromes are *Multiple System Atrophy* (MSA), *Progressive Supranuclear Palsy* (PSP), *Cortico-Basal Ganglionic Degeneration* (CBGD), and *Lewy Body Dementia* (LBD).
- **Secondary parkinsonisms:** The symptoms of these disorders relate to well-defined lesions in the brain from strokes, tumors, infections,

traumas, or certain drugs. Like Parkinson's Plus syndromes, these syndromes are usually less responsive to levodopa. However, if the primary cause of parkinsonism is controlled, these symptoms tend to be less progressive.

In addition to Parkinson's plus and secondary parkinsonisms, *Essential Tremor* (ET) is another source of possible confusion. As the most common movement disorder—as much as 20 times more common than PD—ET's only symptom is a tremor that affects the hands (only while they're moving) but may also affect the head or voice. ET can run in families and is usually benign and non-disabling. The much-admired actress, Katherine Hepburn, may have suffered from ET—not PD.

This Is Your Life—Getting a Second (or Even Third) Opinion

Whatever the diagnosis, if you have concerns, questions, or doubts, then you have every reason to get a second or even a third opinion. After all, you know your body and its symptoms better than anyone else. So if you live within a reasonable distance of a Udall Center (see the sidebar "Morris K. Udall Parkinson's Disease Research Centers of Excellence" earlier in this chapter) or a medical center with a reputation for excellent PD care and research, see whether you can get an appointment and check out what those folks say. Even if you have to travel some distance, the information will be worth the trip.

Another reason to seek a second or third opinion is to find a neurologist you have chemistry with. The doctor who delivered the initial diagnosis may be a fine neurologist with great credentials and experience, but maybe the two of you had no connection and you don't see a partnership with her. With PD, you don't want to be switching from one doctor to another. So, find a doctor that you can build a real partnership with now—one with a proactive and optimistic philosophy about meeting the challenges of living with PD.

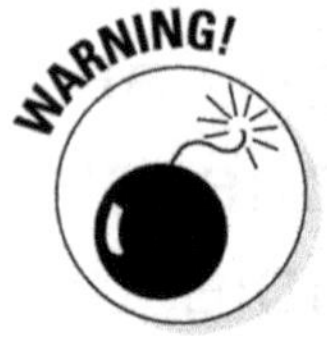

The danger lies in seeking one opinion after another just because you didn't like the first (or second or third) answer—even though, in your heart-of-hearts, you're sure it's true. That's called *denial.* Because you may not want to face the future, you keep running after more opinions, hoping some day some doctor will say you don't have PD.

After a doctor has confirmed the diagnosis (and perhaps another doctor has reconfirmed it), you need to accept it and prepare yourself and your family for the journey. Maybe you've already made significant progress by finding a neurologist that you and your PCP can partner with to maintain and manage your health for the long term.

Chapter 5

You've Been Diagnosed—Now What?

In This Chapter

- Facing your fears about Parkinson's disease
- Establishing your long-term vision and short-term goals
- Caring for the future: Advice for your partner

Okay, it's official—you have Parkinson's disease (PD). In these first days following that blow, no doubt your emotions are rocketing. And like a pinball, they're bouncing moment to moment and hour to hour around those Five Stages of Grief that Elisabeth Kubler-Ross introduced:

- Can't be (denial)
- Shouldn't be (anger)
- Don't let it be (bargaining)
- Why me? (depression)

- IS! (acceptance or at least realization)

A sixth stage to consider in facing a diagnosis of PD is *hope.* You can find some measure of control as you continue toward the future you had already planned—one that did *not* include living with a chronic and progressive illness.

And that's the purpose of this chapter—to help you move beyond those first jumbled emotions of diagnosis toward a clearly focused, take-charge attitude of this disease. In this chapter we first talk you through the emotional steps and then guide you toward healthy goals and plans for coming to grips with PD. We also address your care partner, the one who plans to walk that walk with you, and offer advice for these early months after the diagnosis.

Sorting Out Your Emotions

Depending on your past awareness or experiences with PD, either you have some idea of how your life is going to change or you have no idea at all. In either case, your imagination can get carried away with all the what-ifs.

Stop! This is a new challenge, but it's not so different from other challenges that have taken your life in unexpected directions. Every day people face unplanned events that change the course they thought they were on—job losses, break-ups in relationships, unplanned moves to different locations, the loss of a loved one, hurricanes, and floods. Life happens.

Take a breath. Any challenges that you faced (and survived) in the past (like raising your children, building your career, caring for aging parents, and such) gave you key building blocks and tools to face this new challenge.

Now, give yourself time to:

- Understand that a PD diagnosis is not a death sentence. You have a life to live and choices to make about how you'll face each day, probably for years and even decades to come.
- Believe that past experiences have given you the tools you need to cope with PD.

- Accept the difference between what you can and can't control. Focus on what you can.
- Connect with people who are positive and upbeat.
- Banish negative self-talk ("I can't," or "I won't," and such), and turn the negative to a positive ("I can" and "I will").
- Embrace the joys in your life—your partner, children, friends, work or avocation, love of music, art, sports, and so on.
- Help yourself by helping other people—volunteer, get involved, make a difference.
- Recognize the opportunities you have to educate others, advocate for change (and a cure), make new friends, and know your deeper self.

Basically you have two choices: Define your life as a person with Parkinson's (PWP) or live that life to the fullest—the same as if you'd never been diagnosed with PD.

Dodging denial and meeting your diagnosis head on

When you get the confirmed diagnosis, you and your family—especially your partner—need time to digest the news and react. And the first reaction for one or both of you may be denial. Your partner may become overprotective and treat you as if you're gravely ill. Financial concerns may pop up; your partner may wonder about the costs and sacrifices. Underneath your partner may first feel cheated out of the life you had planned and then angry at such a selfish thought when you're facing a debilitating illness. (For more help in dealing with such difficult feelings, see Chapter 22.)

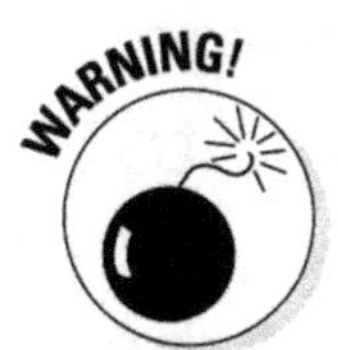

Neither you nor your partner may admit any of these feelings initially. Big mistake. Your fastest route to coping is to work through such feelings together by openly communicating your fears and concerns and then working through possible solutions to each. Following the guidelines set forth in the remainder of this chapter can help.

Denial can take two forms. First, many people who receive the diagnosis of PD—or any other serious illness—soon realize that the early symptoms have been there. Perhaps you dismissed those early warning signs for weeks or even months because you were afraid or didn't want other people to know you had some troublesome symptoms.

The second form of denial comes after you've received the diagnosis. Now the facts are out there. You're human, and no doubt the actual news that you have PD has come as a real blow. *Initially* refusing to believe this is happening is your mind's way of giving you time to gather the necessary strength to go forward.

However, *sustaining* that denial takes an enormous amount of energy—energy that can be much more valuable in facing the actual challenge. Refusing to acknowledge the truth means you're forcing yourself to keep a secret from other people and yourself.

In spite of your denial, deep inside you know this diagnosis is real. You may even be surprised to realize you have a slight feeling of relief because the enemy has a name, and now you can begin to fight it. You can't go back and not have PD. But you can decide how best to move forward.

Allowing yourself to get angry

Anger is an understandable reaction to news like this. The question is: Who's on the receiving end of that anger? The world in general? Your friends and family who've never taken care of themselves like you always have? Your significant other (who you fear—in your current, warped state of mind—may leave you)? God? How about yourself?

Go ahead—rant, rave, and howl at the moon. A little healthy anger is good for you, and certainly you deserve to indulge that anger—within reason. Try these tips for giving anger your best shot.

- Keep the focus on the object of your anger—having PD. It's easier than you may suspect to broaden that focus until suddenly everything and everyone makes you mad.
- Start figuring out ways you're going to get back at this enemy that's attacked your perfectly good life (the same way you'd think of ways to get back at the boss who passed you over for that promotion). For example, you can say to your Parkinson's, "I'll show you that I can still lead my life in spite of the challenges you throw my way!"
- Set limits. When you're overwhelmed by your fury at the

unfairness of this diagnosis, set a kitchen timer for 10 minutes. When the bell dings, you're done—at least for today.

- Find the humor—black though it may be—in this unexpected and unwanted situation and defuse your anger with that humor.

Anger (like denial and a bunch of other normal reactions to news of a chronic, progressive illness) is non-productive *unless* it leads you to fight back. Permit yourself some time to work your way through this news. (For some people, this will be a matter of days; for others it's a couple of weeks.) If the feelings continue longer than that, you need to get some help to resolve the anger. Throughout the course of your PD, you're going to be upset and angry from time to time. Your goal is not to dwell in that anger but to transform its energy into determination to regain control and move forward.

Admitting you're scared

Chances are good that you still don't have a handle on the full impact of this diagnosis. Getting your head around the concept of a lifelong, progressive illness is a pretty tall order, especially in the beginning. It's enough to scare the bejeebers out of anyone! You have so many questions and fears. How do you deal with them?

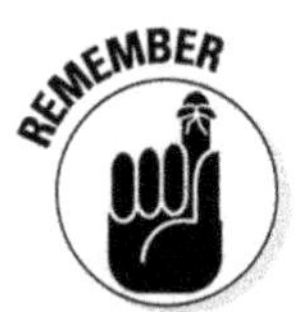

There's no shame in admitting you're scared. The title song from the musical *Cabaret* says, "Start by admitting from cradle to grave, it isn't that long a stay." In other words, life is what we get—no promises and no guarantees. The unknown can be intriguing, exhilarating, or frightening. And certainly, when that unknown is

PD, you may find yourself even feeding that fear through your responses to it.

Instead of further terrifying yourself by reading every case study, article, or book you can get your hands on about PD, place limits on how much information you need and can handle—especially at the beginning. Instead of smiling politely as some well-meaning clerk or neighbor relates his horror story about a fifth-cousin-twice-removed who had PD back in the dark ages, thank him for his concern and leave. Instead of allowing other people to educate you based on hearsay, observations from afar, and an article they read about former Attorney General Janet Reno, educate yourself.

Using the reputable and frequently updated resources listed in Appendix B, you can gather the information you need to become the true expert on what is and isn't possible with PD. Then, when people start telling you about your condition and how to manage your life, quietly but firmly correct them. Trust us; nothing silences a know-it-all like someone who really does know. And nothing helps you get a handle on that gut-wrenching fear like educating yourself on the realities, possibilities, and opportunities for expanding your life—of living with PD.

Getting to acceptance

No one is denying that you need to work through a whole range of emotions, but you can't stay locked in those emotional prisons. When you move through them, you free yourself to fully live your days.

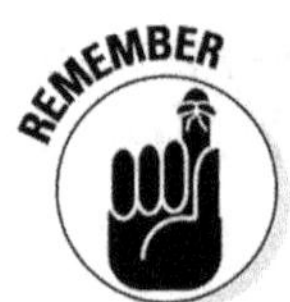

You have a chronic and progressive illness, but

- You have years ahead of you.
- You're still productive.
- You have time to pursue dreams and goals.

- You can live life on your terms if you accommodate PD as *part* of that life, not *all* of it.

How to go about that? Start with these key steps:

- Get the best treatment you can after you have the diagnosis. Part III of this book is all about treatment options, some that you may find surprisingly easy to incorporate into your life.
- Deal with the emotional roller coaster of living with a chronic progressive illness. Chapters 13 and 22 offer tips on facing the depression, anxiety, and other difficult feelings that are part and parcel of living with any chronic progressive conditions.
- Manage your inevitable lifestyle changes and social adjustments with family and friends (and theirs with you). Check out Chapter 7 for tips on who, how, and when to tell about your PD; then look at Chapter 15 for more in-depth advice on maintaining key relationships.
- Protect your unique sense of self-worth and identity. Well, we

could just remind you to read this whole book because our key message in every chapter is that you can live with this condition. In fact, you can have a full and satisfying life—it just won't be the life you thought you were going to have (but isn't that true for most people?).

Sometimes acceptance comes most easily when you turn your attention to the people who love you and have heard your diagnosis. They're wrestling with high anxiety too. Of course, their first concern is for you, but a part of that concern is PD's effect on their relationship with you. How will their lives change with yours? When you acknowledge their fears (as well as your own) and explore that with them, you create an environment of "we're in this thing together" that goes a long way toward sustaining everyone when times get tough. (Tips for ways you can best communicate with other people are in Chapters 7 and 15.)

By taking the lead in figuring out how to live with PD, in many ways you become a mentor. You're the person others look to and trust to show the best way to face this life-changing situation. For many of us, actor Christopher Reeve and his wife, Dana, were the poster couple for finding grace in the face of unspeakable adversity. Think about it: If you built your career as *Superman* and ended up unable to move much less leap over tall buildings, wouldn't you be tempted to feel sorry for yourself? Instead Christopher Reeve found the will and the courage to use his adversity to inspire and motivate people and make a real difference in the world.

No one expects you to become a national icon now that you have PD. But you can become that mentor for people closest to you. Through your attitude and approach, you can set the tone for the way others interact with you and incorporate PD into the relationship.

Taking charge and moving forward

Prepare but don't project needs to be your mantra. The temptation to look ahead and worry about the future can be overwhelming. Our advice: Fight that instinct! Given a diagnosis of a chronic and progressive disease that has no cure, a person's natural tendency is to try and foretell the future. Major mistake!

With PD, every patient's journey is unique, so projecting what may happen can only increase your anxiety. You and your care partner can go crazy, racing around and trying to cover all your possible challenges even before they develop.

The point is that you have a disease that will require—like most health conditions—changes to your lifestyle. For example,

- What will you do if you can no longer manage the stairs in your current home, but the bedrooms (and the main bathroom) are all upstairs?

In Chapter 21, we explore many options for staying in your current residence in spite of obstacles such as this. For example, you may have a room on the first floor that you can adapt as a bedroom; maybe you can convert a half-bath into a full bathroom (with the addition of a shower); or your stairway may be wide enough to accommodate an electric chair lift.

• As your ability to move decreases, how will you handle an emergency such as getting out of the house in the event of a fire?

Even if you didn't have PD, common sense should move every family to have an emergency plan in place. So sit down with the family and figure this one out—for you and everyone else in the household. One solution is to talk to people at your local fire and police department and get their suggestions.

Our guess is that throughout your life (and certainly as an adult) you've planned for the possibility of unexpected changes or events. And even though those plans may come in a year or not at all, you've still considered the options and are prepared to act.

Taking Action

Think of PD as a 400-pound lineman constantly in your face. He's there when you wake up and when you go to sleep. He gets in your way, blocking you when you try to work or play and when your friends come around. Sometimes he's well-behaved, maybe even sitting on the sidelines for a while. But mostly he's charging, blocking, and even tackling to keep you from doing what you want.

How do you get around this lineman? The answer is that sometimes you won't. But other times—most of the time—you can find new and innovative ways to live life on your terms. Managing a chronic illness means you need to give up control over some parts of your life and take control in new ways. Some of those new controls are:

- Educating yourself and your family about your PD
- Developing a long-range strategy for managing your PD

- Turning negatives into positives through creative problem-solving
- Being a real team player—with your healthcare team (see Chapter 6), your care partners, and other PWP

Arming yourself with good information

The key to gathering information is making sure it's trustworthy and evidence-based. The Agency for Healthcare and Research (an agency within the Department of Health and Human Services) recommends these resources:

- **healthfinder** (www.healthfinder.gov) is sponsored by the U.S. Department of Health and Human Services. The site includes links to government agencies, clearinghouses, non-profit groups, and universities.
- **Health Information Resource Database** (www.health.gov/nhic/#Referrals or 800-336-4797) is sponsored by the National Health Information Center. This site offers information on more than 1000

organizations and government agencies that provide health information on request.

- **MEDLINEplus** (www.nlm.nih.gov/medlineplus) is sponsored by the National Institutes of Health (NIH). The site has extensive information from NIH and other trusted resources on more than 650 diseases and conditions.
- **Non-profit organizations** such as the National Parkinson's Foundation and The Michael J. Fox Foundation focus specifically on PD. For a complete list and contact information, see Appendix B.

In addition, try checking with medical libraries in your area (but keep in mind that this information is for physicians, medical students, and researchers—the reading can get fairly technical).

Ignore information from

- Product advertisements that
  - Make extraordinary claims, such as *scientific breakthrough* or *secret formula.*
  - Claim to work for a number of different conditions.
  - Claim the product is available from only one source or for a limited time.
- Well-meaning friends who have
  - Heard of some therapy but can't recall the source.
  - Had a relative who tried *x-treatment.* It worked for that person, so it's bound to work for you!
- Well-meaning strangers who, in their zeal to show sympathy for your condition, rattle off several ideas about treatment.

Jotting down the questions you have

Chances are good that you were pretty numb as you sat in the doctor's office and received the news. (See Chapter 4, where we cover the initial visit with the neurologist.) But now you realize you have all sorts of questions. Or perhaps you asked questions at the time and your doctor offered information, but you really didn't take it in.

Schedule a second appointment (if you haven't already) and let your doctor (or the nurse) know that you want to be able to ask questions and discuss issues that have come to mind since the diagnosis. At that appointment, bring your list of questions (as well as your care partner for that second set of ears) and be ready to take notes. The following questions are a sampling of some concerns you may want to cover.

- What's the technical name of my condition, and what does that mean in plain English?
- What's the *prognosis,* my outlook for the future?
- How soon do I need to make a decision about treatment?
- Will I need additional tests? If so, what kind and when?
- What are my treatment options, and what are the pros and cons of those treatment options?

- What changes will I need to make in my daily life?
- What resources and organizations do you recommend for support and information?
- What resources can your office provide (books, pamphlets, audio or videotapes, and such) that I can review right away?
- And, the question uppermost in your mind: Am I going to die from this?

Establishing realistic and attainable goals

If PD is to be part of your life but not your entire life, then you need a game plan. Fact: If you don't have a plan for dealing with PD, then it will dominate every facet of your life. This section takes you through specific steps toward making and living that plan.

In the world of business, executive teams meet regularly. Their purpose? To plan for the future success of their business. Their process usually follows a three-step course:

1. **Establish a long-term vision.**

2. **Set short-term goals toward achieving that vision.**
3. **Identify and prioritize tasks necessary to attain those goals.** (This is known as the *Plan of Action,* or POA.)

To apply these three steps to PD, the first step (the vision) is already established: to live a productive and satisfying life for as long as possible in spite of PD.

The second step (setting goals) requires you to set aside sentimentality. As much as people wish otherwise, PD (as of this writing) has no cure. So, a goal of being cured is neither realistic nor attainable. As you consider your real goals, remember the following principles:

- Keep them simple.
- Keep them practical.
- Keep them specific.

The third step is the POA. Did you ever see a milk stool, the three-legged variety farmers sat on to milk cows? That three-legged approach is the way you need to think about your POA over the long term because living with PD is not only a physical challenge; it's also a mental and emotional one. And, just like the milk stool, if one leg is missing, the plan will topple.

The following sections provide examples of three goals and their POAs that support a long-term vision for PD.

Goal 1: Maintain maximum physical function

PD has no magic pill. So, after confirming your diagnosis, your neurologist will probably have a number of recommendations that may include management of symptoms with proven medications, physical and occupational therapy, and perhaps a program for diet and exercise.

Although medications and traditional medical interventions may help minimize your symptoms, you enhance your opportunity to achieve your long-term vision when you maintain your best physical condition. On the other hand, if you ignore the doctor's prescription for changes in your lifestyle (such as adjustments to your diet and activity routines or a specific timetable for taking your medications), you compromise your overall vision. (See

Chapter 9 for more about the importance of sticking to your medication schedule and Chapter 12 for a full discussion of exercise and nutrition.)

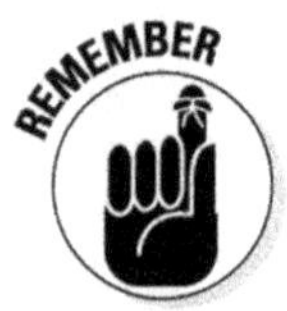

No one has all of the symptoms. Although PD is a chronic, progressive condition, its path varies tremendously from one person to the next. You are unique—as a person and as a PWP. You and your medical team need to keep that in mind as together you select those options (medications, therapies, and lifestyle changes) that have the greatest effect on maintaining your physical function for as long as possible.

Goal 2: Keep your mind sharp

You're certainly going to have a lot on your mind in the days and weeks to come as you and your medical team put together a viable plan for managing your PD symptoms. And you're going to hear a lot of new words—words that PD specialists, PWPs, and their care partners throw around as easily as *apple* or *orange.*

You can refuse to follow that technical PD jargon (and everything else about this intruder), or you can become an expert, someone who actively seeks out background information about PD, understands and uses the technical lingo, and keeps up with the research and new treatment options.

This advice doesn't mean PD has to become your life's work. You have more important (and fun!) ways to spend your time. But remember: Knowledge is power, and seeking out that knowledge exercises your brain. Get started using the resources listed in Appendix B. Getting a grip on PD (what it is and isn't) is a good place to start—but don't stop there.

What are your interests and how did you challenge your mind before you had PD? Are you a sports enthusiast who enjoys statistics and box scores? Do you enjoy brainteasers, like crossword puzzles, jigsaw puzzles, or word games?

Do you love good music, art, and theater?

Continuing to engage your mind in enjoyable ways is as important to your POA as pushing yourself physically. Don't turn your back on the intellectual life you enjoyed before PD.

Goal 3: Embrace the power of emotional and spiritual well-being

Going through a range of emotions post-diagnosis is normal. But anxiety and depression can be viable symptoms of PD as well as viable responses to its diagnosis. Your doctor needs to know if you're experiencing persistent (longer than a couple of weeks) sadness or apathy. (See Chapter 14 for a full discussion of the effects of anxiety and depression in PD.)

Although your neurologist or primary care physician (in consultation with each other) can prescribe medication and professional counseling to help you through these negative emotions, you can also be proactive by

- Acknowledging that these persistent negative feelings are abnormal.
- Finding a support group where you can discuss feelings with other people who

  Perhaps have similar emotions.

  Recognize these emotions as part of the adaptive process in dealing with PD.
- Accepting the support of family and friends as you come to terms with PD and its effects on all your lives.

In concert with your medical team, you can address physical, mental, and even emotional needs as part of your POA. However, one facet of your care plan only you can develop is a plan for your spiritual health. This facet goes beyond faith and religious rituals, although those resources certainly help.

Spiritual health means going inside yourself and coming to terms with your illness day by day. For some PWP, coping comes through challenging activities: participating in sports, continuing to pursue a career, traveling, and so on. If these challenges help you find inner peace and comfort, great!

Other PWP may find spiritual healing in quieter pursuits: a walk in the park or along the beach; music; reading; sitting quietly in a secluded, deserted place. These activities are also excellent choices for maintaining spiritual health.

Take care that your solitude doesn't become a regular hiding place to wallow over your losses. Be aware that seclusion can sometimes lead to depression.

Living your life to the fullest

You can perform a lot of actions to fight PD and its effects. But thousands of PWP believe that a huge part of fighting PD is to approach it as only a piece of their lives. The point is this: Those facets of your life that defined you before you were diagnosed are still there—at least for the most part. If you were a parent before, you still are and your child (children) needs you as much as before. If you had a career that you enjoyed (even loved), don't allow PD to become your new, full-time occupation. If you enjoyed sports, music, and other leisure activities, get creative about finding new ways to enjoy those pastimes. In short, LIVE!

The road will be challenging, but as actor and PD advocate, Michael J. Fox, wrote in his biography, *Lucky Man,* "If you were to rush into this room right now and announce that you had struck a deal—with God, Allah, Buddha, Christ, Krishna, Bill Gates, whomever—in which the ten years since my diagnosis could be magically taken away, traded in for the person I was before, I would, without a moment's hesitation, tell you to take a hike."

Next steps

Getting information you can trust so you can form the questions to ask so you can establish some clear goals for managing this condition—pretty tall order! Consider these three concrete steps that you can take right now to get started:

1. Go online and bookmark the sites listed in Appendix B if you have access to a computer.

These national organizations are your best resource for the latest updates on treatments as well as tips for managing your PD symptoms. Get into the habit of regularly checking in on the sites you find most useful. If the site offers an e-list, sign up.

2. Call the toll-free numbers for the PD organizations if you don't have access to a computer.

Ask them to send you their printed materials and add you to the mailing list for new materials in the future.

3. Keep reading.

Before you turn to the next chapter, take a moment to read

through the following with your family—especially the person who is most likely to be your primary care partner. Even though these sections (scattered throughout this book) are labeled *for the care partner,* try to read them together. The information applies to both of you because you have a responsibility to acknowledge that your care partner has a life beyond helping you manage your PD. (You may also want to check out Chapter 24 for more tips about how to give and receive care and support.)

A Word for the PD Care Partner

In many chronic, progressive illnesses (for example, Alzheimer's disease), family members must increasingly take charge. With PD, however, the PWP can be in charge most of the way. As the care partner, you may want to take over, especially as tasks become more difficult and decisions take longer for your partner to process. But resist that urge. Partnering-in-care is not doing *for*—it's doing *with.*

But where does that leave you as you face your own fears and anxieties about living with someone who has a chronic, progressive condition that won't go away but will color your lives for years to come? Go back and reread this chapter. Everything we suggest for the PWP applies to you as well:

- Sort through your emotions; deal with the anger, the fear, and the realities of how life is going to change (see also Chapter 22).
- Adopt a take charge/move forward/don't look back outlook and start preparing for eventualities that may occur down the road. (You may especially want to read Chapters 20 and 21 about housing options and financial and legal matters.)
- Be proactive. Educate yourself; go to doctor and therapy appointments with the PWP and take notes; become a combination of cheerleader and coach as your loved one faces new challenges.

- Set goals that allow you to maintain a life and identity beyond your role as care partner.

The best support you can offer over the long term is to be a fierce advocate for your loved one's autonomy and independence. The next best way to show support is to take care of yourself and see that your needs are also met. By working together—in partnership—the two of you can take something that could have destroyed you and turn it into a life-experience that enriches you in ways you cannot yet imagine.

Chapter 6

Drafting Your Healthcare Team and a Game Plan

In This Chapter

- Recruiting your professional care team
- Prepping for unexpected scenarios
- Touching base with your care partner

Knowledge may be power, but with today's constant bombardment of information, you need a team of experts that can answer questions and address unexpected situations with the most-advanced procedures.

People with Parkinson's (PWP), like people with other chronic-care needs, must rely on the expertise of several different professionals throughout the course of their illness. In this chapter, professionals and their roles in managing your Parkinson's symptoms are defined. You also take a look at how best to handle hospitalizations, emergency room visits, and other unexpected medical predicaments and complications that are possible for PWP. Last, but not least, your care partner gets ideas for building his own team.

Introducing Your Teammates

Each member of your professional Parkinson's disease (PD) team has special talents and expertise that can help you manage symptoms and maintain normal function and quality of life, often for years following the initial diagnosis. In this section, you discover a list of professionals and their roles in your care, and then you uncover your role in helping these pros perform at their very best.

Lining up the doctors

At least two doctors will help set the course for your care after your PD diagnosis. In addition, you may have other specialists (or you may add them at a later date) if you have other chronic conditions, such as arthritis, hypertension, and the like. The more doctors you have, the more vital it becomes for one doctor (most likely your primary care physician) to take the role of quarterback to oversee and coordinate the plan to meet all your health needs.

Your primary care physician

Your *primary care physician* (PCP) may be a general practitioner (GP) who focuses on family medicine or that person may be an internist who treats adults only. You've probably been seeing this doctor for some time and have built a trust and style of communication that works for both of you. Now that you have PD, you need to talk with your PCP about two things: his willingness to consult and communicate with your neurologist (who'll take the lead on treating your PD symptoms), and how your PD treatment can integrate with your overall healthcare plan.

Your neurologist

Chances are good that your PCP referred you to a neurologist to confirm the PD diagnosis. If so, these two professionals may already have a good working relationship. However, if you went for a second (or even third) opinion and chose another neurologist to oversee your PD care, be sure that these two doctors meet and show a clear willingness to work together. It's also helpful if your PCP and neurologist are on staff at the same hospital in case you need hospitalization or emergency treatment down the road. (For tips on locating and choosing a neurologist, see Chapter 4.)

Other specialists

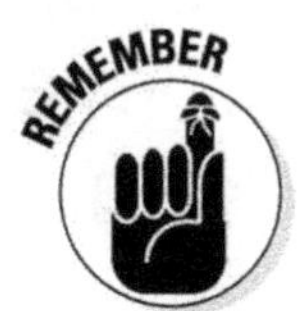

In the event you need to consult with other specialists (a cardiologist, urologist, or the like) for new medical situations that arise, these physicians must work closely with your PCP and neurologist so they're all communicating from the same play book (to continue the sports analogy). Think of these doctors as coming off the bench. When they get into the game, they need to get up to speed on your game plan and their specific roles.

Before you keep an appointment with a specialist ask your PCP (and neurologist, if appropriate) to send the specialist(s) a copy of your most recent records. After your visit with one of these doctors, ask that a copy of the office visit report be sent to your PCP with a copy sent to you at the same time. With this exchange of information between doctors—and by assembling your own file of reports—you enhance the likelihood that everyone is on the same page, working from the same information.

Calling up the therapists

Because PD is a movement disorder that affects your ability to perform basic movements, your physical, occupational, and (possibly) speech therapists are very important. These professionals offer proven methods to enhance and pro-long your control of symptoms, and improve your overall sense of well-being. Their services may or may not be covered by insurance unless your doctor's prescription notes them as *medically necessary* to treat your PD.

Physical therapist

A physical therapist (PT) can teach you how to build muscle strength, increase flexibility, and improve coordination and balance to prevent falls and serious fractures. Techniques may include exercise programs (standard as well as alternatives, like yoga), heat and cold packs, and water therapy (exercises in water).

Your PT can design a program of exercises specific to your individual symptoms and abilities to preserve and even increase your muscle strength and flexibility.

Although exercise doesn't appear to slow the progression of PD, recent studies indicate that exercise may help prevent the orthopedic muscular and skeletal effects of *akinesia* (slowed or impaired ability to move) and lessen *rigidity* (stiff muscles). Exercise helps you maintain balance and prevent falls.

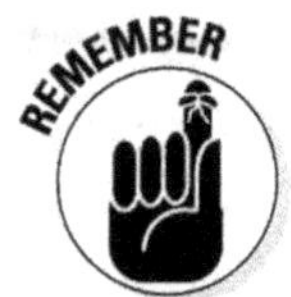

Your PT can't work miracles. If you only exercise when you go to a session with your PT, you're not likely to see ongoing or long-term benefits. When the physical therapy sessions end (or when the time between sessions stretches to two weeks or more), you need to pursue your own regular program of stretching, strengthening, and aerobic exercises if you want the physical therapy to be successful in the long run. See Chapter 12 for a suggested program of stretches and exercises.

Occupational therapist

Essentially, the *occupational therapist* (OT) helps preserve your sense of independence and self-confidence by showing you new ways of performing simple and routine tasks (known in the medical profession as *activities of daily living* or ADLs) that may have become difficult for you. One significant benefit of working with an OT is simply knowing that you can preserve your control (with alternative techniques) when the loss of control seems a foregone conclusion. For example, she may teach you new techniques (such as a *cueing* or a reminder system) and provide assistive devices (such as a special cane) that help you perform certain movements and tasks.

For more information on ways to adapt to your changing symptoms, check out the information in Part III on living with PD.

Speech therapist

Not every PWP needs speech therapy, but if you're experiencing a softened vocal tone, unintentional mispronunciations, or wrong word choices, a speech therapist can help. These professionals can also help if you ever develop swallowing or other throat muscle problems that can come with PD.

If a trained speech therapist isn't available in your area, consider trying a program especially for PWP called the Lee Silverman Voice Treatment or LSVT. For more information about the LSVT Foundation, its programs, and links to other PD groups, see www.lsvt.org.

Drafting other team players

As a PWP, you have your front-line defense consisting of your PCP, your neurologist, and trained movement and speech therapists. But, have you considered the number of other professionals that can help you to manage your symptoms and continue living a normal life as long as possible? Be sure that you include the following care professionals and experts when you're assembling the team.

Pharmacist

Your pharmacist is in the business of knowing medications and their interactions. She knows your current medications, their potential side effects, and the possible impact of any new medication that your PCP or neurologist may prescribe. And, because this is her area of expertise, she's your best resource for answering your questions after you've carefully read the printed information on your prescriptions. (For more information about prescription medicines, be sure to check out Chapter 9.)

Your job? Pick one pharmacy (or chain that shares information among all branches) to fill all your prescriptions and stick with them. Then be sure the pharmacist knows which over-the-counter (OTC) medicines you're taking or considering taking.

Psychologist or counselor

Anxiety and depression are part and parcel of having PD, and they're perfectly normal reactions to hearing a diagnosis of a chronic, progressive condition. A trained and licensed counselor can be a key member of your professional care team. Whether you see this person on a regular basis for *talk therapy sessions* (see Chapter 13 for more on this topic) or just now and then for some emotional unburdening, go ahead and identify this counselor shortly after your diagnosis is confirmed.

Support groups

Throughout this book we tout the benefits of joining a support group—for you and your care partner. You may reject this idea in the early stages. "I don't want to sit around talking to a bunch of strangers or listening to them complain about their PD. I've got my own problems." Wrong! Well, sort of. You definitely have your own problems. But, here's the point you're missing: A support group can help you find ways to cope with those problems.

Many types of support groups are around for PWP and their care partners. Some groups take a broader advocacy approach, while other groups focus more on their members. All support groups should have a trained professional that leads or facilitates the discussions (someone with experience and credentials). For more information, see Chapter 13 or to locate a group in your area go to www.apdaparkinson.org.

Legal and financial advisors

Your PD may eventually affect your ability to make key decisions about finances and legal matters, about the future of your family, and about your own future. Although this problem may never arise, working with an expert as early as possible after your diagnosis to put key documents and plans in order is just smart planning—whether you have PD or not. (For a full discussion of the legal and financial matters that need attention, see Chapter 20.)

Given the complexities of PD costs, drafting an insurance advisor for your team is a wise maneuver. This person can guide you and your care partner through the multitude of questions related to disability (short and long term), Medicare, Medicaid, Health Management Organizations (HMOs), Preferred Physician Organizations (PPOs), Health Savings Accounts (HSAs), and any other alphabet-soup plans that will undoubtedly surface in the future.

Spiritual advisor

Taking a holistic approach—caring for yourself physically, mentally, and spiritually—can give you a jump on managing your PD symptoms. Many people focus on the physical and mental but figure the spiritual will take care of itself. Remember: Your spiritual well being has just as many levels as your physical and mental health. If you have a spiritual mentor that you can tap to join your professional care team, do so early on. This person may be your clergy, someone who's mentored you through other passages, a practitioner of alternative or complementary medicine, or even the counselor that's mentioned in the "Psychologist or counselor" section of this chapter.

Making the cut

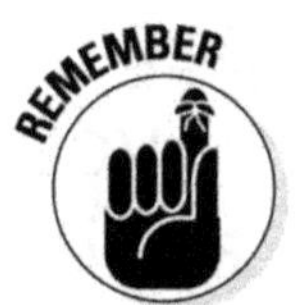

Drafting a team of experts in your battle against PD has benefits well beyond the expertise of each member. When you choose them carefully and treat them with respect, you find these men and women will go to great lengths for you. They even become some of your most enthusiastic cheerleaders, offering support and encouragement, humor, and affection as you confront the challenges of living with PD.

How do you evaluate each member of the team? The criteria are pretty standard—regardless of the profession:

- Does this person have the right stuff—the appropriate credentials and experience—to handle the job?
- Is it a good fit—are you comfortable with this person? Can you talk about anything or ask the silliest question without feeling intimidated?
- Does this person really listen? Is he open to ideas that aren't his own?
- Does this person give you the time you need—especially when your PD may slow your movements, thinking, and ability to put thoughts into words?
- Is this person willing to admit limits to her knowledge and expertise and refer you to someone more qualified to handle a specific issue?
- Will this person be there when you need him?

Working with Your Team to Manage the Unexpected

Stuff happens, and worst-case scenarios happen unexpectedly. Maybe you fall or burn yourself while preparing dinner and end up in the emergency room. Or, despite all precautions, you experience an adverse drug interaction that requires a stay in the hospital. Nonmedical emergencies—a fire, a weather event (such as a severe storm or tornado)—can also crop up. Our advice throughout this book is this: Have a plan in the event something unexpected happens. This doesn't mean you're assuming the worst. You just want to be ready—or as ready as possible.

Establishing an emergency plan

Be prepared—the motto of the Boy Scouts of America is just as useful for PWP and their care partners. You or your care partner may never need to dial 911, but what if...? Why not think in the relative calm of your normal routine and prepare for that possible unexpected event? These next sections provide specific recommendations to help you prepare and then deal with a variety of emergencies.

The home front

Start your emergency plan with home safety by reviewing the tips for accident-proofing your home in Chapter 21. Then consider what to do in case of a medical emergency, such as an allergic reaction or a dislocated shoulder or some other emergency beyond your control—a fire, a flood, a blackout. Who do you call? Where do you go? What do you do?

Your home is unique, just like you, so the best way to prepare for a safety emergency is to contact your local fire department. It may have a program where a firefighter comes out, assesses your home for fire safety, and then offers pointers for handling emergencies. Another resource that offers a checklist for creating your own evacuation plan is available through the American Red Cross at www.redcross.org.

Personal records

Take advantage of the following tips that put you ahead of the panic if a medical or safety emergency does arise:

• Gather this vital information:

- A list of all prescription and OTC medications and a list of any allergies and chronic health conditions you have besides your PD
- Insurance or Medicare numbers
- Your medical history
- Names and contact numbers of your doctors and for an emergency contact person, like your significant other, for example

• Date all this information and update it regularly, especially when you add or discontinue meds.

• Make sure you and your care partner have copies of this info at all times in your wallet or purse and in you car(s).

• Let key others (your employer, a trusted neighbor who may respond to an emergency) know where to find the information should you be unable to direct them.

• Prepare a folder specifically for the emergency room. (People administering care don't have time to read old records.) Include the following pieces of information in the folder:

- All information listed in the previous section, "Personal records."
- A copy of your *advance directive* (a living will and a medical power of attorney), even if the hospital and your doctor already have it on file. If you don't want the medical staff to provide certain interventions or extraordinary measures to save your life, you must provide that information. (See Chapter 20 for more info on these and other legal issues.)

• Prepare a fireproof box with copies of key documents: insurance and Social Security cards; bank and credit card account numbers; wills, powers of attorney (financial and medical), and photos of valuables in case of a fire or weather catastrophe (such as a tornado or hurricane).

• Post critical emergency contact numbers near your home phone. Those numbers include local hospital emergency room, fire department, police department, utility company (for power outages), doctors, pharmacist (in the event of an adverse drug reaction), and a relative or friend to contact.

Easy access

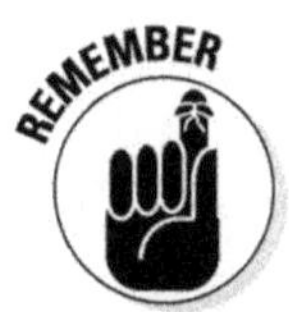

You may never need emergency intervention, but you're better off to be prepared with information that an emergency team can readily access. Take the following measures to prevent glitches when seconds count.

- Distribute duplicate house keys to trusted friends and neighbors.
- Be sure your care partner can access financial funds any time you

may not be able to take financial actions such as writing checks to pay bills or transferring funds from savings to checking accounts as needed.

- If you live alone, get a medical alert system, which enables you to call for help if you're unable to get to a telephone. (Yup, we're talking about that classic TV commercial—"Help! I've fallen and can't get up!")

Decision time

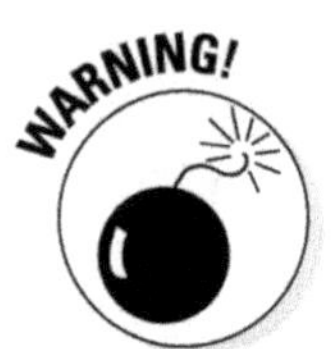

In an emergency, don't waste time worrying whether you should call for help. Risking a little embarrassment rather than your life is always the wise move.

However, if you do need to call for an ambulance or go to the emergency room, be realistic about your expectations. Keep in mind that the

United States has nearly 40 million people with no health insurance; for these folks, the ER doctor is likely their doctor of choice.

Note: The Centers for Disease Control estimates the average waiting time in the ER (if you're not critically injured or ill) is three hours; in cold and flu season the wait can be much longer.

Because of possible delays, you need to

- Speak up if you're experiencing symptoms such as extreme pain, trouble breathing, dizziness, and other signs of distress.
- Tell every ER person who examines or assists you that you have PD (and any other chronic conditions such as diabetes or hypertension) even though someone has taken your history and you know these facts are on your patient information sheet.
- Be proactive. Make sure that the people who treat you are aware of your medications and allergies.

If your situation is serious but not life threatening, call your doctor or the nearest urgent-care or walk-in clinic for faster response and care. And if your doctor does advise you to get to the ER, he can speed up your process by calling the hospital and telling the ER staff that you're on the way.

The hospital stay and its aftermath

If you need to be admitted to the hospital, the cause isn't likely to be your PD. The more likely reasons will be a serious injury (such as a hip fracture or head trauma from a fall) or another heath condition (such as heart problems or diabetes). Regardless, be prepared with the necessary information (see the previous section for suggestions) to make the stay less stressful for everyone.

Leave valuables (checkbook, credit cards, jewelry, and the like) at home. If you must bring them because of an emergency and the haste in leaving for the hospital, hand them off to a trusted family member or friend as soon as possible. Or ask a staff member whether the hospital has a safe place to keep the valuables until you can make arrangements for them.

The same suggestions outlined for an emergency (see the previous section "Establishing an emergency plan") apply for a hospital stay. But, because you'll likely be in the hospital for days rather than hours, you must monitor the orders for your PD medications. The attending physician and the staff may not realize the importance of your PD meds' strict dosing and timing. For example, your neurologist's orders for medication at 8 a.m., noon, 4 p.m., and 8 p.m. may be interpreted by the hospital staff as four times a day over a 24hour period, or 8 a.m., 2 p.m., 8 p.m., and 2 a.m.

I'm not fooling around and I'm not drunk—I have Parkinson's disease

To offset any misunderstandings that may occur during your hospital stay, consider packing a copy of the following note in your bag and showing it to the staff. In spite of its lighthearted tone, the note provides critical information about your care.

To whom it may concern:

First of all, let me say how much I appreciate everything you'll be doing to care for me while I'm here. My care partner and I understand that you have other patients to attend to besides me. In return I ask that you understand some things about me:

- You may have noticed that I'm moving pretty slowly and I probably couldn't walk a straight line if my life depended on it. Am I intoxicated? Nope. I've got this thing called Parkinson's disease.

• Other times you may notice that I seem to be doing just fine—doing normal stuff like brushing my teeth, washing my face, walking around on my own—and then my call bell will light up, and I'll be asking you to please come help me get to the bathroom. What gives? I have Parkinson's, and the medications I take to control it have these *on-off* cycles. One minute I can perform routine things, and the next I need all the help I can get.

• Speaking of meds, I really need for you—and everyone involved in treating me while I'm here—to know that certain medications commonly used in hospital settings can really mess with my PD symptoms. Please check with my neurologist, Dr. _____ at _____, before ordering or administering any new medication—especially antinausea or antipsychotic meds.

• And finally, as long as the subject of antipsychotic is on the table, please be aware that my Parkinson's may cause me to experience confusion, disorientation, and even some interesting misperceptions about where I am and what you're doing. I may also start to hallucinate—fortunately these *visions* I experience are usually benign and silent, so no voices are suggesting that I do you bodily harm. Again please check with Dr. _____ before administering any meds.

That's pretty much it in a nutshell. Having PD and being in the hospital can be a challenge for both of us, but hopefully now that you understand, we'll both have an easier time of it. Thanks for understanding and thanks for your care and concern.

Sincerely,

(Put your name here)

Sometimes your PD meds need to be suspended so new medications for the condition that landed you in the hospital can work. Again, be vigilant about your care. Have your care partner alert your neurologist (or the doctor managing your PD care) as soon as you know you're going to the hospital and insist that the hospital on-call physician (or any doctor who orders the suspension of your PD meds) consults with your neurologist before ordering any changes in medication.

Any time that your medications are being administered *for* you (as in a hospital setting) instead of you taking them yourself, be sure that you or your care partner carefully examine the pills you get. If any of the meds look different from those you take at home, question it. Also, since hospital staff is responsible for administering medications to a number of patients with diverse conditions, there may be a delay in your getting your PD meds on time. If necessary, have your neurologist contact the attending physician at the hospital to discuss the correct medication regimen. Also, make sure the attending staff knows which medications may be *contraindicated* (harmful) for PWP. (Copy the list of red-flag medications provided on the Cheat Sheet at the front of this book and ask the admitting doctor to add it to your file.)

In addition to monitoring your medications, you may have another battle to wage: The hospital staff, even though they're medical professionals, may have limited or no experience with PD and may misinterpret your PD symptoms—on-off cycles, dykinesias, confusion from the stress of a hospital environment, and the like. For example, if a nursing assistant sees you up and mobile at 2:00 and comes back at 3:00 because you want assistance getting to the bathroom, he may think you're just looking for extra attention. For one good idea for heading off any staff resentment or misunderstanding, see the nearby sidebar, "I'm not fooling around and I'm not drunk—I have Parkinson's disease."

More tips for managing the unexpected

Emergencies arise for all kinds of people. But because you have PD, such crises may carry the extra elements of stress and panic. You and your care partner may want to consider taking a basic first-aid course through your local Red Cross or YMCA to better prepare yourselves for unlikely emergencies, such as bleeding, choking, medication reaction, falls, and so on.

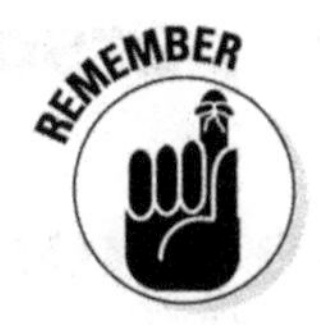

If you need to call 911, be prepared to give the following information:

- Phone number you're calling from
- Address and directions to help the ambulance get there quickly

- Description of the person's condition (breathing? conscious?)
- Your name

In addition, follow these steps:

1. Don't hang up until the emergency operator tells you to.

2. Be sure you unlock the door and turn on outside lights.

Even if it's not night, the lit porch light makes locating the right house easier.

3. If possible, have another family member or neighbor wait outside to direct the emergency personnel.

4. Stay close so you can provide answers to key questions, but let the emergency personnel do their jobs.

5. Gather the information you've prepared (see the earlier section "Establishing an emergency plan") and get ready to go.

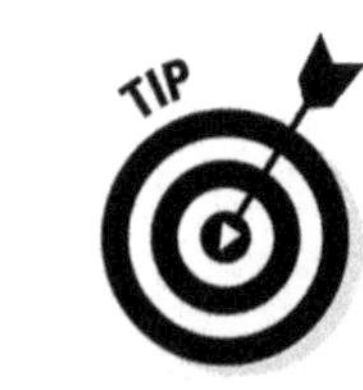

Consider having only cordless phones so you can move around the house (unlocking doors and turning on lights) while you're talking on the phone with the doctor or emergency operator.

A Word for the PD Care Partner

This book has a number of chapters that you may want to read and heed. This is one of them. Putting together a network of professionals that you and the PWP can call upon as issues crop up will make life easier for both of you.

Within this group of professionals, you need to find your own experts—three people you can turn to with your concerns of managing and coping:

- **Primary care physician:** You may have the same general practitioner or internist as the PWP. As long as this physician attends to *your* needs and concerns when you're the patient, that's fine. However, you may want to consider a PCP who isn't involved in your PWP's care. This is your decision, but remember: You need someone to focus on maintaining your physical health and well being.

- **Counselor or therapist:** Being a partner in care can be extremely stressful, especially as the needs escalate. But you'll be better prepared to cope with the unexpected twists and turns along the way if you take time now to connect with a professional who counsels care partners. Don't be stubborn about this. You are at risk for episodes of anxiety, panic, and depression as much as the PWP.
- **Support group and spiritual advisor:** Okay, so we cheated and lumped two into one. But your spiritual health is a vital piece of your ability to partner in care. A support group can provide a safe place to talk about (and let go of) those bad feelings you may be wrestling with (see Chapter 22 for more on this topic). And it has folks who can laugh and share some of

the black humor that comes with being a care partner—they all know, understand, and feel your pain. As for a spiritual advisor, you know yourself best. Your clergyperson, a trusted mentor, your counselor or therapist, and your support-group leader are all good candidates to fill this role.

Chapter 7

Choosing How and When to Share Your News

In This Chapter

- Setting a course with your care partner
- Keeping the story straight: How to share the news with your family
- Sharing with your inner circle: That's what friends are for
- Determining who else needs to know
- Taking the high road: People who overreact and folks who poke their noses in your business

Living with Parkinson's disease (PD) can go well beyond the person diagnosed with PD. Day in and year out, the disease also affects the people who live with, work with, care about, and love the person with PD (PWP). It affects generations—children, grandchildren, and even aging parents (in the case of young onset PD, see Chapter 8), who may be facing their own health challenges.

Everyone has concentric circles of personal contacts. In the closest circles, we have our immediate family (spouse, partner, kids, parents) and perhaps a couple of truly best friends. Next comes a little wider circle—friends we socialize with, extended family, and perhaps a couple of professionals, like our doctor or clergyperson. Further removed from the core of our lives is another group—our employer and co-workers, acquaintances, and neighbors. Deciding when and how to tell each person or group about your diagnosis is an individual decision, one that you have to base on the dynamics of your relationships and your comfort level in sharing this kind of news. But first...

Before You Start Spreading the News

Even if you initially share your diagnosis with very few people, you need to plan how you want these people to react—both immediately and in the future.

Establishing your ground rules

Start by determining your ground rules and the level of support you want. The following categories identify some of the more common PWP stances:

- Some PWP are fighters: They go on immediate offense, take charge, and fight this enemy with every ounce of strength and all the resources they can muster.
- Other PWP take a flight (or more defensive) position: In some ways they choose to ignore the whole situation. Flight folks use their energy and resources to assure everyone (and most of all themselves) that nothing has really changed—life goes on.
- A third group of PWP falls somewhere in the middle, combining facets of fight and flight: Although they want life to continue as normally as possible, they realize

they have to fight back to keep their PD's progression at bay.

Whichever group you're in, you need to think about your ground rules for living with PD. What kind of meaningful care and support can the groups of people in your life offer as you face life with PD? Those who care about you—family members, friends, neighbors, co-workers—naturally want to help. In many cases, they're not sure how to offer that support. You need to explain the ground rules and indicate what will—and won't—be helpful.

Preparing to state your needs

Think through now—alone, or preferably with your care partner (the person who will most likely be with you for the whole journey)—how other people can help. Initially you may need people to listen, to distract you when necessary, and to give you the gift of normalcy just by being themselves.

As your needs become more specific and as you accept the hands-on help of others, you also discover three really important outcomes:

- You empower people by allowing them to contribute something truly meaningful to you.
- You ease some of the responsibility that may have fallen on your care partner's shoulders.
- You prevent yourself from becoming isolated, and you actually increase your ability to take control of situations as they arise.

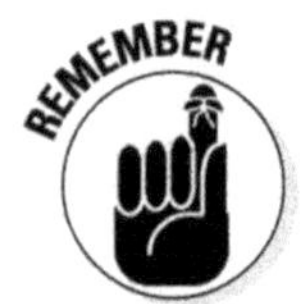

Accepting help is not a sign of weakness; in fact, it's a sign of strength. Acceptance shows you haven't surrendered to the challenges of PD. And when you can't fight the battle alone, you still win because you have people willing to step up to the fight for you.

Meeting the challenge with good humor

We can't say this too often: An upbeat, optimistic attitude is one of your most effective weapons against PD. And right next to it is the ability to laugh—with others, at yourself, and especially at your PD. We're talking black humor here, folks.

Bill of Rights for people with Parkinson's

Declarations of individual rights are nothing new. Perhaps you've noticed *rights* lists posted when you visit a hospital or care facility. But we think it's important that you—the person with PD—know your own inalienable rights. Feel free to edit and add your own ideas to the following list. Then bookmark it and reread it regularly.

I have the right

- To take care of and make decisions for myself for as long as I am capable and to expect my care partners to respect my wishes, should the time come when they speak for me

- To seek help from others as I recognize limits to my own endurance and strength
- To maintain those facets of my life that were part of my identity before my PD diagnosis for as long as possible—even if each task takes three times as long
- To occasionally (and humanly) get angry, be depressed, and work my way through other difficult feelings
- To reject any attempt by others (either consciously or unconsciously) to limit my independence because it'll make life easier for them
- To expect and receive consideration, respect, encouragement, affection, and forgiveness as long as I offer these same qualities in return
- To take joy and pride in my accomplishments—regardless of how small—and the courage it takes to achieve them
- To speak out and demand that new resources and eventually a cure

be found—if not for me, then for those who follow

For example, a diet-center leader famous for her wonderful sense of humor inspired her feeling-sorry-for-themselves clients with the story of her father, a large, barrel-chested man who had always been bigger than life. Then he got cancer and started fading away—literally. One day toward the very end, when he was but a shadow of his former robust self, he said to his daughter, "You know I want to be cremated." She nodded in agreement. "Well," he added, "if I keep dwindling away like this, I think you'll be able to do the job in the microwave!" His daughter was first stunned and then burst into laughter. That's black humor, folks – and it works because it helps you keep your perspective as you face the sometimes tough days of living with PD.

Breaking the News to Your Care Partner

Chances are your care partner was with you when the diagnosis of PD was confirmed. If you learned the news together, then the telling part is done. But the two of you still need to spend some time working your way through the questions of how this diagnosis is going to affect your lives—individually and together.

If your primary care partner is not your significant other (perhaps she's a sibling or an adult child who works, has a family of her own, and lives in another community), give yourself a day or so to digest the diagnosis and think about how you prefer to break the news.

When you're ready (don't wait too long; a day or week at most), try to have the conversation in person and allow enough time to work through the discussion. If you can't talk in person, choose a time when this person isn't distracted by other activities and have the discussion by phone. When you deliver the news, reassure this person that the diagnosis is not life-threatening and you have no need for immediate action. Then set a time when the two of you can discuss your present needs, your needs down the road, and her willingness and capability for fulfilling those needs.

If you have to deliver the initial news by phone, urge your care partner to check out some of the Web sites in Appendix B. Or call the folks at the National Parkinson Foundation at 800-327-4545 and ask them to send copies of their excellent (and free) booklet, *Parkinson's Disease: Caring and Coping* to both of you. (In fact, while you're at it, ask for copies of the entire series of booklets.)

During this sit-down conversation with your care partner, allow enough time to:

- Share immediate emotional reactions—even if you've had a couple of days or a week since you and your care partner heard the news.
- Be prepared for different responses. One of you may react with denial and the other with anger. (Before this discussion, you may both benefit by reading the section on personality differences in Chapter 5.)
- Set down in writing a list of steps to take. Include a tentative timeline for each one based on the tips we offer in the next section.

Resist the urge (by you or your care partner) to leap ahead and take dramatic and life-changing actions such as putting your home up for sale and moving in with your daughter or assuming that you need to quit your job. You have time. You are years—and perhaps decades—from needing to make these lifestyle changes because of your PD.

Telling Your Family

When and how you deliver the news to your immediate and extended family is an individual choice that's influenced by

- The status of individual family relationships.
- Your personal feelings about how soon you want even close relatives to know.

When you're ready to talk to family members, the easiest way may be a family gathering (if geography allows) where you tell all the adult members at once. Everyone can hear the same version, and details won't get distorted through repetition. However, because families are so spread out in today's world, a family meeting may not be possible. In that case, consider arranging a conference call. Again, the goal is to deliver the news to all the adults at the same time.

If you have children, find a place and time to share your news with them before that larger meeting, especially if your PD is of the young-onset variety and your children are still living at home. Your children will make this journey with you; they deserve to have the same time and privacy to digest this news as your care partner had.

Give adults the facts

When you deliver the news to the adults in your immediate and extended family, stick to the basics:

- What PD is
- Whether others in the family are at risk
- How PD is treated
- What your prognosis is

Some family members may have suspected a serious illness of some kind; others may be completely shocked at the news and take it hard. In either case, a good first step is to educate and inform.

PD associations offer a number of basic educational and informational materials for fundamental questions about PD. These excellent materials are listed in Appendix B. Handing out this printed information at a family meeting (or e-mailing it if your family lives elsewhere) gives them a reference for questions after the initial shock wears off. By selecting the same material for everyone, you lessen the chances of that information becoming distorted.

Set a positive tone

After you share the facts of PD with adult family members, consider setting the tone for your emerging new relationships. For example, you can add,

"There's a lot I don't know, but I do know I can live a relatively normal life in spite of my symptoms. The tough part is figuring out how to live it without people feeling sorry for me or treating me differently." With that simple statement you've laid out the ground rules:

- You have PD, but you're still you.
- Most important, you want other people to continue treating you the same. (Okay, so Cousin Fred can let you win a few more poker games and your mother may finally call someone else to get the cat out of the tree each week.)
- How much you say beyond that—symptoms, research, no present cures and such—is strictly up to you and your assessment of how much information this group can handle at the first telling.

When that question of "What can I do to help?" comes up, perhaps the best answer is to make these three points:

- Help me by being yourself and finding ways to continue our relationship as normally and fully as before.

- Help me make sure my care partner maintains a life outside of mine.
- Help me most of all by understanding that I'm still the same person inside. Don't let my PD symptoms scare you or make you treat me any differently.

Don't sugarcoat the situation for kids

Today's children are bombarded with information from every possible angle. Put another way, this generation is far savvier at a far younger age than most adults can imagine. On some level, even very young children can understand that something has changed in their environment. Don't underestimate their capacity for feeling stress and tension, especially when they can sense the undercurrent in the household but no one's talking with them about it.

• Teenagers can usually handle the same information you give the adults. If your teen is especially sensitive or perhaps struggling with other emotional challenges (the break-up of a relationship or not making the sports team, for example), you may want to have the conversation with that teen separately so you can focus on reassuring and comforting her.

• With younger children (or grandchildren), keep details as simple as possible. A terrific resource for telling young children (under age 12) about PD is the book entitled *I'll Hold Your Hand So You Won't Fall: A Child's Guide to Parkinson's Disease* by Rasheda Ali and her father, Muhammad Ali.

• In some cases, children in their middle years (ages 9 to 12) are mature enough to be included with the adults in the general family meeting. But just because they seem to understand and accept the news, don't assume that they don't have concerns or a gazillion questions about how your lives are going to change.

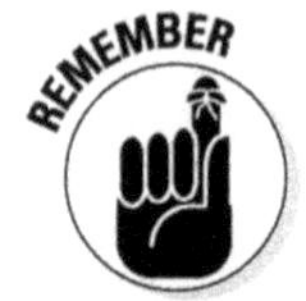

• If the child is your grandchild, decide with the parents the best way to deliver the news.

Regardless of the ages (or seeming maturity) of the children, never forget that they're children; they haven't lived long enough to pile up the life experiences and tools for coping that an adult has. Check in with your children and grandchildren often through positive techniques such as:

- Seeking their help with innovative ways you can cope with certain limits to normal tasks (like dressing) when your PD symptoms hinder you
- Continuing to pursue activities the two of you have always enjoyed—even if you have to find ways to adapt, such as getting a recumbent bicycle instead of riding your old one
- Providing the opportunity (place and time) for them to raise questions and concerns about what your PD means for the future

Giving Close Friends the News

Soon after you break the news to your family, consider how and when to tell your closest friends. Again several issues are at play here, including the fact that friends may have already noticed your symptoms and discussed their concerns with each other. They may not have brought their concern to you directly because they didn't want to intrude.

How and when you choose to tell this group depends in part on the nature of the group. In other words if your close friends are also close with each other, then inviting everyone over to your house and telling them all at the same time may be best. The advantage is that everyone hears the same words (although they may process them differently) at the same time directly from you. In addition, they can see your response to the diagnosis—hopefully upbeat and optimistic—at the same time. And they can all hear the ground rules for how you want them to respond to your diagnosis.

In cases where you have close friends who are not close with each other or friends who live in other places, you may want to tell each individually. If so, try to do it face to face (or at least by phone—not e-mail) so the person can see and hear how you're handling the diagnosis.

Consider providing the same helpful information (fact sheet and list of Web sites) that we identify in the two previous sections so your friends can pursue questions that may occur after you tell them.

Friendships can be critical to your overall sense of control and well-being when you're living with PD. Unfortunately, a lot of PWP make the mistake when they get the diagnosis of pulling away from their friends or denying their need for that support (tangible support like cutting the lawn or intangible support like just being there to listen).

When PWPs (or their care partners) react as if the support is an insult or a statement of the PWP's incapacity, they make matters worse. This reaction can have a snowball effect because the friend who wanted to help feels rejected (even embarrassed) at apparently adding to your stress. Before you know it, those treasured friendships (along with the normalcy and pleasure they brought your life) have disappeared.

As soon as you and your care partner are ready to go public with your news to friends, take control and set the tone by doing the following:

- State your needs regarding your approach to PD. For example, tell them you understand that they may want to rush in and start helping you (preparing meals, handling the household and yard chores, and such), but the best support they can offer is to help you maintain as normal a life (and relationship) as possible for as long as possible.

- Appreciate any offer of support and help (even if you shudder to think that they believe you need that help).
- Be prepared to suggest alternate ways they can be a part of your network of support and caring.

Another way to think of outside help is to consider your care partner and his soon-to-be-filled-to-capacity schedule. By maintaining a normal routine with friends and associates, you give your care partner a break to pursue life aside from PD.

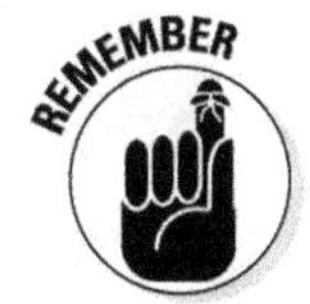

When you respond to your friends' invitations to activities you enjoyed before PD with "I can't...," they may stop offering and gradually get on with their own lives. Instead, try an attitude of "I'd love to [play cards, bike, meet you at the coffeehouse]. Help me figure out how we can make that happen." Then you can brainstorm options together.

As Lance Armstrong (the seven-time Tour de France winner and cancer survivor) has said, "C'mon, man. *Everything's* an option."

Widening the Circle: Informing Others

On the outer fringes of those concentric circles we describe at the beginning of this chapter are those people who play a role in your life but not a vital or intimate one (neighbors, community group associates, professionals you rely upon, and so on). Breaking the news to this last circle of contacts (with the possible exception of your boss and co-workers; see Chapter 16 for the specifics on that special group) is not a responsibility that you need to feel compelled to do right away—or ever. Basically, your condition's really none of their business.

On the other hand, don't underestimate the unexpected support and management resources that may come from one of these people. For example, your barber or beautician may offer to make a house call as your symptoms change. Or your neighbor may be happy to be on call for emergencies when you're alone and your partner's at work.

When the timing seems right during the first months following your diagnosis, let these people know you have PD. Only you can decide how much information they need or what kind of support and response they may provide. But, as with anyone you tell, be prepared to set the tone for their response, to correct misinformation they may have about PD, and to appreciate their concern and support however they express it.

Handling Sticky Conversations

Having said that, we need to get real here. Some people (and they may be in your closest circles) are more hindrance than help when they hear you have PD. One type simply can't handle bad news of any sort, so you end up spending a lot of time and energy comforting and emotionally supporting their (mostly unfounded) fears and anxieties. Another type believes they have all the answers even though they have zero real knowledge about PD. They, too, can use up your resources of energy and good humor as you try and educate them to the realities of living with PD. Consider these tips for handling those sticky situations:

- For people who simply can't cope with difficult news, consider being prepared with a specific request. You can ask, for example, "You're such an avid biker, would you be willing to bike with me once a week? My doctor tells me that exercise, especially now in the early stages, is really important, but I'd rather not go out alone."

If this person is a close friend or family member, you may want to speak with him separately and acknowledge his obvious fears and anxieties. Then let him know that he can be most helpful by trying to remain upbeat and positive—at least in your presence.

If all else fails, allow such people an initial period of mourning over your news. Then insist that they get over it or else you'll have to limit your contact with them. This is not about these people. You're the one with PD and, bluntly stated, you just don't need other people bringing you down.

• For the well-meaning folks (even strangers!) who see your tremor or some other PD symptom and start telling you the story of their uncle's wife's brother who also had PD, you need a different tactic. No doubt such people mean well, but they'll never be part of your care team. This empathy and advice (or showing off!) is about them, not you.

Don't allow unwanted advice or comments to upset you. Of the two of you, *you* are the expert at PD. Acknowledge their effort to help, and then walk away.

Chapter 8

Special Advice for Those with Young Onset Parkinson's Disease

In This Chapter

- Noting similarities and differences of YOPD and traditional PD
- Fleshing out problems unique to YOPD
- Incorporating financial security into the plan
- Refining the PD care partner's role

When it comes to Parkinson's disease (PD), no one's more famous than the popular actor Michael J. Fox. The twinkle in his eye and his legendary self-deprecating humor—even about life with PD—make him less the celebrity and more the national support-group leader for millions of people with

Parkinson's (PWP) and their care partners.

In a 2006 interview in *AARP, The Magazine,* Fox reported that as many as 40 percent of the 60,000 new PD cases each year involve someone younger than age 50. This figure alone blows holes in the myth that only old people get PD. The fact that Fox was first diagnosed in his 30s shines an even brighter light on the growing numbers of young and active people who face this challenge.

The cause of *young onset Parkinson's disease (YOPD)* is as debatable as the cause of traditional onset PD (see Chapter 2). But what isn't debatable is the fact that it hits people in their prime, plays havoc with their established roles (spouse, parent, adult child of aging parents), derails rising careers, and over-rides plans for the future.

In this chapter we take a look at the specific issues facing people diagnosed with YOPD. When the information is the same for any PWP, we refer you to other chapters in the book. But if you're 30, 40, 50, or not yet 60 and have PD, this chapter's for you.

Comparing YOPD to Traditional Onset PD

The term *onset age* means when symptoms first appear—not when a diagnosis is made. If the onset age is earlier than age 50, the diagnosis is usually YOPD. (In very rare cases, PD symptoms appear before a person reaches the age of 21; the term *juvenile Parkinson's* distinguishes it from traditional or YOPD.)

Two excellent resources for information specially aimed at people with YOPD are Young Onset Parkinson's Association (YOPA) at www.yopa.org and The Michael J. Fox Foundation at www.michaeljfox.org, where you can sign up to receive regular *Fox Flash* e-mail bulletins. These periodic updates cover upcoming foundation activities and provide valuable tips and information for PWP and their care partners.

How they're the same

PD is chronic, progressive, and (at least at this writing) incurable regardless of your age and when you get it. On the positive side, it's possible to live for many years—in some cases a regular lifespan—in spite of having PD. It's possible to continue to work, to raise a family, to see children marry and have children of their own, and to enjoy many of the same activities you enjoyed before being diagnosed.

How they differ

YOPD and traditional onset PD differ in three basic ways:

• People with YOPD are less likely to experience the dementia (memory problems) or balance problems that affect people whose PD begins when they're older. Part of the reason for the difference is that older people are more likely to have multiple conditions (such as Alzheimer's, a series of small strokes, or adverse medication interaction) that affect memory and balance.

• People with YOPD may experience a condition known as *dystonia* (unusual muscle cramping, aches, or abnormal movement in a particular area of the body such as a foot or shoulder). For reasons that still aren't clear, older patients seldom experience dystonia but tend to have *tremor* (shaking), a symptom that's less common for a person with YOPD.

Although dystonia is well recognized as the possible first symptom of YOPD, your diagnosis may be delayed if your doctor isn't familiar with such PD symptoms in younger patients. According to the Young Onset Parkinson's Association, the number of people with YOPD may be significantly under-reported for the very reason that many people experience early symptoms for years before they get to a doctor who considers PD as a possible diagnosis.

• In general, people with YOPD appear to respond well to antiparkinsonian medications, yet side effects (such as *dyskinesia*—uncontrollable movements) may affect them more quickly than older PWP.

In an article for the American Parkinson's Disease Association, Lawrence I. Golbe notes that people with YOPD experience two specific medication-related problems more than older PWP: early wearing-off of the medication benefits and on-off fluctuations (when PD meds lose their effectiveness so symptoms reappear before the next dose is due).

Many people with YOPD (and their doctors) elect to postpone treatment with antiparkinsonian meds as long as possible to avoid some of these escalated symptoms and side effects. ***Note:*** Research shows no clear evidence that early withholding of therapy has long-term benefits.

Faster or slower? What's the prognosis?

The jury's still out on the pace of progression for people with YOPD. However, more advanced therapies may eventually postpone the progression of symptoms for a longer time—perhaps adding years to the person's relatively normal life.

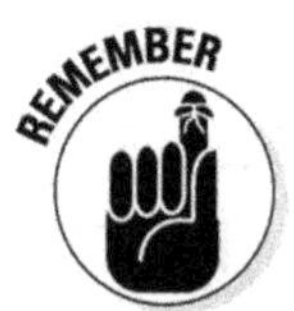

PD—regardless of the age of onset—affects each individual differently. As with any health issue, your physical and mental health at the onset of PD (and your fight to maintain that well being through a balanced diet and regular exercise program) can have an enormous effect on the prognosis. Nothing is carved in stone regarding the progression of symptoms—no matter how old or young you are when they start.

Facing the Special Challenges of YOPD

If you have YOPD, the most difficult challenge may be the very fact that you're young. You had planned a life packed with many goals, and one of them was *not* living with a chronic and progressive condition!

Most people in their young adult years tend to see themselves as invincible. They may take steps to ensure financial security for their family and themselves in the unlikely event that something bad happens, but they really don't consider it a possibility.

But, now it appears that the *unlikely* event has happened: You've been diagnosed with YOPD. And it's standing directly in the way of the life you've planned. At first you can see no way around it. But you know better. You know something this scary, this bleak can enrich your life in many ways.

Stop for a moment and consider other times when you faced what seemed like an impossible challenge. How did you respond to that challenge?

Maybe it was a basketball game when your team was down by a point with only seconds to go and you were at the line for two free throws. Maybe it was a far more serious situation like financial difficulties or the possibility of losing your job. Maybe it was when you needed and wanted to prove yourself to someone you admired and respected. Whatever the challenge, you took some mental steps early on to face the threat or achieve what you wanted.

In this section we give you the mental steps to help you get through this diagnosis and come out on top—again.

Getting an accurate diagnosis

The diagnosis of YOPD is based on the same cardinal signs used to diagnose PD at any age:

- Tremor at rest (trembling when body part is not engaged in activity)
- Rigidity (muscle and joint stiffness)
- Bradykinesia (slowed or impaired ability to move)

- Postural instability (impaired balance)

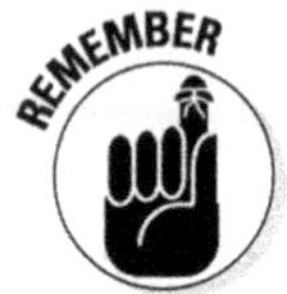

Cases of YOPD tend to present less often with tremor and more often with bradykinesia, rigidity, and abnormal muscle cramps (dystonia) that frequently affect one foot.

When a person develops PD at a young age, the doctor must make sure that the patient doesn't have another disorder that can mimic parkinsonism (see also Chapter 4). Your doctor should always check for two rare diseases in particular: *Wilson's disease* (which requires a different treatment) and *Dopa-responsive dystonia* (DRD), which has a prognosis very different from PD.

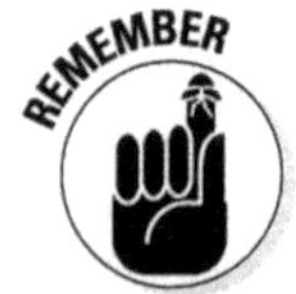

The genetic element (see Chapter 2) seems to be more prevalent in YOPD than older PD patients. In some cases, the doctor may order a test for *Parkin* mutation, which is more frequent in YOPD. If you agree to have this DNA test, be sure you ask to see a certified genetic consultant in order to discuss all the implications (emotional and practical) of this test for you and your family.

Handling the diagnosis: A positive attitude is the best offense

Get ready for a ride on the emotional roller coaster after you get the diagnosis. Your initial reaction may range from disbelief to denial to anger to all of the above and then some. Your mind may rocket from image to image—will you see your kids grow up, graduate, and marry? Will you be able to work and support yourself and your family? What about the dreams you had of traveling, starting your own business, running that marathon? What about those words *no cure?*

Give yourself some time to mourn the fact that your life does not—for the moment—seem to be headed in the direction you had hoped. And then get on with it. This is the life you've been given. Everyone has to deal with challenges and tough choices at some point in life. PD is yours.

Because you're under 50 (even under 40), you have young onset PD, which has no cure—yet. However,

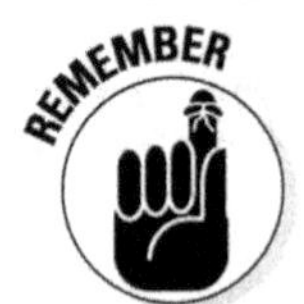

• Researchers have already developed proven techniques and therapies for managing and treating symptoms.

• You can maintain function and a relatively normal lifestyle over a period of years and—in your case—possibly decades.

• You will not die from Parkinson's disease

• Much of the life you imagined is still within your reach. The odds are very good that you'll

- See your children grow up, graduate, marry—and have children.
- Continue working for years to come and even realize the dream of starting a second career.
- Travel. Why not? (The marathon may be a little trickier.)
- Get very good at finding ways to adapt PD to goals that are really important to you.

And the best defense is a good offense

Okay, so you've taken time to digest the diagnosis and you have the attitude thing going. Now what? Take a look at the following sections to keep moving in the right direction.

Brain power

You initial response may be to run to the library or computer and look at every statistic you can find on YOPD. What were the odds that you'd get PD? What's the likely prognosis in years?

What percentage of PWP your age are able to keep working, see their children grow up, have sex?

Mark Twain said there are three kinds of lies—lies, damned lies, and statistics. You can choose to believe the statistics and project them onto the rest of your life or you can refuse to be a statistic. You can determine that you're unique and that you'll custom design (with your care team—see Chapter 6) your PD management for you—and only you. But the immediate challenge is to get to work educating yourself (and your family and friends) about this diagnosis.

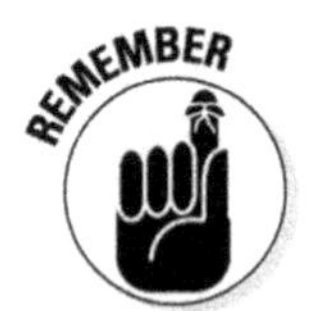

You've already taken a positive step by reading this book! It's chock-full of chapters offering information for anyone living with PD—young or not-so-young. After you've read it (and, of course, shared it with people close to you!), keep it handy. As you make this journey with

PD, use this book as a guide to the resources you'll need along the way.

Carpe diem: Seize the day!

The overriding emotion you may feel early on is a sense that you've totally lost control of your life. But you can only lose control if you surrender to it—if you choose to hand it over to someone else and simply follow other people's orders. There's a better approach to PD for you and your care partner—one that gives you the best chance of living the life you planned before the diagnosis.

Take charge of this thing—the same way you'd attack any other unlikely event (like losing your job or your home being damaged by fire). Life can hand you bigger problems than PD—really! Unlike people facing a terminal illness, you have time and a reminder to be proactive and do what matters most now, not some day.

Without going all the way to Pollyanna-mode, consider the advantages of a can-do and optimistic outlook:

- The very fact that time becomes more precious can instill the determination not to waste an hour or a day.
- Close relationships can be strengthened—marriages, parent-child connections (yours as a parent and yours as the child of aging parents).
- Genuine and dedicated friends will stick; hangers-on will not (and you may be surprised at who's who in the bunch).
- New people—interesting and stimulating, understanding and fun—come into your life.
- There's nothing like a progressive illness to make you get off your butt, take that trip, write that novel, or go back to school.
- You now have the opportunity to work with other people to make a real difference in the lives of millions. How many people do you know who can say that?
- In some ways you're getting a fresh start—the chance to change you. Suddenly you understand in a very real way that life *is* finite.

Staying on track in your career

A question that's bound to be at the top of your mind is whether or not you can continue working. On so many levels, your ability to pursue a career, run a business, or maintain financial security is integral to living the life you envisioned. Be sure to read Chapter 16 for a full discussion of PD in the workplace.

One of the key messages you want to send to your employer, co-workers, and yourself is that the prognosis of YOPD is good. With proper management of PD symptoms through exercise, diet, and medications, your career can be good to go for years to come. When your neurologist, physical therapist, and nutritionist fully understand your job's requirements, they can structure your care plan (and timing of meds when you begin taking them) to provide optimal function when you need it most.

Before you sit down with your employer to discuss your diagnosis and its possible effects on your work, plan ahead by

- Exploring options such as flexible hours or telecommuting. If your employer makes such options available to other employees (like new parents or regular part-timers), then you're not asking for special consideration.
- Thinking through the demands of your specific job and how to handle them. Anticipate the questions (and doubts) your employer may have about your ability to continue.

If you think it's necessary, ask your neurologist to prepare a letter that explains the status of your PD in relation to your work.

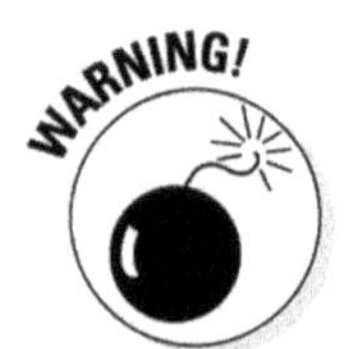

Stress can pack a double whammy when it comes to maintaining your job and career because stress comes with the territory in many (make that *most*) jobs and can do a real number on your YOPD symptoms. Take a look at Chapter 16 for ways to manage stressful situations in the workplace—this is a huge step toward successfully maintaining your position for years to come.

Dealing with PD's impact on relationships

Now that you have PD, your diagnosis can become the two-ton gorilla in the room, sitting squarely between you and other people—if you let it. When you fear that your lover, child, best friend, or co-worker can't see you because PD's in the way, then take the initiative. Make sure these people remember that you're still you! By addressing PD issues that may affect your most important relationships, you can remove that gorilla from the room.

Your role as a spouse or significant other

The roles you and your partner have settled into may undergo quite a make-over as your PD progresses. Fortunately, this progression usually occurs over a period of years with ample time to adjust. But that delay doesn't mean you can't or shouldn't prepare for necessary changes. In other words, begin communicating now. Communication and patience are your best resources for adapting later to these inevitable changes. These are some examples:

- If your tremor worsens and you've been chief handyperson for the household, how's that going to work out? Talk about ways that you can manage the task with more time, or use this opportunity to teach a child how to wield a hammer.
- If small, cramped handwriting is an early symptom of your PD and you're the lead check writer and bookkeeper, can that continue indefinitely? Maybe you can pay bills online or install software to print

out checks that you only need to sign.

- If you've been the family's gourmet cook but now you take hours longer to turn out one of your signature meals, then you (and those around you) need to practice patience by allowing for the extra time you need. Then again, you may consider graciously (and willingly) accepting some help.

Don't rush into changes before they're necessary. Do take time to plan with your partner the ways that you can adjust certain tasks or roles before you give them up.

As your symptoms progress and your medication timing switches unexpectedly into on-off mode, your spouse or significant other may find it tough to believe you're suddenly struggling with a task that you managed fine just a minute earlier. Be honest about what's going on. Acknowledge that it looks like you don't want to do this task, but—for now—you really can't. Communication and patience are paramount here!

Another common concern when you have YOPD is the question of intimacy. Okay, to put it bluntly—you're wondering about its impact on your ability to perform sexually. The answer: If you experience a change in your sexual desire, performance, or pleasure, a host of underlying causes are possible. Some of the more common ones are:

- Side effects of medications
- Effects of certain cardiovascular conditions (high blood pressure, circulatory problems, reduced blood flow, heart disease and such)
- Impact of other conditions such as urinary incontinence, menopause for women, or prostate problems for men
- Effects of depression, stress, or anxiety
- Symptoms common to PD (tremor, stiffness, on-off episodes,

dyskinesias and such) that can affect movement (not to mention the mood!)

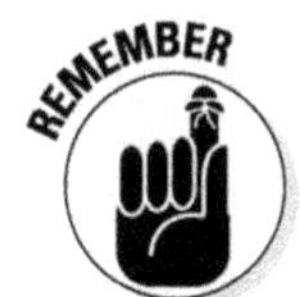

PD may cause sexual dysfunction, but this symptom usually occurs several years into the progression of the disease, and other symptoms (including those listed above) can play a role. Don't simply assume that a change in your desire for intimacy or ability to make love is a normal part of PD. Solutions are available, so talk to your doctor and look at Chapter 19 for more information on sexual dysfunction.

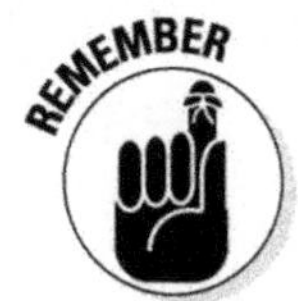

Intimacy means more than the act of making love. Think about the progression of your relationship. Maybe it began with flirting and progressed to the sheer romance of the courtship before you two decided you were in this for the long haul. Maybe you surprised your partner with an unexpected romantic gesture—flowers for no reason, holding hands at the movies, the funny card, or handwritten note. Rekindle those little moments that led to falling in love and the commitment of a long-term (or even lifetime) relationship.

Maintain a sense of humor. Surely even at your healthiest you had those moments—embarrassing, silly, laugh-out-loud times when it all went hay-wire at a critical moment. Plan to roll with them. Shared laughter can be incredibly sexy.

Your role as a parent

How life may change for you and your kids will depend on their ages when you're diagnosed. If they're very young, you can keep the news simple and guide your children as they grow up and your symptoms progress. By the time they reach their middle or high school years, living with a parent who has PD will seem so normal that it'll be their friends' parents who seem different.

If your children are older (middle or high school) when you're diagnosed, communication may be more difficult. At this age your children are dealing with a lot already. They're trying to locate their own sense of identity among their peers and within the family unit, they're trying to live up to adult expectations, and they're facing ever-escalating pressure to make the right choices. No wonder they shut down sometimes!

Now you come along and deliver the news that you have PD—a disease they may have heard about but one that they may have some real misinformation on. Depending on their age and your relationship, your children may or may not ask questions, but don't assume that they have none. On the other hand, dole out information carefully. You may hear "TMI!" (too much information) from your teen when you start throwing around terms like *bradykinesia, substantia nigra,* and such.

If you have teens or middle-schoolers, you may want to ask for help in researching information. They're undoubtedly proficient on the computer. Give them a focused PD topic to research and ask them to share it with the family. For example, put them to work locating and bookmarking the best PD Web sites for the family. What organizations can they find? What are the strengths of each site? By proactively including your children in a management plan for your PD, you take away a lot of their fear and distress that can come from being left out of key discussions and decisions.

Your role as a friend

If you're fortunate enough to have a network of close friends—even if that network is only two or three people—you have a fabulous resource for coping with your PD. Friends can listen when you really don't want to burden your spouse or significant other. And they can take your focus off PD to get you back on the track of living the life you'd planned. Friends can make you laugh and let you cry. They can push, shove, and irritate you until you'll do anything to get them off your case. They can admire your courage, wonder at your ability to contain this beast, and celebrate each passage—just as they did when you didn't have PD, and just as you've done for them.

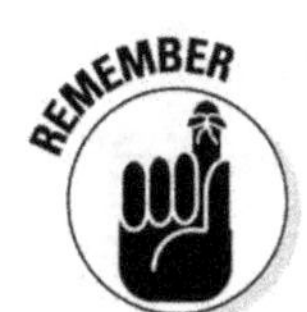

Friendship is a two-way street. Your friends can only be there if you let them, and they'll be there for the long term only if you let them know you'll do the same for them. For more ideas on PD and friendships, see Chapter 15.

Your role as a co-worker/employee/employer

By some estimates, up to one-third of PWP (at any age) are actively employed. As the news of your diagnosis spreads at work, your co-workers will probably take one of two positions: Some will immediately come forward, express their concern, and ask what they can do to help; others will pull back, take a let's-see-how-this-goes position.

As with all your relationships, this one is yours to manage. Frankly, your best bet is to let people know that you have PD (after you've told your employer). Otherwise the rumor mill is going to be the messenger. Consider sitting down with members of your department (with your supervisor's approval) to give them some brief, basic facts about YOPD. You can then ask these co-workers to use these facts to squelch rumors they may be hearing.

If you're the employer (or department head), be aware of immediate employee concerns for you *and* for themselves. What does your PD mean for the future of the business and their job security? Again carefully prepare by anticipating questions and concerns (from good employees seeking other positions or ambitious staffers eyeing your position) for you and your business.

Whatever your job, you need to realistically assess (and reassess regularly and frequently) your ability to handle the job. Your greatest barrier will be stress, and the greatest stress comes when people around you clearly question your ability to do the job. For ways you can address this problem and the related challenges of PD in the workplace, see Chapter 16.

Your role in the community

Over time your PD becomes more and more difficult to disguise. Even if you can manage the outward symptoms like a tremor or impaired movement, the stress of trying to keep it a secret can drain you. But why expend so much energy to keep people in the dark when they may become unexpected sources for support and outright help?

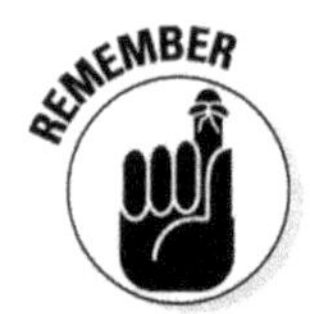

Maintaining (or instigating) community relationships isn't just about the personal returns. When you volunteer at your child's school or join in for a charity walk or bike event, you're making a better world for others—and that's empowering. You're not this poor PWP; you're someone who chooses to take advantage of an opportunity to make a real difference for yourself and the community around you.

Speaking of community action, the Parkinson community—national, regional and local—is well organized and a great place to get involved. By taking an active role in advocating for more research dollars, better therapies, and eventually a cure, you empower yourself and other PWP. Not a marcher or the outspoken sort? Not a problem. Check out www.parkinsonaction.org or any of the national organizations listed in the appendix of this book for ways you can get involved behind the scenes.

The Dollars and Cents of YOPD Financial Planning

Definition of *terrifying:* The experience of a person in the prime of life getting news that he has a chronic and progressively debilitating illness. Although people with YOPD can hope for a cure in their lifetime, basing their financial futures on such a pipedream is, unfortunately, unrealistic.

Realistically you'll live with PD for many years to come, years that may include getting married, raising a family, sending kids off to college, securing the future for your partner, caring for aging parents—a host of emotional and financial challenges. Our suggestion? Regardless of your economic status, take your partner and get to a financial planner now (see Chapter 21 for tips on choosing one) to help you plan for the future.

If you're in debt now, you need a plan to manage that debt and end it as quickly as possible. If you have plans for major financial commitments (such as buying a car or home or sending your child to college), you need to ask yourself whether such plans are still viable.

Financial planning is one of those tasks where preparing for the worst scenario is the wisest move. You may ask, "But what if I never need to put the plans in action?" The best answer is a different, more challenging question: What if you *do* need to?

If you haven't already done so, take time to ask the big questions:

- What are my current health insurance plan's benefits?
- What hospitalization, disability benefits, and programs may be available through my work?
- What are the benefits and limitations of the COBRA program if I have to stop working?

- What long-term care insurance program can I (or my partner) benefit from?
- Am I eligible for that program?

Connecting with other YOPDers

"I have plenty of friends," you say, "so I don't need to connect." Oh, but you do. You have a condition that usually strikes people decades older than you. You have a chronic, progressive condition that's going to impact every facet of your life. On top of that, you have this life—of work and relationships and social events and community functions and.... So, you're going to have times over the coming months and years when the very person you need to talk with is someone who understands what it means to have YOPD, someone who's been there, who's still there—someone who can tell you to knock it off, stop wasting precious time, and get on with your life when you start feeling sorry for yourself.

So where can you find these people? If you're really fortunate, a

YOPD support group is close enough for you to conveniently attend meetings. If it isn't, then check with the facilitator of any PD support group that meets in your area to see how many of the participants have YOPD. If that fails, ask your neurologist whether she treats other YOPD patients. If she does, perhaps names and contact information can be exchanged.

Your best resource may be the Internet. One established organization specifically for YOPDers is Movers and Shakers at www.pdadvocates.org The Parkinson Action Network at www.parkinsonsaction.org is another great place to connect with PWP of all ages. The National Parkinson Foundation at www.parkinson.org sponsors an annual conference for YOPDers and their families. In addition, chat rooms and other sites offer people with YOPD a chance to connect—even in the wee hours of the morning. Two such sites are www.braintalk.org and www.plwp.org.

The point is that you (and your care partner) can connect with others your age that understand and have experienced or are experiencing many of the same frustrations you are. Your friends and family members may be terrific—supportive and concerned—but how can they possibly understand the full impact of YOPD? Not even your neurologist can fully appreciate what it means to have PD in the prime of your life.

Connecting with YOPDers isn't about giving up on friendships that have sustained you (and that still sustain you). But connecting with other YOPDers can lessen your sense of isolation and provide you with resources and news to manage your symptoms in a variety of situations. Another person with YOPD may not become your new best friend—but then again, don't rule out the possibility.

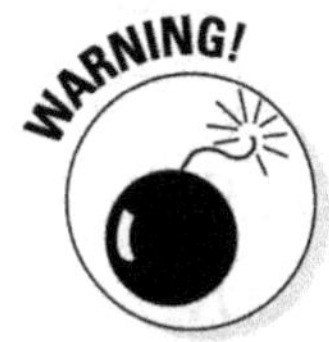

If you have no insurance, talk to your financial planner immediately about options that may be available in your state or through federal programs. If the financial planner can't answer your questions or provide information in a timely manner, find another planner!

In addition to your financial planning, take the following measures to help your medical providers:

- Establish a *durable* power of attorney for healthcare decisions as well as financial decisions.
- Write a living will or advance directive; make sure you distribute copies to every doctor who treats you and carry a copy with you in case you need to go to the hospital or emergency room.
- Be sure that the people you appoint to speak for you know what you want them to say and do!

For a more detailed discussion of legal and financial concerns that need your attention sooner rather than later, turn to Chapter 20.

A Word for the PD Care Partner

When you discover that someone you love has a condition that takes that person's functions and abilities, your instinct may be to go into full caregiver-mode and take charge. Please resist that urge! The person you love is exactly the same person that he was before the diagnosis. PD doesn't change a person overnight. In fact, the changes are gradual enough for the two of you to take the time to adapt, prepare, and plan.

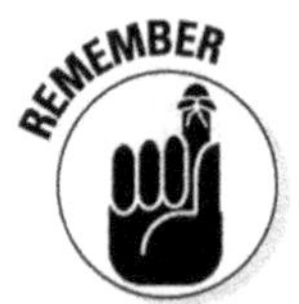

But you don't want to run away either. Throughout this book we talk about the fight-or-flight response to tough situations. If you're a person who takes flight (backs away and finds reasons to become disengaged), then you need to reassess that instinct. The person you love and are devoted to needs you—your support and understanding—in the early going, and she may eventually need more of you as her spokesperson and advocate.

If you're a fighter (a person who takes charge or refuses to lose), you may need to dial it down a notch or two. Although you're the care partner, the operative word is *partner.* You're not in charge; you don't have YOPD. Contribute and discuss options—yes. Coax and encourage—absolutely. Defend your right to a life beyond your partner's PD—positively. But in the final analysis, the person with PD has the right (as well as the ability) to decide how she wants to face this challenge. It's called *patient autonomy* and it's the very foundation of medical ethics.

Part III

Crafting a Treatment Plan Just for You

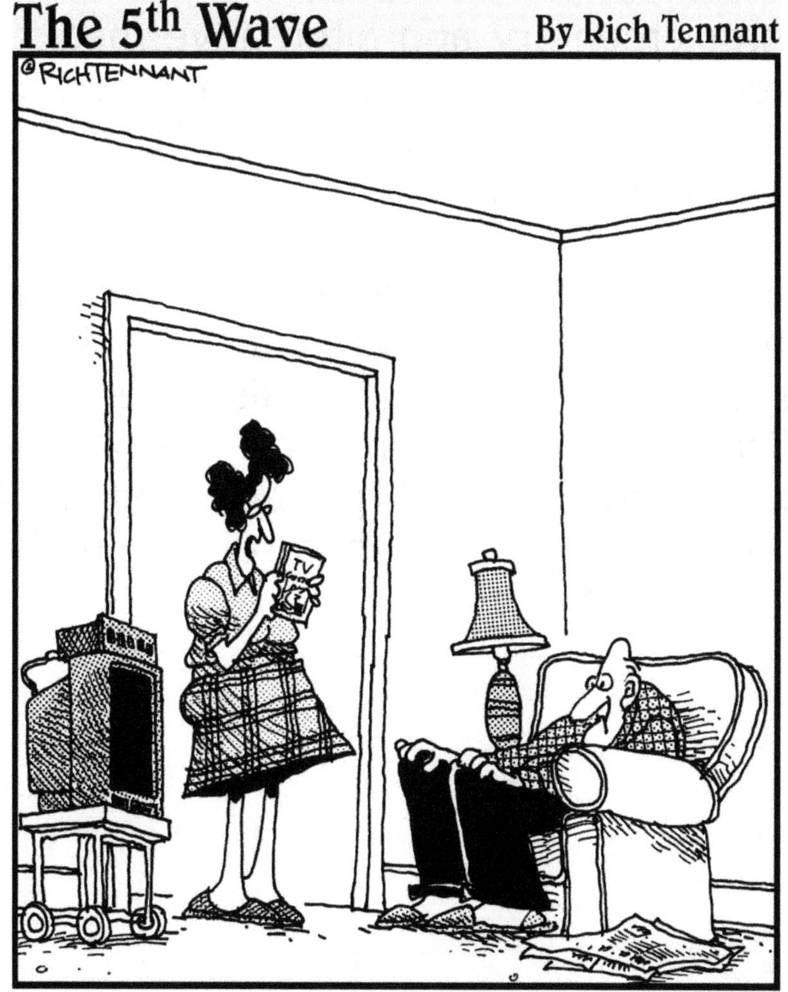

"Well Dad, if you're feeling down why don't you watch some TV. Let's see, there's 'Silent Killers', 'When Puppies Attack', and 'War of the Worlds.'"

In this part...

You can explore the variety of options available to treat your PD and help manage symptoms. These include medications and surgery as well as complementary and alternative medical treatments. Our chapter on diet and exercise includes an illustrated program of stretching and strengthening exercises that you can take to your doctor or physical therapist for review. Finally we have a chapter on clinical trials where we discuss the pros and cons of participating in such projects and what you need to know before you make a commitment.

Chapter 9

Managing PD Symptoms with Prescription Medicines

In This Chapter

- Grasping the lowdown on meds for PD's motor symptoms
- Minimizing those non-motor symptoms
- Getting (and staying!) squared away on your meds

Your Parkinson's disease (PD) diagnosis will include treatment options for managing your symptoms. If you have no symptoms of functional disability at the time of your diagnosis (in other words, if the PD isn't interfering with your ability to live your normal life), then your doctor will most likely prescribe programs like exercise and nutrition counseling, a support group, and, of course, regular visits to his office to monitor symptoms and any signs of progression.

As your symptoms begin to affect your work, social, and routine activities, your doctor will likely add *pharmacologic* therapy (prescription medications) to the treatment plan. In this chapter, we look at the most common medications for managing symptoms, some that have been around for decades and others that are relatively new to the scene. We also pass along some suggestions for staying on top of your medication regimen.

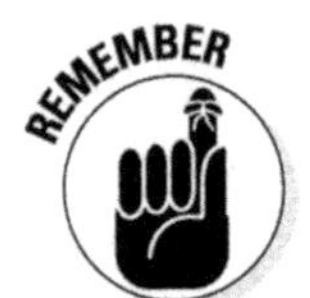

Because PD has no cure at this time and there is no means of preventing its progression, the treatment goal is to manage the symptoms, postpone their progression, and minimize the onset of new symptoms for as long as possible.

Managing Motor Symptoms with Proven Prescription Medication

In managing your symptoms, your doctor may prescribe a variety of medications to help prolong your current level of function. The medication may be available only as a brand-name drug (meaning it's still under patent protection), or it may be available in the generic form (meaning the patent has expired). Brand drugs are usually newer, more expensive, and possibly more beneficial than generics.

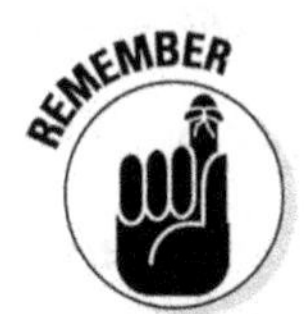

All medications for PD have one goal: to restore brain concentration of dopamine to near-normal levels. To achieve this goal, your doctor may prescribe one or more pills with different mechanisms of action (similar to different foods that we routinely use to restore sugar levels in our body, such as pasta, fruit, and sweets). The number of pills doesn't necessarily correlate to the gravity of the disease!

Almost 40 years after its introduction, the combination of *levodopa* and *carbidopa* (usually prescribed under the brand name *Sinemet*) is still the preferred treatment for most people with Parkinson's (PWP). The following sections cover the components of this medication and the role each one plays.

L-dopa—The gold standard

The most effective prescription medication to date for controlling PD symptoms is *levodopa* (often abbreviated to *L-dopa*), which brain cells use to produce more *dopamine,* the neurotransmitter that PD reduces. Producing more dopamine permits relief for PD symptoms such as stiffness, tremor (shaking), facial mask, cramped handwriting, slow movement, and impaired gait (walking).

Historically, L-dopa was administered alone, which caused a whole list of side effects including nausea, loss of appetite, vomiting, lowered blood pressure (leading to dizziness and possible falls), and rapid heart rate. Because these side effects were so significant, researchers almost dropped L-dopa from the regimen before they discovered the advantages of prescribing it with its now-conventional partner, *carbidopa.* Coupled with carbidopa, L-dopa can almost completely control PD symptoms for a *honeymoon* period of two to eight years.

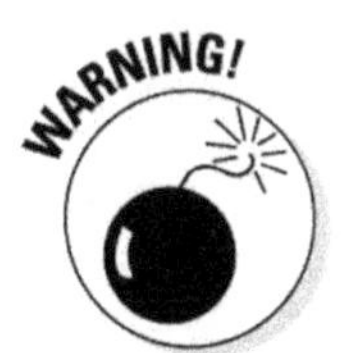

Unfortunately, 50 percent of PWP develop motor complications after 5 years of levodopa therapy; virtually all of them experience a decline in the benefit of levodopa after 10 to 15 years of therapy.

Carbidopa—L-dopa's companion

Any time the treatment seems worse than the condition, researchers look for ways to make the treatment more palatable for the patient. Carbidopa's main purpose is to offset the serious and uncomfortable side effects of levodopa without causing side effects of its own. In addition, carbidopa

- Allows your system to absorb the essential vitamin B6
- Lessens the amount of levodopa you need to control symptoms

When your symptoms do require medication, the prescription will probably be a low dose of carbidopa/levodopa. The prescription includes two numbers—usually 25/100. The first number refers to the amount of carbidopa and the second is the amount of levodopa. Your doctor monitors your symptoms on this low dose (usually taken at regular intervals three to four times a day). If you experience side effects, he can double the amount of carbidopa in your prescription. As the symptoms of PD progress, your doctor may increase the dosage and shorten the periods between doses.

Two other formulations for this medication are:

- The controlled-release (CR) form of Sinemet, which prolongs the effect of levodopa
- The orally disintegrating tablet (ODT) form of carbidopa/levodopa(brand name *Parcopa*)

With ODT delivery systems, you place the tablet on your tongue and it melts (like a mint) in a matter of seconds without water.

Entacapone—Another bodyguard for L-dopa

Recently a new class of drugs, *catechol-O-methyl transferase* inhibitors (COMT-I), has been added to PD therapy. COMT-I blocks the enzyme 3-O-methyldopa and allows even more levodopa to reach the brain. (Imagine levodopa with two body guards—carbidopa and *entacapone* or *tolcapone* (see the following paragraph)—to shelter it from dangerous enzymes on its journey toward the brain.) Other advantages of adding COMT-I to L-dopa are

- Longer duration of the L-dopa effectiveness
- Potential for reducing the dosage of carbidopa/levodopa
- The possibility of managing *off* times more effectively (See "Tracking the on-off fluctuations of your meds" later in this chapter.)

Entacapone (brand name *Stalevo*) is a new L-dopa therapy that combines the COMPT-I with carbidopa/levodopa. This three-in-one combination makes dosing easier because you take one pill, not two. Another COMT-I, *tolcapone* (brand name *Tasmar*), is available but has some limitations associated with liver toxicity.

Other effective prescription medicines

Your doctor may prescribe other medications in addition to your carbidopa/levodopa to better manage your symptoms. We cover the most common classes of these companion drugs in the following sections.

Dopamine agonists (DA)

Unlike levodopa, which is transformed into dopamine, *dopamine agonists (DA)* imitate the characteristics of dopamine. Your doctor may recommend that you try a DA before prescribing Sinemet as a first-line treatment in order to delay the complications associated with the use of levodopa over the long haul. (See the previous section "L-dopa—the gold standard" for more about Sinemet.) DAs have been in use for two decades with proven effectiveness in treating PD symptoms. But their use may be limited by troubling side effects, such as daytime sleepiness, low blood pressure, edema (swollen feet), vivid dreams, and, on occasion, hallucinations.

Four dopamine agonists are available. Older generation drugs (bromocriptine and pergolide) are rarely used because of possible cardiac side effects. But newer generations of DAs (including *pramipexole* and *ropinirole*) offer effective management of symptoms with relatively fewer side effects.

Of the four DA medications available, studies haven't proven one to be more effective than another. Therefore, if you have an unfavorable response to one DA, ask your doctor about trying a different one to see whether it's more successful.

Monoamine oxidase inhibitors (MAOI)

This class of drugs works by interacting with monoamines, chemicals in the brain that transmit messages between nerve cells. Of the three monoamines (dopamine, serotonin, and norepinephrine), dopamine is the focus for PWP because it controls messages related to movement.

Although MAOI has two subtypes (Type A and Type B), only MAOI-B is used to treat PD. Its fundamental task is to inhibit the *oxidation* (burning) of dopamine, which clears the dopamine from the *synaptic space* (the tiny space between brain cells where chemical messages are exchanged). As a consequence, more dopamine is available and PD symptoms improve.

Interestingly, MAOI-B may provide an additional benefit by acting as a kind of neuroprotector (see Chapter 2), possibly slowing the progression of PD and delaying the need for carbidopa/levodopa therapy.

The original drug from this group is *selegiline,* which doctors still prescribe for the early stages of PD because it provides some control of PD symptoms. A new formula of orally disintegrating selegiline *(Zelapar)* has recently been introduced with a lower incidence of side effects and a once-a-day dosing schedule. The most recent drug in this class to receive FDA approval is *rasagiline* (brand name *Azilect*), also taken once a day for the treatment of early PD. For PWP in the moderate to advanced stages, a combination of selegiline and L-dopa can improve symptoms.

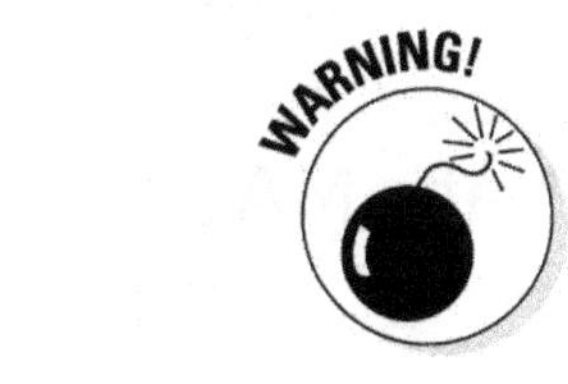

The downside to MAOIs is their potentially serious effect on blood pressure, especially when the patient is taking other medicines that also affect blood pressure. Take these precautions to avoid serious problems:

- Be sure all doctors know you're on this medication and always check with your pharmacist before using:
  - Over-the-counter (OTC) products such as cold-cough remedies (especially those including *dextromethorphan*) and diet supplements
  - Prescription medicines such as antidepressants that increase serotonin levels
- If you're scheduled for surgery, be sure the anesthesiologist knows you're taking rasagiline because anesthesia combined with the MAOIs can cause a dangerous drop in blood pressure.
- Be aware that MAOIs can cause abnormalities of blood pressure known as *tyramine* (or cheese

effect) when the patient is eating aged cheese or drinking red wine.

Consult your doctor if you have additional questions about the serious side effects of MAOIs.

Transdermal patch—A new delivery system

In most cases, prescribed medications come in a tablet or capsule form. But researchers are working on other ways to get the drug into your system with improved effectiveness, fewer side effects, and a shorter waiting period before the drug takes effect.

As one example of such research, at this writing the Food and Drug Administration (FDA) is in the process of reviewing a *transdermal* (skin) patch for the delivery of rotigotine, a dopamine agonist. You apply the patch to your skin (back, shoulder, or abdomen) once a day. The advantage of the patch is its consistent delivery of medication throughout the day. Consistent delivery of the dopamine agonist helps smooth out the amount of medicine you receive unlike the peaks and valleys that occur when taking tablets or capsules multiple times each day. This new method may improve symptom control and reduce side effects. Patches for the delivery of levodopa are also under study.

Amantadine

Amantadine is another older medication that doctors occasionally prescribe in early stages of PD because it can provide some benefit before levodopa is needed. Exactly how amantadine helps relieve symptoms isn't clear. In fact, it was originally (and continues to be) a treatment for the flu, but scientists serendipitously stumbled on its potential PD benefits. Most recently doctors have noted amantadine's benefits in managing *dyskinesia* (the writhing, twisting of the body) that may occur after long-term levodopa therapy.

Keeping the names straight

Your doctor has a growing arsenal of medications with which to treat your PD symptoms. Table 9-1 provides a handy reference for their generic and brand names.

Table 9-1: Generic and Brand Names of Common PD medications

Class of Drug	Generic Name	Brand Name
Carbidopa/Levodopa		
	Carbidopa/levodopa	Sinemet
	Carbidopa/levodopa controlled-release	Sinemet CR
	Carbidopa/levodopa/entacapone	Stalevo
	Carbidopa/levodopa orally disintegrating tablet (ODT)	Parcopa
Dopamine Agonists (DA)		
	Bromocriptine	Parlodel
	Pergolide	Permax
	Pramipexole	Mirapex
	Ropinirole	Requip
	Rotigotine (transdermal system)	Neupro

COMT Inhibitors		
	Entacapone	Comtan
	Tolcapone	Tasmar
MAO-B Inhibitors		
	Selegiline	Eldepryl
	Selegiline ODT	Zelapar
	Rasagiline	Azilect
Others	Amantadine	Symmetrel

Treating Non-Motor PD Symptoms

PWP must deal with a whole range of symptoms—only some of which involve movement. In the chapters that follow, we discuss in detail the PD symptoms of depression and anxiety and symptoms that may occur as your PD progresses. (See Chapters 13 and 19.) However, if any of the following non-motor symptoms become disruptive to your routine and life, talk to your doctor about medications that may be helpful:

• **Dizziness or changes in blood pressure when you stand after lying down or sitting:** Report this to your doctor! Treatment may include changes in habits (such as increasing fluid intake or wearing support stockings) or a change in medications.

• **Increased saliva or swallowing problems:** Again, your doctor needs to know about this because it may be a side effect of a medication or it may be the progression of your PD. Either way, don't ignore it!

• **Sleep disturbances:** The disease itself and some of your antiparkinsonian meds can cause sleep disturbance. Ask your doctor whether a sleep aid may be helpful. In some cases where sleep disturbances are especially troublesome, a more specific sleep study may be indicated.

- **Pain, cramping, or dyskinesia:** These symptoms are often worse at night or bedtime. A change in your evening dose of Sinemet (higher or lower) may solve the problem, or ask your doctor whether anti-inflammatories (such as ibuprofen), muscle relaxants, or dopamine agonists may help.
- **Nausea, stomach upset, constipation, and heartburn:** These symptoms may be part and parcel of your medication routine. Talk to your doctor about when, how often, and to what degree of discomfort these symptoms occur.
- **Urinary frequency or urgency:** Conditions other than your PD (such as prostate hypertrophy) may be at play here. Talk to your doctor if you experience any change in urinary habits, especially if you experience pain or any sort of discharge with urinating.

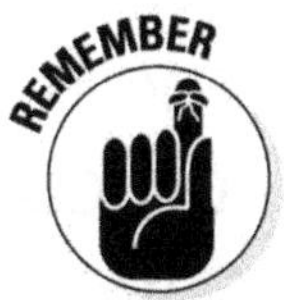

If you're seeing another doctor or taking medication for high blood pressure or another chronic condition, be sure your neurologist and all doctors consult with each other before prescribing new meds for you.

Using Your Medication Safely and Effectively

As a person with PD, you need to pay close attention to your medication timing and dosing. You also need to be aware of changes in performance and function (mental or physical), especially if such changes seem to relate to your medication routine. In short, you need to

- Take an active role in monitoring your medications and the results you get (or don't get) from them.

- Inform your doctor and pharmacist of any side effects, new symptoms, or worsening of current symptoms.

This section covers the important ways you can work with your doctors and pharmacist to maintain a healthy regimen with your meds. We also pass along some advice for keeping track of your meds and their effectiveness with your PD symptoms.

Partnering with your doctor and pharmacist

Work with your neurologist to review *all* your medications from time to time. Be sure to include any OTC products you take regularly. And remember to pay special attention to any dosing changes or new prescription meds another doctor may have ordered.

When your neurologist and other doctors write a new prescription for you, ask the following questions:

- Why are you prescribing this medication at this time?
- What results should I expect after I begin taking this medication?

- How soon should I expect positive results?
- How should I take the medication—timing, dosing, with (or without) food and so on?
- What side effects might I experience?

Keeping the costs of meds under control

If the cost of your medications is overwhelming, you may be eligible to receive some of your prescription medications for a reduced cost or even for free. The American Parkinson Disease Association (APDA) partners with a coalition of health providers, pharmaceutical companies, patient advocacy groups, and other organizations to help you get the medicine you need. Call 888-477-2669 or go online to www.pparx.org for full details on eligibility. You can also check with your state Office on Aging or go to www.benefitscheckup.org or www.needymeds.com for more information.

- What side effects should I notify my doctor about immediately?
- What side effects would require me to get to an emergency room or call 911?
- What does the medication cost?
- Can I get the same benefits a less expensive way?

For example, Stalevo is convenient but can be expensive. Taking Sinemet and Comtan separately may save money.

- Are any interactions possible between the new medication and other prescription or OTC meds that I'm already taking?

When you get the medication the first time, be sure the pharmacist prints out and reviews the prescribing information sheet with you. (If you don't have a regular pharmacist, ask your neurologist to recommend pharmacies in your area that she respects and communicates well with.)

Before you leave the pharmacy:

- **Ask questions if anything on the information sheet raises a red flag for you.** For example, if a side effect of the new med is low blood pressure and you're taking medication to manage high blood pressure, how will the new drug affect it?
- **Check the label to be sure you can read it and that you have received the right medication according to your doctor's instructions.** If a substitution has been made (a generic for the brand your doctor prescribed, for example), ask the pharmacist to call the doctor to be sure the switch is okay.
- **Open the package and look at the medicine, especially if it's a refill.** If the pill or tablet doesn't look like the med you've been taking, immediately bring that question to your pharmacist's attention.

Mixing prescription and OTC medications

Pick up any magazine these days and you'll likely find an article touting the advantages of some herbal supplement or vitamin. Or maybe a friend recommends some OTC product for your heartburn, headache, or cold symptoms. The question is: How will these commonly used products interact with your prescription meds—especially your antiparkinsonian meds?

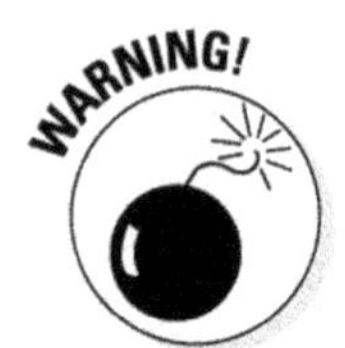

Anyone who takes a prescription medication to manage or treat a chronic illness needs to vigilantly read labels on all OTC as well as prescription products for potential interactions. Call the primary care physician or neurologist and talk to the pharmacist before taking the meds to let these professionals help you decide if this med is right for you.

Common signs of potentially dangerous drug interaction include accelerated or slower heart rate, diarrhea or constipation, heartburn, nausea or cramping, fever, skin rashes or unusual bruising, dizziness, confusion, loss of appetite, or abnormal fatigue. If you experience any such side effects, contact your doctor. If side effects are severe—or a doctor is unavailable—call 911 or get to an emergency room.

Note: Ask your doctor whether grapefruit juice can have an effect on your medications. Studies have shown that grapefruit juice can interfere with the liver's ability to break down some medicines—especially prescription drugs.

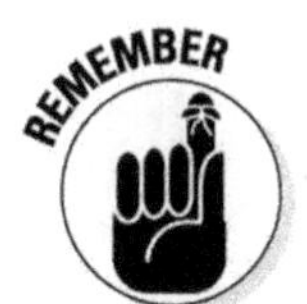

Balancing the benefits of medications against their potential side effects is delicate. In partnership with your doctor, determine what combination works best for your lifestyle and quality of life. The goal is to keep you *in* control—as opposed to *under* the control—of your meds and your PD.

Setting up a routine for managing your meds

Being human, we have a tendency to ignore or bend the rules, especially when it comes to faithfully following a medication regimen. We skip doses, miss the timing by a couple of hours, cut the dose to save money, and even share prescription meds with other people (because it did so much good for us).

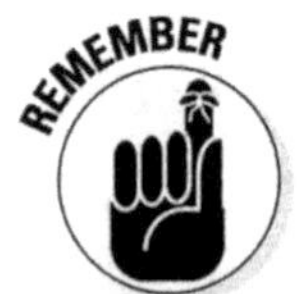

With PD, taking medicine and taking it in the prescribed and timely manner is critical. And, because you probably take more than one medication for PD (not to mention the meds you may take for other conditions such as high blood pressure), timing is indeed everything.

As your PD progresses, you may experience memory problems, so it's enormously important that you figure out now how you're going to remember to take your meds. This section offers suggestions for both organizing your medication regimen and remembering it.

Three keys to avoid problems with your medications:

- Make sure one (and only one) doctor (your neurologist is the best choice) oversees all your medications, including OTC vitamins, supplements, or herbal remedies.
- Choose one pharmacy (or one pharmacy chain that maintains your records regardless of where you are) to fill all your prescriptions.

• Take a list—if not the actual meds—to every doctor's appointment (including dentists, podiatrists, and so on) and to the hospital or emergency room if you need to go there.

Hospitals use several medications to combat nausea following anesthetic that are *contraindicated* (or *not to be used*) for PWP. These drugs not only worsen PD symptoms but can actually produce Parkinson-like symptoms in people with no diagnosis of PD. For a complete list of these drugs, see the Cheat Sheet in front of the book.

You also need to get organized at home—where you most likely take your meds. You've probably seen or even used those plastic pill-containers that organize meds by day (or even by dose throughout the day). Some of these containers come with a beeper that signals the time for a dose. Other varieties have large sections to accommodate several pills or larger pills.

Consult with your pharmacist on the best choice in medication organizers for your purposes. Think about your daily activities:

- Are you home all the time?

If you are, then one large, multi-sectioned container may be a good choice.

- Are you at work when one dose comes due?

Then a smaller pocket container or one with the reminder alarm is a good choice for that dose.

Establish a regular time (the same time and day every week) for loading the meds into the proper container. Then place the container(s) in the most obvious place to remind you. (For example, you may want your morning and bed-time meds next to your toothbrush.)

Tracking the on-off fluctuations of your meds

As if multiple motor, cognitive, and other symptoms of PD aren't enough, the common PD medications can also affect the course of the disease. Read any PD article or get into a discussion with any PD patient or care partner, and sooner or later you hear the terms *wearing off* and *on-off.*

The *wearing-off* effect may appear when the PWP has been on the same dosage for some time. Over time, the positive effect of the med simply wears off before the next dose. In that window between the end-of-dose benefit and the delivery of the next dose, the PWP may experience heightened symptoms of PD, such as tremors, difficulties with balance and coordination, and so on. Such incidents commonly occur after a relatively long *honeymoon,* when the antiparkinsonian meds effectively control the symptoms. The usual solution is to shorten the time between doses, increase the dose, and/or add other meds.

The *on-off* phenomenon (which is fairly unique to PD) refers to the PWP's ability to perform common physical activities one minute and then be totally incapable the next minute, all within the same dosing cycle. Another way of looking at this phenomenon is that the wearing off effect loses its predictability so PD symptoms emerge without warning. Some PWP actually refer to the sensation as someone flipping a switch. Usually this effect occurs when the PD is in the advanced stages.

We recommend that you track your on-off fluctuations after they begin by noting the following and reporting your findings to your doctor:

- The time the meds start wearing off in relation to your next scheduled dose of medicine.
- The exact symptoms that reappear.
- The frequency of the off-period. Is it every dose or just now and then? If it's now and then, is there a recurring pattern?

Finally, *dyskinesia* (involuntary movements) is another treatment-related symptom that may become apparent as the disease progresses. Movements may range from dance-like to irregular and jerky motions, and they usually occur when the medication dose is at its height.

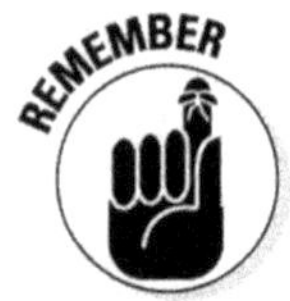

For friends and family, this seemingly random ability of the PWP to act normal one minute and need help the next minute may appear calculated, to gather sympathy or manipulate other people. But the cause is simply not known. Recent theories link the continued loss of dopamine-producing cells and years of drug therapy as a possible cause. Both the PWP as well as family and friends must understand that this on-off effect isn't within the PWP's control, isn't a deliberate attempt to gain sympathy, and may not respond to a change in the medication routine.

Chapter 10

When Surgery Is an Option

In This Chapter

- Sizing up your chances for successful surgery
- Checking out the advances in surgical options
- Stepping through the deep brain stimulation process
- R & R: Life with your DBS

As Parkinson's disease (PD) progresses, medications often lose their effectiveness; sometimes they cause, rather than alleviate, problems for the patient. In these instances, surgery may bring much-needed relief and even restore some level of normalcy to the patient's functions and life for many years. In this chapter, we explore current surgical procedures and raise the important questions for you to ask before deciding to proceed.

Deciding Whether You're a Candidate for Surgery

First things first: Of the many people with Parkinson's (PWP), which ones are more likely candidates for surgery? The following questions are a general guide to help you understand your chances for a successful outcome from surgery.

- Have you successfully used antiparkinsonian medications (primarily L-dopa therapy) for several years?
- In spite of an optimal medication regimen, are you experiencing increasing freezing episodes (sudden difficulty in moving), on-off fluctuations (shortened time between response to meds and time for next dose), and dyskinesia (twisting motion—a major side effect of taking the antiparkinsonian meds)?
- Is your tremor so severe that medication can't control it?

Of course, your age, past medical history, and general health are always considerations before deciding to undergo surgery, but you're more likely to benefit from surgery if you answered "Yes" to all of the above questions.

Note: Unfortunately, PWP whose main issues involve cognitive loss, impaired balance that doesn't respond to L-dopa, poor speech *(dysarthria),* or swallowing problems *(dysphagia)* are less likely to be helped by surgery.

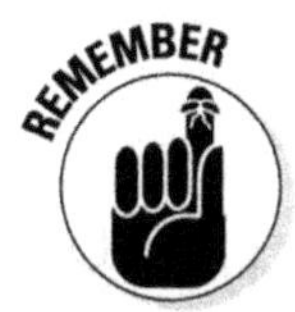

Even if you appear to be a prime candidate, you have a great deal to consider before deciding whether surgery's right for you. Most importantly, remember that you may experience relief—even significant relief—of some symptoms, but your PD will progress. In particular, symptoms that surgery can't address (such as autonomic dysfunction or cognitive decline) may still be a factor in the progression of your PD.

On the other hand, if certain symptoms (like tremor, bradykinesia, dyskinesia, rigidity, and on-off fluctuations) have begun to rule your life, surgery may buy you some much-needed relief and time to enjoy a higher quality of life. This isn't a decision you or your doctor should make lightly.

Weighing Your Surgical Options

At this writing, surgical options for treating PD are virtually limited to *deep brain stimulation* or DBS (see section below). But scientists continue to seek new procedures that may prove more effective in controlling symptoms or stopping them altogether, allowing the patient to remain symptom-free for a period of time. (See the sidebar "Stem Cell Research: The Controversy" later in this chapter.)

Deep brain stimulation (DBS)

The new standard for surgical treatment is a process called deep brain stimulation. Since the FDA approved DBS in 2002, over 25,000 PWP have had the procedure. In addition, DBS can effectively treat other neurological conditions such as essential tremor and dystonia (See Chapter 4 for more information.) Follow-up studies have shown consistent benefits for up to five years. However given the relatively recent introduction of DBS to PD therapy, the long-term safety and effectiveness of this procedure is still being studied.

According to a 2004 report from the University of Florida Movement Disorders Center, of 174 PWP referred to the center as candidates for DBS, only eight met the criteria that indicated they could benefit from the procedure. Proper screening by a medical team experienced in DBS is essential.

During the DBS procedure, a specially trained surgeon implants a *neurostimulator* (a battery-operated device similar to a pacemaker) to send electrical stimulation to those areas of the brain that control movement. The procedure follows these steps:

1. The surgeon drills a small hole in the skull and then inserts an electrode (called a lead), positioning it in a targeted area of the brain.
2. The surgeon then inserts an implantable neurostimulator (sometimes called a pulse generator or IPG), or battery pack, under the skin in the area of your collarbone.
3. In a procedure that takes place two to four weeks after the implant of the lead, a thin, insulated wire (called the

extension) connects the battery pack to the lead.

4. Your neurostimulator is then programmed to send signals appropriate to your individual condition and symptoms. (Several sessions may be necessary to get the programming right for you.)

Advantages of DBS include:

- The possibility to tune the device at any time in order to maximize benefits and minimize side effects
- A significant reduction in the amount of medication you need
- Significant relief from the troublesome side effects (such as dyskinesia) of those medicines
- The possibility of reversing the procedure in the future if a new, more promising procedure becomes available

Downsides of DBS include the following:

- This is still brain surgery with potentially severe—though rare when DBS experts perform the surgery—complications, including the potential for brain hemorrhage (bleeding).

• DBS isn't intended to stop the progression of your PD, although long-term studies are needed to clarify the long-term benefits of DBS.

• Two significant factors you must consider are cost and proximity to the center where the procedure is performed.

Find out in advance whether your insurance covers the cost of DBS. Also make plans for making the trips to and from the DBS center for follow-up visits.

Lesion procedures

Procedures such as *pallidotomy* and *thalamotomy* were the earliest surgical procedures to relieve PD symptoms.

- Pallidotomy destroys (or *lesions*) the *globus pallidus* (a part of the brain that becomes overactive in PD) in an effort to restore movement control.

- Thalamotomy is a similar surgery aimed at controlling tremor by surgically destroying a selected portion of the brain's thalamus.

Despite some encouraging results in the 1980s and 1990s, doctors recommend these lesion surgeries much less frequently today because benefits tend to regress after five years. In addition, serious side effects (such as difficulty in speaking, poor balance, and cognitive dysfunction) are possible, especially if the surgery is on both sides of the brain. Unlike DBS, these procedures are not reversible and will probably prevent the patient from taking advantage of more effective surgeries in the future.

However, for a small number of patients, this procedure may be more appropriate. Candidates include patients with poor access to programming and continued follow up after DBS, patients with higher risk of infections from a foreign body, and patients that—for one reason or another—can't have a stimulator.

Gamma knife surgery

Gamma knife surgery is an alternative technique for pallidotomies and thalamotomies in PWPs. Not a knife at all, the gamma knife is actually a machine that uses powerful, focused beams of radiation to precisely target the specific area of the brain. The procedure is usually on an outpatient basis, takes under an hour, and uses only local anesthetic. According to a study from Emory University in Atlanta, although lasting benefits in some patients have been reported, gamma knife surgery may have a higher complication rate than has previously been indicated due to delayed onset and under-reporting of changes.

Looking to the future: Surgical possibilities

Scientists are working on improvements to DBS, focusing on such details as a smaller and longer-lasting battery pack or a battery pack in the electrode so everything operates as one unit in the scalp. Another possibility is providing branch leads in the stimulator that network to various parts of the brain that control movements.

Stem cell research: The controversy

Until scientists can prevent the loss of or repair damage to dopamine-producing brain cells, PD will continue to be a chronic and progressive disease. This is where the controversial topic of stem cell research comes into play. Actor Christopher Reeve was an outspoken and tireless advocate for stem cell research, believing it was the only hope for people with brain or spinal injuries. Other spokespeople in favor of stem cell research include former first lady Nancy Reagan for Alzheimer's disease, Mary Tyler Moore for juvenile diabetes, and of course, Michael J. Fox for PD.

The debate is not only scientific but ethical. Scientists have ample evidence that cell transplantation may be the key to curing or preventively treating millions of people suffering from various conditions. In a nutshell, stem cell research focuses on transplanting renewable cells to replace lost or damaged cells due to problems such as chronic and progressive conditions, brain or spinal injuries, and the like. However, as researchers begin using human subjects to test the cell-transplant models already proven in animals, the need for a renewable supply of stem cells from human fetuses creates a heated debate.

Opponents' primary argument is that these cells are part of a viable fetus; therefore taking them is the same as aborting a human life. Further, they argue that scientists have no real evidence that cell transplants will work, especially in diseases like PD, where the root cause is unknown. People in favor of stem cell research argue that stem cell research isn't limited to finding cures; it focuses on the larger arena of understanding, preventing, and treating disease more effectively.

Scott Stern, associate professor of management and strategy at Northwestern University's Kellogg School of Management sums it up this way: "To stop stem cell research now because there are no immediate applications would be like stopping work on transistors in 1947 when their main application was considered as a potential hearing aid."

For more information on the stem cell debate, go to www.parkinsonaction.org or www.michaeljfox.org.

Beyond DBS, researchers hope to prevent, stop, or even reverse the death of dopamine-producing cells through advances in gene therapy and cell regeneration. (See the sidebar in this section, "Stem cell research: The controversy.")

Undergoing Deep Brain Stimulation

Brain surgery is pretty scary, but it certainly places a whole new light on managing PD's symptoms and living a full and functional life for as long as possible. Keep in mind that this surgery is elective—it's *your* call, not the doctor's.

Note: Because DBS has virtually replaced all previous types of surgeries to treat PD, we focus on it in the remaining pages of this chapter.

Asking the right questions before DBS

Regardless of what your doctor tells you, this decision is yours to make. So take time to educate yourself (and your family), and consider this surgery from all points of view.

Before making a decision, take advantage of the following suggestions:

- Read the literature your doctor offers, and educate yourself fully about the procedure, the benefits, and the risks. Get written information about possible complications and risks. A primary question to ask is, "Can DBS make my PD worse?"
- Meet with your neurologist and the neurosurgeon. As with any potential

surgery, ask questions and expect definitive answers about the risks and worst case scenario. (For example, less than 5 percent of patients will experience serious complications, such as stroke or bleeding, from DBS surgery, but a slightly higher percentage may develop an infection at the implantation sites.)

- Ask the neurosurgeon what percentage of his total practice are DBS procedures. Also ask whether the surgeon has ever been sued for mal-practice related to a DBS procedure and how many procedures he has performed.
- Ask the neurosurgeon who will follow up with you after the implant. Does he collaborate with an experienced programmer and movement-disorder specialist to manage the settings on your neurostimulator? Is he part of an established DBS program or does he work on his own?
- Ask your neurologist (or your support-group facilitator) to introduce you to two other patients

who have had the procedure—at least one of whom is a few years postsurgery. Talk to those patients about their experiences before, during, and after the surgery.

If you decide to go forward after weighing all the pros and cons of surgery, read on so you and your family know what to expect.

Passing the presurgical tests

Before your procedure can be scheduled, you need to pass several presurgical tests. These tests are fairly standardized and usually include a general medical examination to be sure you're healthy enough to endure the stresses of surgery; neuropsychological testing to be sure you don't have dementia and are emotionally and mentally prepared; brain imaging tests (such as an MRI or CT scan); and the usual blood tests, electrocardiogram, chest X-ray, and such.

Ironing out the details

After successful preliminary testing, the next step is scheduling the procedure. DBS is never an emergency, so the surgery date should be based on the surgeon's schedule and availability but also on your (and your family's) convenience.

Before the doctors get to work on your brain, cover the following two issues:

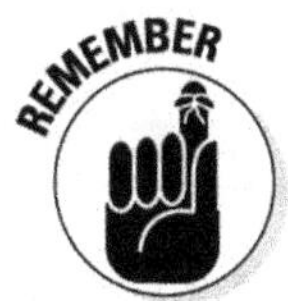

- Everyone involved in the surgery and postsurgical care needs to be aware of your medications (for PD and anything else). Be sure a clear plan is in place for managing all your medications (including those for other conditions, such as high blood pressure or diabetes) during post-surgical care and throughout your recovery.

> See the Cheat Sheet inside the front cover for a list of common post-surgery drugs that can be a real problem for PWP in the postsurgical recovery period.

- Make sure your family knows when and where they can expect to see the doctor following surgery.

Knowing what to expect during and after surgery

Okay, everyone's in place and ready to go. The day of surgery isn't too pleasant, but then surgery's rarely a walk in the park.

For three to six hours, you'll be under local (or possibly no) anesthetic, off your medication, aware of your surroundings and the doctors, and experiencing the full range of your PD symptoms. The good news is that you'll be so integrally involved in the procedure—answering questions from the surgeon and other people as they work—that you'll probably be less aware of the discomfort than you imagine.

(Prior to surgery, your doctor can provide printed information and a full description of the procedure).

Because DBS requires precise work, your head will be in a helmet-like contraption that attaches to your skull and the operating table to ensure that your head remains still throughout the procedure. (Sounds like something out of a sci-fi or horror movie, but in most cases, the only complaint is a post-surgery headache.)

The steps necessary to implant the neurostimulator are precise and demanding. Fortunately modern technology has special brain-imaging equipment that permits your surgeon to calculate the precise coordinates of the targeted area deep in the brain. In addition, most centers proceed to *map* your brain activity by recording the electrical activity of different groups of cells encountered during the journey from the surface to the depth of the brain. In fact, every area of the brain has a distinctive electrical *language,* which allows the surgeon to match the initial coordinates with the proper area activity. (Someone has compared this process to a tourist traveling blindfolded through Europe trying to identify his position based on the local language.)

After the lead is in place (see the previous section "Weighing Your Surgical Options" for more about this process), your surgeon may implant the battery and extension wire at the same time or wait up to a week before connecting the system.

Compared to implanting the electrode, connecting the system is child's play:

1. While you're under general anesthesia, your surgeon makes a small incision near your collarbone and inserts the implantable pulse generator (IPG) in a pocket formed under the skin.
2. Next, he runs a small wire from the IPG under the skin up your neck and behind your ear to connect the IPG to the DBS lead in your scalp.
3. Finally, your surgeon closes the incision with stitches or staples.

Hospitalization for DBS surgery is usually two to three days. For more complicated surgeries (when postsurgery confusion, infections, or other complications occur), the stay may be longer. In most cases, however, recovery is a matter of resting for a number of reasons: to get past the emotional and physical exhaustion that can be a part of any surgery; to rest after the possible slight headache (because of the helmet apparatus); and, in some cases, to reduce the mild confusion. Most DBS patients are able to leave the hospital the morning following the procedure.

Most routine postoperative conditions clear up after the first day. The stitches or staples in your scalp will be removed by your doctor a week or so after your discharge. The IPG (battery pack), which is usually implanted two to four weeks later, will be visible as a slight bump in your chest (especially if you're slender), but you don't feel the wires or apparatus as they work.

Programming DBS into Your Life

Surgery of any type takes a lot out of you. There's stress and anxiety from anticipating the procedure, exhaustion from the procedure itself, and suspense and concern about whether it worked, whether it was worth the trouble. This section helps you anticipate your life after your DBS surgery.

Changes you can expect

Following DBS surgery, your neurologist determines the best time to begin reducing your medication. But first, your neurostimulator must be programmed. This process may take one long session *(initial programming session)* and several outpatient visits, because just as you have unique responses to medication, you may have unique responses to the stimulator.

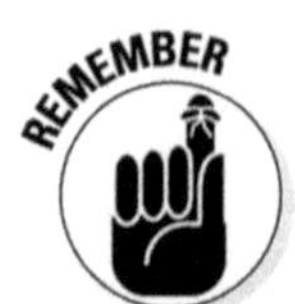

You may not realize the benefits of DBS for weeks or even months, although most people experience some effects the same day the unit is programmed. Tremors and dyskinesias are usually the first symptoms to respond. Be patient as your doctor works with you to balance the settings on your stimulator with your medication regimen.

During this sometimes-exasperating process, you may have some temporary discomfort, such as minor shocks or muscle spasms. These symptoms are related to adjusting and programming the neurostimulator and should be brief. Before you leave the office after a programming/adjustment session, your doctor may want you to wait an hour or so, just to be sure you're okay with the new settings.

Warning signs you need to heed

Although you may experience some discomfort and unusual symptoms as your neurostimulator is programmed, let your doctor know whether you experience any of the following symptoms after implantation or between programming sessions:

- Shocks or tingling sensations
- Numbness or spasms, especially in the face or hands
- Impaired balance or dizziness
- Slurred speech
- Blurred or double vision
- Depression
- Dykinesia-like movement

As you go about your normal routine, take these precautions:

- Ask for a hand-check when you go through security while traveling. If the electromagnetic field of the security equipment causes your stimulator to shut down, you can turn it back on with a handheld remote. Not to worry: Airport security personnel are accustomed to travelers who have implants such as a defibrillator or pacemaker.

- If you play sports, carefully rethink any high-level contact sports like basketball. Repeated direct blows to the implant or connections can cause harm or the need for replacement.
- At home, try to stay away from microwave ovens (while they're in use) and be aware of the magnetic strip that keeps the refrigerator door shut. Swiping it near your chest may inadvertently turn off your neurostimulator.
- Check with your neurologist before any doctor orders imaging tests such as an MRI or CT scan for you. The test may be perfectly safe for you, but it doesn't hurt to be sure.
- Other common warnings are provided in the patient-information manual you receive. Review them in detail with your treating physician or programming nurse.

Chapter 11

Considering Complementary and Alternative Medicine Therapies

In This Chapter

- Noting the distinctions: Alternative versus complementary therapies
- Grasping options for your mind and body
- Choosing the right CAM professional
- Spiriting the right approach

Medication and surgical procedures are only two of the options for treatment of your Parkinson's disease (PD) symptoms. Increasingly the healthcare profession is embracing the benefits of some complementary and alternative medical treatments.

This chapter helps you understand the differences between complementary and alternative therapies so you can sort through the various options and weigh the potential benefits of each. It also helps put you in touch with reputable practitioners if you decide to expand your treatment plan.

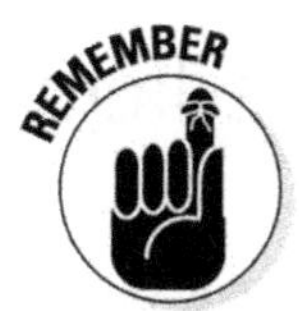

Don't underestimate the importance of diet and exercise to your success in managing your PD symptoms. These topics are so vital that they get their own discussion (see Chapter 12). In this chapter, though, we look at therapies you may have heard of but never considered as viable complements or alternatives to the conventional plan you expect your doctor to recommend.

What's in a Name? CAM Therapies Defined

Techniques, medicines, and therapies that take a holistic (mind, body, and spirit) and unconventional approach to the treatment of disease are often called *complementary* or *alternative medicine* (CAM) therapy.

Alternative medicine usually refers to approaches (yoga, T'ai Chi, acupuncture, special herbal remedies, diets, and the like) that aren't standard in Western society but are quite common in Eastern societies.

Complementary therapies, on the other hand, include techniques and approaches (physical, occupational, and speech therapy; modifications to diet; regular exercise, and such) that are more familiar to Western societies.

Alternative treatments often *replace* more conventional treatments, and complementary therapies *augment* conventional methods.

Although alternative and complementary treatments may work in tandem with more traditional medical treatment, they usually haven't passed (or even been required to pass) the rigorous, scientific, evidence-based tests that conventional medicines and treatments must navigate for the Food and Drug Administration's (FDA) approval.

However, in 1998 the National Institutes of Health (NIH) established the National Center for Complementary and Alternative Medicine (NCCAM) because of

- The growing popularity of alternative and complementary therapies.
- The need for establishing standards for practitioners.
- The need for a respected resource for validating information and conducting research on their benefits.

NCCAM focuses on four key areas:

- Research
- Training and career development for researchers working on projects related to alternative or complementary treatments
- Public outreach and education
- Integration of CAM treatments with conventional medicine

You can find information about specific therapies on the NCCAM Web site www.nccam.nih.gov or by calling (888)644-6226.

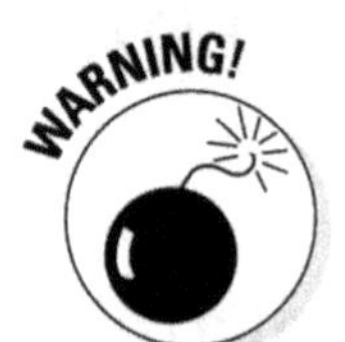

Before you consider any alternative or complementary therapy, talk with your neurologist and make sure the therapy is from a licensed, certified practitioner. (See the section "Finding the Best Practitioner" later in this chapter for tips on determining the right practitioners.)

The following section explores the major categories of CAM treatments available today.

Debunking the myths about treating PD

PD treatment has a number of urban myths that surface from time to time about what does and doesn't work. Often these falsehoods are from credible sources (such as members of your support group or even articles in respected, usually trustworthy publications). The Internet is another prime source for such rumors. For these reasons, remember to seek and confirm information by asking questions of your doctor or other trusted healthcare professionals (such as your pharmacist). And use only reliable PD information resources, such as those listed in Appendix B.

The following are some of the more prevalent myths floating around:

- Levodopa is toxic. (Actually it's been working for PWP for over 40 years.)

• Levodopa will stop working after a while. (No, but symptoms may escalate, causing you to need stronger, more frequent dosing.)

• You die from PD. (How you're going to die is as much a mystery now as it was before you were diagnosed—could be a car accident, lightening, a heart attack, and so on.)

• You're definitely going to be in a wheelchair. (Keep in mind that PD is unique to every person. Your chances of being in a wheel-chair are probably higher than some PWPs and far lower than others'.)

• You're definitely going to be demented—a vegetable. (PD has no definites. As for being a vegetable? Just focus on eating vegetables and stop predicting the future.)

• My children will have PD. (Go back and read Chapter 3—right now.)

• You can't eat proteins while taking levodopa. (Ah, the protein myth—see the section "The protein factor" later in this chapter. Meanwhile, eat your protein.)

• Surgery doesn't work for PD. (Right, it may not work for some people, but it does work in combination with prescription medications for many others, and you may be one of them.)

• You can cure PD with alternative therapies such as glutathione and nicotinamide adenine dinucleotide, NADH. (We've said it before and we'll say it again—PD doesn't have a cure yet.)

• And our personal favorite: You can cure PD with foot massage. (We're not even going to comment on that one.)

As you can see, each myth has a little bit of truth. Remember, somewhere along the way you were told: If something sounds too good to be true, it's probably not true. So when someone tries to sell you the snake-oil-of-a-cure, or a concoction that reverses symptoms, or a plan that halts PD's progression, just walk away. Your best weapons against this web of half-truths? Be informed, keep up with new research, and ask questions.

Introducing Your Options

The concept of any therapy other than traditional medical methods (medications and surgery) may be new to you. And one of the beauties of reading up on these various CAM options before you talk to your doctor about them is that you can do so in the privacy of your own home.

In this section, we introduce you to several of the more prevalent therapies. Before taking any action, though, be sure you discuss with your neurologist the potential of such therapies for helping your PD symptoms. (Then again, maybe your neurologist has suggested one or more of these techniques, and you're reading this section because you [wisely] want to get a better idea of just what you're in for.)

East treats West: Acupuncture and other traditional Chinese medicine

For centuries Western medical experts considered Eastern medical techniques to be experimental at best and quackery at worst. But much of that attitude has changed dramatically in the last decade. Traditional Chinese Medicine (TCM) is founded on the concept of *qi* (or *chi*), when the person's natural flow of energy is in balance. This system includes forms (such as exercise, herbal remedies, acupuncture, and massage) that work with identified energy points in the body.

Perhaps the most familiar TCM is acupuncture. This therapy usually requires a series of appointments by a trained and licensed therapist who inserts sterile needles (about the size of a human hair) into a part of the body believed to affect the area needing treatment. Although acupuncture has not been shown to relieve PD symptoms, it may help persons with

Parkinson's (PWP) who experience cramping, stiffness, pain, or sleep disturbances.

In 1997, the NIH noted the increased use of acupuncture by a growing number of physicians and other medical professionals in the United States for relief or prevention of pain.

Ohhh! Ahhh! Experiencing body-based CAM therapies

Treatments that manipulate or move various parts of the body (such as muscles and joints) are considered body-based CAM therapies. Major examples of this category are chiropractic and osteopathic therapy and body massages.

Chiropractic and osteopathic therapy

Chiropractors focus on the structure of the body as it relates to the function, preservation, or restoration of various parts. ***Note:*** In chiropractic literature you may find some poorly defined theories that relate PD to previous head and neck traumas, which then suggest neck manipulations to treat (and cure!)

the disease. Given that these assumptions are criticized even within the chiropractic profession, the role of chiropractic therapy in PD is unknown at this time.

Osteopathic medicine is a more-conventional medical system based on the principle that all the body's systems work together. When one system is affected, then other systems are likely to be affected as well. The hands-on techniques of some osteopaths to manipulate various body parts are considered a CAM therapy.

Massage

Many people associate massages with a ritzy spa or salon. But many medical professionals view regular massage therapy by a trained and certified therapist an important complement to conventional medical care. Massage can help relieve some of the stiffness and muscle contractions common in PD by

- Increasing blood supply to the muscles.
- Increasing range of motion.

- Stretching the muscles for greater flexibility.

The bonus to these physical benefits is the mental payoff: reduced stress and anxiety. You and your care partner may find that regular sessions with a massage therapist are a great way to relieve stress, build a sense of well being and calm, and improve circulation.

Massage is also a good form of relaxation. Under the right circumstances, it offers an environment conducive to meditation and centering. See the next section, "Exploring mind and body options to relieve tension, stress, and anxiety," for more about these benefits. You can also check out *Massage For Dummies* by Steve Capellini and Michel Van Welden (Wiley) for more info.

Therapeutic massage and other CAM therapies may be covered by your insurance if your doctor prescribes them as medically necessary.

Exploring mind and body options to relieve tension, stress, and anxiety

Mind and body therapies rely on the mind's ability to influence physical function and symptoms. They include meditation, creative outlets (as in music, art, or dance), and so on.

Employing relaxation and meditation techniques

Living with a chronic and progressive illness takes a lot out of you. Combine that reality with life's thousand other pressures (like work, relationships, financial security, crime, the weather, and such) and you have a prescription for stress. So when you have PD, finding ways to eliminate tension from your mind and body makes especially good sense.

You can have planned relaxation without going anywhere, hiring anyone, or paying any money. It's a simple matter of finding a quiet place to focus totally on you for at least 15 minutes twice a day. At the end of that time, close your eyes, hum a mantra, or sit cross-legged on a pillow—it's totally up to you.

Start by being aware of your *physical* tensions. Slowly and softly breathe in and out as you relax each muscle group one at a time: forehead, neck, shoulders, arms, hands, fingers, torso, hips, thighs, calves, ankles, feet, and finally toes. As you become more aware of your body relaxing, you have a better idea of where you tend to store that stress and tension (for example in the neck and shoulders, the fingers, or perhaps the jaw). Soon you'll be able to consciously relax those areas beyond your planned relaxation sessions.

Another tool is meditation, which you can use when your tension is not only physical but also mental and emotional. It can take many forms; consider the mantra-chanting practice of Zen meditation or the visualization techniques that follow recorded prompts to imagine (visualize) a calm, peaceful setting.

If you've never tried meditation, the Mayo Clinic recommends these tips to help you get started:

- Select a form of meditation that fits your lifestyle and daily routine and works with your fundamental beliefs.
- Set aside the time. If 15 minutes twice a day seems too much, start with 5 minutes and work your way up to longer sessions.
- Forgive your slips. If your mind wanders, recognize it. Then come

back to your focus on relaxing and calming your mind, body, and spirit.
- Experiment until you find the timing and method that works best for you.

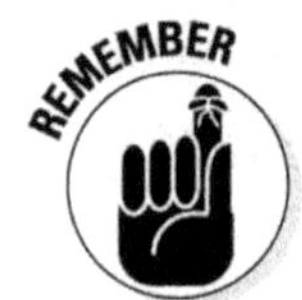

In combination with relaxation, meditation can reduce stress for mind and body. But, like all complementary and alternative practices, meditation should supplement—not replace—your doctor's traditional therapies.

Getting in touch with your creative side

Quilting. Woodworking. Gardening. Knitting. Playing an instrument. Dancing—by yourself or in a group. Writing poetry or stories. Journaling. Everyone has a creative side. And, as one sage said, "If something is worth doing, it's worth doing badly." You may not be Picasso or Mozart but you can find pleasure in creating something unique. Who knew that such pleasure could be good therapy as well?

At the 2006 World Parkinson Congress in Washington DC, one of the most popular areas was a wonderful art exhibition by dozens of PWP. To supplement the display, there were delightful performances by musicians, poets, story-tellers, and others. Some of the work was good enough to be in a fine gallery or shop, but the real beauty was in the obvious joy and delight of the artist in creating it. To see examples of the exhibit, go to www.pdcreativity.org.

Take these steps to get your creative side in gear:

- Find a new or return to a former hobby, art, or craft that appeals to you. Establish a regular time to pursue it—an hour every evening or once or twice a week if time is tight.
- Consider taking lessons at a local art center, community center, or shop. You can enjoy the dual therapy of creativity plus socialization.

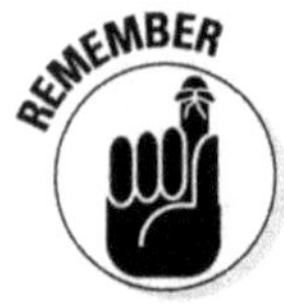

Letting those creative juices flow isn't about being good. It's about finding pleasure, escape, and relief from the daily grind of managing your PD symptoms. Just say "Ahhh!"

Staying active via alternative exercise

Postural instability (the loss or impairment of your natural ability to hold yourself upright and maintain balance) can be a major problem for PWP. The greatest danger, of course, is falling. But a close second is the fear of falling that causes you to overcompensate for these off-balance positions, further jeopardizing your stability. One of the benefits of regular physical activity is realizing that alignment, stability, and balance are vital to our overall well being and independence.

For PWP, Eastern exercise programs may be as beneficial, if not more so, than the traditional, strenuous Western types. Eastern exercise therapies tend to be performed slowly and focus on stretching motions that can enhance flexibility. These Eastern methods aren't for everyone, but if you haven't been off the couch and gotten real exercise in a while, you may want to consider this variation.

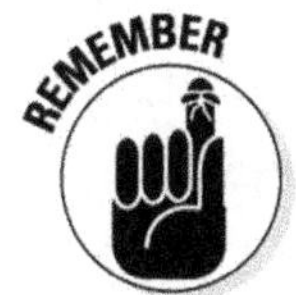

Check with your doctor before beginning any exercise program—conventional or alternative.

T'ai Chi

This ancient, low-impact Chinese exercise combines measured breathing with slow, dance-like movements that develop flexibility, enhance cardiovascular well being, and improve balance. Although books and instructional visual aids are available, the best way to get started is by working with a trained professional to understand the proper moves and breathing combinations. Check with your local community center, senior center, or health club for classes in your area. *T'ai Chi For Dummies* by Therese Iknoian (Wiley) can provide a solid introduction.

Yoga

Another exercise program that incorporates stretching and balancing exercises in a slow, rhythmic pattern of movement is yoga. Forget the painful-looking, pretzel-like positions you may have seen on television or in movies. Yoga—properly done—combines stretching with breathing and meditation to achieve a greater sense of physical, mental, and spiritual balance.

As with T'ai Chi, yoga classes have levels from beginner to advanced and different styles of teaching. For example, some instructors focus more on the physical movement; others distribute the focus between the physical, breathing, and mind exercises.

If possible, find an instructor who can and will modify the traditional yoga positions and movements to accommodate your limitations. For example, if getting up and down from a mat is difficult, perhaps you can do a modified version of the movements while sitting in a chair. *Yoga For Dummies* by Georg Feuerstein and Larry Payne (Wiley) is a great reference for beginners.

Delving into dietary, protein, enzyme, and vitamin options

Although Chapter 12 has a detailed discussion of diet and exercise, the subject of complementary therapies also involves dietary issues. Because each person plays an active, participatory role in such therapies, this section provides information about CAM diets and diet supplements.

Diet—The usual rules apply

You know the drill. With or without PD, a healthy lifestyle includes a diet rich in fruits and vegetables but low in sugar, fats, and highly processed foods (*white* foods like white bread, white flour, white rice, and such). You also want to avoid foods that have been exposed to pesticides and other toxins. (Stick with organic fruits and vegetables even though they're more expensive—you're worth it!) As we mention in Chapter 2, overexposure to pesticides and herbicides (common in nonorganic farming) may be a contributing factor in the onset of PD. For additional help, consider asking your doctor to recommend a trained nutritionist.

This professional may suggest a diet high in anti-oxidants (green leafy vegetables and the like) because ongoing studies indicate that such a diet may be beneficial for PWPs. Another diet-specific concern is whether you're getting enough calcium (osteoporosis leads to softer bones, which lead to breaks from falls). Finally, studies have shown that the intake of protein in combination with antiparkinsonian meds can be a problem for some PWP. For more on the protein factor, see the next section.

The protein factor

A common PD myth is that protein in a PWP's diet is not good. Although you certainly don't want to remove protein from your diet, your doctor or nutritionist may recommend that you limit protein intake to particular meals and take your anti-PD meds (in particular levodopa/Sinemet) on an empty stomach.

As your PD progresses, you may experience the on-off phenomenon (your meds start to wear off sooner and symptoms reappear more rapidly between doses) that's common among PWP who've taken Sinemet for several years. Some studies indicate that diets rich in protein may negatively affect the brain's ability to absorb Sinemet if meals and dosing aren't properly coordinated. In fact, levodopa is an amino acid (the building block of every protein); a high protein intake at the same time of your medication dose may compete with the absorption of your precious medications. Taking levodopa 30 to 45 minutes before meals can avoid the problem.

CoQ10 and other over-the-counter supplements

CoQ10 (coenzyme Q10) is naturally produced by the body, but it decreases with age and in people with certain chronic conditions such as PD. Available as a dietary supplement, this enzyme may slow the progression of PD for some PWP.

In 2006 the NIH announced plans to enroll recently diagnosed and early-stage PWP in a study to determine whether exceptionally high doses of this over-the-counter (OTC) enzyme may indeed affect the progression of PD. "We're looking for the aspirin of Parkinson's disease," stated Diane Murphy, head of Parkinson's research at NIH. Although some patients already take CoQ10 (with the guidance of their neurologist, we hope), the NIH dosing plan is much higher than the recommended OTC dose.

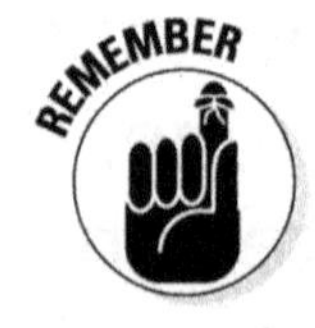

Also under study are minocycline (an anti-inflammation antibiotic available only by prescription), and creatine, an energy-boosting dietary supplement. The fact that the federal government and medical community continue to sponsor such studies is a clear indication of their willingness to consider the possibility that PD may be better managed with the use of a combination of therapies rather than a single magic bullet.

Vitamin supplements

Taking vitamins that maintain your recommended daily levels is important for PWP. For example, a good multivitamin—one that includes the key B vitamins that are so important for brain and nerve health—is a good choice. Calcium with vitamin D helps prevent osteoporosis, which is a common concern for PWP, and calcium with magnesium can play a role in relieving muscle cramps. After running some standard blood tests, your doctor may make specific recommendations. Be sure to ask your doctor about continuing the vitamins and supplements you used before your diagnosis and about adding new ones.

Several studies have looked at vitamin E as a way to prevent the onset of PD or slow its progression. The most important was the DATATOP study, a ten-year controlled trial that found no benefit in slowing or improving the disease with the use of very high doses of vitamin E. Indeed, a recent report in the American Academy of Neurology's journal stated: "Vitamin E is probably ineffective in the treatment of PD." Moreover a recent analysis of medical literature warned that high-dosage vitamin E supplementation may actually increase mortality. In other words, too much of a good thing may not be a good thing.

On the other hand, scientists have found some protective qualities in the vitamin E in foods such as green leafy veggies, whole grains, and nuts. Mahyar Etminan, a lead researcher for the Centre for Clinical Epidemiology and Evaluation at Vancouver Hospital in Canada cautions that "this is an interesting hypothesis, but it needs to be validated." Of course, eating a diet rich in natural sources of vitamin E is always a good idea for your overall health.

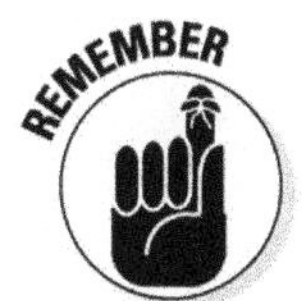

In general, no regimen of vitamins has shown the ability to reduce or control PD symptoms. However, because one theory about the cause of PD (see Chapter 2) involves the oxidation of free radicals, it is possible that anti-oxidants (like vitamins C and E) may reduce the levels of these free radicals and, therefore, provide some benefit.

Interestingly, a trial that combined vitamin C and E supplements in people with early PD showed a delayed need for drug therapy (L-dopa) by an average of two and a half years. However, more studies are needed to confirm these findings. Similarly, because PWP can be prone to bone loss, your doctor may prescribe (especially for women patients) a calcium supplement or a prescription medication for preserving bone mass. See *Osteoporosis For Dummies* by Carolyn Riester O'Connor and Sharon Perkins (Wiley) for more about this connection.

Finding the Best Practitioner

Keeping in mind that managing PD over the long haul is a team effort, be sure you talk to your neurologist about the potential benefits and pitfalls of alternative or complementary therapies you're considering. Your doctor may take a "no harm, no foul" attitude and not actually support the idea. Or she may suggest specific therapies for you to try or avoid.

Adding CAM therapy to your PD management plan requires you to carefully choose the person who'll administer that therapy. The following tips can help you in that search:

• If your neurologist endorses the idea, ask for recommendations.

• Be sure this person has received training from a respected source and passed the exams necessary to earn the appropriate degree or license.

• Acupuncturists and herbalists specializing in the use of herbs as medicine should be licensed.

Consider adapting the checklist for finding a neurologist (we provide this in Chapter 4) to guide your choice of alternative medicine practitioners.

After you've selected a practitioner, you still have a number of questions. On your first visit, ask:

- What benefits can I expect from this therapy?
- What are the risks associated with the treatment?
- Does it have any special benefits or risks related to my PD?
- What are the side effects?
- How many sessions or how long will I need to have the treatment to achieve the expected results?
- Does this treatment have any conditions that are contraindicated (to be avoided)?
- What is the cost per session?
- Will insurance pay?

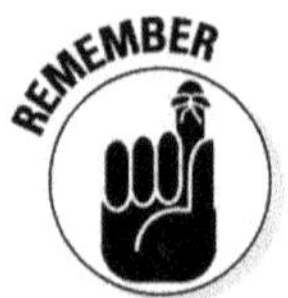

You're not married to a specific practitioner. If you're uncomfortable with the treatment or the practitioner as the sessions proceed, then stop and talk the problem out. If you aren't satisfied with the response, move on.

Considering Your Approach to Life: It Too Can Help ... or Hinder

You know the difference between the eternal pessimist (who always expects the worst) and the forever optimist (who's over the top, always anticipating the best). Somewhere in the middle is the realist (as well as a bit of an idealist, philosopher, and activist) who accepts that bad things do indeed happen to good people. This person faces adversity and then looks for ways to get life back on track.

Celebrities like Lance Armstrong, Christopher and Dana Reeve, Michael J. Fox, Muhammad Ali, and others come to mind. But chances are good that you know people within your circle of family, friends, and co-workers who also fit this positive profile. As a PWP, you're going to benefit most from this glass-half-full-and-things-could-be- a-lot-worse philosophy.

Three characteristics that most survivor-types have in common are

- A *positive* attitude.

- The ability to laugh even at the unfairness of life.
- A spiritual core that's as well-tended as their physical or mental health.

The way you approach life—and all its joys and adversities—can play an enormous role in how successfully you live that life. The very fact that you bought this book and are reading it tells us that you're a survivor and a fighter. Our message to you is that we're right here with information and ideas that can help you successfully find ways to live a full and fulfilling life in spite of having PD.

The therapeutic power of positive thinking

Life has no guarantees. But a lot of people live life more fully by rolling with the punches and taking a positive, can-do approach.

So, how do you deal with a diagnosis like PD? How do you face the progressive symptoms and side effects of the medicines? Believe it or not, the one factor that remains in your control throughout this journey is your attitude. You can expect the worst or you can fight back by choosing to live life fully and positively—as if you had never heard that diagnosis.

As a matter of fact, for some people the diagnosis creates this shift in attitude. Discovering that they have PD turns their world upside down, so now they focus more intently on the positives. The realization that life is finite after all can be a real turning point for you—if it comes with the determination to live every day to the fullest. (And if your faith tells you that God doesn't test you more than you can endure, then you can start believing that higher opinion *and* start honing those survival capabilities!)

Laughter—Still the best medicine

Face it: When you laugh, you feel better. Your outlook improves—if only momentarily. You may even feel better physically. Consider the angry, depressed man who had just gone through brain surgery. He told his wife he didn't want any visitors. But when she ran into several close friends at the elevator and told them, "Not today," the friends still insisted. "We'll only stay a moment," they promised. Within moments the woman heard the welcome sound of laughter—her husband's. As the visit went on and the friends worked their magic, that laughter couldn't be repressed.

Open up to life—Physically, mentally, and spiritually

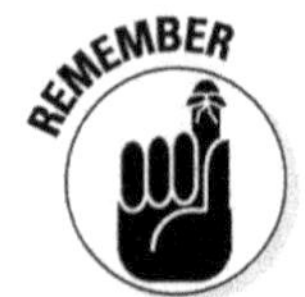

When you face a chronic and progressive illness day after day, you understandably have times when you just want to burrow under the covers and hope it all goes away. Resist that temptation!

Because we address your physical and mental well being throughout this book, this section looks at one other dimension, your spiritual needs, and how meeting those needs can enhance your life.

Spirituality is that core inside you where your sense of well being and survival reside. For some people, organized rituals of religion can be a part of this core, but rituals can't be all of it; for other people, rituals and religion play no part at all.

Your spiritual core is also where you store your self-identity. Your body may shake and twist and your mind may play tricks with your memory and concentration, but your spirit is still there. A relative of a PWP who was in the later stages said it well: "I just believe that he's still in there somewhere, that his spirit is still aware and fighting to let us know."

Like your PD, spirituality is different for every individual. But one way to begin focusing on your spiritual well-being is by using your senses to their full effect. Consider the following suggestions:

- Listen—to a sermon, an inspirational reading, a concert, water flowing, wind in the trees, rain on the roof, your innermost hopes and dreams
- Look—at the people who surround you, love you, and care for you
- Touch—by taking a friend's hand; petting a dog or cat; hugging a loved one; stroking a leaf, a rock, a child's hair
- Smell—freshly cut grass, an autumn fire, cookies straight from the oven
- Taste—the bitter as well as the sweet

- Savor—the unique tastes, sounds, sights, scents, and feelings that form the wonders of your life

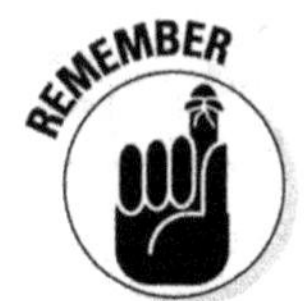

Tapping into your spiritual side takes the same focused effort as your physical and mental needs. And your willingness to push yourself on all three levels can pay off in ways you never thought possible.

Chapter 12

The Key Roles of Diet and Exercise

In This Chapter

- Eating to live versus living to eat
- Improving mobility through exercise and activity
- Getting (and staying) physical
- Empowering the mind and spirit

You've heard it since you were a child—eat right and exercise! But, for people with Parkinson's (PWP) and their care partners, the importance of proper diet and a regular program of exercise can't be overemphasized. The benefits go well beyond physical fitness to bring relief from the general stresses of living with a chronic, progressive disease. In addition, a good diet and regular exercise help fight off the anxiety and depression that can accompany Parkinson's disease (PD). With or without PD, you owe it to yourself to be as fit—physically, mentally and spiritually—as possible. How else are you going to participate fully in life?

In this chapter we show you that good health isn't about training for a marathon or depriving yourself of foods you love. It's about making the choices that give you the best chance of living well and pursuing the pleasures of your life for many years—in spite of PD.

The Joy of Good Food—Diet and Nutrition

According to the National Institute of Aging, the combined effects of not making the right food choices and not being physically active make up the second largest underlying cause of death (behind smoking) in the United States. Often the element most absent from the diets of Americans is *nutrition,* foods that provide the proteins, carbohydrates, vitamins, minerals, hydration, fiber, and—yes—fats that the body needs to operate at its best. Add to that fact that PD medications and symptoms can significantly reduce the pleasures of eating, and you have a situation ripe for disaster.

This section isn't about losing that extra twenty pounds; it's about making the best food and nutrition choices to maintain optimal health as you fight the progression of PD.

Balance is the key

As a PWP, you have to perform a real balancing act when it comes to your diet. Along with the ready-made factors that impact nutrition and diet (like age, gender, and physical fitness), you have to deal with the nutritional sideshows of PD. For example, side effects of medications may include loss of appetite or even nausea. As your PD progresses, swallowing and constipation can become issues. And you may have side effects from medications for other chronic conditions, such as high blood pressure, diabetes, or arthritis.

Finding the proper balance between a healthy diet and these PD issues may require the help of a professional, so your neurologist may prescribe a consultation with a nutritionist or dietician as part of your treatment plan.

If not, go ahead and ask him for a referral.

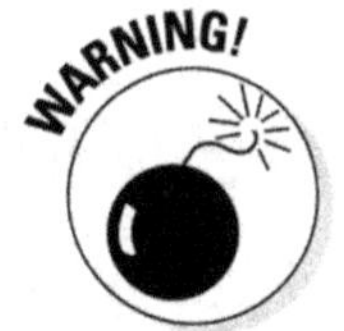

Keep in mind that timing the dosing of your medication (see Chapter 9) with meals is very important, especially for meals that include significant servings of protein. Protein—although essential for a balanced diet—can compete with the absorption of your antiparkinsonian meds. The usual recommendation is to take medication at least 30 minutes before meals unless you experience nausea or *dyskinesia* (uncontrolled twisting writhing motions) after taking your medications. If nausea is the problem, your doctor may recommend you take a low-protein snack, such as juice or saltines, with your meds. If dykinesia occurs, slowing the absorption by taking your anti-PD meds at mealtime may be exactly what you need. Be sure you and your doctor discuss the timing of meals and medications to offset this problem.

Banishing the bad and embracing the good-for-you foods

No doubt you've seen the food pyramid—which is now a bar grid—recommended by the U.S. Department of Agriculture. (See www.mypyramid.gov.) And you probably know you should hold your intake of fats and oils (not to mention desserts) to a minimum and spend most of your calories on fruits, veggies, whole grains, and dairy. (By the way, a banana split does not count in your fruit and dairy allowance!)

But this is your life, and presumably you're prepared to fight this PD that's parked like a tank in your designated space. A nutritionist or dietician can be a real help, showing you how to adapt your needs to your lifestyle. You tell her how you normally eat—on the run, in your car, at home standing at the kitchen counter, or seated with the family at the table, in fine restaurants, or fast-food joints. You reveal your food weaknesses—hate veggies, love bread, and such. Then the professional works with you to build a food plan that fits your lifestyle and your likes and dislikes.

Focus on these key issues when you start rearranging your pyramid:

- **Water, water, water!** Flavor it with a slice of lemon or a little fruit juice if you can't take it straight, but six to eight big glasses every day. (And, no, soda, coffee, and tea don't count.) Caffeine beverages may increase *diuresis* (your amount of urine output) and, as a result, cancel your efforts to hydrate your body. ***Note:*** Some studies have shown that caffeine may reduce the risk of PD for some people, so caffeine in moderation probably won't hurt—and may help.
- **Fiber** (whole-grain breads—not the mushy white stuff—brown rice, and whole-wheat pasta). In fact, stay away from white foods in general. Green leafy vegetables, whole grains, and nuts are rich natural sources of vitamin E that

may have a protective effect against PD (see Chapter 11).

Whole grain breads must be refrigerated, but white bread isn't. (White bread is so devoid of actual nutrients that even bacteria won't eat it. That's a pretty good clue.)

- **Bone-strengthening nutrients (calcium, magnesium, and vitamins D and K).** Think dairy products and, believe it or not, exposure to sunlight (a vitamin D source). Also, regular exercise (we discuss this later) can help you keep bones strong, maintain balance, and prevent the falls so devastating for PWP.

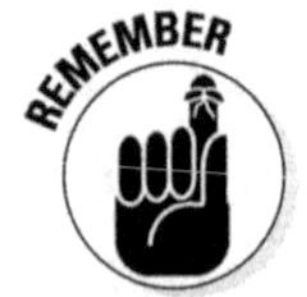

Although your doctor may recommend adding supplements (such as a daily multivitamin, iron, or calcium pill) to your regular diet, the key word here is *supplement.* Such products are no substitute for a nutritionally balanced diet.

But good-for-you foods can actually be more delicious and easy to prepare than you imagined. One example is the fabulous fruit smoothie: Throw berries, half a banana, a cup of fat-free yogurt, and some ice cubes in a blender. Add a teaspoon of ground flax seed for fiber, turn the blender on high, pour the milkshake-like concoction into your car mug, and you're good to go (Smoothies are also great for preventing the constipation associated with PD medications.)

Food as celebration

If, like millions of Americans, you've fallen into a rut with the when, what, and where you eat, think about spicing those meals up. The following is our list of ideas for making meals more of a celebration than an afterthought:

- Choose your setting to match the menu, the mood, and the season—dining room, kitchen table, inside, outside; at home or at a sidewalk café.
- Set the table, even if it's just for one.
- Think *S.H.E.* when cooking at home—simple, healthy, and engaging.
- Try adding special (non-salt) seasonings and flavorings to spice up your food and make it more enjoyable.
- Be adventurous and try new dishes you've never tasted when eating out.

Request a soup spoon when ordering items like rice or small veggies (peas, corn, and such). A large spoon makes these foods easier to manage if you have a tremor.

- Savor food with all your senses—the vision of healthy food presented well; the smells, tastes, and textures; even the sounds of laughter and conversation interspersed with clinking dishes and glasses.

Food is life—and as a PWP, you understand the importance of celebrating every moment.

Use It or Lose It—The Healing Power of Exercise and Activity

Plenty of research backs up the fact that regular exercise can do wonders for your health. Consider that

- Exercising regularly boosts the power of neurotransmittors in your brain to enhance your mood and your ability to see life in a more positive light.
- Exercise can relieve the muscle tension from your body's natural instinct to lock up in the face of challenges or battles.
- Exercise can enhance your self-image, which can lead to

greater self-assurance and confidence, which can lead to a greater ability to deal with life's stresses.

Talk about a win-win!

In addition, PWP who exercise regularly seem to experience a milder and less-progressive disease process. In fact, exercise may be as good for brain function as it is for heart and weight factors. Recent laboratory experiments on animals have shown that physical exercise can potentially reduce the rate at which brain cells die. Further studies are under way to see whether regular exercise can actually slow the progression of PD.

Many exercise programs can benefit PWP. The Performance Centers of Wheaton Franciscan Healthcare in Milwaukee, Wisconsin designed the following exercises specifically to stretch and strengthen the key muscle groups for optimal flexibility and balance. Your doctor and physical therapist may fine-tune these exercises to match your specific needs, but this chapter gives you a good starting point. Begin the routine with the stretching exercises and repeat them during the cool-down period after the strengthening exercises.

The principles of a stretching/flexibility exercise program for PD are the same as those for sports-medicine rehabilitation:

- Listen to your body.
- Avoid joint pain during exercise.
- Forget the Vince Lombardi adage: No pain, no gain.
- Remember, for joint or other pain after exercise, "Ice is nice; hot is not."

Because PD frequently develops in a person's later years, other bone and joint conditions may already be present such as *osteoarthritis* (wearing of joints) and *osteoporsis* (thinning of the bones). So before you begin any exercise therapy, get the approval of your doctor and a prescription to work with a trained, experienced physical therapist.

A stretching program to enhance flexibility

The following exercises are designed to enhance your flexibility. With your doctor or physical therapist's initial guidance and ongoing monitoring, do the exercises every day, even twice a day.

If you also do strengthening exercises (such as the ones in the "A strengthening program to build muscle and stabilize joints" section later) or an aerobic activity, such as walking, bicycling, swimming, or working out on a treadmill, use these stretching exercises to warm up and cool down.

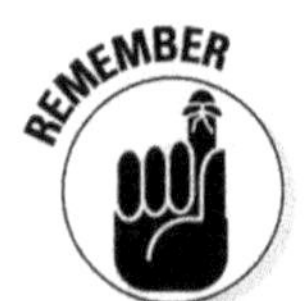

Stretching should be slow, smooth, and gentle. No bouncing allowed! And if it starts to hurt, listen to your body and ease up.

Neck stretches

Begin your routine by gently stretching the muscles in your neck, head, and shoulders.

The Chin Tuck

To perform the Chin Tuck:

1 **Looking forward, tuck your chin by pulling it in—a little like a turtle (see Figure 12-1).**

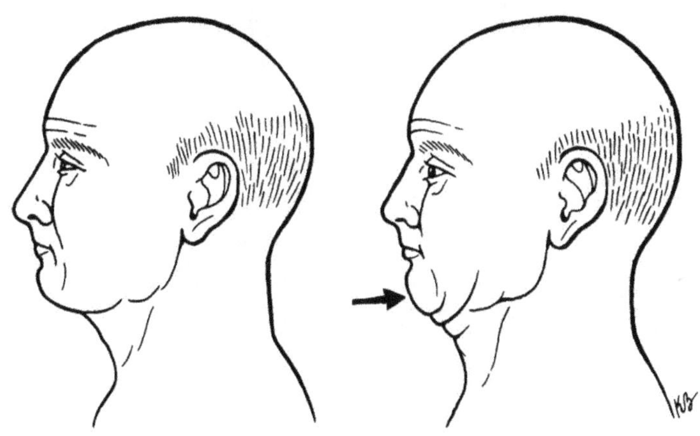

Figure 12-1: Chin Tuck

2 **Hold your chin in the tucked position for five seconds.**

3 **Untuck your chin and relax.**

Repeat this exercise five to ten times.

The Head Turn

To perform the Head Turn:

1. Looking straight ahead, slowly turn your head to the right until you're looking at the wall or view to your right (see Figure 12-2).

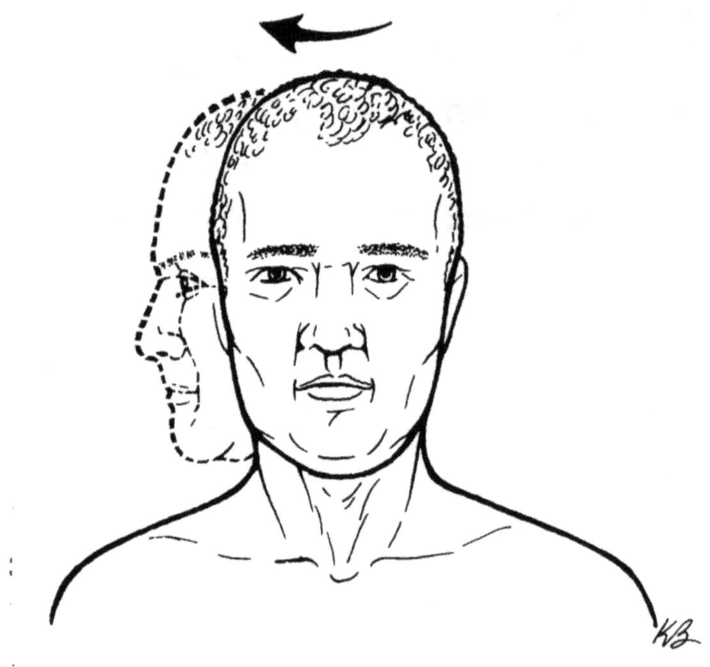

Figure 12-2: Head Turn

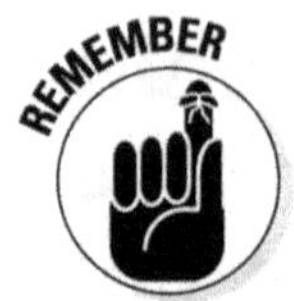

Don't force the movement; at first you may only be able to turn your head slightly to the right or left; with practice you'll become more flexible.

2. Hold the position for five seconds and return to center.

3. Repeat Steps 1 and 2, this time turning to your left.

Repeat this exercise five to ten times on each side.

The Head Tilt

To perform the Head Tilt:

1. Looking straight ahead, bend your head to the right as if to rest your head on your right shoulder (see Figure 12-3).

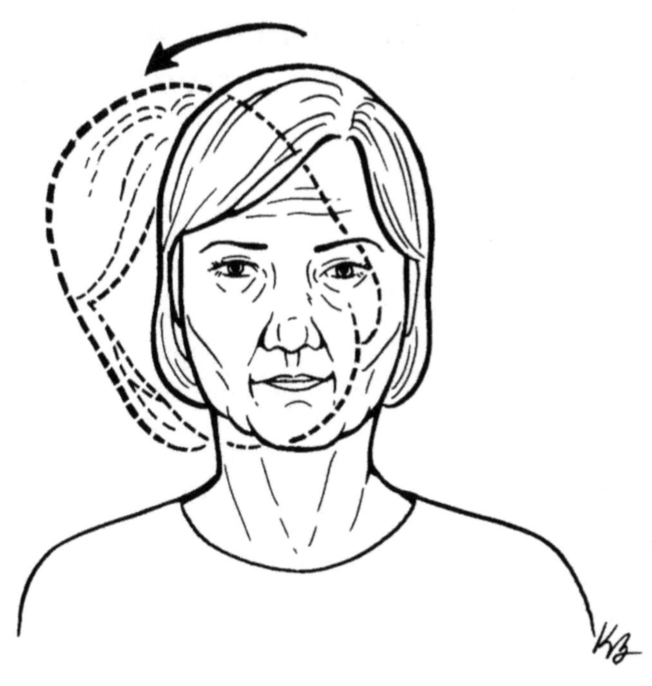

Figure 12-3: Head Tilt

Don't raise your shoulder—let the stretch of your neck do the work.

2. Hold the position for five seconds, and raise your head back to straight ahead position.

3. Repeat Steps 1 and 2, this time bending to your left side.

Repeat this exercise five to ten times on each side.

The Shoulder Roll

To perform the Shoulder Roll:

1. **Standing tall and looking straight ahead, lift and roll both shoulders back in a circular motion five times (see Figure 12-4).**

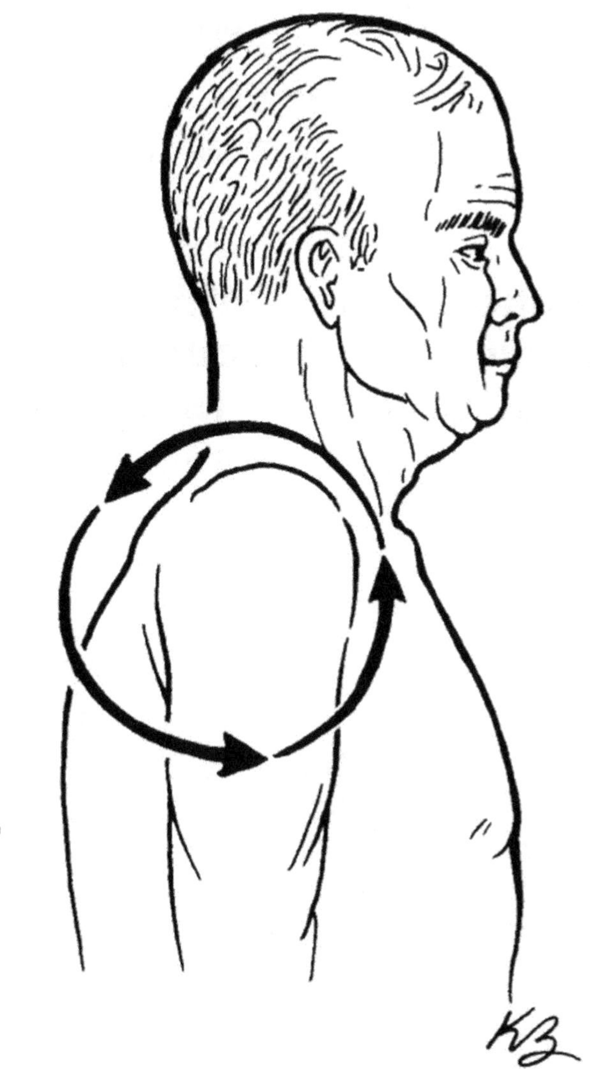

Figure 12-4: Shoulder Roll

2. **Relax.**
3. **Lift and roll shoulders forward in a circular motion five times.**
4. **Relax.**

Repeat the backward and forward rolls five to ten times each.

The Chest and Shoulder Stretch

To perform the Chest and Shoulder Stretch:

1. **Standing tall and looking straight ahead with arms at your sides, pull your shoulder blades together (see Figure 12-5).**

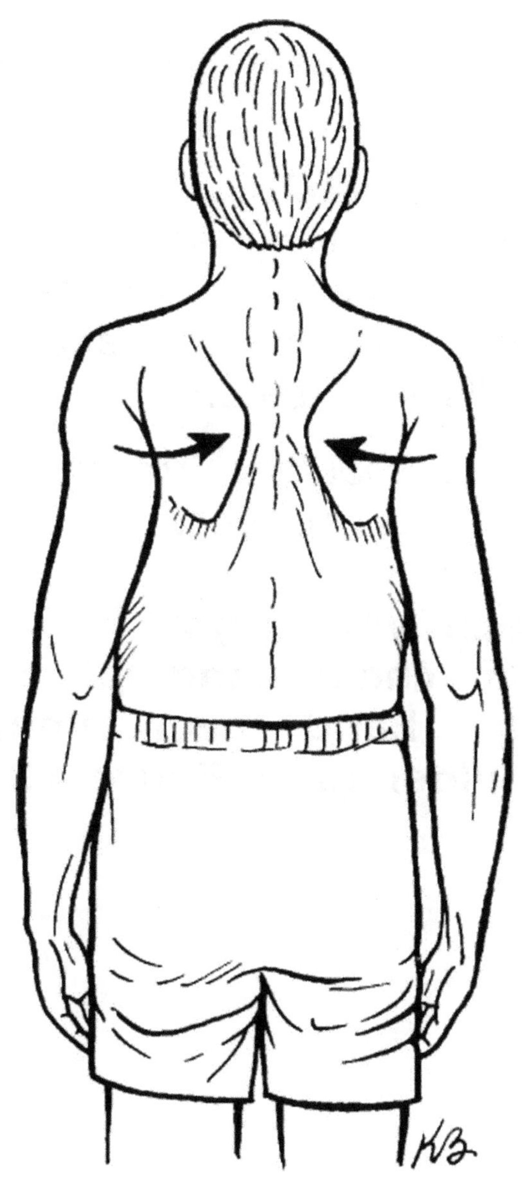

Figure 12-5: Chest and Shoulder Stretch

2. **Hold for five seconds, and then relax.**

Repeat this exercise five to ten times.

Upper body stretches

Use the following stretches before and after your regular exercise routine to lengthen your muscles and prevent muscle pulls and tears.

The Posterior Shoulder Stretch

To perform the Posterior Shoulder Stretch:

1. **Reach your right arm across your chest, and place your right hand over your left shoulder (see Figure 12-6).**

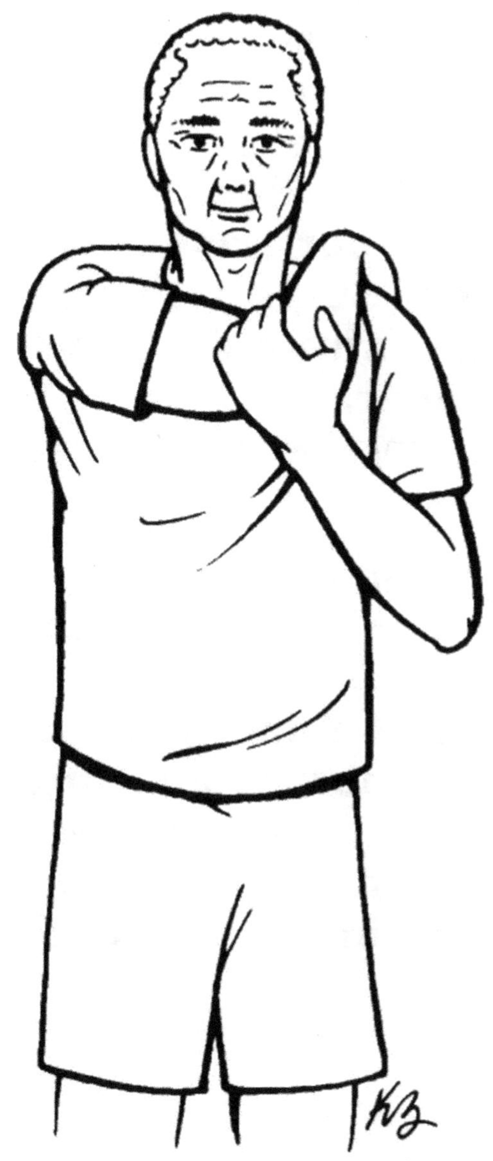

Figure 12-6: Posterior Shoulder Stretch

2. **With your left hand, grasp your right elbow and apply light pressure to the elbow, moving your right arm closer to your chest.**
3. **Hold for five seconds, and return your arms to your sides.**
4. **Repeat Steps 1 through 3, this time stretching your left shoulder.**

Repeat this exercise five to ten times on each side.

The Anterior Shoulder Stretch

To perform the Anterior Shoulder Stretch:

1. **Reach behind your back and clasp your hands, interlocking your fingers and keeping your arms straight, with elbows turned in (see Figure 12-7).**

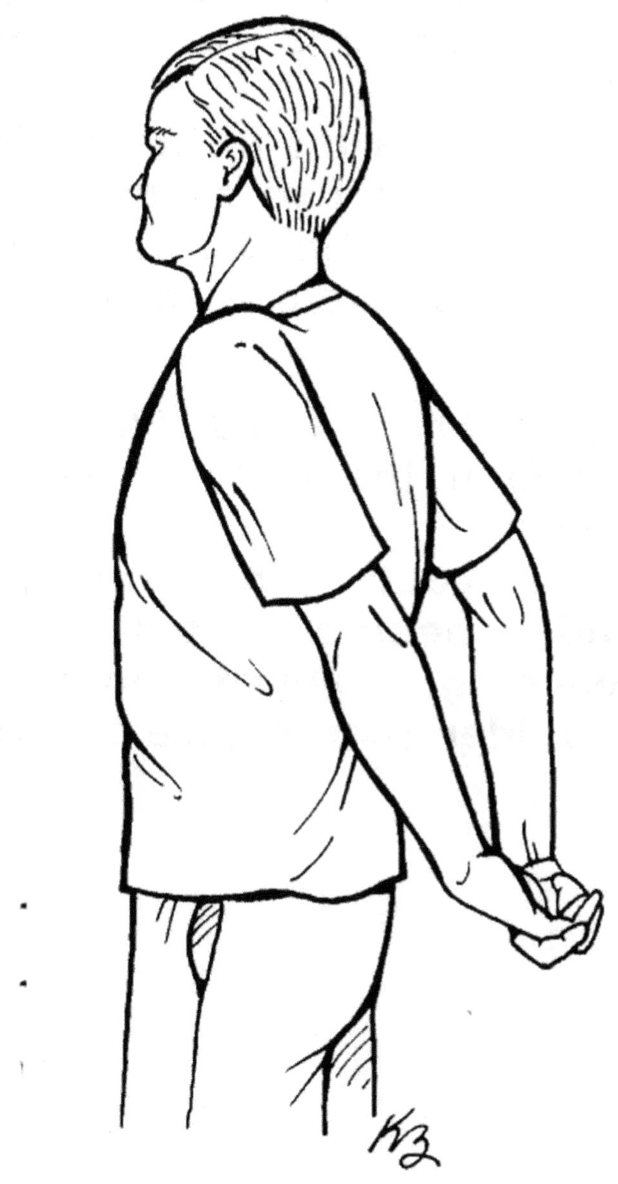

Figure 12-7: Anterior Shoulder Stretch

2. **Lift up your arms until you feel a stretch (not pain) in your shoulders and across your chest.**
3. **Hold your arms in the elevated position for five seconds.**
4. **Lower your hands, and relax.**

Repeat this exercise five to ten times.

The Posterior Shoulder Side Stretch

To perform the Posterior Shoulder Side Stretch:

1. **Raise your right arm above and behind your head, reaching toward your left shoulder (see Figure 12-8).**

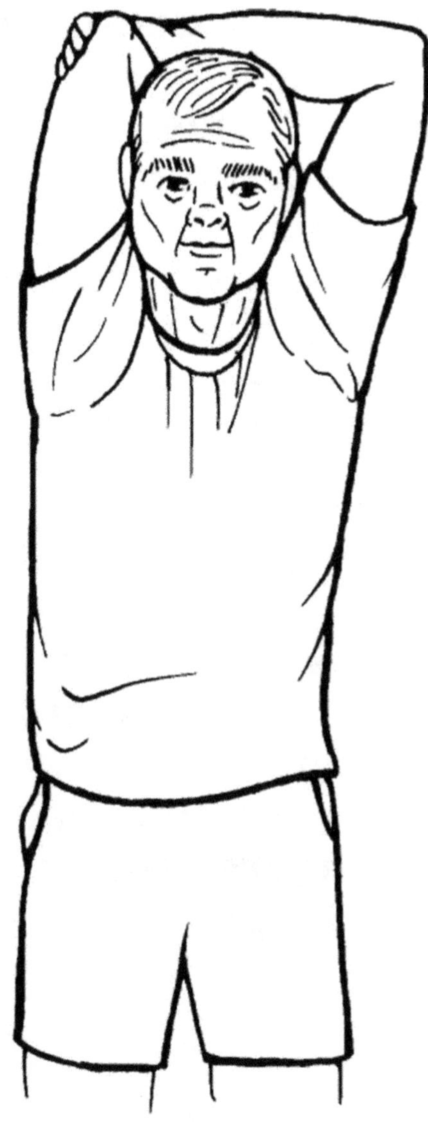

Figure 12-8: Posterior Shoulder Side Stretch

2. **With your left hand, reach behind your head and pull your right elbow gently in toward your head.**
3. **Hold for five seconds and relax, returning your arms to your sides.**
4. **Repeat Steps 1 through 3, this time stretching your left side.**

Repeat this exercise five to ten times on each side.

The Wrist/Forearm Stretch

To perform the Wrist/Forearm Stretch:

1. Extend your right arm straight in front of you, fingers pointing toward the floor.

2. With your left hand, gently pull your fingers and hand down (see Figure 12-9a).

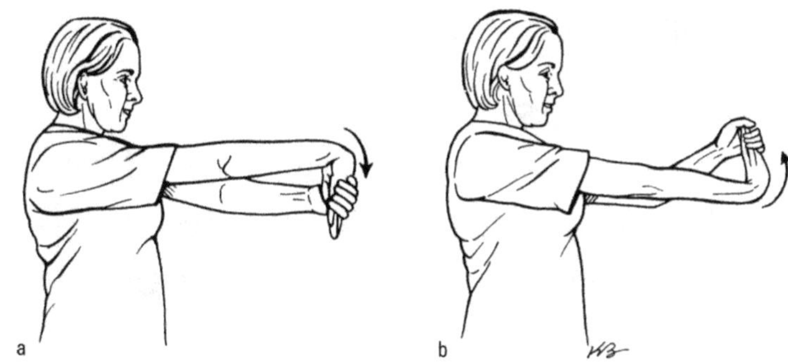

Figure 12-9: Wrist/Forearm Stretch

Your arm should remain extended.

3. Hold for five seconds, and then release your fingers.

4. Repeat Steps 2 and 3 five to ten times.

5. Flex your right wrist back so your fingers point to the ceiling.

6. With your left hand, gently press your fingers and palm back toward your forearm (see Figure 12-9b).

7. Hold for five seconds, and then release your fingers.

8. Repeat Steps 1 through 7, this time extending your left arm and stretching your left wrist and forearm.

Repeat this exercise five to ten times on each side.

Leg stretches

These stretches work on the hips, legs, knees, and ankles. As with any stretch exercise, they're good before and after your strengthening or aerobic routine to prevent muscle-strain tears and pulls.

The Hamstring Stretch

To perform the Hamstring Stretch:

1. Sitting on the floor with your right leg straight out in front of you, bend your left leg so the bottom of your left foot rests on the inner thigh of your extended right leg (see Figure 12-10).

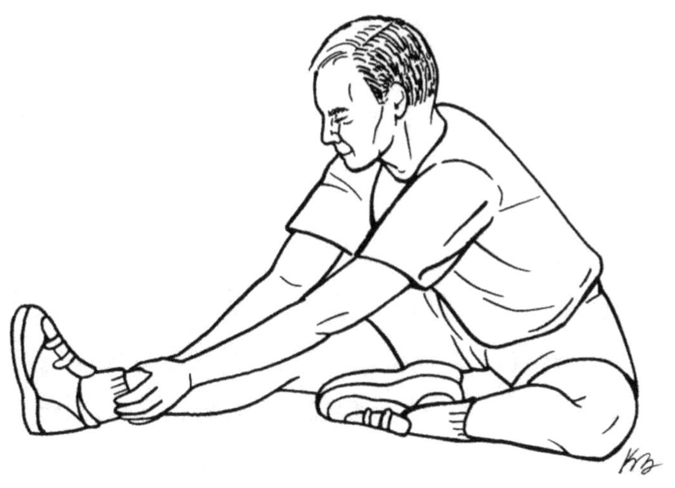

Figure 12-10: Hamstring Stretch

2. With your hands on your outstretched calf or ankle, slowly bend forward from the waist, keeping your back straight.

Don't bounce. Stretch only until you feel a mild (non-painful) stretching sensation in the back of your thigh.

3. Hold the stretch for five seconds, and then relax, releasing your calf or ankle and returning to the upright position.

4. Repeat Steps 1 through 3 five to ten times with your right leg.

5. Repeat Steps 1 through 4, this time extending your left leg and tucking your right leg.

Do five sets of five to ten repetitions each per side.

The Quadriceps Stretch

To perform the Quadriceps Stretch:

1 Standing beside a table, place your left hand on the table for balance.

2 Bending your right knee, grasp your ankle with your right hand and pull your foot backward toward your buttocks (see Figure 12-11).

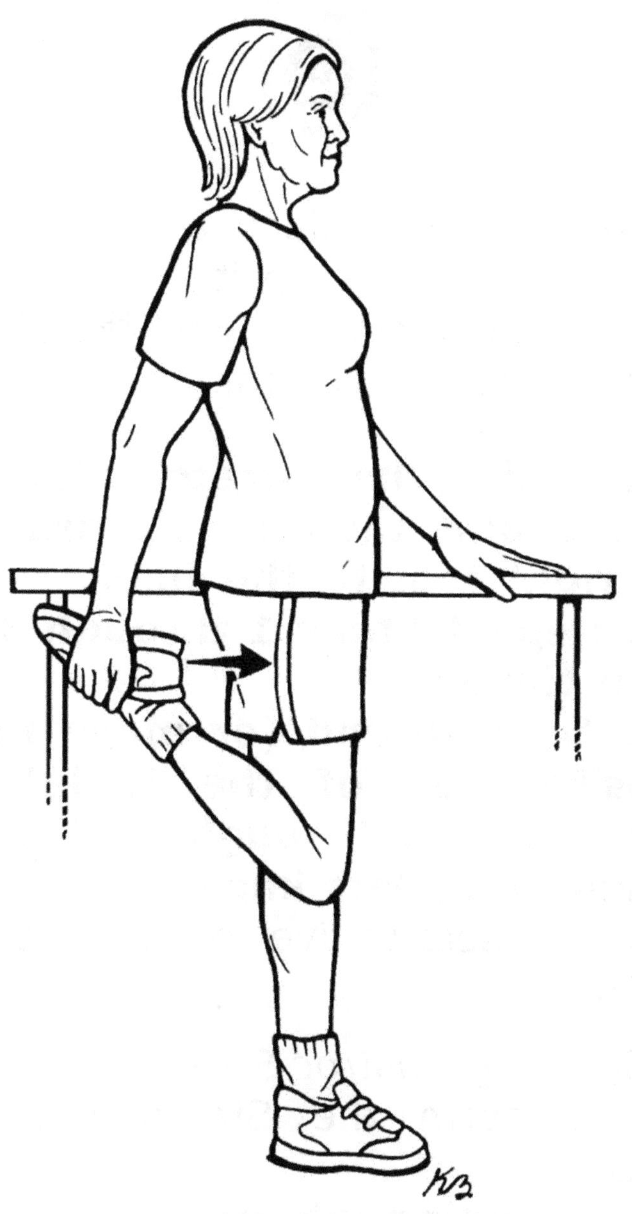

Figure 12-11: Quadriceps Stretch

You can also place a belt around your ankle and grasp it.

Don't lean forward. Feel the stretch in the front of your thigh.

3. Hold the stretch for five seconds and then relax, returning your right foot to the floor.

4. Repeat Steps 1 through 3 five to ten times.

5. Turn around (or move to the opposite side of the table) and repeat Steps 1 through 3, this time bending your left knee.

Do five sets of five to ten repetitions per side.

The Standing Gastroc Stretch

To perform the Standing Gastroc Stretch:

1. Standing about 2 feet from the wall, lean forward so flattened palms are against the wall.

2. Keeping your left foot planted, bend your left knee as you step backward with your right leg; lean forward into the wall until you feel a stretch in your right calf (see Figure 12-12).

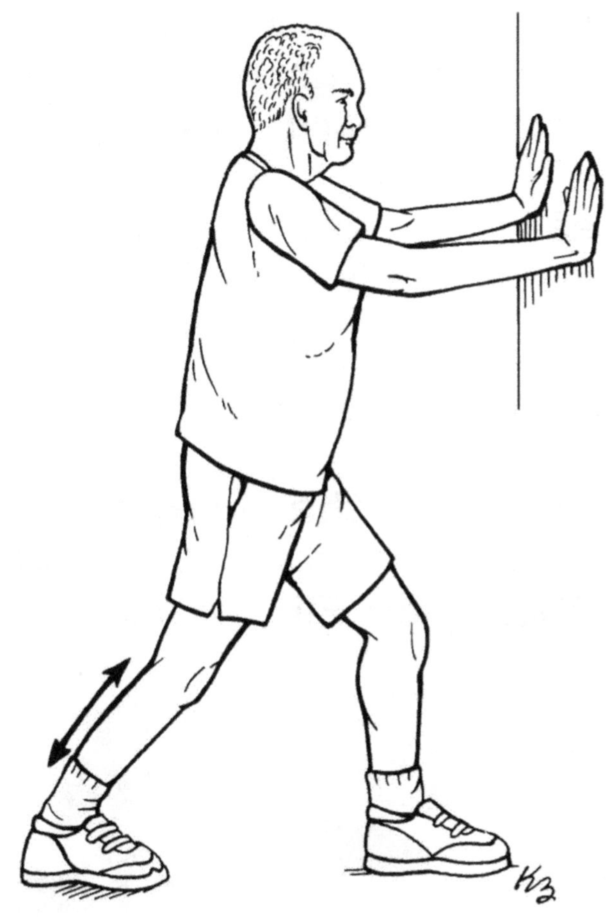

Figure 12-12: Standing Gastroc Stretch

Your right leg should remain straight, with your heel on the floor and your toes turned slightly outward.

3. Hold for five seconds and then relax, bringing your feet together.

4. Repeat Steps 1 through 3 five to ten times.

5. Repeat Steps 1 through 4, this time bending your right knee and stepping backward with your left leg.

Repeat this exercise five to ten times on each side.

The Inner Thigh (Groin) Stretch

To perform the Inner Thigh (Groin) Stretch:

1. Sitting on the floor, bend your knees so the soles of your feet face each other (see Figure 12-13).

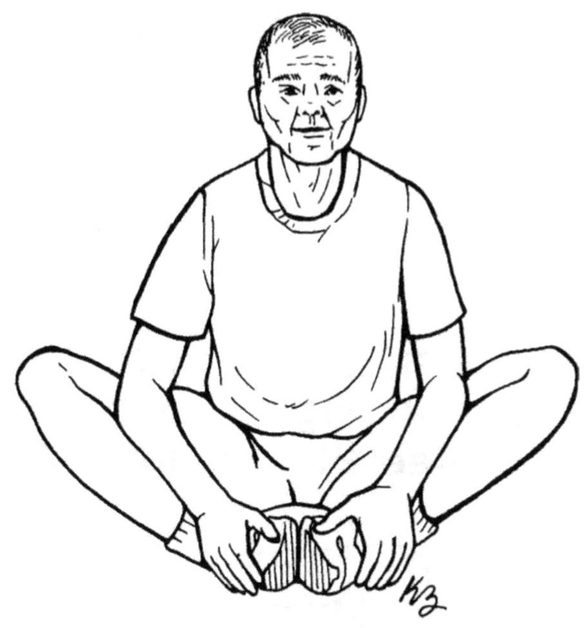

Figure 12-13: Inner Thigh (Groin) Stretch

2. Cup your hands around your toes, and gently press down on your thighs with your forearms until you feel a gentle stretch in your inner thighs.

Don't bounce your knees—stretch only until you feel a slight pulling sensation in your inner thigh.

3. Hold for five seconds, and then relax.

Repeat this exercise five to ten times.

Lower back stretches

The following stretches can protect your back from injury and help you maintain flexibility.

Knees to Chest

To perform the Knees to Chest Stretch:

1. **Lying on your back, slowly raise your right knee to your chest (see Figure 12-14).**

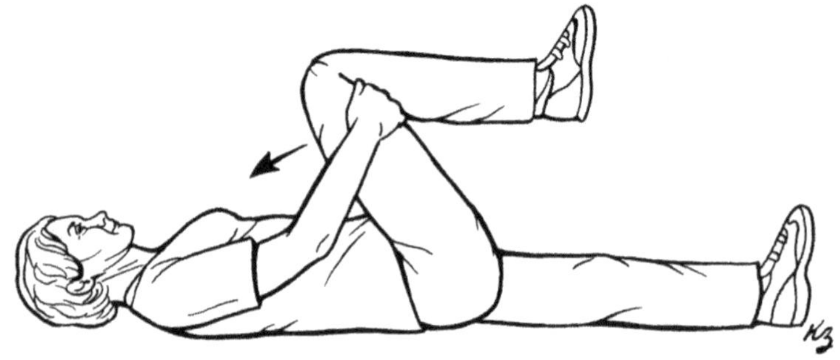

Figure 12-14: Knees to Chest

2. **Use your hands to hold your knee to your chest; you should feel the stretch in your lower back.**
3. **Hold this position for five seconds and then relax, returning your right leg to the floor.**

4. **Repeat Steps 1 through 3 five to ten times.**
5. **Repeat Steps 1 through 4, this time bringing your left knee to your chest.**

Repeat this exercise five to ten times on each side.

Bridging

To perform the Bridging Stretch:

1. **Lying on your back with your arms at your sides, bend your knees so your feet are flat on the floor (see Figure 12-15).**

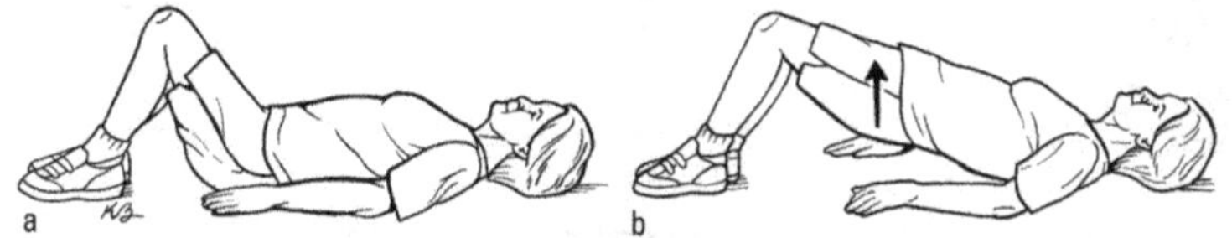

Figure 12-15: Bridging

2. **Tightening your stomach muscles, slowly raise your buttocks until even with your knees.**
3. **Hold this position for five seconds and then relax, lowering your buttocks to the floor.**

Repeat this exercise five to ten times.

Alternate Arm and Leg Lifts

To perform the Alternate Arm and Leg Lifts Stretch:

1. Lying on your stomach, extend your arms over your head.

2. Tightening your stomach muscles, simultaneously raise your *right* arm and your *left* leg 3 to 6 inches off the floor (see Figure 12-16).

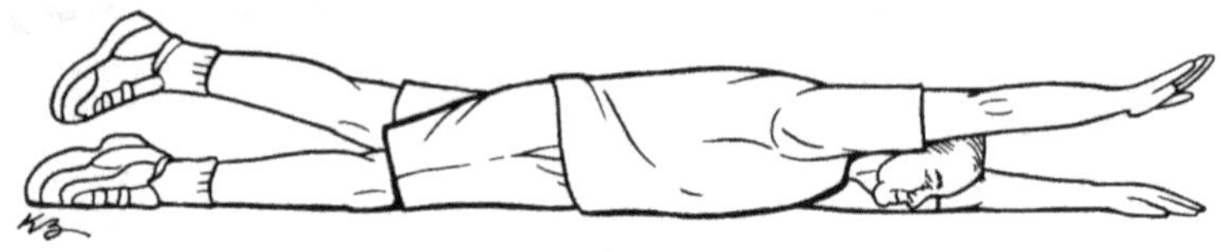

Figure 12-16: Alternate Arm and Leg Lifts

Keep both arms and both legs straight.

3. Hold this position for five seconds and then relax, returning both limbs to the floor.

4. Repeat Steps 1 through 3 five to ten times.

5. Repeat Steps 1 through 4, this time raising your *left* arm and *right* leg.

Repeat this exercise five to ten times on each side.

Standing Extension

To perform the Standing Extension Stretch:

1. **With both hands on your lower back, bend as far back as is comfortable (see Figure 12-17).**

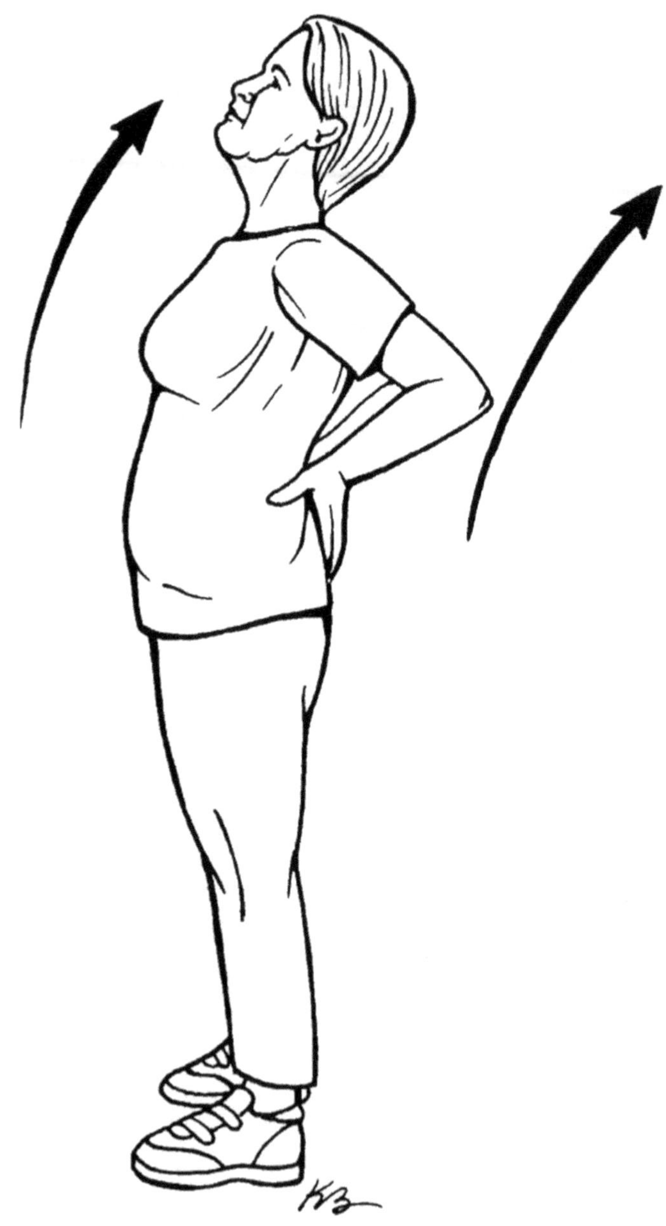

Figure 12-17: Standing Extension

2. **Hold this position for five seconds and then relax, straightening to the upright position.**

Repeat this exercise five to ten times.

A strengthening program to build muscle and stabilize joints

Although stretching is key to maintaining flexibility, don't ignore the benefits of strengthening your muscles—especially the muscles you need for maintaining balance and postural stability. You can perform the following shoulder and leg exercises three to five times a week to help maintain strength in these key areas.

Shoulder strengthening

The following exercises strengthen the shoulder area, especially the rotator cuff muscles (where your shoulder and arm connect). Your physical therapist can provide the stretchy exercise bands as well as help you adjust the tension and size to your needs. Or you can purchase a five-foot length of rubber tubing at a hardware store or athletic supply shop (they call it a *sports cord*). For some of the exercises, you also need a large bath towel to stabilize your arm.

Internal Rotation

To perform the Internal Rotation Exercise:

1. **Attach a band to a doorknob that's even with your elbow, and be sure the door is solidly shut.**
2. **Standing three feet from the door with your right side toward the door, grasp the band with your right hand, bending your arm at the elbow.**
3. **Place a rolled towel under your right arm, between your arm and right side of your body to stabilize your arm (see Figure 12-18a).**

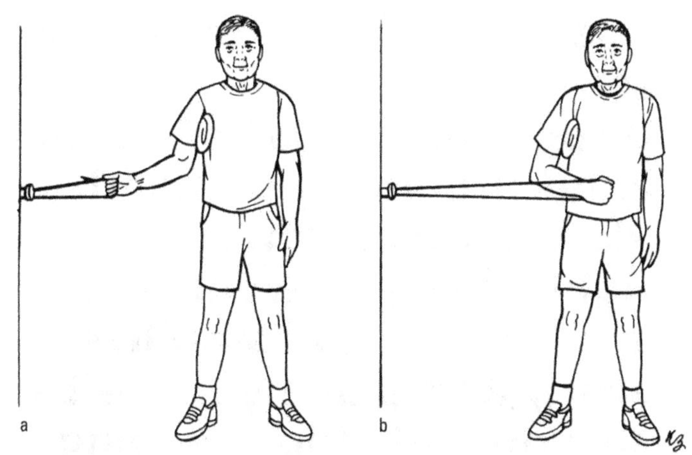

Figure 12-18: Internal Rotation

4. **Pull the band slowly across your body, rotating your arm and shoulder inward (see Figure 12-18b).**
5. **Slowly return your arm to its start position.**
6. **Repeat Steps 1 through 5 five to ten times.**
7. **Turn around so your left side is toward the door (move the towel under your left arm), and repeat Steps 1 through 5, this time extending your left arm.**

Repeat this exercise five to ten times.

External Rotation

To perform the External Rotation Exercise:

1. **Wrap the ends of a sports band around each hand.**
2. **Place a rolled towel under your right arm (between your arm and chest to stabilize your arm), and place your left hand on your left hip, keeping your right hand close by (see Figure 12-19a).**

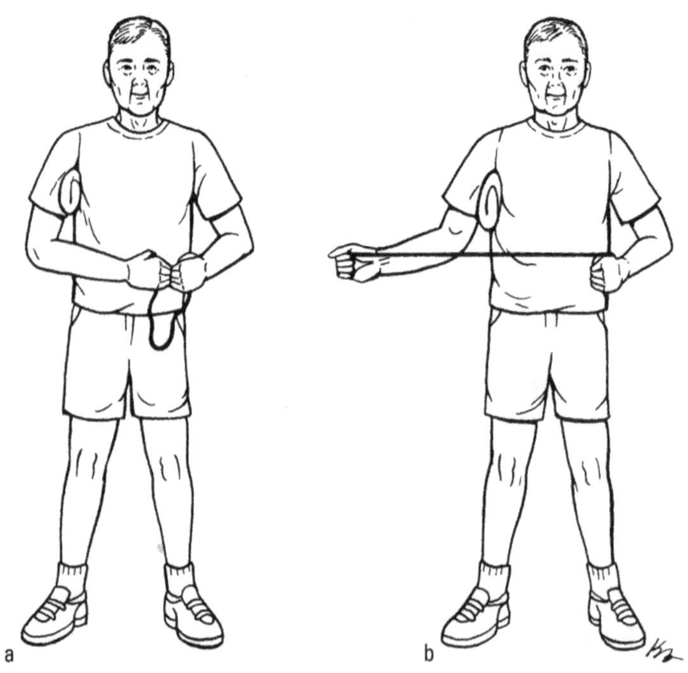

Figure 12-19: External Rotation

3. **With your right hand, slowly pull the band across your body, rotating your arm and shoulder outward (see Figure 12-19b).**
4. **Slowly return your arm to its start position.**
5. **Repeat Steps 1 through 4 five to ten times.**
6. **Repeat Steps 1 through 5, this time extending your left arm. (Don't forget to place the towel under your left arm.)**

Repeat this exercise five to ten times.

Extension Pull

To perform the Extension Pull Exercise:

1. **Attach a band to a doorknob that's even with your elbow, and be sure the door is solidly shut.**
2. **Stand facing the door (about 3 feet from the door) with the band in your right hand (see Figure 12-20a).**

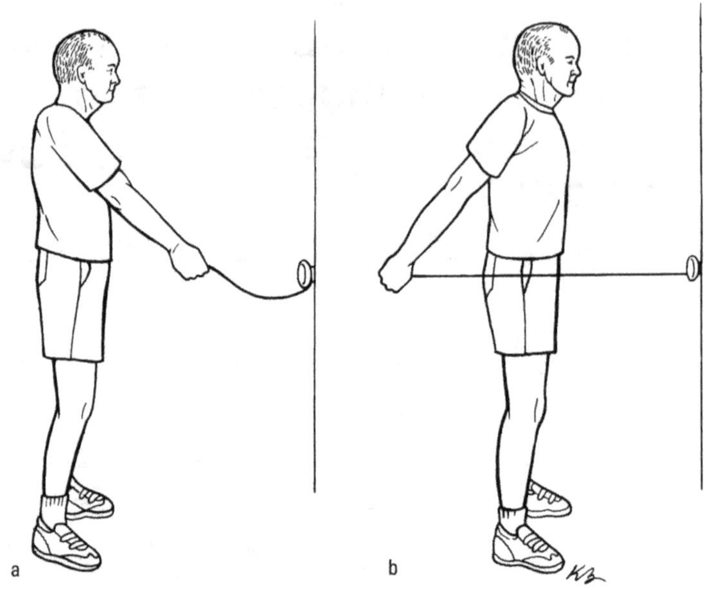

Figure 12-20: Extension Pull

3. Starting with your arm straight and forward, pull the band back by slowly lowering your straightened arm until it's at your side (see Figure 12-20b).
4. Slowly return your arm to its start position.
5. Repeat Steps 1 through 4 five to ten times.
6. Repeat Steps 1 through 5, this time extending your left arm.

Repeat this exercise five to ten times.

Flexion

To perform the Flexion Exercise:

1. **Place one end of an exercise band under your right foot and hold the other end in your right hand (see Figure 12-21a).**

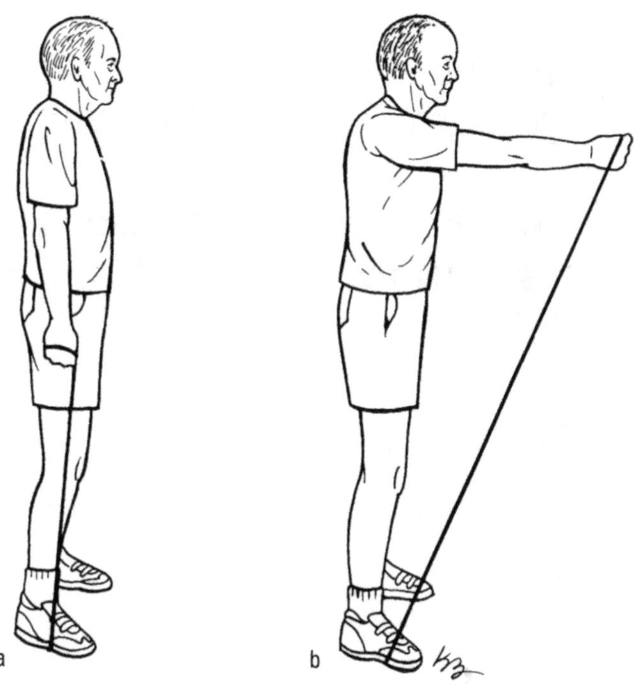

Figure 12-21: Flexion

2. **With your thumb on top of the band and your elbow straight, raise your right arm forward until it's level with your shoulder (see Figure 12-21b).**

3. **Slowly return your right arm to its start position.**
4. **Repeat Steps 1 through 3 ten times.**
5. **Repeat Steps 1 through 4, this time extending your left arm.**

Repeat this exercise five to ten times.

Horizontal Pull

To perform the Horizontal Pull Exercise:

1. **Hold the band with both hands at shoulder height (see Figure 12-22a).**

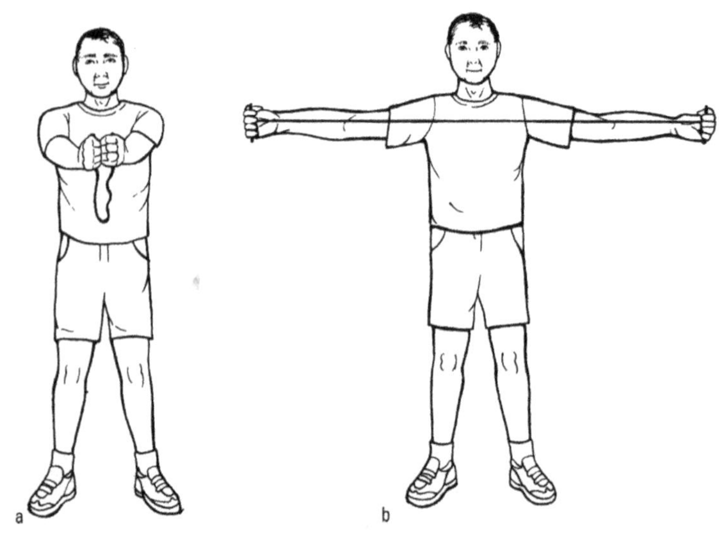

Figure 12-22: Horizontal Pull

2. **With your hands close together, extend your arms out in front of you and slowly stretch the band out until your arms are wide open (see Figure 12-22b).**
3. **Slowly bring your arms back together.**

Repeat this exercise five to ten times.

Leg strengthening

Your muscles are the stabilizers for your joints. Exercises that stretch and strengthen the muscles surrounding your hips, knees, and ankles can prevent injury and possibly improve balance. Perform the following exercises at least three times a week.

Straight Leg Raise

To perform the Straight Leg Raise Exercise:

1. Lying on your back, prop yourself up on your forearms, and slightly bend your left knee; keep your left foot flat on the floor.

2. Tightening your right leg's front thigh muscle, raise your right

leg 8 to 10 inches from the floor (see Figure 12-23).

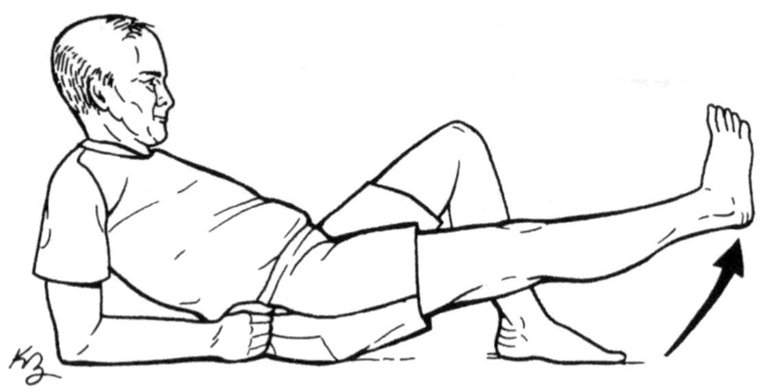

Figure 12-23: Straight Leg Raise

Keep the extended leg straight and knee locked as you perform the exercise.

3. Slowly return your right leg to the start position.

4. Repeat Steps 1 through 3 five to ten times.

5. Repeat Steps 1 through 4, this time bending your right leg and raising your left leg.

Repeat this exercise five to ten times.

Hip Abduction

To perform the Hip Abduction Exercise:

1 **Lie on your left side with both legs straight.**

2 **Slowly lift your right leg toward the ceiling to a comfortable height (at least 5 to 10 inches), keeping both legs straight (see Figure 12-24).**

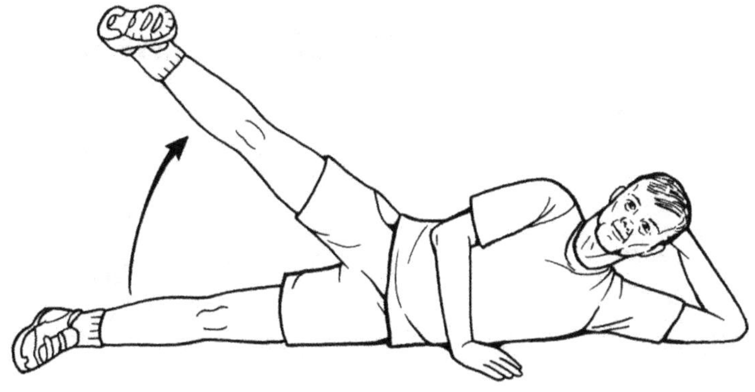

Figure 12-24: Hip Abduction

3 **Slowly lower your right leg.**

4 **Repeat Steps 1 through 3 ten times.**

5 **Turn to your right side and repeat Steps 1 through 4, this time lifting your left leg.**

Repeat this exercise five to ten times.

Hip Adduction

To perform the Hip Adduction Exercise:

1. **Lying on your right side with your right leg straight, bend your left leg at the knee so your left foot is flat on the floor in front of your right thigh or knee.**
2. **Keeping your right leg straight, raise your right leg off the ground 5 to 10 inches (see Figure 12-25).**

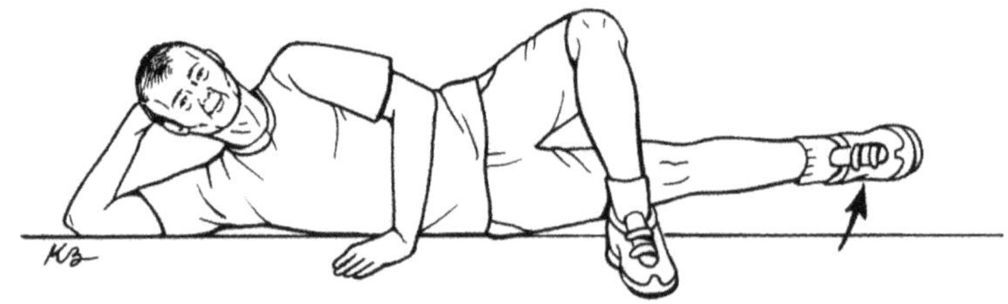

Figure 12-25: Hip Adduction

3. **Slowly lower your right leg to its start position.**
4. **Repeat Steps 1 through 3 five to ten times.**
5. **Turn to your left side and repeat Steps 1 through 4, this time lifting your left leg.**

Repeat this exercise five to ten times.

Hip Extension

To perform the Hip Extension Exercise:

1. **Lie on your stomach with both arms bent and under your chest.**
2. **With legs straight, and knees locked, tighten the muscle in your right thigh and lift your right leg 8 to 10 inches off the ground (see Figure 12-26).**

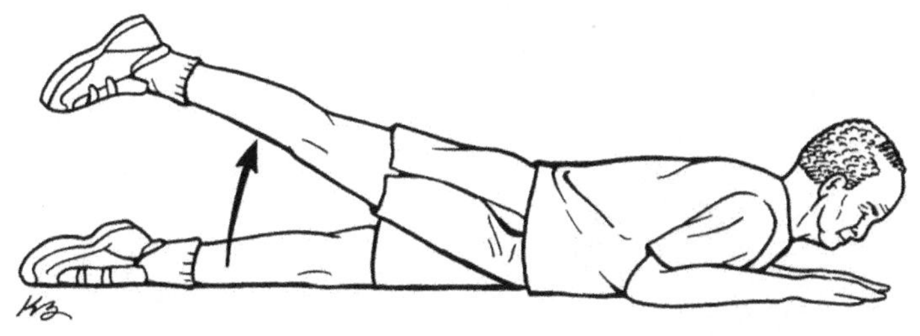

Figure 12-26: Hip Extension

3. **Slowly lower your leg back to the ground.**
4. **Repeat Steps 1 and 2, this time lifting your left leg.**

Repeat this exercise five to ten times.

Wall Slide

To perform the Wall Slide Exercise:

1. **Standing 12 to 16 inches from the wall and facing away from the wall with your feet shoulder-width apart, lean back against the wall.**
2. **Slowly lower your buttocks toward the floor as far as you can, but no more than your thighs being parallel to the floor (see Figure 12-27).**

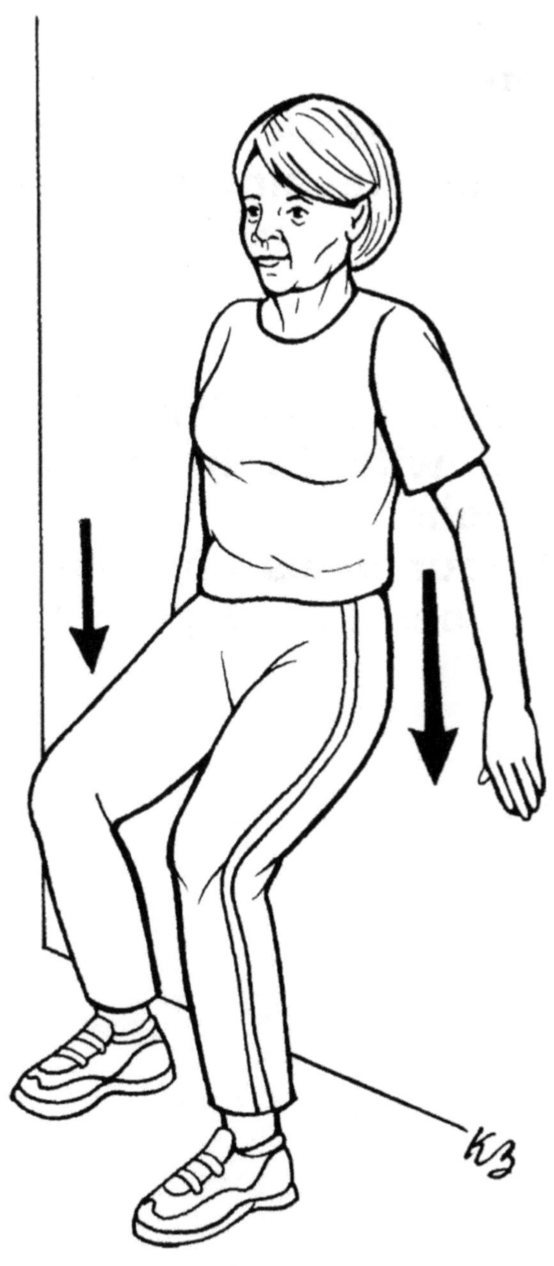

Figure 12-27: Wall Slide

3. **Hold this position for five to ten seconds.**
4. **Tighten your thigh muscles and slide back up to a standing/leaning position.**

Repeat this exercise five to ten times.

Toe Raise

To perform the Toe Raise Exercise:

1. **Stand with both feet flat on the floor.**
2. **Lift your heels and rise up on your toes (see Figure 12-28).**

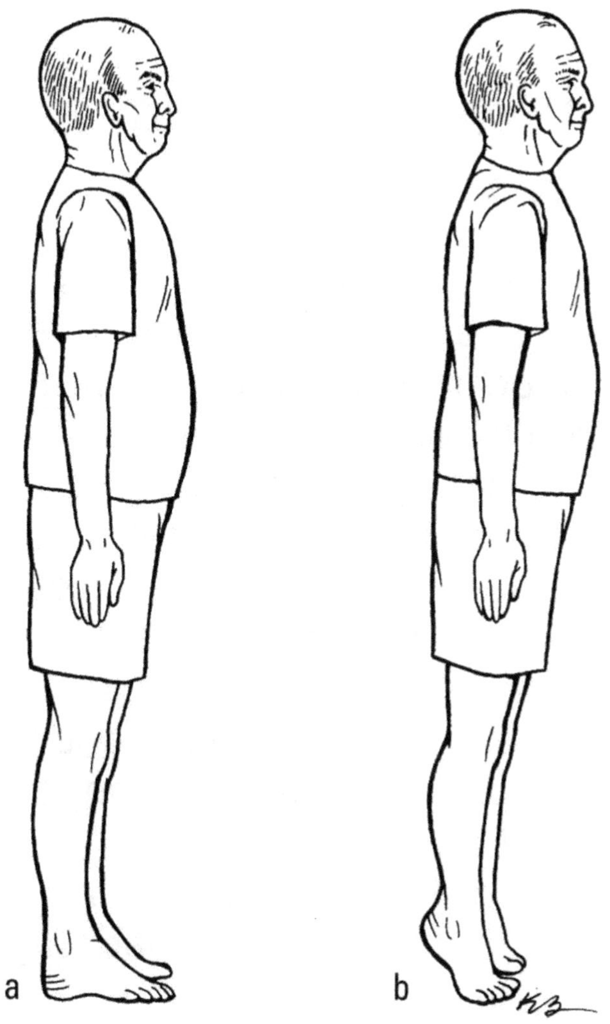

Figure 12-28: Toe Raise

3. **Hold this position for five seconds.**
4. **Lower your heels back to the floor.**

Repeat this exercise five to ten times.

Other exercise programs that can help

After you've mastered the stretches and exercises in the preceding sections, you may be ready for a program that's more challenging and yet specifically structured for PWP. Many national PD organizations consider regular exercise so essential that they've created a variety of programs and tools to help you get started. Some of these aids are listed below. For more options in programs and equipment, be sure to check out Chapter 23.

Two programs available through the Parkinson's Disease Foundation (PDF) are:

- *Motivating Moves for People with Parkinson's:* In this program developed by movement specialist Janet Hamburg, participants sit while doing the exercises. The program is available in either VHS or DVD format.

- *The Exercise Program:* This tool by Dr. E. Richard Blonsky and a team of physical therapists specializing in rehabilitation therapy comes with audio instruction tapes and a binder with illustrated exercise cards.

Call 1-800-457-6676 for more information on either program.

The American Parkinson Disease Association (APDA) has free booklets entitled *Aquatic Exercises for Parkinson's Disease* and *Be Active: A Suggested Exercise Program for People with Parkinson's Disease.* For information, call 1-800-223-2732 or look online at www.apdaparkinson.org.

Structured exercise is important in maintaining flexibility and physical function, but equally important is maintaining an active lifestyle. Read on for ways that you can use daily physical activity to enhance your well being.

Beyond a Structured Exercise Program—PD and Physical Activity

Finding ways to redefine ourselves—especially following life-changing events such as career changes, retirement, the end of a relationship, or a diagnosis of PD—is not new to most adults. But when circumstances change the way we define our satisfaction and happiness, we either adapt or choose a less-than-satisfactory mindset, which may include depression and self-pity. Far better to work at rediscovering our identity with new resources for pleasure and purpose.

The saying "Quality trumps quantity in life" may not resonate for everyone. But if you have a PD diagnosis, then you have a choice: Bury your head in the sand or get out there and live each day to the fullest.

Enjoying recreation

Physical activity, or recreation (see how that word is really *recreation?*), differs from exercise because recreation usually provides an element of immediate pleasure, accomplishment, or revitalization that structured exercise may not. For example, if you garden, think about the pleasure of seeing the results of your hard work. In a similar way, biking and canoeing allow us to be physically active while taking in the fresh air and scenery.

But recreation goes beyond simple physical endeavors; it includes contact with other people and opening ourselves to new experiences and information. When we were kids, we called it *playing.* But adults can still play, even when they're facing grown-up stuff like PD.

Keeping up with routine roles and activities

Chances are good that you played multiple roles before getting the diagnosis of PD. Take a moment to list them: son/daughter, spouse/lover, friend/companion, parent/grandparent, employee/employer/co-worker, community leader/volunteer. How about the roles you played at home? Cook, gardener, decorator, financial manager, handyman/woman.

Ask yourself whether you think some of these roles are no longer possible. For example, do you think you can't keep up with your current job (see Chapter 16) or do you withdraw from social functions because you don't want pity from friends and family (see Chapter 15)? Maybe you don't cook anymore because the tremors make a mess. Or maybe you're afraid of making a mistake in the checkbook, so you've handed over the finances to your significant other.

Now take a good look at Chapters 2 and 3 to see whether you find a cause or symptom of PD that says you have to start peeling away pieces of your life and abandoning vital relationships. We'll wait.... Did you see it? Ah hah! We knew you wouldn't!

This is a good time for you to re-evaluate those activities you may have assumed were no longer possible—employment, volunteer work, and social activities, such as card playing, sports, and the like. The harder you work to maintain your normal routine and activities, the less likely your PD will dominate your life.

True, you may need to make some adjustments in physical activities to accommodate your PD. For example, you may find that sports requiring more lateral (side-to-side) movement, such as golf and ping pong, are easier for you. Or, if you were a marathon runner, think about race-walking or just plain walking. One PWP, Parky, biked over 42,000 miles in a ten-year period by switching to a recumbent three-wheel trike. (See www.inevergiveup.org. for more about his story.) His motto: "Let's take the PARK out of Parkinson's."

The point is that you do have choices and you can take charge instead of allowing assumptions to dictate your routine. Work with your doctor and other members of your professional health team to determine the right physical activities for you.

The same advice for physical activities applies to activities that engage you mentally and spiritually. This next section suggests ways to incorporate mental and spiritual activity into your daily life.

Exercises for the Mind and Spirit

Okay, you're exercising regularly and maintaining an active and productive lifestyle. Caring for the physical body is huge for you and for those people who make this journey with you. But be sure you give attention to the mind and spirit. What's happening inside your head? For that matter, what's going on with your care partner—that person (or persons) who's been with you from the moment you were diagnosed with PD?

In fact, many PWP develop apathy, a condition defined by

- Reduced interest and participation in routine activities
- Lack of initiative
- Difficulties in starting or sustaining an activity
- Lack of concern for events and people around them

In other words, the mind and spirit seem to simply give up.

Apathy in PD is more likely a direct consequence of *physiological* changes in the brain than a *psychological* reaction to the disability. As a result, this condition is different from the other psychiatric symptoms and personality changes associated with the disease (such as depression and anxiety—see Chapter 13). In addition, PD apathy can trigger major frustration for that person's care partner especially when the care partner sees that he's working harder at keeping the PWP active and involved than the PWP is.

Basically you can approach your life's uncertainties in two ways: Devote your efforts to worrying and trying to change the situation, or devote your energy toward living the most fulfilling life you can. Although you can't control the progression of your PD, you can control your choices:

- To exercise or not
- To remain engaged in the community or not
- To set a tone for your friends and family that you may have PD but it does not have you
- To wake up every morning and make good choices all over again or not

Choices for the person with PD

Just as proper diet and exercise are the best choices for maintaining your physical health, they're also your best weapons for maintaining the health of your mind and spirit. People who walk, bike, or run often report that they do their best thinking then; they're working out mental and emotional issues as well as physical ones.

These are some exercises you can make a part of your daily (or at least weekly) routine:

- Take time out for daily spiritual renewal (see Chapter 11). Meditate, pray, read inspirational books or poetry, take a walk, attend religious services—whatever gives you a sense of renewal.
- Challenge your mind. Work a crossword or Sudoku puzzle, play along with a TV game show (preferably one that actually requires some mental effort), read a book.
- Learn something new. Take a class at the local college or community center, ask a friend to teach you a craft or new sport, attend a lecture, watch a documentary. Then share your new ideas with someone else.
- Get involved in your community by taking an active role in a cause or organization that you think is

important: the local library, a museum or historical site, national projects with local chapters (such as Habitat for Humanity).

- Create a legacy for your children and grandchildren. Write or record your family history, research the family tree, organize photo collections into albums that truly tell the story of your family's past.
- Partner with your partner to find activities you both can participate in and maintain the activities you both enjoyed before your diagnosis. Go to that play, that ballgame, that festival.
- Join a support group—preferably one for PWP—where you can interact with other people who fully understand the problems you and your care partner are facing.
- Accept that life with PD has no more certainty than life before PD. Turn to the *Bill of Rights for the Person Living with Parkinson's* in the front of this book. Tear it out, read it, and put it where you'll see and read it every day.

Choices for the PD care partner

As the care partner to someone living with PD, you also live with it. It affects your daily life in ways you had never imagined or planned for. A person in your shoes may want to abandon pieces of her own life to take care of the partner. And the most likely piece to fall by the wayside is your own physical health. You eat (or maybe don't eat!) as a reaction to your worries rather than as a source of nourishment. And when you add the responsibilities of caring for someone with PD to your full calendar, something's gotta give; the most likely candidate is your own regular exercise. *Stop!*

Before you go any further, take a moment to consider the following:

- Someone you love has PD and will *eventually* need help.
- You partner is managing fine with the present treatment plan. You understand that this plan can last for years by monitoring the disease and using medications.

- You have a choice:
  - Project the worst as you try and control the future by making life-changing decisions right now.
  - Make reasonable plans and preparations by educating yourself about options and then living the life that's still reasonably normal.

If you elect the second option, congratulations! Plan to familiarize yourself with the information in other sections of this book, especially Parts 4 and 5. Now, about *your* body, mind, and spirit. Start by following the same guidelines we suggest in the "Exercises for the Mind and Spirit" section. Then read the Bill of Rights for the PD care partner in Chapter 19.

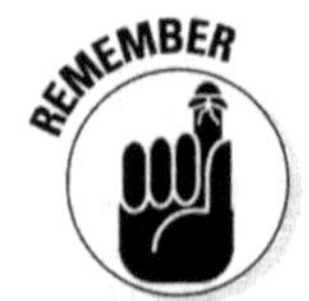

You don't have PD. You have a life beyond caring for this person—just as the PWP has a life beyond living with it. Mental and spiritual well being for each of you depends on maintaining normalcy as long as possible. The greatest danger is surrendering your potentially good and happy years to anxiety and depression, which can be a major factor with PD. Check out Chapter 13, where we address that concern in depth.

Chapter 13

Combating Anxiety and Depression

In This Chapter

- Getting on top of the downside: Anxiety, depression, and apathy
- Looking for help in all the right places
- Thinking positively for you and your care partner

You've gotten some bad news: It's Parkinson's disease (PD). At the moment, you don't know a lot—about the disease, about its impact on you and those you love, about so many questions. You're trying to come to terms with a diagnosis that means your life has changed and will keep changing as the years roll by. Of course, you have anxious moments—maybe some full-blown panic attacks. And news like this doesn't exactly put a smile on your face or a lot of sunshine in your outlook. When reactions like these last for a short time and then pass, that's normal human behavior.

On the other hand, feelings of anxiety, panic, and depression that persist for days, weeks, or even months are not normal. And for people living with Parkinson's (PWP), the anxiety and depression can be complicated by their PD—a combination of living with a chronic, progressive illness *and* the neurochemical changes occurring in the brain.

This chapter looks at the ways PD plays a part in the onset of anxiety and depression, and we provide a host of proven solutions—some of them admittedly a little unorthodox—that can bring you relief.

Recognizing the Mental Downside to PD

Anxiety and depression are serious—but treatable—medical conditions that can affect your quality of life and ability to function as you adapt to living with PD. And a number of circumstances (like stress, side effects of meds, and lifestyle changes due to PD) can trigger an episode that sends you reeling.

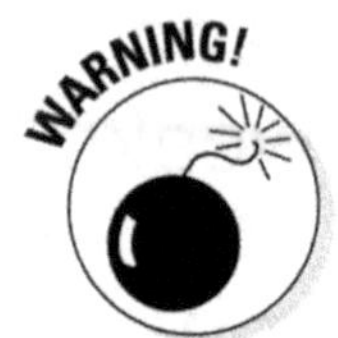

Don't take the symptoms of anxiety and depression lightly, and—just as important—don't postpone getting to the appropriate professional for treatment! (See the section "Finding and Accepting Help" later in this chapter for specifics about professional help.)

Anxiety is normal—to a point

Some situations naturally warrant anxiety and worry (the meeting with the boss, for example, or giving a major presentation or party). However, when the panic, terror, and outright impending doom aren't relieved by time, accomplishment, or common sense, something's wrong. Are you normally easygoing, self-confident, and optimistic?

If you suddenly (and regularly!) find yourself dealing with dread or disproportionate fear, these feelings need attention.

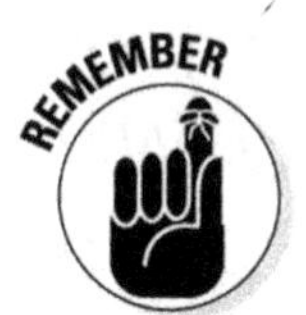

Research studies confirm the following facts about anxiety for PWP:

- It affects up to 40 percent of PWP.
- It can be one of the first symptoms that make the PWP seek a doctor's care.
- It often goes hand in hand with depression.

Identifying the source of that anxiety

Anxiety can be brought on by any number of circumstances and generally takes one of several forms:

- ***Generalized anxiety disorder (GAD):*** A condition in which the person lives day in and day out with an underlying sense of worry that something will go wrong, but the worry has no real basis.

- ***Social phobias:*** When that persistent worry focuses on a specific situation or circumstance related to the social environment (such as a fear of failure or of interacting with other people).
- ***Panic attack:*** When anxiety strikes unexpectedly, suddenly, and hard. Usually a panic attack comes complete with major physical symptoms (such as a racing heartbeat, shortness of breath, and even chest pain). In fact you may think you're having a heart attack.

Circumstances leading to anxiety may include a particularly unsettling and stressful event (such as a diagnosis of PD); personality traits (such as low self-esteem and poor coping skills); or the presence of an additional mental condition (such as depression).

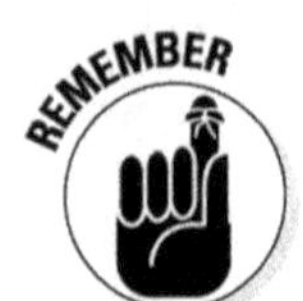

One way to identify the circumstances that cause anxiety is to be mindful of your own *fight-or-flight*

mechanism. (*Fight-or-flight* is the most common reaction when people face situations that bring on stress, anxiety, or outright panic. In other words, they either stand and fight or take off.) Think of the times when you faced that choice. For example, if your boss confronted you about a missed deadline and you simply accepted his blame, that's flight. But if you listened and then explained exactly why the delay was unavoidable, that's fight.

So as a PWP, what sets off your fight-or-flight alarm? How persistent is it? Is your first instinct usually to take action, find answers, seek knowledge? (That's fight.) Or do you wait for others to direct you? (That, of course, is flight.) It's perfectly understandable that you'll have times when you just want to crawl under the covers and let somebody else live with PD for a while. But the more you adopt the fight mentality, the more likely you are to maintain independence and control over your life.

Measuring your level of anxiety

Although doctors use professional tools to diagnose anxiety, a short self-evaluation of your symptoms can help determine whether you should seek professional help. Which feelings in the following list do you experience on most days and for much of the day?

- Anxious or nervous
- Afraid (for self or others)
- Out of control
- Panicky or jumpy
- Short of breath or pounding heart
- Dizzy or faint
- Flushed or sweaty
- Unable to concentrate or take action
- Unable to remember
- Sensing impending doom

If you answered "Yes" to five or more of these symptoms, talk to your doctor. You may be suffering needlessly from anxiety.

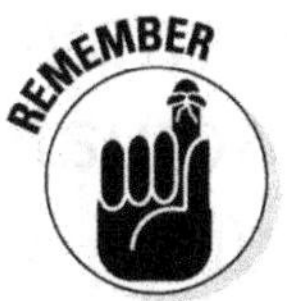

Anxiety disorder includes additional categories such as post-traumatic stress disorder and obsessive-compulsive behavior disorder, but these are less common among PWP.

Depression—More than just sad and blue

According to the National Institute of Mental Health, depression can strike anyone, but PWP may be at greater risk. This section can help you consider your symptoms and determine whether it's time to take action.

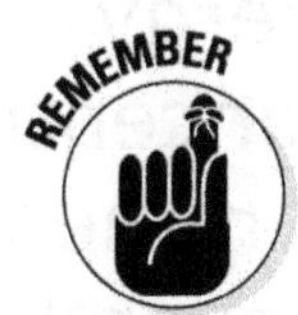

Keep in mind that some PD symptoms (such as the masked facial expression, slow movement, and lack of energy) can actually be symptoms of depression—and vice versa. But when these symptoms accompany anxiety, apathy, or loss of interest or pleasure in activities and relationships, consider the possibility that you have a *treatable* mental health condition.

Recognizing the symptoms

The National Institute of Mental Health lists the following as symptoms of depression:

- Persistent sad, anxious, or empty feelings
- Feelings of hopelessness and pessimism
- Feelings of guilt, worthlessness, or helplessness
- Loss of interest and pleasure in hobbies and activities
- Fatigue, feeling slowed down, or decreased energy
- Difficulty concentrating, making decisions, or remembering
- Insomnia or oversleeping
- Appetite or weight gain or loss
- Restlessness and irritability

- Thoughts of death or suicide; suicide attempts
- Crying, especially over little, seemingly incidental issues

Ask yourself these questions

Although we definitely don't recommend self-diagnosis or treatment, ask yourself these ten questions if your feelings (mental and emotional) concern you on a daily basis:

- Are you discouraged or sad?
- Are you moody or irritable?
- Are you feeling isolated or lonely?
- Have you lost interest in activities you can still do?
- Have you pulled away from interactions with friends and family?
- Is your outlook affecting your ability to work, make decisions, or make choices?
- Has your mood affected your sleep (for example, sleeping more in the day or not sleeping at night) or energy level?
- Have you experienced changes in appetite and weight?
- Have you lost interest in sex or intimacy with your partner?

- Have the people you trust suggested that you seem depressed?

If you've answered "Yes" to five or more of these questions, you need to raise the possibility with your doctor that you may need treatment for depression.

Dealing with apathy and lack of motivation

Many PWP develop *apathy,* a condition defined by

- Reduced interest and participation in routine activities
- Lack of initiative; having difficulty starting or sustaining an activity to completion
- Indifference or a lack of concern
- A flattening of affect (the mind and the spirit seem to give up on all emotions: good, bad, pleasant, or painful)

In addition to these symptoms, the PWP's apathy can trigger frustration in family, friends, and the care partner. When those around an apathetic person begin to realize that they're working harder at fighting your PD than you are, the tendency is to think that the person suffering from apathy doesn't appreciate their efforts or help. The end result can be that family and friends gradually go back to their own lives, leaving the person with apathy (and the care partner) more isolated and in need of help than before.

Apathy can be associated with several neuropsychiatric illnesses (such as Alzheimer's dementia, PD, and stroke). In PD, however, apathy is more likely a direct consequence of physiological changes in the brain and lack of dopamine than a psychological reaction to disability. Although professionals can distinguish apathy from psychiatric symptoms and personality features (particularly depression and anxiety), it's not an easy task. Consider these subtle but distinguishing characteristics:

- Like people with depression, apathetic patients may be sluggish, quiet, and disengaged. They may talk slowly or not at all.
- Unlike depressed patients, apathetic PWP deny being sad, feeling guilty, or having suicidal thoughts.

Recognizing apathy and differentiating it from depression in PWP is important because the medical treatment for the two conditions may be different. Patients with apathy are not lazy and may respond to a series of strategies that include gentle encouragement to initiate activities as well as schedules and routines to keep them busy.

For example, consider a PWP who's always loved going to the ballpark. When his best friend invites him to a major league game for his birthday, he says he wants to stay home in front of the television. But when the friend insists, they go to the park, and the PWP has a good time all day. However, he immediately turns the television back on when he returns home.

Ask your primary care doctor or neurologist about the differences between apathy and depression and what symptoms you (and your care partner) should watch for in either case.

Finding and Accepting Help

You may have experienced depression or anxiety before the onset of PD, or your first episode may come after the diagnosis. But the chicken-or-the-egg question doesn't really matter. What does matter is that the symptoms (see the previous sections) are unnecessary hardships when you're dealing with PD.

Ask your doctor to recommend a consultation with a mental health professional who'll work closely with your doctor to assess your depression in the context of your PD.

Taking medication may help

In most cases, PWP tolerate antidepressant medications well. But medications can take weeks to have a real effect, and the right medication can take trial and effort. As a result, many doctors recommend a combination treatment plan that may include or take the place of antidepressants. Combo possibilities include

- Talk therapy (the services of a professional counselor)
- Changes in diet, exercise routines, and sleep habits

Before you take any medication (prescription or over-the-counter) to treat symptoms of depression or anxiety, be sure your prescribing doctor is fully aware of all your other medications. Some over-the-counter (OTC) supplements can interact in a negative or even harmful way with your other medications.

Seeking a professional counselor

Your doctor may recommend a professional counselor who helps you talk through the feelings and fears that are at the foundation of your depression or anxiety. In looking for the right counselor, keep in mind the different categories:

- **Psychiatrists:** Medical doctors with training (at least four years) beyond their medical degree. These doctors are board-certified by the American Board of Psychiatry and Neurology and licensed in the state where they practice. They can prescribe medications and coordinate a total care plan for any mental or emotional health issue.
- **Psychologists:** Counselors with a master's degree (MA or MS) or a doctoral degree (PhD or PsyD) in psychology and/or counseling. Psychologists are board-certified by the American Board of Professional Psychology and licensed by the state where they practice.

  Psychologists are less focused on biological causes of depression and anxiety and more focused on treating your symptoms.
- **Clinical social workers:** Counselors who are licensed or certified by the state and usually hold a masters degree in social work and/or counseling. Some social workers have advanced

training in psychotherapy and may have the title of Licensed Clinical Social Worker or LCSW.

- **Other counselors** include
- **Psychiatric nurses or clinical nurse specialists** (CNS) who are registered nurses (RN), with additional training in psychiatry
- **Family therapists** who hold a title or degree but focus primarily on counseling within the context of a family group
- **Pastoral counselors** who, in addition to religious training, have training in counseling

Finding a counselor

Therapy to treat depression, anxiety, or a mental or emotional condition should be a collaborative process. More than with any other healthcare professional, you need to feel a real sense of trust and rapport with this person.

Keep in mind that your therapist will push you to examine and confront sometimes unpleasant and even painful issues. She's not trying to be mean, but she is trying to get you past roadblocks that may hamper your ability to accept PD in order to live a fuller, more satisfying life.

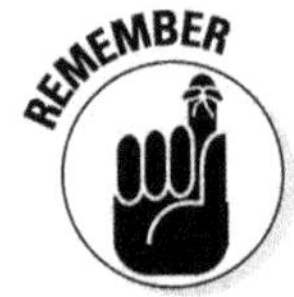

Any mental health professional has the ethical (in some cases, legal) responsibility to keep your therapy discussions confidential *unless* you threaten to cause harm to other persons or property.

Choosing the right counselor for you

In addition to checking his credentials and experience, take time to really consider the connection you'll have with this therapist or counselor. The following are key steps to follow:

• Be sure your primary care physician (PCP) has already ruled out medical causes for your depression or anxiety symptoms.

• Consider specifics (such as the therapist's age, gender, ethnic or religious background) that may be important to you and make those known when you ask for referrals.

• Get at least two (and preferably three) referrals from your primary care doctor, neurologist, or support group facilitator.

• Be sure to consider location. You're going to see this person on a regular (perhaps weekly) basis over several months. The last thing you need is an inconvenient journey to and from the appointment.

• At your first appointment

• Ask the same questions you ask your other specialists. (See Chapter 6 for these questions.)

• Be prepared to describe the symptoms that led you to seek help.

• Listen to the therapist's possible plan for treatment (medications, talk therapy, or both).

Listen for language like "in cases like yours..." that suggests a generalized rather than a customized approach to therapy. If this one-size-fits-all seems to be the therapist's approach, keep looking.

- After the first appointment, keep in mind that a genuine trust and connection with this person is key to successfully conquering your symptoms. Give yourself time to think about the first meeting—what went well and what disturbed you—before keeping a second appointment.

Check with your insurance provider (or Medicare/Medicaid if appropriate) to find out what services are covered.

If your insurance provider doesn't cover mental health services (or only covers a portion), ask the therapist whether he has a sliding fee scale based on income.

Sharing the emotional journey with a support group

A support group can be a real lifesaver for many people with a chronic, progressive condition (and their care partners). Through these gatherings, you can hear about valuable coping skills and keep up with the latest myths and bona fide medical advances. Generally, each group has a facilitator with professional experience in working with PWP and their care partners. This objective, outside facilitator has the following responsibilities:

- Keeps the discussion moving
- Doesn't allow a few outspoken participants to highjack the meeting so quieter personalities fade into

the background (and eventually leave the group)

- Covers the logistics: Meeting place and time, special speakers or programs, and notices of meetings

The most successful groups determine their own personality and style. The following are examples of group formats:

- Participants talk about PD news and personal updates. They support one another emotionally and offer ideas for coping.
- A speaker presents a specific topic for discussion.
- The group has a political focus, such as getting Congress to allocate research dollars that will put PD on the front burner for finding a cure. (See information on the Parkinson's Action Network in Appendix B.)
- Some groups include all of these formats, alternating support with specific programs and advocacy projects.

PWP and their care partners are indeed fortunate to have a number of national organizations that offer support groups through their regional or state chapters. To see whether such a group is available in your area, check www.parkinson.org or www.caregiver.org.

Two other possible resources are the community education and outreach department of your local hospital or the local PD exercise class we describe in Chapter 12.

If your area has zero groups specifically for PWP or their care partners, consider starting one. See the sidebar "Building a support group: From *me* to *we* in five easy steps" to get started.

Whether you join an established group or start one yourself, support groups can enrich your life beyond anything you can imagine because you

- Connect with people who truly understand the challenges of living with PD.
- Have the opportunity to laugh and cry together.
- Can advocate for better treatments and a cure.
- Can make an enormous difference for yourself and for those who love and care for you.

Building a support group: From me to we in five easy steps

The steps for starting a PD support group are relatively simple:

1. Ask your doctor or neurologist to tell other PD patients and their care partners that you're interested in organizing a group.

Provide cards with your contact information for the doctor to give to interested PWP. These people can then contact you (not the other way around).

2. Gather the following information:

• Ask your local hospital or home care agency whether they have anyone qualified and willing to facilitate the group.

• Find out whether your local library, book-store, coffeehouse, or medical clinic has a room available for 10 to 12 people for two hours once a month at no charge.

3. Consider initially combining PWP and care partners in the same group.

As the group grows, you may hold separate meetings for the PWP and care partners.

4. When at least four people have expressed interest, call an organizational meeting and ask these people to invite other PWP or care partners.

5. At the first meeting:

• Have nametags and perhaps light refreshments.

• Ask attendees to briefly introduce themselves and state what they're looking for in a support group.

• Establish the working details for the group: when and where to meet;

how often; for how long; dues, if any, to cover cost of refreshments or mailings; and programs or format style of the group.

• If possible, ask an experienced support-group facilitator to lead this meeting.

• If you don't have a trained facilitator, consider professionals speakers to lead the first several meetings. Then alternate the leader role and assign responsibilities (meeting room, program, and participant notifications) for the next three months.

• End the meeting by checking everyone's contact information and allowing time for people to socialize and get to know each other better.

Making lifestyle changes to improve your point of view

Two words: exercise and diet. (But you can check out Chapter 12 for a few more words.) It's no secret that research shows how regular exercise and a properly balanced diet can work wonders for your health. But just in case you need a refresher on some of those wonders, did you know that exercise can

- Boost the power of neurotransmitters in your brain to enhance your mood and your ability to look at life more positively?
- Relieve muscle tension when your body's natural instinct is to tense up in response to a challenge?
- Enhance your self-image, which leads to greater self-assurance and confidence, which increase your ability to deal with negative stress?

Not a bad return on an investment of only 30 to 60 minutes a day!

As for diet, start with a simple choice like lessening stimulants (such as caffeine and chocolate) that can contribute to your anxiety. Ready to kick it up a notch? Educate yourself about the mind-enhancing powers of certain food groups. (For more information on diet and nutrition, see Chapter 12.) When you combine these power foods with regular exercise, you have the right formula to make an enormous difference in your emotional state of mind and self-image.

Alternative therapies (such as relaxation and meditation) and mind-exercise programs (such as T'ai Chi and yoga) can also be enormously effective in relieving the symptoms of anxiety and depression. See Chapter 11 for more info on each of these techniques.

Don't worry—Be happy

No doubt you'd like to remind us that PD isn't exactly humorous. But at least one of us (the author with PD) knows all too well that finding humor in the mishaps and misadventures with PD is no different from finding humor in other life challenges (like the impossible in-law or the service people who don't show up and then don't give much service when they do get there).

The following sections provide a few tips for ways you (and your partner) can fight anxiety, depression, and apathy.

Just say the word

One PWP came up with the acronym *S.O.F.A.* (as in "Get off the sofa") to remind himself that anxiety, apathy, and depression were dangerous areas for anyone with PD. *Sadness* can lead to *Obstructions* (of physical and mental abilities) that lead to a *Fall* (the danger for any PWP), so the only cure is *Ambition* (to get moving—physically, mentally, and spiritually). This acronym may not work for you, but try one of your own—a password that empowers you and your care partner when anxiety and depression start to rear their ugly heads.

The crème' de la comedy

Renowned essayist and editor Norman Cousins pioneered the idea of laughter as medical therapy. In his book, *Anatomy of an Illness,* Cousins describes how he watched hours of classics like the Marx brothers and *I Love Lucy.* As a result of his and other researchers' work, laughter is now a respected therapy that supplements mainstream medicine.

It's not all about you: Ways to look beyond your PD

One sure way to get past the poor-pitiful-me piece is to focus less on yourself and ramp up your attention to other people. This simple change can also remind other people to stop viewing you as someone with an incurable condition and start seeing you as the vital, loving, and giving person you've always been.

Fresh out of ideas? Not surprising. But, hey, that's why we're here. Pick any one of the following and see what happens:

• If a clerk or service person gives especially good service, tell him and then tell his boss.

• Offer to trade seats on a bus, train, or plane to let a family or couple sit together—even if you end up with the dreaded middle seat.

• Find old pictures of family members, frame them, and send them to the person with a note that recalls what the photos mean to you.

• Look beneath the surface. When a friend's in a crummy mood, know that it probably goes well beyond the surface. Acknowledge that she seems to be having a bad day and ask if there's anything you can do to help.

• Pass along a good book you've just finished or make special scrapbooks or family recipe books for the children in your family.

• If you're a gardener and need to divide your perennials, offer the new neighbor some plants from your garden. (They can do the digging!)

• Put an extra coin in an expired meter.

- Call the clerks and other service people that you regularly see by name.
- Take a treat to your co-workers, even if you have to buy rather than bake it.
- Use the magic words, "Please" and "Thank you," and make a big deal out of someone going the extra mile for you.

Focusing on other people—caring for and about them—is possibly the simplest way to move beyond your self-pity and angst about PD. Of course, it's not a cure for clinical depression or anxiety, but caring for others is a major first-step in changing your destructive, negative self-talk to something far more positive and life-affirming. Bottom line? It is indeed better to give (care and concern) than to receive (pity and avoidance).

Did you hear the one about...

At your next support group meeting, suggest the group indulge in some laugh therapy for 15 to 20 minutes by sharing funny incidents. After all, who else can understand the ridiculousness of trying to shave (if you're a man) or pulling on a pair of pantyhose (if you're a woman)? Who else but PWP can laugh out loud and not seem cruel when you describe yourself hurrying to catch an elevator?

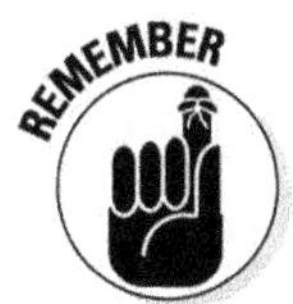

The humor you find in PD is, of course, bittersweet, but don't permit the bitter to overpower the sweet. Choosing to laugh at yourself—and the frustrations and mishaps with PD—offers a healthy dose of the absurd that'll work better than any pill. The ability to laugh can work miracles.

Tapping into the power of positive thinking

The ability to enjoy life—to be content—is often bound up in the need to be in control. But how much can anyone really control? The next hour, day, or year? Nope. The only control you really have lies in how you choose to react to life's circumstances and challenges. And when you choose to react with a sense of humor and a positive life outlook, research suggests three possible benefits:

- You'll greatly reduce your physical and emotional stress and greatly enhance your relationships with other people.
- Your outlook will be contagious. By setting the tone (as we suggest in Chapter 5), you can help your care partners (professional and personal) accept the diagnosis and move forward with you.
- You'll have an aura of self-confidence that also inspires people around you (who may be tempted to nurture or baby you) to step back and let you take the lead. They'll be more inclined to make decisions *with* you than *for* you.

Your attitude can very well be the difference between taking control of this disease and allowing PD to control you. How much better to hear people marvel at your incredibly upbeat and positive attitude toward PD than to hear them talk in tones of pity and sympathy!

So how can you change a glass that's half-empty into a glass that's half-full? More to the point, is it even possible to change it, given your PD diagnosis?

Optimists tend to believe that good things do happen and bad things are just temporary challenges. Fortunately, enhancing your optimistic side is within reach. Check out these tips for becoming more optimistic:

- Find the joy—in work, in relationships, in everyday stuff like preparing a meal, cleaning, repairing something, getting dressed, and meeting the day head-on.

- Surround yourself with people who are positive, upbeat, and optimistic.
- Commit random acts of kindness (not original to us, but we like the sound of it!) by looking beyond yourself to the needs of others (see the sidebar, "It's not all about you: Ways to look beyond your PD."
- Accept and work through situations you can control; let go of those you can't. (Does the word *serenity* come to mind?)
- Be aware of your reactions. Banish negative self-talk ("I can't," or "I never..."), and look for underlying traits you admire (or even love) in the family members and friends who irritate you.
- At the end of every day, write or tell yourself three good things (okay, they can be really little) that happened that day.

As Garrison Keillor, author and host of the popular radio program, *Prairie Home Companion,* once said, "They say such nice things about people at their funerals that it makes me sad that I'm going to miss mine by just a few days."

A Word for the PD Care Partner

Given the nature of depression, anxiety, and apathy, it's most likely that you—not the PWP—will need to be vigilant about recognizing symptoms and getting help to break the cycle. These are a few actions you can take:

- **Pay attention.** Look at the PWP's body language. Listen to what she says (or doesn't say). Sure, that mask (lack of facial expression) or stooped posture may be a result of PD, but is something else at work here? If the person you love seems persistently uninvolved and disinterested in the normal routine you two once enjoyed, those clues need your attention.
- **Don't be afraid to ask questions.** Your PWP may have a logical but curable reason for appearing to be depressed, apathetic, or anxious. Through gentle questioning, maybe you can get him to admit his concern so the two of you can talk about it (and address it with his

doctor). On the other hand, if his answer to all your questions is something like "There's nothing wrong," he may have more troubling him than he can manage. In that case, you can:

• Offer information from PD Web sites (see Appendix B) and books like this one that clearly demonstrates how such feelings are common for PWP and can be treated.

• Suggest that he talk to his neurologist about his emotions and ask whether these unusual feelings are treatable.

- **Talk to the experts.** If the PWP refuses to address your concern that he may be depressed or suffering from anxiety or apathy, contact the neurologist yourself and ask for help. Or ask the care partners in your support group whether they've dealt with these issues. If they have, ask for some suggestions on how you can follow through.

Don't forget to take care of you

Being the primary care partner for a PWP will—over time—become a natural piece of your life. Before you realize it, the role is more than a daily routine; it's part of your identity. "That's Joan Sutton. Her husband has Parkinson's," someone may say, implying that your husband's condition somehow identifies you as well.

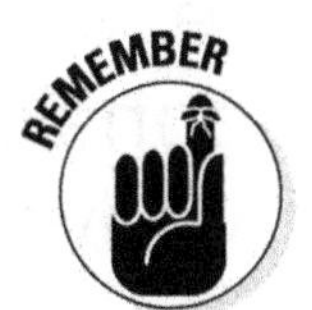

The processes of partnering in care and caregiving requires constant adjustment. Understandably you'll have days (and weeks) of exhaustion, frustration, and depression. But, interspersed will be moments of such high drama, joy, and sharing that you find the will and energy to fight on. You make an enormous difference for the PWP. The support and care you provide is vital, important work.

The danger comes when you try to do it all (or at least more than you should), and you burn out. The signs of burnout aren't that different from depression (see the earlier section, "Depression—More than just sad and blue"). Decide now to watch out for these signs and give yourself permission to take a break, hand off some of the responsibility to others, and most of all, have a life of your own.

Positive steps you can take

We recommend the following ways to help you hang in there:

- **Identify and nurture your personal support system.** You need people to be there just for you—to listen to and comfort *you.* You're dealing with a host of feelings including grief and bereavement. If you feel so isolated that you can't think of anyone to talk to, you need to consider seeking some counseling. Ask your primary care doctor to recommend a counselor, or perhaps your clergyperson is able to help.

- **Join a support group!** We can't stress this enough. The underlying cause of depression in care partners is a sense of isolation. The people you meet in a support group don't replace your best friends, but they do give you a place to vent and share PD war stories.
- **Give yourself a break**—an actual physical break—every day if possible. Use your support network to come in and take over for an hour. Take this time for yourself. Go for a walk, watch a movie, grab some coffee. Don't use your personal time for tasks like paying the bills or calling the insurance company.
- **Keep your priorities straight.** Your health is vital to the PWP, so exercise, eat a balanced diet, and

maintain your own social interactions and activities.

Chapter 14

Clinical Trials and Your Role in the Search for a Cure

In This Chapter

- Defining clinical trials
- Understanding the process
- Weighing the pros and cons of participation
- Knowing where and how to begin
- Making an informed choice about participation

It's one thing to say that a new drug or treatment works in a monkey or mouse, but it's quite another to take that next leap and declare the product safe and effective for people. Research scientists make that leap by conducting *clinical trials* (experiments) that use human volunteers.

Okay, interesting, you say, but not exactly a priority for you at the moment. But maybe it should be. Why?

Because you can make a difference—for yourself and for those who follow you down this path of Parkinson's disease (PD)—by getting involved. Want to know how? Read on.

What Is a Clinical Trial and Why Should You Care?

Clinical trials (also called *clinical research studies*) answer certain questions related to a specific health condition. They're also an important hurdle before new therapies for the treatment, management, and cure of a disease can be approved and marketed. Without such trials, therapeutic advancement is impossible. But eventually these studies require human participation. That's where you and other people living with Parkinson's disease (PWP) come in.

Recently major PD organizations have formed an alliance to build awareness of clinical trials among PWP. In addition to making more persons with PD (and their physicians) aware of clinical trials for treatments—and even a cure—these organizations offer some good reasons for participation:

- If more people living with PD volunteer to participate in a trial, the testing and marketing periods (on average 12 to 15 years) can be cut in half, a whopping 6 to 7 years shorter.
- If the testing and marketing periods can be cut, then new therapies can be available sooner and at a lower cost. (For you curious souls, the average cost to bring a single new medicine to market is approximately $800 million.)

The statistics tell their own story. According to a presentation at the 2006 World Parkinson's Congress, only 1 percent of PD patients participate in a study compared to 5 percent of the total cancer community. Although both stats seem small, the National Cancer Institute estimates that, if they can double the number of participants in clinical trials for cancer, many studies can be completed in one year (rather than the current three to five years). Simply doubling the numbers can have an enormous effect on the researchers' and the industry's ability to understand PD (its causes and course), find advanced treatments, and make those treatments available sooner.

But, before you volunteer, you need to understand how clinical trials work as well as their benefits and risks. The following sections explain this process.

Taking a Close Look at the Process

This section explains in a nutshell how the clinical trial usually unfolds. Like most topics in the world of medicine and science, the subject of clinical trials comes with its own unique vocabulary, so we clearly define each term when we introduce it.

First, to get a clinical trial underway, a team of research scientists must determine the general category of their clinical trial. Their options include

- **Interventional trials:** Scientists test experimental treatments and drugs or new ways of using existing therapies with groups of patients under controlled conditions.

- **Observational trials:** Researchers study a specific health issue (such as aging or stress) with a large group of people in their natural home, work, or community setting.

Note: In this chapter we discuss only an interventional trial, but you may participate in either type of trial for PD.

Next, the team applies for approval from an Institutional Review Board (IRB) to conduct the clinical trial. The IRB is a group of physicians, statisticians, researchers, community advocates, and others that meets independently of the research group and ensures that the trial protocol is ethical and that the rights of study participants are protected.

After the IRB approves the trial, the team follows the study's *protocol* (roadmap), which outlines the process, establishes timelines for completion of each step, and describes the profile of participants. The research team evaluates the safety and effectiveness of the trial drug, but the protocol specifies safeguards for monitoring the overall health of participants throughout the trial.

Researchers conduct studies in phases.

- Phase 1 usually tests the therapy on a small group (20 to 80) of healthy volunteers to assess potential side effects and risks.
- Phase 2 tests the therapy on a larger group of people (100 or more) who have PD and evaluates the effectiveness and side effects of the therapy.
- Phase 3 tests the therapy on at least 500 volunteers with PD and compares the new therapy with therapies currently available.

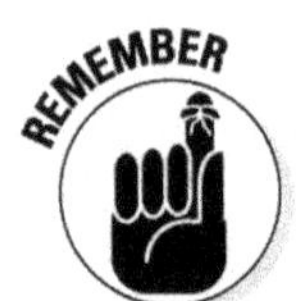

Although trials may go through several stages and take years to complete, they're still the fastest, safest way to discover and test any new treatment, medicine, and medical device before these products are available to the general public.

In every trial the research team establishes certain qualifiers for selecting participants. These are the *exclusion/inclusion guidelines* for the study. For example, the study may include people over the age of 60 but exclude anyone under that age. Or, if liver problems are known side effects of the drug, then individuals who already deal with liver problems are excluded. Criteria can cover gender, age, even weight or geographical location. Such guidelines are included in the trial's description.

After participants are selected (that's you!), they sign a document of informed consent (which we discuss in more detail later in the chapter in "Considering the Benefits and Risks Before Signing on") and are assigned to a *treatment group* (where everyone receives the same form of treatment). The study may include one group for the experimental drug, one for an existing drug that's the current preferred treatment, and one for a *placebo.*

A placebo is a medicine with no active ingredients—no way of medically effecting change either for better or worse—so your symptoms remain unchanged. (You may have heard people talk about the *placebo effect,* meaning the observed effects arise from the patient's expectations rather than from the treatment itself.) In clinical trials, researchers want to remove that placebo factor from the equation. However, as many as 30 percent of patients who receive a placebo in a trial report improvement. This result seems to be especially true in PD because the just the possibility of getting a better medicine can create the expectation of a reward and liberate *dopamine* (the chemical in your brain that controls movement). This placebo effect is one reason that research for PD is so difficult and takes so long.

In other words, trial participants usually go into one of two treatment groups: participants who receive the real treatment or drug and participants who receive a treatment that only *looks like* the real deal but doesn't have any of the active ingredients.

Double-blind studies are the preferred design for testing new therapies today because they assure objectivity throughout the study. In double-blind studies, participants don't know which treatment group they're in, and the researcher doesn't know which group is getting the test therapy. In *single-blind* studies, only the participant or the researcher (but not both) knows which group is receiving the placebo and which is taking the actual drug. In *open label* studies, both the doctor and the study subject know what drug is administered.

Clinical trial researchers must adhere to the strict standards of the Food and Drug Administration (FDA), the government bureau that monitors trials and approves research to move on to the next stage. After the trial progresses through its stages and is successful, the FDA signs off, and the new treatment (or medicine or medical device) becomes available to the general public. (There's a lot more red tape involved, but you get the gist.)

Considering the Benefits and Risks Before Signing on

By taking part in a clinical trial, you're

- Taking that proactive role that we've encouraged throughout this book.
- Gaining access to new therapies before they become available to the general public.
- Contributing to the cure for a disease that you wouldn't wish on your worst enemy.
- Getting the expert attention of scientists and healthcare professionals.

These benefits are fairly impressive but, of course, they come with risks, and those can be major. Although major risks are rare, you still need to know what you may be up against before you sign up. These are some possibilities:

- The treatment may have unforeseen side effects.
- The experimental treatment may not work for you.

- The trial may have costs associated with participating—travel to and from the trial site, for example.

Before you decide to participate in a trial (assuming you meet the needs of the study and have been invited to participate), you'll be asked to sign a document of informed consent. This document is your agreement that you've received the key information about the clinical trial (its purpose, how long it will last, what's expected of you, and the names and contact information for the research team). Your signature on this document also indicates that you're aware of the risks, potential side effects, and potential benefits of the treatment. Take your time. Talk the document over with your family, your doctor, and even your attorney to get a full picture of what you're agreeing to. ***Note:*** If the document has way too much *fine print,* ask for a *large print* version—literally and figuratively.

The informed consent is not a contract or legally binding document for you or the company/institution conducting the trial. You have the right to with-draw from the trial at any time you choose. But keep in mind that participation of people like you brings us closer to a cure—faster.

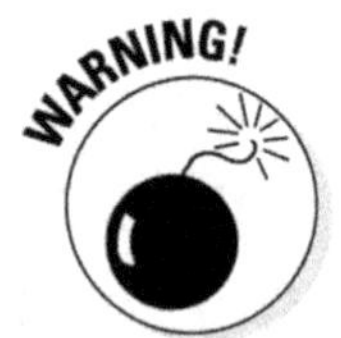

Although the informed consent is intended to protect the patient, you're still responsible for understanding all you can about the trial before agreeing to participate. You must ask the important questions such as what happens (to your body and brain) during the trial and, more importantly, what the risks are and how the team handles any adverse reaction. Answers to these questions are especially important if you're participating in a study for surgical treatment of PD.

Taking the First Steps into Volunteering

To volunteer, you first have to know where to look. Clinical trials start all the time all over the country. The key is to find a trial that's convenient for you, that's actively enrolling participants, and that you and your doctor believe may help your individual situation. Ready to get started? Read on.

Finding clinical trials for PD

The most efficient way to shop for clinical trials is the Internet. Two excellent Web sites are www.PDtrials.org and www.clinicaltrials.gov. Both sites give you important base information about locations of trials, exclusion/inclusion criteria, and other facts that can help you rule out certain studies right away. If you don't have access to a computer, ask a friend who has one to help you, or go to your local library and ask the librarian to assist you in browsing these sites.

Also you can call PD Trials at 800-801-9484 and request to be on the mailing list for periodic information and updates related to PD trials and studies.

Volunteering to participate

Volunteering to participate in a trial is not as simple as volunteering at your local library or school. Each study or trial works under a strict set of guidelines and standards, and participants must meet certain specific criteria. These restrictions assure that new therapies are tested under the most appropriate conditions to prove or disprove the study team's theories.

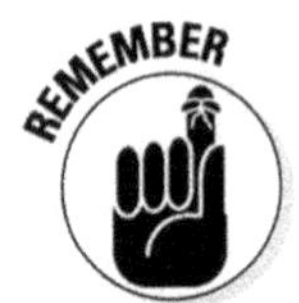

Don't get discouraged or take it personally if your application is denied. Keep trying to participate because the future of new treatments (and perhaps one day a cure) needs you!

These are the steps you need to take to be part of a clinical trial:

1. Find a trial through the resources we list earlier in this section.

2. Read the description and record the number that begins with NCT (the official assigned trial number) and all contact details.

3. Call or e-mail the contact; include any initial questions you have and request more detailed information about the study or trial.

4. Discuss your interest in volunteering for this trial with your neurologist and your family; if possible, talk with people who've participated in past clinical trials.

5. If you don't qualify for a certain trial (or the trial has the full quota of participants), ask the coordinator to stay in touch.

The trial may need more participants as it moves forward, or the contact person may become aware of other trials that better match your profile.

6. Keep a record of your calls, e-mails, and conversations, noting dates and responses. Make follow-up calls if you haven't heard back from the coordinator in a

timely manner—within two to three weeks.

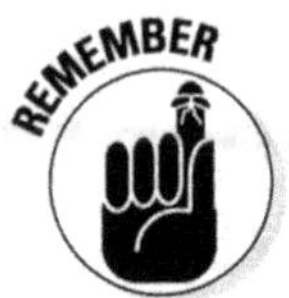

Trial coordinators are juggling many calls and details, so be patient about a reasonable response time. On the other hand, be persistent and ask when you can expect a response.

Why prescription drugs cost so much

Unless you've been living on another planet for the last decade or so, you already know that prescription medications don't come cheap. Of course, we can assume that pharmaceutical companies are not in business for the good of mankind—at least not entirely. These companies are businesses and, by definition, they want to make a profit. ("But do they need to make such a *large* profit?" you ask. The answer depends on who you ask. All we're going to say is that, in America, capitalism remains king.)

Seriously though, the journey to discover and develop new therapies for treating disease is long, costly, and fraught with uncertainties. Nearly half of all new medicines and therapies come from laboratories and clinical studies in the United States. The system may be cumbersome, but it works.

European countries often get bogged down by each country having its own approval protocol; a drug readily available in one country may be years away from approval for distribution in a neighboring country. That situation would be like taking the approval process away from the FDA in the United States and handing it over to the individual states. In that case, the drug you need may be approved for distribution in California, but you live in Maine, where it's still three years away from final approval.

Think of it this way: Every purchase has a value beyond its

dollars and cents cost. Ask yourself what the value of a new therapy for PD means to you and your family. Ask yourself the value of finding a cure. Like those ads for the credit-card company: a prescription that relieves symptoms—$xx; a new medical device that enhances movement—$xxx; a cure for PD—priceless. Keep in mind that your health and safety through the course of that journey is also priceless.

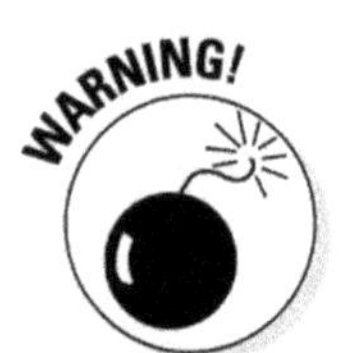

Never volunteer for a trial just because you think you may get *free* medicines because you may end up in the placebo group. And always question any trial that offers you significant monetary reward if you join. Payments for expenses and medical care are one thing; pay-outs to get you in the door are something else entirely and should raise a huge red flag. Similarly, if your doctor seems overly anxious to *sell* you the idea of participating, you need to question the doctor whether he's receiving an incentive from the trial sponsor to recruit patients.

Asking Important Questions Before Committing

An invitation to participate or an approval of your eligibility for a study doesn't obligate you to sign up. Before you make that decision, gather as much information as possible. Address your questions directly to the research team even though many of the answers are in the informed consent document (check the "Considering the Benefits and Risks Before Signing on" section earlier in this chapter for more on this document). We suggest you ask the questions in person, not over the phone or via e-mail, so you can judge for yourself exactly how on board they are with the information in the informed consent. Most people can't imagine buying a car or home without meeting the dealer or realtor face-to-face. Participating in a clinical trial can be far more important than a car or a home.

For that meeting with the team, come prepared with your questions in writing. Bring someone along to act as scribe so you can focus on listening and assessing the unspoken responses of the team. Better yet, bring along a tape recorder and record the meeting so you can play it back later as you make your decision.

In a face-to-face meeting, you want to ask:

- **What's the purpose of the study?** According to the National Institutes of Health, studies may be conducted for one or a combination of reasons:
    - Testing experimental drugs or approaches to therapy

• Testing to determine ways to prevent disease

• Testing to discover new ways of diagnosing a disease

• Testing ways of detecting a specific disease

• Testing ways that patient comfort and quality of life may be improved in chronic illness

- **Who's sponsoring the study?** Sponsorship for a clinical trial can come from a variety of sources including pharmaceutical companies, private foundations, universities and medical centers, biotech companies, or even the government. When you know the sponsor (read that as *funding source*), you can better determine whether it's a reputable and reliable source with the funds necessary to see the research through in spite of any glitches along the way.
- **Who's conducting the study?** The members of the research team should be well qualified to manage the study and safeguard the health and well being of participants during the study. Because the study team

has been approved by the IRB (see the earlier section "Taking a Close Look at the Process"), you may want to ask this question simply to better identify the role of each member.

- **Why does the research team believe the therapy or research question will be helpful or effective in the treatment or management of PD?** The answer should cover information about previous studies. Perhaps they've already tested animals; maybe researchers in another country have tested (or even used) the therapy.
- **In what ways does this therapy differ from the current treatment regimen for PD?** The answer can help you gauge whether the difference between your current therapies and the new drug or treatment is substantial enough to warrant your participation in the test.
- **What tests and treatments will be performed in the course of the study?** With this answer you

start to get specific information about their expectations of you.

- **Where will those tests and treatments be administered?** The convenience of the study site is important because you need to be there during the course of the trial. An important follow-up question is, "How often will I need to come to the site?"
- **During the study, who will be in charge of my PD care and my general healthcare?** The answer should make it crystal clear that someone is going to take charge of your general care during the trial.
- **Will hospitalization be necessary at any time during the trial?** If the answer is yes, be sure to ask about the length of stay, where you'll be hospitalized, and who'll pay the bill.
- **What are the risks—potential side effects—of the treatment or study?** One of the primary reasons for the trial is to determine the risks and side effects. Still, the team has some idea of what they anticipate, and you should know

these facts before you agree to participate.

- **How will your current treatment be affected during the trial?** You need to know whether your current medication regimen for managing your PD symptoms will be interrupted, changed, or stopped altogether during the study.
- **How long will the trial last?** Trials can last for a matter of weeks, months, or even years (usually the longer trials focus on quality-of-life issues). The research team needs to be clear about the time this study will take, but only you can decide whether the time is reasonable for you.
- **What will it cost and who will pay?** You can reasonably expect expenses directly related to the study to be covered during the course of the study. In addition, you may receive a stipend for some indirect costs, such as mileage to and from the study site. You should not expect the study to cover the costs of managing your general health. In other words, a study for

a new PD therapy probably won't include payment for that dental crown you've needed.

- **Under what circumstances would the trial or study be stopped?** Trials may be stopped for any one of several reasons. In the most serious circumstances, the government can stop a trial because side effects and risks become too common and serious. In another case, a company may halt a trial because a competing drug has been approved and is coming to market. Follow-up questions here are: "How will participants be notified if a trial is stopped?" and "What follow-up can participants expect?" For example, will there be regular (as in quarterly or annual) check-ups to see how you're doing and will you have a contact person in the event of a change in your reaction to the medication or therapy down the road?
- **After the trial's complete, will you still have access to the trial therapy if it's worked for you?** Especially if you're participating in

an early phase of the trial and the new therapy seems to make a difference for you, you want to know that you'll be able to continue taking the medicine or receiving the treatment.

- **What if you agree to participate but you change your mind after a few weeks?** You always have the right to leave a study. Ask this question to understand how your decision to leave in the middle of a study may affect the overall results.

As you collect the information and ask any follow-up questions, pay attention to details such as how they refer to you and other participants; you want to be the *patient, subject,* or *participant* and never the (heaven forbid!) *number.*

Following this interview, check with these people before you make your final decision about volunteering:

- Your doctor(s) to discuss the potential benefits and risks of participation.
- Your family to discuss any reservations they may have.

- Your attorney to review the document of informed consent.

As you weigh your decision, remember that you're a key stakeholder in this process. Don't be a passive participant; instead, take your place at this table as an equal player. The research team may have the degrees and fancy titles, but you're the key to that treasure—finding new and more effective therapies for PD and, one day, its cure.

Part IV

Living Well with PD

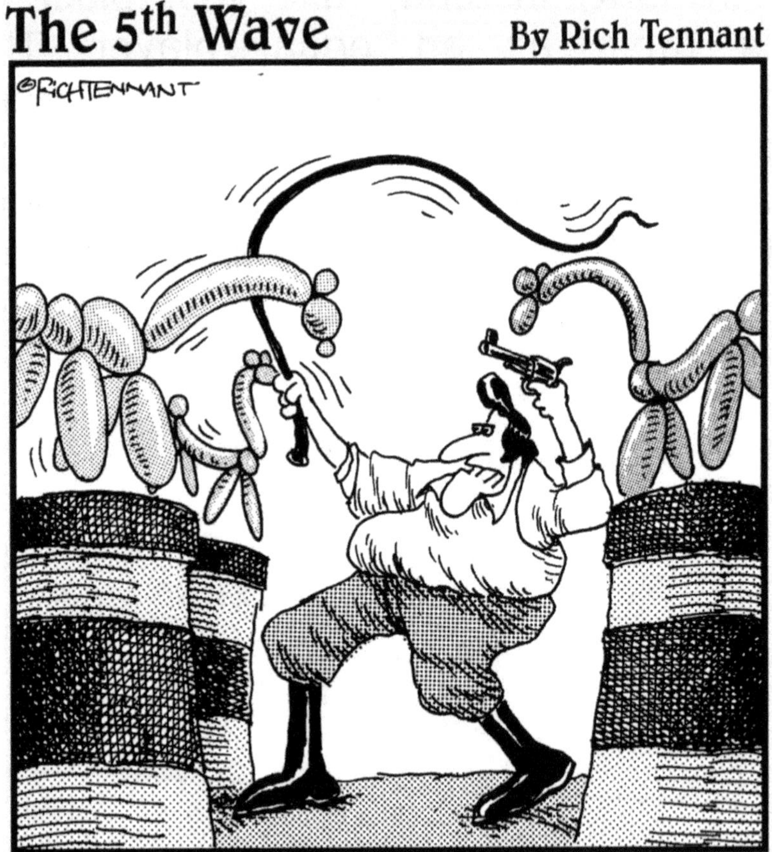

Attempting to reduce the stress in his life to help his Parkinson's disease, Waldo 'Whip' Gunschott goes from being a wild animal trainer to a wild balloon animal trainer.

In This part...

Having Parkinson's disease may well change your lifestyle, but it doesn't have to be a life sentence. In this section we explore ways that you can maintain the relationships and activities that give your life meaning and purpose. We also pass along ideas on the best ways to manage your PD on the job. Last but not least, we take a look at adapting and adjusting to the changes that a progressive condition can bring.

Chapter 15

Maintaining Healthy Relationships

In This Chapter

- Renewing your relationship with your significant other
- Keeping kids—young and old, near and far—in the loop
- Maintaining close ties with the grandchildren
- Accepting help from your first family
- Letting friends be friends
- Keeping your sense of self

Your relationships with family and friends (as well as those you'll create with healthcare professionals, support group members, and others along this journey) can hold the key to successfully managing your Parkinson's disease (PD) symptoms over the long haul. In sharp contrast, shutting yourself off from people or permitting those who have loved and supported you to drift away can only make matters worse—for you and for them.

But your relationships will change. The shifts you see in balance and roles will be healthy for and vital to maintaining a full, productive life. In this chapter, we take a more in-depth look at these key relationships. After seeing how your PD can affect each of these relationships, we offer suggestions for bringing those relationships back in line so that you (and the other people) understand that your bond hasn't changed just because you have PD.

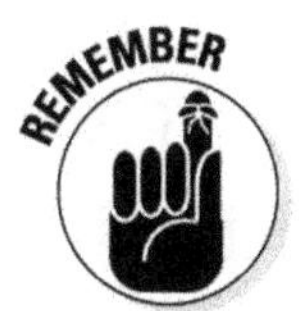

Normal is a relative term in life. With any luck, it includes the people and activities that bring satisfaction and contentment to your days. But having PD doesn't mean you need to start from scratch on a new definition of *normal*—the fundamentals are still there. Although you do need to get creative as you adapt your routines to PD, you don't need to abandon those people and activities that brought you happiness before your diagnosis.

Life, PD, and Your Significant Other

Your relationship with your significant other is likely your most important and cherished relationship. This person is the one you can trust with your deepest (and sometimes most unpleasant) feelings and thoughts; who'll be there in spite of your anger, fear, and bouts of self-pity; who'll laugh with you when your performance of some task borders on the ridiculous. This person is the one who'll act as your advocate when speaking for yourself is difficult, who'll remind you that you both have lives outside of PD, and who'll affirm that you're the same person you always were. This person is your primary care partner and, perhaps one day, your caregiver.

Sharing the journey

When one partner in a relationship gets a diagnosis of PD, that diagnosis may seem to be for both of you. Both lives will be affected every day. But how the two of you face that fact and prepare for the inevitable changes can be the difference between strengthening your relationship and straining it to the breaking point. The good news is that for most couples, facing a challenge like PD as partners actually strengthens the relationship.

If this relationship is new and relatively untested by life's normal challenges, be sure each of you knows what living with PD will likely mean. And if the relationship is longstanding but was beginning to show signs of wear and tear before the diagnosis, both of you need to face that at the outset.

Sharing the PD journey is bound to put an extra strain on the relationship—at least part of the time. In either case (that is, new but untested or established but shaky), seek the counsel of a trusted and objective third party before leaping into full-blown care-partner mode. If it's not a good fit with your significant other, you need to discuss what role your partner can manage and then decide who else in the family or close circle (perhaps an adult child, sibling, or extremely good friend) can step up.

When you get the confirmed diagnosis (see Chapter 5), each of you needs time to digest the news and react. And the first reaction for one or both of you may be denial. Or maybe your partner will become overprotective and treat you as if you're gravely ill. Underneath your partner may first feel cheated out of the life you had planned and then angry at such a selfish thought when you're the one facing a debilitating illness. Financial concerns may pop up; your partner may wonder about the costs and sacrifices involved.

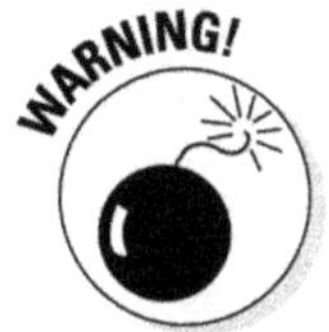

Neither you nor your partner may admit any of these feelings initially. Big mistake. (Again, check out Chapter 5 for more specific information about the pitfalls of the early days after diagnosis.)

Warning! Trouble ahead!

After you've both had time to let the diagnosis sink in, you need to prepare to face some common pitfalls that can result when one partner has PD and the other remains healthy. Here are three of the most common:

- **Changes in the dynamics of your partnership:** With PD in the equation, roles can shift. For example, now that you have PD, your wife's job is more important than ever because your health insurance is through her employer. Understand that this puts added stress on your partnership. Not only is she facing a new role as your care partner, but she's also facing the stress of performing her best at work so her job (and that vital insurance) is secure.

At the same time, your traditional role as the head of the house and breadwinner (if you bring home the larger paycheck) is also stressed. You both need that paycheck, but how will your PD affect your ability to perform at work and for how long? (See Chapter 16 for a full discussion of PD in the workplace.) Your best bet is to prepare for such role changes by talking them through—with a counselor if necessary.

- **Co-dependency (not a good thing):** Co-dependency occurs when your care partner is more invested in managing your PD than you are. The danger here lies in your partner abandoning major pieces of his own life in order to take control of the situation, to fulfill what he perceives to be your needs and wishes. When his perception and your needs don't jive, resentment quickly follows.

He resents doing his best but not being appreciated (plus he's surrendering pieces of his own life to offer you this unappreciated gift!). You resent fighting as hard as you can to maintain independence and autonomy, and you feel guilty for adding to your partner's anxiety and frustration by refusing—however gently—to accept his solutions.

- **"But everyone else manages so well" syndrome:** Remember Jackie Kennedy after the assassination of JFK? In the face of this unspeakable personal tragedy, she held a nation's hand through the sheer force of her grace, courage, attention to detail, and devotion to her children.

Spousal care partners may remind you of Jackie Kennedy and her remarkable achievements. These men and women seem to do it all—and do it with style. She works full-time, cooks, cleans, does the yard work, manages the finances, provides the most complex level of personal care for her partner, deals with the professionals, and maintains an active family and social life. And the most annoying part is that she does it all with an aura of serenity and calm that's intimidating to say the least.

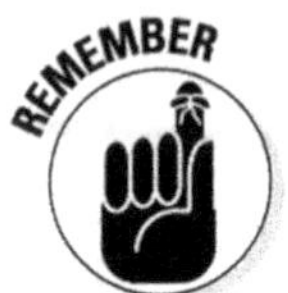

Beneath the most serene surface lie whirlpools of unspeakable pain, anxiety, and even anger and resentment at the havoc PD is wreaking. Even Jackie Kennedy's calm façade cracked behind closed doors. Just like super-partner, you and your partner do your best and that's more than enough in most cases to sustain the partnership during this difficult time.

The next section offers a couple of concrete suggestions for avoiding the pitfalls and getting on with living life.

Avoiding the pitfalls

In any life-partner relationship, certain passages come with the territory: transitions, such as children growing up and going on to lives (and families) of their own; lifestyle changes, like a bigger house, a better job, retirement, and downsizing; and tough times, great times, chaotic times, and calm times. Through it all, you and your partner have formed your own unique ways of managing each passage. Now you face life with PD. It's one more challenge—but a big one, and one that'll affect the rest of your lives.

Here are two keys to avoiding the pitfalls in your partnership while managing the stresses and strains of living with PD:

- **Communication and caring=coping:** You'll both have times when you struggle to adapt to the changes caused by PD. Your partner may feel stressed by all the extra responsibility. As the PWP, you may be depressed and anxious for good reason. Take time to talk it out, to state your needs, to listen to your partner's concerns—even if you can't immediately solve the problem. If you're seeing a counselor to manage depression and anxiety (see Chapter 13), ask that person for tips for improving communications during especially stressful times.

- **Mutual respect—the foundation of successful relationships:** Think about all the reasons the two of you teamed up in the first place. You loved her bubbly outgoing personality—so different from your shy, quiet demeanor. She loved your take-charge-in-a-crisis style. The activities that gave you individual identities also strengthened you as a couple. You aren't clones; you complement (complete) each other. Now one of you has PD and the other has been cast in this new role of care partner. Just as you adapted in the past (when the kids came along or one of you changed jobs), you can do that again.

Few relationships remain stagnant (at least those that survive and thrive don't). So chances are good that the dynamics of your partnership would have changed and shifted whether or not you had PD. So, don't permit yourself (or your partner) to stress out about the possible changes you'll face as the years pass. And for heaven's sake, don't allow PD to keep you from enjoying the intimacy that comes with living in a loving partnership.

Keeping the magic alive—Sex and intimacy in spite of PD

For some couples, one of the most challenging shifts can come in the area of intimacy. You and your partner can either surrender to a loss in this area or you can get creative and find new ways to share your love.

Humans take a certain amount of pride in their physical, mental, and even emotional attractiveness. The diagnosis of a lifelong, debilitating condition can play havoc with a person's sense of self, and it can be especially devastating for his or her sense of sexuality. The relationship you may have enjoyed with your significant other for years—even decades—suddenly comes under question. Can I adequately satisfy the needs of this person I love? Is this person humoring me by pretending that nothing's changed? Why don't I feel like being intimate even though I love this person? Doesn't this person deserve a *whole* lover?

Okay, just stop it. Take a moment to get the facts before you leap to unfounded (and, in some cases, unnecessary) conclusions. These are the facts:

- When sexual needs and desires change, the root cause usually responds to medication or other therapy. Check first with your primary care physician to see whether the cause is treatable.
- If the change comes on the heels of the diagnosis—well, duh! You just got some tough and depressing news. Talk about a mood crasher!
- As a matter of fact, depression and anxiety may well be symptoms of

your PD (see Chapter 13), so your sexual concerns may result from the disease itself. And what about those prescription meds for depression? Read the label. Most likely they list sexual dysfunction as a side effect.

- Certainly people with PD may experience performance anxiety, given the facts that PD is a movement disorder, and good sex often involves coordination and flexibility.
- Women's fluctuating hormone balance in the perimenopausal years can affect desire. Women with PD should be sure their gynecologist and neurologist work together to regulate hormone replacement and antiparksonian medications.
- Unfortunately the effects of PD can play havoc with self-image. The *mask* (inability to show facial expression) is one example. Struggling to manage basic grooming (shaving your legs, styling your hair, putting on make-up) can also make a woman feel less than desirable.

- If you're male, you may experience episodes of erectile dysfunction—another sideshow of PD—because the brain needs to work with the body for you to maintain an erection.

So what to do? Well, you don't want to ignore any problem that may have a solution. And sexual dysfunction is one of them. Let your doctor know because treatments are available. For example, if depression is behind your change in sexual interest, counseling may be the answer.

And for both your sakes, talk to your partner. Your partner may be having problems as well. For example, when faced with a loved one's diagnosis, some partners leap light years ahead to the day (that may never come) when the loved one can't function at all. As a result, your partner goes into serious protection mode and tries to avoid any activity that he or she thinks may cause you more stress (and that includes sexual relations).

Yes, you and your partner may need to explore new ways of being intimate. Gee—experiment with new ways to kiss, to hold each other, to touch, to.... Sounds like a good thing!

Retaining personal space for each of you

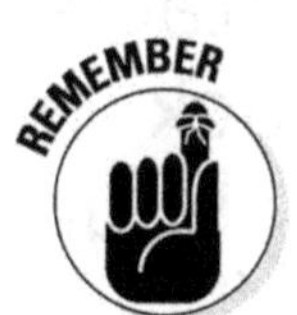

Receiving a diagnosis of PD may draw the two of you even closer together, but don't make the mistake of abandoning your individual activities and contacts. As much as you love and cherish each other, you still need some personal space from time to time. The richness of relationships is often rooted in the fact that each has interests (and friends) that are unique.

> You may share news about these activities and people with each other, but you both accept that this is *my* activity or *my* friend and that's okay.

In these early weeks, you have a lot to take in (tests, doctor's appointments, therapy sessions, and such). But if your partner has enjoyed a weekly card game or volunteer activity for years and hasn't been able to get back to it for months now, this is a problem. And *you* need to lead by example. Take stock of those individual activities and contacts you've let slide and get them back on your calendar. Then insist that your partner do the same.

A second time that you and your partner are in danger of surrendering your personal space occurs when your PD symptoms become more troublesome. As your need for assistance and care escalates, your partner may become so entrenched in caring for you that her own physical, mental, and emotional well-being is jeopardized. Make it your job to prevent that problem from happening. Prepare in advance for ways each of you can protect your life beyond PD. This strategy isn't an act of selfishness; in the long run, this separateness can bring the two of you closer and enrich the life you share. (Check out Chapter 23 for more ways to care for your care partner.)

PD and Kids—Adult or Younger

For people with Parkinson's (PWP) who have children, the change in your relationships will depend in part on the age of your children. A person with young onset PD (see Chapter 8) may have very young children. But if your PD was diagnosed later in life, your children may have children of their own (your grandchildren) who will also need your attention. Regardless of their age, children can become confused or alarmed when they hear that a parent has PD. Some of that initial response comes from a knowledge base (or lack of one) about PD and its progression. And some of the response can be normal self-concern about life changes now that a parent is ill. In either case, you need to reassure your children and include them as you and your care partner make decisions that may affect their lives.

Addressing their fears about the future

"What if they need to use my college savings fund for Mom's medical bills?"

"I thought we'd have more time before I needed to be there for my parents."

You and your significant other need to discuss early on how to deliver the news of your diagnosis to your children (see Chapter 7). After you tell them, look for obvious and not-so-obvious reactions, such as withdrawal or slipping grades when she was an honor student before the diagnosis. If you see mood changes (such as increased irritability) or personality changes (your little extrovert suddenly becomes quite the introvert), talk it out. You may consider taking your preteen and teenage children with you to the next neurologist's appointment so they can raise their own questions. Or consider going with your child for some talk therapy with a counselor.

Regardless of your children's ages, your positive outlook and sense of humor will go a long way toward reassuring them that life won't change much just because you have PD. As time goes by (years—not weeks) and the PD becomes more difficult to control, your children will adapt with you.

In the following sections, we give you some tips on discussing your PD with your children, both young and adult.

When your children are young

If your children are very young (under age 10), keep your information simple. But if young children ask questions or change their normal behavior toward you, then those concerns need your attention. Just be careful not to blow problems out of proportion. For example, your child's very simple concern, "Can I catch Parkinson's like a cold?" may have an easy answer, "No."

Middle-schoolers (ages 10 to 13) need a more direct approach. Kids today can get a lot of information through the Internet. The problem is when they check sites that scare or worry them. Consider giving these children an assignment; put them in charge of staying on top of and reporting the PD e-news from the trusted sites listed in Appendix B. A specific assignment like this can help a child feel a part of the solution. It's vital that you avoid allowing children of any age feel as if they're being kept in the dark.

Teenagers (ages 14 to 19) are fully capable of participating in a family discussion (see Chapter 7) and plan of action for managing household changes. When included from the beginning, teens are more likely to take ownership and responsibility for additional chores or tasks. Whenever you and your partner reassess the plan and discuss necessary changes, include your teen.

A great way to empower children who are struggling with a parent's illness is to encourage them to raise funds for a national organization that's searching for a cure. Maybe your child can participate in a run or bike ride and ask for donations. How about a lemonade stand? Kids like action. Help them take an active (and proactive) role to raise awareness or money for research.

When your children are adults

Adult children may live at home, nearby, or miles away. They may be single, married, have children of their own, have promising and demanding careers, be in college or graduate school, or have a combination of these. The point is that they've moved on (even if they're still in your house) into lives of their own. You're a part of that life but not in the way when they were younger.

After your diagnosis, chances are good that your adult children feel (even if you don't) the roles have shifted; they may now consider taking care of you instead of the other way round. Such ideas can make for some interesting relational conflicts. Your best tactic is to clearly demonstrate through words, actions, and—most of all—attitude that you do need their support and concern but you're still fully capable of deciding how you'll live with PD.

If you don't ask, they won't help

Maybe your natural instinct as a parent is to protect your kids from worrying about you. If you constantly respond to your children's concern with, "We're doing fine," then don't be upset when your kids take that at face value and get on with their lives. But here's a news flash—they're probably worrying anyway *and* frustrated that you won't let them help. Give them a chance to help by stating your needs! (Check out Chapter 7 for more on this step.) The worst result is that you'll be disappointed by the reaction. The best result is that your child steps up to the plate and delivers a solid hit by taking on some chore, visiting more often, or bringing the grandkids to see you more often.

When they live nearby

Adult children who live nearby can be a blessing for you and your care partner—especially when your PD progresses and you can use a little more help. Establish some new family traditions, like potluck or ordered-in dinners once a week for you, the kids, and grandkids. This ritual can

- Help your children and grandchildren adapt to the impact of your symptoms on your normal life
- Open the door to the more intense regular contact down the road

Because PD tends to progress slowly, you'll probably read the signs that your symptoms are getting worse. (For example, your meds may not work as well and routine tasks become a struggle.) When you recognize these new limits on your abilities, consider a family meeting (see Chapter 10).

The following suggestions can help you in that meeting:

- Offer specific ways your adult children (and older grandchildren) can pitch in.
- Clearly demonstrate that you appreciate their busy schedules.
- Start small. For example, can your grandson cut the lawn? Can your daughter cook up a casserole once a month for the freezer?

Ask yourself whether you would have been willing to commit to this responsibility when you were your kids' ages. Would you have cheerfully taken on additional weekly tasks? Would you have put this ahead of everything else on your schedule? If the answer to these questions is "No," then perhaps your ideas about what and how much responsibility your children can handle is overly optimistic. Far better to start out with smaller, less time-consuming tasks such as loading the dishwasher or taking out the garbage and then add more responsibility as time (and your PD) progress.

The goal: Involve your adult children almost from the beginning so that, as your needs escalate, they are already a part of the routine. Be sure you include them in the decisions and planning. Ask for their opinion and input. The decision is ultimately yours, but including your children in the discussion permits them to feel a vital and valued part of the whole process.

If some adult children live nearby and some live farther away, don't take the assistance of nearby children for granted. In many families, visits from far-away kids and grandkids are a cause for celebration, but in-town children who provide regular hands-on help (at some personal sacrifice) also need to feel appreciated. Call your in-town daughter specifically for the purpose of thanking her after she's rearranged her schedule to do something for you. Comment on how much you appreciate something specific that each of your children (in-town and out-of-town) does for you when you're all together.

When they're far away

Adult children who live far away may suffer some guilt from not being available. When they visit, you may want to plan some major project (changing the storms and screens, cleaning the basement, or painting the kitchen) so they become a part of that hands-on care routine. You want them to realize that they're not your guests—they're your children. Even though they can only offer sporadic hands-on help, you still need them to come through for you and your care partner.

Be sure to include these adult children in family meetings and conferences (even if only by e-mail or phone). Ask for their input and include them as you come to a decision. In short, distance can shut down lines of communication even with today's cell phones, computers, and such. Make a personal commitment to keep all your adult children in the loop. They need to hear your news, including major decisions or changes, from you (or your care partner)—not from a sibling.

PD and Grandchildren

Your first step with your grandchildren is to consult with their parents before you talk with them about your PD. How do the parents want you to handle their children's questions? What have the parents told your grandchildren already, and how did they tell them? After you know those answers, show your grandchildren through your interactions that nothing has really changed. You are still Grandma or Grandpa. Keep your routine with them as normal as possible.

If you've played games or gone apple-picking with them in the past, keep that up. If those tasks aren't possible for you now, find new activities. Perhaps make a game of doing your exercises with your grandchild. Or go to the apple farm and buy the apples, bring them home, and make applesauce with your grandchildren. Most of all, reassure them with simple but honest answers to their questions, and let their parents know whether you see signs that your grandchildren are holding questions or concerns inside.

Children are wise beyond their years and extraordinarily tuned in to the moods and vibes of the adults in their world. They may not fully understand what's going on, but they know when you're upset, sad, depressed, or angry. And more often than not, they mistakenly think they're to blame or that your mood has something to do with them.

We're not suggesting you fake a happy-go-lucky attitude around the young ones. But don't sell them short. You're the adult here. You know when your frustration causes you to lash out or withdraw. Pay attention to your reactions and to the reactions of the child you're with and speak up. "Sorry I snapped at you. Sometimes I just get so frustrated when I can't do the things I used to do. Do you ever feel sad like that?" Now you've opened the door to a dialogue with the child and perhaps to a conversation that can reveal some of their own angst about your PD.

Children and grandchildren of all ages can be good medicine. Their curiosity and sense of adventure can be contagious in a good way. Their belief that they're indestructible and immortal can be inspiring. The way that kids pack 40 hours of activity and energy into a single day can serve as an important reminder: This is the day we get—live it or lose it!

PD and Parents and Siblings

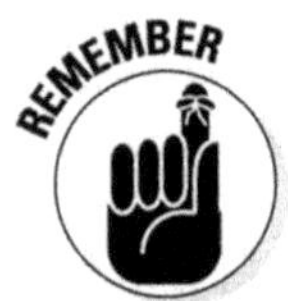

If you have children of your own, you realize that nothing's as terrible as discovering that your child has an incurable and progressive condition. Regardless of your age, you will always be your parent's child.

If the parent-child relationship is such that you can confide in your parent, allow your parent to play the role of mentor and counselor as you face this new challenge. Seek advice for balancing the demands of PD with your other life responsibilities. A good way to start this discussion is to remind your parents of difficult challenges they've faced over the course of their lives.

However, if your parents are more emotionally fragile and thrown by the news of your illness, your role may become one of reassuring them rather than relying on them. But, because you really don't need more emotional responsibility at this time, consider asking a sibling to reassure Mom and Dad. This arrangement can be especially helpful if your brothers or sisters are looking for ways they can offer you support and tangible help.

Considering parents and siblings, remember that you have a longstanding history with these people. If you never could please your mother or if your brother always had to live up to your example, those facts have colored the way your family interacts. Don't make the mistake of expecting the foundations of your relationships to magically change simply because you have PD.

Over the course of your life each of you has found ways to adapt to those unique interactions. Perhaps you handle your Mom's apparent disappointment in you by simply enduring her comments and moving on. Good choice. Likewise your brother's sense of insecurity (and inferiority) is his issue—not yours. Be sympathetic but understand that he's no more likely to step up now than he has before.

If your sister or brother becomes your primary care partner, the two of you need ground rules about the relationship just as if your care partner were your spouse or significant other. For example:

- You both need to acknowledge and then set aside the familial roles you may have assumed throughout childhood. For example, if she always played the big sister role and you followed her lead, that relationship needs to change. The way you choose to handle life with PD is your decision, and she needs to be willing to follow your lead.
- You both need to face the fact that you're adults, which means you've

probably gone in different directions philosophically and may have different approaches to a variety of issues.

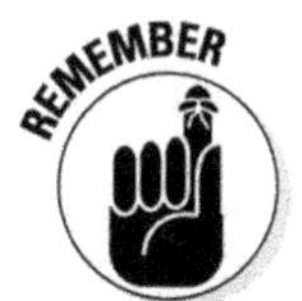

Having said that, you need to focus on the reasons having your sister as your care partner makes sense: She brings strengths to the table that you counted on when the two of you were growing up. You've chosen her for those strengths. She's agreed because your history tells her that she can work with you the same way the two of you faced challenges together as children.

For people diagnosed with young onset PD (see Chapter 8), the chances are very good that your parents are still living. If your parents' health is compromised and you're providing some care for them, you and your care partner need to consider how best to incorporate your dual role as adult child with PD and caregiver for aging parents into an already busy life.

PD and Close Friends

No matter what your friendships are like, there's nothing like a chronic, progressive, and eventually debilitating condition for sorting out friends who'll be there from those who'll eventually drift away. And discovering who's who in this process is usually surprising. The guy you thought would be there no matter what may not handle the idea that you can't enjoy the vigorous sports activities the two of you have always shared. Even though you assure him that it may be years before that happens, he doesn't hear you. Meanwhile a co-worker you've always seen as a casual acquaintance (nice to have a beer with after work and such) steps up, intuitively understanding how to be helpful but not intrusive for you or your care partner.

The following suggestions help you make this transition with your friends as smooth as possible:

• **Tell it like it is:** Friends may want to help but don't know how. And, like everyone else, they'll take their lead from you. If you repeatedly assure them that everything's fine and reject their efforts to understand PD and figure out how to help, then shame on you. And if you shut them out with self-pity, depression, and a nobody-can-help attitude, don't be surprised when they drift away.

It's all in how you look at it

At the foundation of your ability to maintain healthy relationships is your ability to maintain a healthy sense of self. With respect to PD, you certainly have an impressive roster of celebrities to emulate (Muhammad Ali and Michael J. Fox to name the most obvious). But, to understand the importance of this sense-of-self on a personal level, go to a PD support group meeting and look around.

Joan sits over there in a corner. Diagnosed two years ago, her symptoms are well controlled with medication. Yet Joan is always looking for the downside; her conversations project a dire future. She likes to report disastrous cases, like the person who fell, hit his head, and became demented almost overnight. (Take this opportunity to move on as quickly as possible!)

You notice Charlie in another part of the room. He's had PD for over a decade. His hand shakes uncontrollably at times, he has trouble swallowing, and you have to lean in close to hear him. But you discover that he still runs his own business, attends social functions with his wife, and is an active volunteer in the fight to find a cure for PD. He's telling a story about his latest doctor's visit:

"Doc asked whether I had vivid dreams ... and whether I was in my dreams," he says. "I told him I was in my dreams, and I didn't have PD—just me moving freely with no tremor."

You ask Charlie what the doctor said about that and Charlie replies, "He said I must have one whopper of a positive outlook!"

You can be Joan, you can be Charlie, or you can be someone in between. The choice is yours. No doubt Charlie has his bad days. But how he's chosen to get through those days is worth finding out.

• **Treat me the same:** Okay, you don't want to lose your friends, but you also don't want them treating you any different. Tell them that. Be open to their questions. Give them the facts. Seriously consider their suggestions for treatments, doctors, and such before you reject them out of hand. Let your friends know you'll have good days and bad. And then decide together how they can best support you.

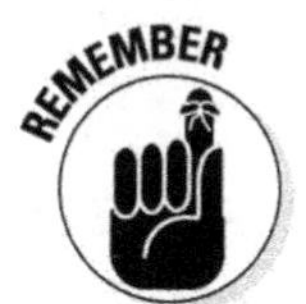

• **Lend me an ear:** Friends are terrific at playing the role of confidante for you and your care partner. And, by the way, we hope you and your care partner have one really good friend (not the same one!) that you can trust to hear you vent, whine, and feel sorry for yourself now and again.

• **Know their strong suits:** Recognize that some people are good listeners and counselors and others need to offer hands-on help. Surely you know these folks well enough to know the difference. So when the inevitable question of "What can I do to help?" arises, be prepared with concrete and specific ideas—just as you try to with your children and other family members.

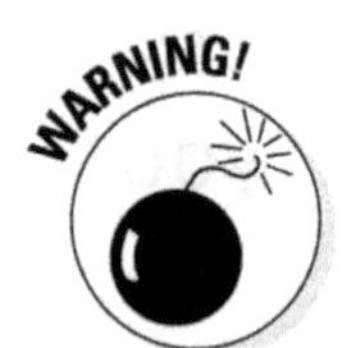

• **Keep a balance:** Beware of accepting too much help. Some people (friends and family) may start strong, practically smothering you with their help. But the odds are good that these people will over-promise and under-deliver, eventually burning out. By the same token, the more you permit other people to do for you—especially early on—the less you push yourself to remain active and independent for as long as possible.

And Then There's YOU

Having Parkinson's is a life-changing situation—one that will continue to affect you for the rest of your days. But are you a PD patient, or are you still the same active, involved, in-charge person you were before you had PD? You can choose to allow a diagnosis of PD to dominate your daily routine even in the early stages or you can take the proactive approach—doing what it takes to adapt PD to your lifestyle.

Consider these two questions: How many hours do you average each workweek? Between what times do those hours occur? For most people, the answer to the first question is between 40 and 60 hours, and the second answer is between 8 a.m. and 6 p.m. So, one way to look at adapting PD is to focus on those daytime hours and how to use them in meaningful ways.

Although you certainly can't schedule your PD symptoms, the basic idea of adapting PD to fit your lifestyle has some merit. You're still the same person you were before you got diagnosed. Your life's activities may need to change over time—just as they do for everyone with or without PD. But for now, your normal routine is probably still viable.

As a matter of fact, you may be able to get back to some activities you had dropped when your PD symptoms went untreated. Perhaps your stiffness and slowness can be partially relieved through physical therapy and a regular exercise routine (see Chapter 12). Maybe those feelings of anxiety, persistent sadness, and depression that you thought were job-related are treatable with therapy and counseling (see Chapter 13). And maybe your hand tremor can be managed with medication (see Chapter 9).

The point is that you and those around you had a life before you were diagnosed, and you still have that life. You may have to accept changes, but your ability to participate in those activities that gave your life purpose and meaning are still possible.

Chapter 16

PD in the Workplace

In This Chapter

- Get ready, get set: Understanding your work potential
- Timing is everything
- Approaching your boss with the news
- Checking in with Human Resources
- Getting the right word out to co-workers
- Tapping into private and government programs that can help

Adapting to life with Parkinson's disease (PD) works best when you can partner with other people. We hope you're already partnering with your healthcare team (see Chapter 6) and your primary care partner (along with your family and friends—see Chapter 15). The third angle of this partnering triangle is your partnership with your employer and co-workers, a relationship that permits you to stay on the job and takes into account your employer's need to run the business effectively. In this chapter, we offer some ideas for delivering the news and building the workplace version of that team-oriented partnership.

Don't assume that our suggestions are exactly right for your situation. Every employer-employee relationship is unique, just as your PD is different from other people's PD. You know the specific climate that surrounds your work-place, and only you can decide the best approach for telling your employer that you have PD.

Doing Your Homework

If there's one message we pound home in this book, it's this: Your best course of action in all facets of managing your PD is to prepare, prepare, and then prepare some more.

That advice is never more true than when you're about to tell your employer that you have a chronic and progressive condition. And those words are exactly (and probably only) what your boss is likely to hear. Therefore your job is to prepare to fight that misperception with every resource you can muster.

Before you tell your employer, you have homework—and yes, we do mean you! In broad strokes (with details to follow), here are your assignments:

- Put together an honest assessment of your position requirements and whether or not you can continue to fulfill them.
- Discuss your job responsibilities with your neurologist and get a medical evaluation of your ability to perform those duties.
- Research what the company can offer to accommodate your changing needs and has offered other employees in the past (such as a different workstation configuration or a flexible schedule so you can work when your symptoms are well managed or work from home).

- Familiarize yourself with options that may be available through the Americans with Disabilities Act (ADA) or other government programs.

Honestly assess your ability to continue in the job

Before you start spreading the news that you have PD to your boss and co-workers, decide how and if you'll be able to continue working. To do this, you first need a clear understanding of your job requirements and performance demands. You and your neurologist both need this information so you can honestly assess your ability to continue in the job as your PD progresses. For example, if your job requires fine hand-work and you already have a significant tremor in one hand, you can't ignore this problem.

Keep in mind that PD progresses at different rates for different people and neither you nor your doctor can really predict its course. However, two ways to acquire the information you and your doctor need in order to make the best possible assessment are:

- Reviewing the written job description from when you were hired
- Taking advantage of recent or upcoming performance review sessions where your employer restates the expectations and requirements of the position

If you didn't receive a printed job description or your next performance review isn't in the near future, then consider asking for an informal conversation with your supervisor—especially if she's not the same person who hired you. Her expectations for your performance may not be the same as your former supervisor's were. Keep the meeting informal and conversational. If you say something like, "I wonder whether you'd give me a written, detailed description of my position," you're going to raise all sorts of red flags (especially if you've been working there for some time already).

If you have no job description and can't have a chat with your immediate supervisor, take time to think through the tasks required of you—physical, mental, and emotional (stress-related). Be as specific as possible.

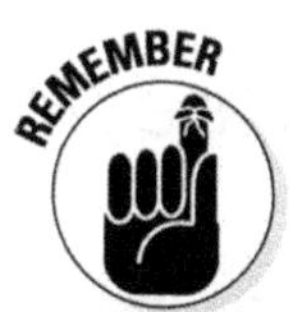

This is the time—*before* you sit down with your supervisor to deliver the news that you have PD—to be brutally honest. For now, no one else is asking these questions or listening to your answers. But if you try and fudge the answers when you know your PD's already making some tasks difficult, you're only harming yourself.

Ask yourself the following questions:

- Do you have a desk job, a manufacturing job, or something more physical?
- How many hours a week are you scheduled?
- How much overtime or work at home do you typically have in a week?
- What are the physical demands of the job (Standing most of the time? Sitting at a computer? Moving around—perhaps teaching small children—much of the workday? Traveling? Needing fine motor control?)
- What are the mental demands of the job? (Quick decisions? Complex problem-solving? Coordinating the efforts of several other people?)
- What are the stressors of the job? (Bottom line expectations of employer? Deadlines? Balancing several projects at the same time?)
- What are the emotional challenges of the job? (Supervisor is in over his head, making your job harder? Working in healthcare with patients who are ill or infirm? Balancing the demands of your job with your role

as a spouse or parent and your PD symptoms?)

- And finally, do you see your schedule getting less intense? More intense?

At your next appointment with your neurologist, discuss your job requirements and how to adapt your PD symptoms—those you're experiencing now and those that are most likely to occur over the next year or so—to the demands of the job (and vice versa). Take notes. If you think your employer may have safety concerns but your doctor indicates that you can continue the job, ask your doctor for a letter stating that you're capable of performing the tasks in question.

Consider options that may be available

Depending on the size of your company, you may have an entire list of options to help you stay on the job and perform effectively—or you may have no options at all. If you work for a larger company, your employer may be able to offer flexible hours, job-sharing, working from home one or two days a week, or a reduced workload (which, of course, may have a reduction in pay).

But even the small business owner may still have some options. For example, if you work in a restaurant that's busiest at breakfast and lunch, your employer has little leeway for adapting your hours. But is it possible for you to work a later shift when the restaurant has fewer customers to serve?

Think outside the box. Your employer's not the only one responsible for devising options for you. The employee who needs to be on the job by seven but struggles with getting up, dressed and out the door in time to meet that start time may need to get up an hour earlier and talk to his doctor about adjusting the timing on his medication routine to accommodate his early morning start time.

If you work for a larger company, you probably received an employee hand-book as a part of your new hire information. As part of preparing to tell your boss about your diagnosis, dig this employee handbook out and read it. Better yet, go to the company's internal Web site and get the latest version. If your company (or the company your care partner works for) provides group insurance for employees, read those policies. Make notes so that in the meeting with your boss (and eventually the person from Human Resources, HR) you have a firm understanding of the company's policies regarding special accommodations or coverage for short- or long-term disability.

Deciding When to Disclose Your Diagnosis

Although PD is progressive, it isn't one of those you've-got-six-months-to-live situations. You have some time to tell your employer about your PD. On the other hand, you also want to choose the best time for your specific situation. We help you make that all-important decision in this section.

From your perspective

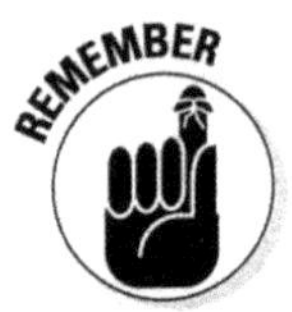

Only you can decide the appropriate time to tell your employer. The goal is to minimize the fallout from sharing this kind of news.

Consider the effects of these two scenarios:

- You rush in to your boss's office within days of the diagnosis and announce that you have PD.
- You withhold the news until your symptoms become more difficult to control and begin to affect your performance.

In the first case, the danger lies in your employer (and co-workers) viewing you *and* your performance differently. In other words, well before your PD symptoms have any effect on your ability, other people may perceive a problem and attribute it to your PD. Inadvertently you may be labeled and pigeon-holed (possibly passed over for a better position) because of other people's misperceptions.

In the second scenario, you may think you're controlling your symptoms, but your news comes as no surprise to your employer or co-workers. If your boss has been aware of a change in your performance for some time, she may wonder why you took so long to come forward. Worse, if facial *mask* (lack of facial expression) is one of your symptoms, she may have interpreted that symptom as disinterest or apathy and then attributed the decline in your performance to that misinterpretation.

If your supervisor has expressed concern about your recent job performance (via questions like "Is everything all right?" or "How's everything going at home?" or even at a more formal review of your performance), that's a good hint that he's concerned about you and the work he needs from you.

Depending on your job, it may be years before your PD has any real impact. In the meantime, make use of the initial days and weeks following your diagnosis to accept that you have PD and that it's going to be a factor in every facet of your life, including your work. (See Chapter 5 for more specific ideas on getting through those first weeks after diagnosis.)

If you know that safety will eventually become an issue, stay ahead of the curve by considering other positions within the company that you can handle as your PD progresses. If training for such positions is available, take it to maximize your options. Prepare and plan ahead.

From your employer's perspective

Keep in mind that bosses can't look at a situation in isolation. Employers must consider how your situation affects other people and, yes, ultimately, the bottom line. This fact of life may seem harsh, but the point of opening a business is to make enough money to reinvest in the company's future and keep the business going. Most employers want very much to maintain good employees. If you're a person who delivers on the job and adds value to the company, your employer will probably be eager to help you stay on the job for as long as possible.

If safety is relevant to your position, your employer can't put the company, you, or your co-workers at risk. And in this case, the bottom line isn't about making a profit; it's about security for you, your co-workers, and your families.

The first person to tell at work is your immediate supervisor (and then the folks in your HR department). In rare circumstances, employers can be short-sighted when it comes to supporting employees in tough personal situations. Maybe you and your supervisor already have an adversarial relationship, so you're concerned your PD will tip the situation over the edge.

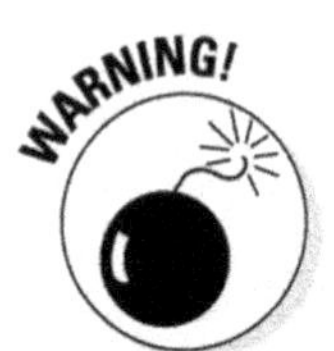

In such cases you may be tempted to go around your superior and seek out someone in the company that seems more supportive. But this plan only makes the problem worse and can actually backfire on you. Your supervisor may resent being passed over and make it more difficult for you to convince other people that you're still a valuable asset to the company.

Telling Your Boss

Okay, the moment's at hand. It's time to deliver the news of your PD to your employer. Here are some steps to consider:

1. Request a meeting.

This can be informal if you and your supervisor have a relationship that permits you to say, "Do you have 20 to 30 minutes today or tomorrow? I need to talk to you about something." If the request needs to be more formal, follow the company process for requesting and scheduling a meeting with your supervisor or manager. Allow at least 30 minutes for the meeting.

2. Prepare and practice your talking points—those key points you want your boss to hear after you've said, "I have Parkinson's."

Keep the points short and simple. This is no time to try to educate your boss about the intricacies of PD. Ideally, you'll take a positive and proactive approach. For example, you may say, "I've been diagnosed with Parkinson's disease." (Allow time for a short response—hopefully a sympathetic one.) You continue, "The good news is that progression is slow and my doctor agrees that it may be some time—even years—before symptoms really have an impact."

3. Demonstrate that you've done your homework.

Your boss may hear very little after you say, "I have Parkinson's." And inevitably he'll start thinking of its short- and long-term impact on the business. This may be a good time to offer him a simple fact sheet about what PD is (and is not).

This is also a good time to produce a copy of any letter your neurologist has provided that states your ability to continue in the job.

Follow up with a few simple comments that demonstrate the effort you've already given the situation: You've reviewed the job description and performance expectations set out for your position; you've met with your doctor and gone over the demands of the job; and your doctor has given you the letter. This is where all your homework and advance preparation pay off, but keep it short and simple. You don't want to inadvertently raise red flags by saying something like, "And as for the travel piece of my job, well, I'm pretty sure that won't be a problem as long as the travel doesn't increase."

Note: You don't want to come off as threatening or adversarial at a time like this; you don't want the message to be, "I have PD, and I know my rights." Instead, say something like, "I know this raises all sorts of questions, but I'm confident that together we can find answers and solutions that will allow me to continue to contribute effectively."

4. Maintain a positive and can-do attitude throughout the meeting regardless of the response you get from your manager.

Understand that your manager is going to need some time to take this all in, so don't agree to any firm offer or accommodation your supervisor may offer off the top of his head at this initial meeting. Acknowledge any such offer as a possibility but one that you should both discuss after he's had time to digest the news—the same way you needed some time to digest your diagnosis.

You know that having PD is a challenge but not a deal-breaker when it comes to your ability to contribute. Your job in this meeting is to demonstrate through your can-do attitude that this is just one more challenge you can conquer.

5. Address the subject of co-workers at some point in the meeting.

One suggestion is to meet with the members of your immediate department and give them the news. Show your manager a brief fact sheet that answers frequently asked questions about PD. (One excellent handout is available online at www.ninds.nih.gov/disorders/parkinsons_disease.) Tell your employer that, with permission, you want to tell these co-workers about your diagnosis, give them the fact sheet, and ask them to help squelch rumors or misinformation as the news spreads.

6. Let your manager know that you'll be contacting the HR department to gather information about your benefits and options.

7. Thank your manager for his support and concern and ask whether the two of you should set a time to meet again or you should wait to hear from HR. Then get back to work.

Getting the Facts from HR

Your HR department can provide answers to most questions related to your insurance options and work options if you're no longer able to do your job. But just as you prepared for your meeting with your manager, prepare a list of questions for this meeting, and be ready to write down the answers (or get printed materials that provide the information).

The Americans with Disabilities Act—your golden parachute—maybe

According to the Equal Employment Opportunity Commission (EEOC), the

Americans with Disabilities Act (ADA) gives civil rights protections (similar to those for race, color, sex, national origin, age, and religion) to individuals with disabilities. The ADA prohibits discrimination in all employment practices: job application procedures, hiring and firing regulations, promotion opportunities, benefits, and compensation.

The broad protection given by the ADA sounds very promising. But keep in mind the fine points as well—points that can affect your rights under the law. Examples are:

• If your workplace employs fewer than 15 people, you may not be covered under this legislation.

• As a person with PD, your disability must "substantially limit major life activities such as seeing, hearing, speaking, walking, breathing, performing manual tasks, learning, caring for oneself, and working."

• You must be qualified to fill the requirements of the job, and your employer maintains the right to establish performance and production standards that all employees must meet, disabled or not.

The ADA further requires your employer to consider whether you can continue to do your job with certain "reasonable accommodation." Examples of this requirement include special products (such as voice-activated computers), changes that make your existing workspace more accessible, or restructuring the job itself.

Because every disability and its effect on an employee's ability to do a specific job is slightly different, keep the following suggestions in mind:

• Your employer will rely on you to speak up and suggest possible solutions. If you don't have a suggestion, do some research and work with your employer to find one.

• Understand that the company is expected to pay for any equipment or necessary accommodation, but your employer isn't required to provide an accommodation that causes an *undue hardship* on other employees or the business. If cost is a factor (and you can afford it), you may consider offering to pay part of the cost.

• The ADA doesn't give you a free ride. Your employer can hold you to the same standards of performance and production as people without disabilities. You have a responsibility to be honest with yourself and your employer about your ability to meet those standards.

We strongly urge you to

• Become familiar with the pros and cons of the ADA for your situation.

• Not assume an adversarial or threatening attitude with your employer when it comes to applying ADA regulations to your situation.

Managing your PD is a team effort between you and your health team, you and your care-partnering family and friends, and you and your employer.

For more information about ADA, call 800-514-0301 (voice within USA), 800-514-0383 (TTY), 202-514-0301 (outside USA) or check out www.ada.gov.

When you meet with your HR representative, you're actually on a fact-finding mission. You're not necessarily going to act on any of the following factors right away, but you need to clearly understand your employer's policy related to:

- Disability
- Early retirement
- Availability of any pension/401K funds
- Government programs, such as COBRA
- Health savings accounts (HSAS)
- Social Security disability benefits
- Medicare and Medicaid
- Any available state health insurance pools

The Americans with Disabilities Act (ADA) can be a real resource of options as your PD progresses. But be aware that the ADA doesn't apply to all employers, and it does have limitations. (See the sidebar, "The Americans with Disabilities Act—your golden parachute—maybe.")

Positioning the News for Co-Workers

The type of job you have and the people you work closely with will influence what and how much you tell your co-workers. Here are two possible scenarios:

- You are in a management or supervisory position and have several people who report directly to you. After you've told your boss (and gotten his agreement that you need to break the news to your team), call a meeting of your group. Keep it informal. (In some business settings, this meeting is called a *huddle,* like a football team huddling to get the play before going into action. The huddle's a great analogy for the kind of atmosphere you want to create for delivering this news.) Consider taking these steps:

- Deliver the news. Do it with humor, if possible, but keep it direct and simple.
- Hand out the simple fact sheet about PD (see the earlier section, "Telling Your Boss").
- Lay out the ground rules for what aspects may change, but emphasize that it will be business as usual—you're still a team.
- Offer some guidelines for how you expect your team to handle any gossip or rumors they may hear about you or PD. (Remind them that they can squelch any such nonsense using the simple facts you've provided.)
- Let your co-workers know that they can come directly to you with any concerns or questions, assure them that you are most definitely still you, and send them back to work.

- You're part of a close-knit group whose ability to succeed relies on everyone pulling her weight. Your teammates react to the news with one of two attitudes: "Poor Mary. How will she manage? What can I do to help her?" or "Poor me" (as in "This is going to end up meaning more work for me."). Be prepared for either reaction by:
  - Maintaining that same upbeat, can-do attitude you demonstrated when you told your boss
  - Offering the fact sheet and stating outright that, according to your doctor, you're going to be around for years to come
  - Assuring everyone that you're not expecting special considerations from them and you'll continue to pull your weight on the team

The manner in which you deliver the news of your PD to your manager and co-workers forms their attitude as they carry that news forward. If you're positive and upbeat, they're more likely to assure others that you have a real handle on it. And that image is exactly the one you want to project to everyone.

Taking Steps to Protect Your Income

Working people have a variety of ways to protect themselves and their dependents if they can no longer work. The following list describes the more common methods.

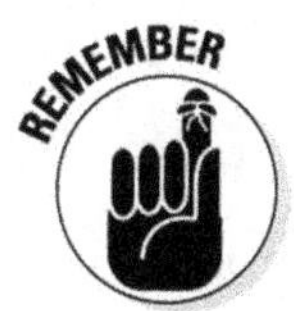

Although this list provides general definitions of a variety of options, we aren't recommending any one of these programs. If you need to leave your job and rely on other sources for your income, consult with a qualified financial planner or counselor (see Chapter 21).

- **Income-generating plans:**
  - **Employer Disability Plans:** Such plans can be short- or long-term, and eligibility

requirements differ from one employer to another. In general these plans allow employees to purchase short- and long-term disability insurance as a part of their overall company-sponsored benefit package. If you need to leave work because of a disability, the plan pays you a percentage of your salary while you're disabled. Some plans pay that full percentage even if you're also eligible for and receiving benefits from Social Security (see the next bullet); other plans may prorate their payments based on what you receive from the government. (For specific information of disability benefits, talk to your HR department.)

- **Social Security Disability Plans:** This segment of Social Security is different from the more common retirement benefit payout. Two programs are available: Social Security Disability Insurance (SSDI) and Supplemental Security Income (SSI). Both programs have stringent eligibility requirements.

SSDI is for people with an established work history; the amount received is determined by that history and specific earnings.

SSI is based on financial need and serves people with little work history and very limited financial assets. (For more information on becoming eligible for either program, call 800-772-1213 or go to www.ssa.gov.)

- **Insurance coverage options:**

    • **The Consolidated Omnibus Budget Reconciliation Act** (COBRA): This option permits employees who lose their employer-sponsored benefits to pay out-of-pocket for the same health insurance coverage they received while working. The normal period you can pay for coverage is 18 months after you leave unless you're determined to be disabled, in which case you can extend coverage to a total of 36 months. (For more information, talk to your HR department.)

    • **Long-Term Care (LTC) insurance:** LTC insurance plans

provide coverage for care necessary to help a person with the basic activities of daily living, such as bathing and dressing. Benefits are usually available for a range of settings—the home, an assisted-living facility, or a nursing home.

A growing trend among employers is to offer an LTC insurance option as a part of the employee benefit package. If your company provides this option and you haven't taken advantage of it, check into it again. If you aren't eligible, your care partner may be. (For more information on LTC insurance, talk to your HR department or call your state Office on Insurance.)

- **Medicare:** People under the age of 65 can qualify for Medicare (the federal health insurance and drug coverage plan). For current information on qualifying if you aren't yet 65, call 800-633-4227 or go to www.cms.hhs.gov. (For a more complete explanation of the Medicare program, see Chapter 21.)

- **SHIP Programs and Medicaid:** Every state has some form of a State Health Insurance Counseling and Assistance Program (SHIP) to help its citizens find the best insurance options regardless of the person's financial or health situation. In addition, every state offers Medicaid, the federally funded and state-managed program that provides health services based on financial need. (For more information on Medicaid in your state, go to www.hcfa.hhs.gov/medicaid.)

Chapter 17

Adjusting Your Routine as Your PD Progresses

In This Chapter

- Easing into new routines and daily rhythms
- Keeping the family up to date and in focus
- Befriending your friends
- Going public *and* enjoying it
- Making room for R&R
- Going forward with your care partner

In the early months after the onset of your Parkinson's disease (PD) symptoms, you may be surprised how little accommodation your symptoms require. In fact, if your doctor's recommended regular exercise and a balanced diet and you've followed her advice, you may be feeling better than you have in some time. Your symptoms may actually be more of an annoyance than any real concern. Now that you think about it, you may have avoided going to see the doctor for that reason—the symptoms weren't really interfering with your routine.

As time goes by, however, your symptoms will become troublesome enough to affect your life and routine—perhaps significantly. But this doesn't mean you can't live a full and active life. In this chapter, we offer tips for managing your symptoms—even as they worsen—*without* letting PD be the driving force in your life.

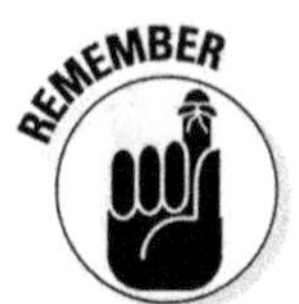

You're the same person you were before the diagnosis. You hold the same importance to your family and friends and retain many of the talents and skills you developed through your life. You may need to adapt—doing activities a different way, at a slower pace, or even with the help of others—but nothing about your essential identity has changed.

Exploring Ways to Make Daily Activities Easier

You can take a number of positive and proactive steps to keep your daily routine from overwhelming you. In this section, we look at some key ways that you can stay in control—as long as you're willing to adapt and not dig in your heels with a my-way-or-the-highway attitude!

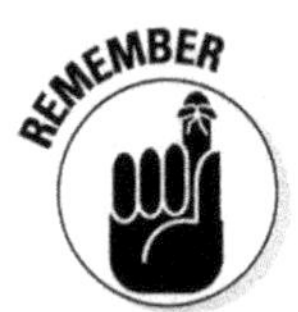

Do not allow other people's expectations or your own internal demands to direct your activity. The added stress of trying to compete or live up to last year's successes (big and little) can have an adverse effect on your overall health. Stress and performance anxiety can actually inflame your symptoms and incapacitate you even more—at least momentarily.

Timing your activities

The main difference in your life now is timing—it can be everything. Your ability to understand when you can and can't do something may be the key to continuing many (or most) activities you've always enjoyed. We're not talking about timing your meds (which you and your doctor need to work out together) or your activities for your *on* times (see Chapter 9). We're talking about accepting and understanding that *everything* is a matter of time. You take longer to get ready to go places and longer to get from here to there. You take longer to do a task (like dressing or brushing your teeth) that you used to knock off in a matter of minutes.

Even if you take four or five times longer, you're still independent. It's important that you continue to perform these basic activities with little (if any) help for as long as possible.

Those around you—family, friends, employer, co-workers—also need to understand this need for extra time. Working out an appropriate time schedule for tasks you perform personally or on the job is important. Be realistic. If you used to take 15 minutes to do something, you may now need an hour.

Reserving your energy

Accept that your energy is limited and must be conserved and used wisely. This attitude can help protect your right to live independently and fully for as long as possible. Some days you'll just be downright pooped, unable to complete the list of activities you'd planned. So what? Are you saying you never fell short of completing an ambitious list *before* the onset of your PD symptoms?

Yeah, right. Everyone overestimates the potential for accomplishment from time to time. You're just wise enough to say, "Okay, I'll tackle that tomorrow—or the next day."

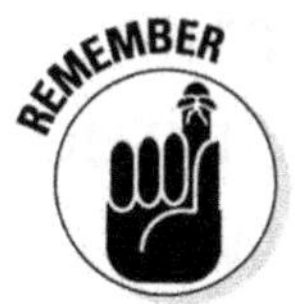

Approach each day with an I-don't-have-to- do-everything-but-will-do-as-much-as-I (and my PD)-can attitude. These are a few more tips to help you manage your energy bank:

- Take the time to think through the demands on your schedule each day; prioritize the list by what you need to tackle and what you can put aside for later.
- Schedule important tasks for when you're at peak-performance.
- Discuss with your doctor the advantages of regular exercise and diet changes for improving your levels of energy; implement his suggestions.

Taking tips from other PWP

Your ability to manage basic tasks may vary greatly from hour to hour and depend on where you are in your medication dosing cycle. But the ingenuity of 1.2 million people with PD (PWP) in the United States and a history of nearly two hundred years can provide you with more than a few tricks to make your life with PD easier. The following sections share ways other people with Parkinson's (PWP) maintain independence in spite of their symptoms.

Your occupational therapist (OT) can offer ideas and explain proven techniques for adapting your routine to accommodate your symptoms. Appendix B also recommends a number of resources and devices available to make life easier.

Strategizing

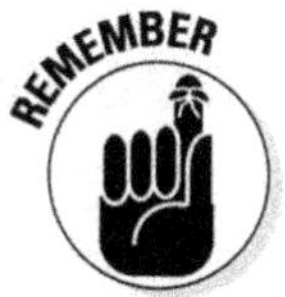

Your determination to be as independent as possible—no matter how long a basic task takes—begins with curiosity and imagination. Take advantage of these general tips to make each day run a little more smoothly:

- Try to approach each situation as a separate challenge and break each task into individual steps. Focus on one step at a time. Try to start with the simplest one; after you've conquered that, move on.
- Keep in mind that timing is everything—coordinate the timing of these tasks with your medication routine to avoid *off* symptoms (see Chapter 9) that can make each step even more frustrating.
- Let your partner know that the difficulties you face are as frustrating for you as they are for

her, but it's important that you continue to try. Discuss ways she can help without taking away your opportunity to do as much as you can. For example, your partner can put toothpaste on your toothbrush and leave it out for you. Or while you shower or bathe, your care partner can remain nearby in case you need help; she can also lay out your clothing for the day.

Grooming

Personal grooming is probably so much a part of your day that you barely think about all the individual tasks. Brushing your teeth, washing your face, shaving (if you're a man), applying makeup (if you're a woman), and combing your hair are routines you've performed for decades.

But now your symptoms are making these simple tasks next to impossible and even exhausting. Are you at the point where you need to ask for help? Not necessarily. Give these proven techniques a try:

- Sit down instead of standing—you'll not only conserve energy but also lower the risk of losing your balance and falling.

- Prop your elbows on the counter to steady your hand and support your shoulders as you shave or apply makeup.
- Use electronic appliances—razor, toothbrush, and so forth—that do a lot of the work for you.
- Try a hairstyle that's easier to manage and dries quickly without a hair dryer. In a pinch, try one of the dry-shampoo products available at drug-stores or beauty supply shops.
- Treat yourself to a weekly (or bi-weekly) shampoo and styling at a discount hair salon or local beauty school. (This tip is also great therapy for relieving stress!)
- Suggest a certificate for a professional manicure or pedicure when people ask for birthday or holiday gift ideas. Or check with a local beauty school for a less-expensive session with a student.

Other people respond more positively to the person who takes an interest in the way she looks. And looking your best empowers and keeps you in control of your own destiny. So make the effort—put your best face and foot forward every day.

Dressing

Before your PD symptoms started getting in the way, you probably never thought about the many balance and flex movements that are necessary just to put clothes on.

Before you begin breaking down this task into manageable steps, take the time to go through your closet and assess your wardrobe. Are the clothes easy to put on and take off? Consider these suggestions:

- Look for pieces with closures that are easy to manage. Try an elastic waist in place of a button and zipper, for example.

- Consider replacing the buttons on a favorite shirt or blouse with magnetic snaps or Velcro closures.
- Consider having the buttons sewn closed when clothes are loose or stretchy enough to pull on over your head.
- Use elastic shoelaces (or shoes with Velcro closings) to avoid tying your shoes.

Avoid clothing items that only make life more difficult for you, no matter how much you love them. For example,

- Stay away from fabrics that tend to cling or stick to other fabrics (flannel, velour, corduroy, and such).
- Avoid sweatpants that have elastic at the ankles.
- Get rid of bedroom slippers (use non-skid socks like hospitals have), and avoid heavy-weight shoes (wingtips, for example).
- Women: Abandon pantyhose in favor of knee-highs or socks, and forget the high heels.

Think through the steps of dressing—from choosing what to wear to putting on each item—and allow plenty of time. These tips make the tasks easier:

- Prepare the night before: Choose your clothing and lay out all the pieces (from underwear to accessories).
- Sit on a sturdy armchair (not a rocker or the edge of the bed) and use the arms for support as you dress.
- Have a small footstool close at hand to provide support when you put on socks and shoes.
- Lie down on the bed if that makes it easier for you to put on certain items such as pants or socks.

Try to look your best—it can make a difference. When you look good, you feel good—or at least better. Some days you may think, "What's the point of getting dressed? I'm not going anywhere and no one's going to see me." Yes, you are going places—even if it's just around the house. And your family (and any friends who happen to stop by) are hardly *nobodies.*

Bathing and showering

Bathtubs and showers can be falls waiting to happen, so your first step is to make them as safe as possible. Your OT can help assess the need for safety bars, tub mats, shower chairs or stools, non-skid rugs, and such. (Read more about OTs in Chapter 6.)

The next step is to determine whether your normal bathing routine still applies. For example, when you consider the extra effort a shower or bath takes with PD, is your former daily routine realistic or even necessary? ***Note:*** One symptom in the mid-to-later stages of PD is excessive perspiration. If this is the case, at least a daily sponge bath is indeed necessary.

Because of the danger of falling, never attempt a shower or bath when you're home alone. Although you may want the privacy of managing this routine on your own, your care partner or someone in the family should be close enough that you can call for assistance if you need it. (Besides, what's so bad about having someone else wash your back?)

Whatever schedule you and your care partner decide is best, these additional tips can make bath time less stressful:

- Cut down on trips that can drain precious energy by gathering everything you need (soap, towels, shampoo, robe, and such) in one place—perhaps a plastic container in the bathroom can keep it all together.
- Check that the bathroom is free of drafts and that the water temperature is comfortable. Your bath time should be a pleasant, relaxing time, not a time when water that's too hot or too cold surprises you and can lead to a dangerous loss of balance or a fall.
- Undress and, using the techniques you practiced with your OT, get into the tub or shower. If your

neurologist hasn't prescribed occupational therapy and you're beginning to struggle with such movements as getting in and out of the tub, ask for an OT referral. The OT can come to your home to work with you. In the meantime, be safe. Let your partner assist you in and out of the tub or shower, or plan to take sponge baths.

- Take your time—the sensation of washing yourself should be a pleasurable one. If holding onto a bar of soap is difficult, consider using a bath mitt, which is a glove-like washcloth that's available at most drugstores. And speaking of soap, go easy on the bath oils. They can make the shower or tub floor slippery (even with a rubber safety mat). Better to rub on bath oil as part of the drying process after your bath.
- Dry yourself thoroughly when you've finished. Again, take your time. Apply any lotion or cream to dry or chafed skin, and put on your robe. In fact, a thick terrycloth robe is a super way to dry yourself when the

flexibility needed to towel dry becomes more difficult.

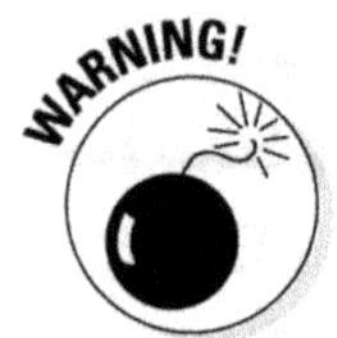

Don't attempt to get even partially dressed in the bathroom; the danger for falling as you attempt to dress in such close quarters is huge. Put on your robe and go back to your bedroom to dress, following the guidelines in "Dressing," earlier in this section.

Thinking outside the box

You may have heard the old joke about the patient who says to the doctor, "Doctor, if I follow your treatment, will I be able to play the piano?" When the doctor says, "I don't see why not," the patient replies, "Great. I always wanted to be able to do that."

Dr. Gary Guten—yes, the guy whose name is on the front

cover—had battled PD over a decade when it occurred to him that playing the piano may be a way to maintain flexibility and coordination in his fingers and hands. Over the years, Gary—an orthopedic surgeon, marathon runner, and expert in the field of sports medicine—has found several innovative ways to meet the various challenges of his PD. Taking up the piano is just one more *therapy* he's devised to deal with the advancement of symptoms.

In the process, Gary and his teacher developed various techniques—like placing 2-pound weights on Gary's wrists to help steady his hands and creating a system for remembering notes and reading music. After several weeks of lessons and practice, Gary joined 20 other students (average age of 13) to present his first recital. As Gary said, "At my age and at this stage of my PD, what else could I do to earn the applause of 75 people?"

Early in his PD, Gary discovered that ski-pole-like hiking sticks (available at www.exerstrider.com) help him maintain an even stride and balance, allowing him to walk with rhythm and relative confidence. He also discovered that lateral twisting movements (from side to side) are easier than straight-on movements. As a result, he plays golf and ping-pong (which use a lot of lateral movement) to remain active—and athletic.

You may not be an athlete or a musician, but Gary's advice is to remember the words of the famous writer Gilbert Keith Chesterton: "If a thing is worth doing, it is worth doing badly." Like Gary, you and your healthcare team can get creative about what works for you in the fight to maintain your balance, mental alertness, and independence. By keeping a there-must-be-a-way attitude while you hold onto your optimism and good humor, you may have won half the battle against advancing PD.

Personal hygiene

One symptom PWP can develop as their PD progresses is urinary incontinence (see Chapter 18 for a discussion on the impact incontinence may have on your PD). This problem is not only a health concern but also a real hygiene issue due to the potential for odor. Of course, your first step is to discuss these problems with your doctor. Also consider these tips:

- Try using one of the disposable products (such as sanitary pads available in varying degrees of thickness) on the market today. Many of these are far more discreet than wearing an adult diaper product.
- Make certain that the pathway to and from the bathroom is well-lighted and free of obstacles. Or ask your doctor to prescribe a portable commode that you can place near your bed to avoid trips to the bathroom at night.
- Keep moist towelettes, disposable pads, and other products within easy reach in your bathroom so you can clean yourself as needed.

- Keep a few pre-moistened disposable wipes and an extra set of clean underwear and clothing in a plastic bag in your car, in a bag, or in a backpack for whenever you go out, just in case.

Maintaining the Family Dynamic

Collaborative management is a relatively new term in managing the symptoms of a chronic condition such as PD. In medical circles it applies primarily to the healthcare team (see Chapter 6) that helps you plan for and manage your PD symptoms. But it's also a useful term for families that need to include a chronic and progressive condition into their daily routines. The elements of collaborative management within a family unit may include:

- **Defining** the issues to be managed (medical, mental, and physical health) as well as the emotional impact of PD on the PWP and the family. For example, if the PWP's been the family's chief financial manager, this is a good time to train another family member in the details of managing the finances, paying the bills, investing and saving, and so on.

- **Targeting** each issue by establishing realistic goals, achievable objectives, and a satisfactory plan of action for the PWP and the family. Goals can be simple and short-term such as planning a family trip. If the PWP has always handled the planning, preparations, and details, then other members of the family need to step up and define ways they can take on some of those tasks.
- **Supporting and encouraging** the PWP's autonomy and independence through medical interventions, lifestyle changes, and emotional support systems so the PWP and her family can maintain as normal a routine as possible. Often a family member will respond to the PD diagnosis by jumping in and trying to do everything for the PWP. Because that person wants to deal with this challenge through action, find ways she can contribute. For

example, maybe she can prepare a salad or side dish for dinner while the PWP—an accomplished cook—makes the rest of the meal just as she did before PD.

- **Monitoring** (through ongoing and open communication) the status of the PWP's role within the family unit and the family's ability to adapt to the presence of PD. Regular weekly or bi-weekly family meetings (see discussion of initial family meeting in Chapter 7) can accomplish this goal and provide a safe haven for members to voice concerns. The agenda starts with an update from the PWP. Then other family members engage in a round of *concerns and joys* in which each person can talk about possible needs or red flags and then mention something that is working well or has brought special delight since the last meeting.

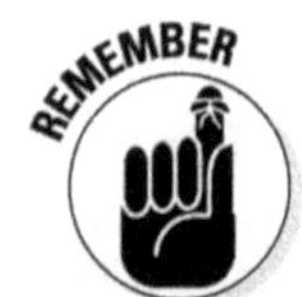

As much as the challenge of living with PD may appear to be all about you, in fact it affects every family member. Whenever you have these family gatherings, make sure that *you* listen to your family's honest concerns (and sometimes outright frustrations). Acknowledge the concern, focus on the specific issue rather than the emotional overtones, and, opening the discussion to everyone, seek the best solution together.

Socializing with Friends

Every circle of friends has the person or persons who drive the social calendars of getting together, going places, calling, e-mailing, and the like. Each circle also has people who wait to be called, e-mailed, and the rest. Before your diagnosis, which role did you play? Were you the extrovert or the introvert? The social butterfly or the hermit?

If you're an introvert by nature, maybe the friends you counted on to call and set up get-togethers seem to have turned into a bunch of loners. If you were the social cheerleader of the group, maybe you've dropped that ball now that you have PD—not wanting to impose yourself and your symptoms on your friends.

Get over it! If your friends are real, they're waiting for you to show them the way. If the usual extroverts seem to be hanging back, call them and clear the air. Chances are they've been hanging back while trying to figure out what you want. If you were the social leader, get back in the game. Call the old gang together and have an open discussion about your PD, how you're handling it, and most of all, how you hope *they'll* handle it. Then get back to doing whatever you did together before your diagnosis.

Whatever activity you decide on, do not make your PD the focus of (or reason for) getting together. The purpose here is to bring the relationships back to some semblance of normalcy. After your friends see you in action and enjoying the activities you've always enjoyed (maybe with a bit more effort and a little less speed), they'll relax and the friendship can move forward.

Going Out and About in the Community

You may as well get used to it. You'll have times when total strangers stare at you with pity (or worse, disgust), children point and snicker, and people even cross to the other side of the street to avoid passing you on the sidewalk. Some people will misread your balance symptoms as intoxication. Others may read your facial mask and lack of expression as a sign of mental illness or not being very bright. (This is fairly obvious because the person speaks ver-r-ry slowly and loudly as if instructing a small child or a non-English speaker.)

You can choose to take this ignorance and lack of good manners personally, or you can choose to understand that this stranger is the one with the problem—and then get on with your day. In either case, what do you care about the opinions of strangers? Are you going to permit people like that to stop you from living normally? Aha! We didn't think so. The following sections provide some tips for maintaining your activity in the larger community.

Attending public events

Try to schedule your medication timing and dosing to your greatest advantage during the planned outing. (Talk to your doctor about your plans and let him suggest any modifications to your normal dosing routine). If you're going to a play, movie, concert, ballgame, or restaurant, some simple steps may help:

- Call ahead to get answers about accessibility (ramps not stairs, seat on the aisle if preferred, room for a wheelchair if necessary, and so on).
- Get plenty of rest before the event.

- Allow plenty of time to get ready.
- Arrive early so you can be seated and settled without rushing.

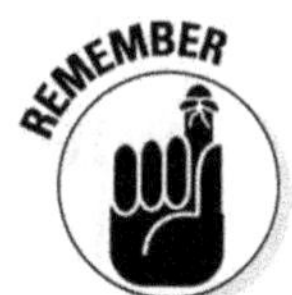

Social outings should be as enjoyable for your care partner as they are for you. This is not the time for you to try and prove your independence. For example, if helping you get ready (such as putting on your shoes for you) allows more time for your care partner to get ready, accept the help—*appreciate* the help. If using a wheelchair makes life easier and the occasion less stressful for your care partner, use a wheelchair. Think of this acceptance not as a surrender of your autonomy but as a gracious way of caring for your care partner.

Traveling

Taking a trip requires careful planning to make the trip a pleasurable experience rather than a hassle. As with everything else, when you consider taking a trip, break it down into more manageable steps:

• Choose where you'll go. At this point in your PD journey, what's realistic (a theater tour of NYC?) and what's not (scaling Mt. Everest?)? Talk to a travel agent about special tours available for folks traveling with a disability.

The Web site www.travelconsumer.com/disability.htm provides links to special topics (such as recreational vehicles [RVs], tour groups for people with special needs, and cruises) and a link to *Travelin' Talk,* a network of people with disabilities around the world who are in regular contact and gather firsthand information about accessibility in a particular area.

• Figure out the transportation. Plane, bus, car, train? Or maybe all of the above? If you go by car, you and your travel companions are probably well aware of your limitations and needs. If you're taking a plane, train, or bus, contact the company well in advance to discuss provisions they offer special-needs travelers.

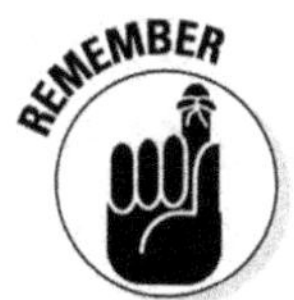

• Be very specific about your needs. For example, you may need your seat to be close to the bathroom. On the other hand, navigating the entire length of a jumbo jet as you board just so you can be close to the economy-class facility may be more trouble than it's worth. Ask whether you can have a seat closer to the front and permission to use the closer facility in business or first class. ***Note:*** If you'll be using a wheelchair—not a bad idea to conserve energy as you get from place to place within airports and train stations—the carrier needs advance notice.

• Select your overnight accommodations carefully. You may love an old, historic bed and breakfast, but is that realistic if you have to navigate stairs (which in old buildings can be steep, winding, and narrow!)? If you're fine with a traditional hotel and it publicizes *accessibility* for people with special needs, do not take them at their word. Call and ask specific questions. For example, does the bathroom have grab bars and a walk-in shower (not a shower in a tub)? Are the doorways wide enough to accommodate a wheelchair or walker?

• Plan to get out and about. Most tourist attractions in major cities around the world are well-prepared to accommodate visitors with special needs. But often the trick is to locate those entrances, facilities, and other special services. Call ahead and gather complete information about available services. Then on the day of your visit, call again and let the staff on duty know that you're on your way. (You may want to call the day before to give advance notice.)

If you or your traveling companion holds a membership in the museum or site, call the member-services department and let them know you're planning a visit. They may be able to offer you and your party more than the standard accommodations for special-needs visitors.

- Be prepared—just in case. Emergencies happen even on vacation, so take the following suggestions seriously:
- Always hand-carry your medications, don't put them in your baggage.
- Always take along an extra supply (two to three days' worth) of your medications *and* their prescriptions in case you have to replace medications.
- Always carry a list of your medications (including over-the-counter products) and the emergency information listed in Chapter 9.

- Ask your neurologist to recommend a colleague in the place you're visiting (or check online at www .aan.com for a complete listing of certified neurologists worldwide).

Volunteering—The double blessing

Giving back to your community and making a real difference in the lives of other people pays double dividends. Not only are you contributing to the betterment of society—locally, nationally, or globally—but you're permitting yourself to turn your attention away from your own problems.

Whether you were an active volunteer before your PD or never had the time because of work and family responsibilities, now is the time. When you give of your time and energy in spite of your own challenges, you inspire other folks and give them hope. If you can manage your PD *and* mentor a troubled teen or manage the volunteer program for the blood drive or coordinate a fundraiser for your church, then you move other people to action.

And that's something. As one song says, "You can hang a life on that."

And speaking of getting involved, don't overlook this golden opportunity to really make a difference for yourself and other PWP. See Chapter 24 for ways you can build awareness of and increase knowledge about PD locally or even nationally. The national PD community is active, organized, and inspiring—not to mention a great deal of fun.

Taking a Breather—Respite for the Weary

Living with a chronic, progressive condition (and living with someone who has such a condition) can become stressful and even overwhelming as the months and years go by. The warning signs are right there:

- Communication problems, like increased frustration, irritability, short tempers
- Physical symptoms, like stomach upset, shortness of breath, headache

- Unhealthy lifestyle behaviors, such as overeating or not eating enough, increased smoking or alcohol use, sleeping too much or too little
- Emotional symptoms, such as depression, anxiety, feelings of deep anger or sadness

The trick is not to lose control of these symptoms before you take action. But the real trick is to plan regular respite for yourself and your care partner—separately and together—as part of your daily routine. (Even the lowest-paid laborer gets fifteen-minute breaks a couple of times a shift!) In addition, you and your care partner need to consider the following:

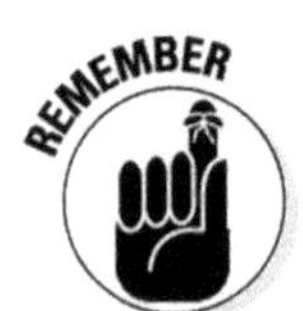

• Your diagnosis doesn't require the two of you to be joined at the hip. You had separate activities before (and probably enjoyed telling your partner about the experience). That arrangement shouldn't change simply because one of you has PD.

• You both need to identify (in some cases, *remember*) the ways you individually relaxed and found respite before PD. Perhaps your partner spent an afternoon with the grandchildren. Maybe you had a regular card game. Maybe each of you gave time to a favorite charity.

• Try to plan vacation-type respites together. You'd be surprised how the travel industry has begun to accommodate the special needs of travelers like you. Check out the Web sites we list in the "Traveling" section earlier in this chapter.

If long-distance traveling becomes more stressful than fun, then perhaps going on *vacation* in your own community is a possibility. Ever notice how much you enjoy the special sites and events of your community when you have out-of-town company? Treat yourself—move to a hotel or accessible

Bed and Breakfast for a few days; eat meals out at restaurants you've been meaning to try; visit a tourist attraction such as a concert, play, or sporting event, and buy souvenirs for the grandkids. Just remember to pace yourself and get the rest you need to enjoy the *trip.*

• As your PD progresses, you may find that you don't have the freedom to physically *get away.* Respite for you may come in the form of alternative and complementary therapies such as meditation or yoga, which we discuss in Chapter 11. And you may be surprised to discover how regular exercise can also be a respite therapy (see Chapter 12).

A Word for the PD Care Partner

Watching your loved one struggle to perform simple tasks can be frustrating and even emotionally painful for you. You may instinctively want to do what-ever you can to make the task easier. That compassion certainly isn't bad, but you really need to fight the follow-through.

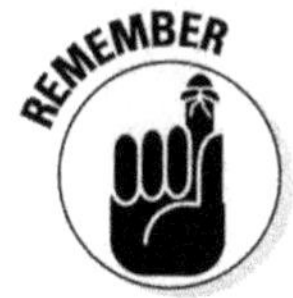

Managing the symptoms of PD means the PWP must fight to maintain as much movement, flexibility, and independence as possible for as long as possible. If you permit yourself or your loved one to give up on an activity that she can still do, you're actually (in a small but significant way) accelerating the process for real hands-on care.

Instead, discuss ways you can help without taking away her ability to manage on her own. For example, show your complete confidence in her ability by assuming she will be the one behind the wheel (as usual) when the two of you go out. At the local coffeehouse, if the PWP's tremor makes you shudder every time she tries to transport a cup of coffee from the counter to the table, *ask* if you can carry it for her. If she refuses, accept that.

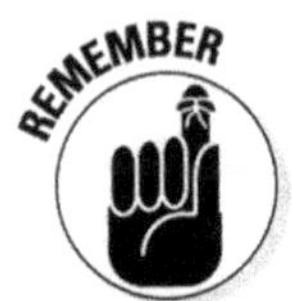

Respite is vital for you and the PWP as you face the progression of current symptoms and the onset of new ones (see Chapter 18). Take advantage of available support so you can care for yourself without guilt. You have every right to do this. Those supports may include:

- Family and friends who assume the role of primary care partner for brief periods while you take a break
- In-home or respite care or adult day care programs (see Chapter 20) when care partnering becomes caregiving

Part V

Coping with Advanced PD

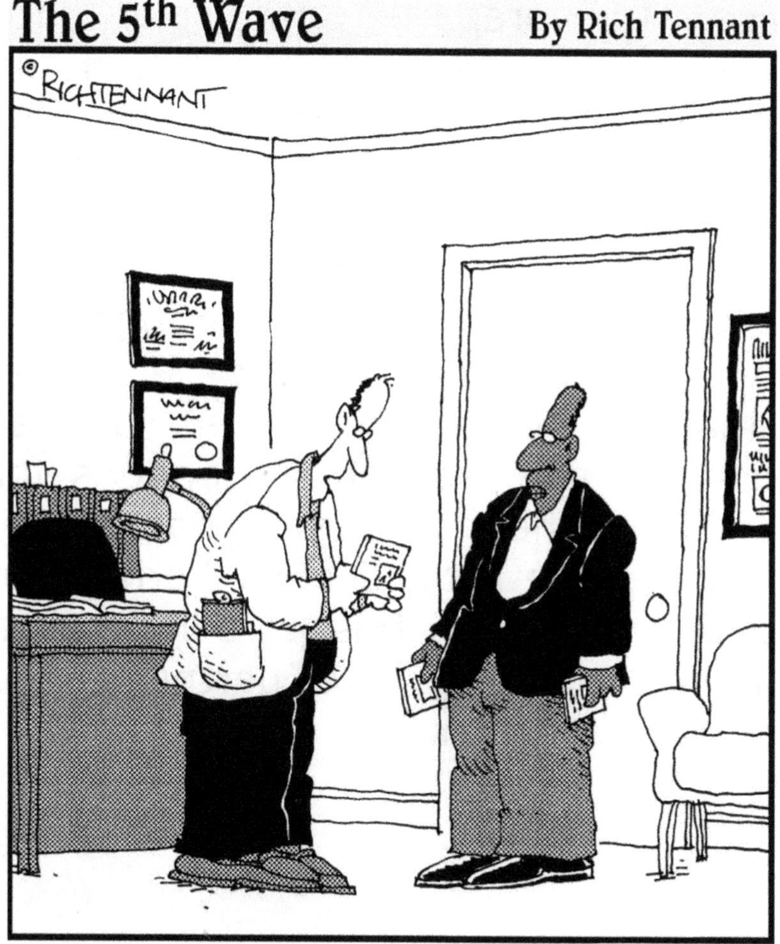

"I Know – when you want a particular haircut, you bring the barber a picture. But this is vocal surgery – bringing me CDs of Pavoratti isn't going to work the same way."

In this part...

Over the years you and your care partner will continue to adapt your lifestyle to the demands of PD. So it's wise to prepare and plan for circumstances that may come in the later stages. The chapters in this part help you do just that. In this part we look at the financial and legal matters that everyone (even people who don't have PD) needs to work through. We give you information that helps you remain in your home for as long as possible, and we set out options for the time when staying at home may no longer be a good idea. Perhaps of most importance, this part includes a chapter about a care partner's role shift to caregiver.

Chapter 18

Facing the Progression of PD Symptoms

In This Chapter

- Timing (of meds) is everything
- Slaying the dragons (eight of them anyway): Handling those new or increasing symptoms
- Refining your offense: Stay in control

Sooner or later the time will come for you to accept that a progressive disease like Parkinson's disease (PD) is reluctant to remain in the background of your life. In this chapter, we tackle the symptoms that may be brand new for you—perhaps even unexpected. Or maybe you've been dealing with some of them already. Our suggestion? The best defense is a good offense: Decide to fight back by:

- Discussing any changes in your condition with your neurologist
- Exploring options for additions to your current treatment or therapy
- Preparing for lifestyle changes that may become necessary (such as relying on a cane or walker or changing your living space arrangements)

On the follow pages, we look at PD symptoms that usually occur later and we also suggest some realistic ways to combat these symptoms.

Noticing Changes Caused by Your Meds

You may face a couple of challenges after you've been on meds that control your PD symptoms for a while.

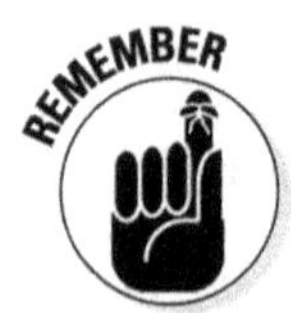

The first medication-related challenge is *wearing-off,* which occurs when your medication can't control symptoms over several hours. In this case,

- Symptoms simply return earlier than usual, initially on a predictable basis (for example, you notice the symptoms return half an hour or an hour sooner than they used to).
- An unfortunate evolution (the *on-off syndrome* discussed in Chapter 9) occurs where you can't predict the length of symptom control from one dose to the next. Some people with PD (PWP) get to know the pattern and may elect to simply live with the *off* times rather than increase medication.

Another challenge brought on by the meds is *dyskinesia,* that twisting, writhing movement (see Chapter 9). Dyskinesia is the result of a complex interaction in the brain between the disease progression and the chronic administration of dopamine medication. As a result, dyskinesia

- Usually appears after you've been on the meds for some time

(somewhere between two and ten years)
- Affects PWP in varying degrees that range from mild to severe, depending on the progression of their disease and their dose of levodopa

Your neurologist may be able to lessen or control your dyskinesias through a change in your medication routine. If the situation becomes intolerable, your doctor may suggest DBS surgery. (See Chapter 10.)

The best way to help your doctor control your symptoms is to keep a diary of the symptoms, including the time of medication intake and the time you feel the symptoms begin to return.

Doctors treat on-off problems in a variety (or combination) of ways:

- Prescribe medication doses closer together
- Add a second medication
- Increase the dose to reduce wearing-off or reduce to control dyskinesia

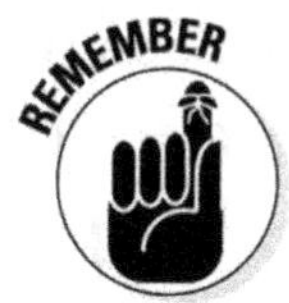

Whenever you notice a different reaction to your antiparkinsonian medications, talk to your neurologist before making any changes in your dosing routine on your own.

When Communication Becomes Difficult

For PWP, *dysarthria* (problems with speaking clearly, understanding, reading, writing, telling time, or using numbers) can be especially disheartening. These problems in communicating can become downright depressing and frustrating. The following sections break down two major problems: vocal and written communication.

The challenge to vocal expression

You can recognize changes in your normal communication by paying attention to the dynamics of a conversation. Consider the following scenarios:

- People (not just your significant other) seem to be leaning in or straining to hear and understand what you're saying. They do a lot of nodding and smiling but don't appear to comprehend your ideas.
- People often ask you to repeat what you just said or to speak up.
- People seem to be talking over you or finishing statements for you.
- You're frustrated from a normal conversation because you're asked to repeat yourself, or worse, you're ignored.

Do these situations seem all too familiar? Try to minimize these frustrations by asking your family and friends to do the following:

- Be patient and look directly at you when the two of you are talking.
- Try to conduct conversations away from background noises such as televisions, car radios, or other competing conversations.
- Keep in mind that your *mask* (lack of facial expression) doesn't reflect your level of interest in the conversation. (See Chapter 3 for an earlier discussion of this symptom.)

You can help yourself, too, by taking care of your voice:

- Take a deep breath and project, without straining or shouting.
- Allow time to rest your voice.
- Slow down if your words come out too fast.

- In any case, use it (talking, reading aloud, and singing). Use it or lose it!

As symptoms progress, you may want to seek help outside of yourself and your care partner. We help you explore your options in the following sections.

Speech pathologists

Speech pathologists (specially trained speech therapists) have the training and tools to improve symptoms or delay their worsening by using therapy in conjunction with your medication regimen. Your therapist can assess your needs, design a program of exercises to help strengthen your voice, and offer tips for making communication a more productive and pleasant experience.

If you have no speech professional in your area, consider ordering one or more of the following tools:

- *Parkinson's Disease: Speech and Swallowing:* A free booklet from the National Parkinson Foundation that includes exercises to help you strengthen vocal and facial muscles.

(Available online at www.parkinson.org or call 800-327-4545.)

- *LSVT (Lee Silverman Voice Treatment) Alive!:* An interactive vocal exercise video. (Available at www.lsvt.org or call 888-606-LSVT [5788].)

Special devices

Several devices (such as message boards or more complex voice-activated software for your computer) can also help by amplifying your voice or making communicating easier. ***Note:*** These devices can be expensive and awkward to carry around and use. Your speech professional can advise you on these tools or you can contact the American Speech-Language and Hearing Association (ASHA) at www.asha.org or 800-638-8255.

Amplifiers that you wear to facilitate communication are also available. Also, to improve communication via telephone, phone companies offer special equipment at very low prices and at no cost for customers who qualify. For more information, contact your phone provider.

Handwriting—Telling the story of your on-off cycles

Micrographia is characterized by writing that starts out normal-size but becomes increasingly smaller and more cramped. This symptom may appear early in the progression of your PD, later, or not at all. When medications are managing symptoms well, handwriting may appear normal. But as medications wear off and the PWP gets closer to the next dose, the fine motor skills may be compromised. When this happens, your writing may start strong and normal but quickly trail off into small, cramped letters and words.

Consider these tips to help you compensate for the writing challenges:

- Ask your neurologist to have you write a sentence and then repeat that exercise at each check-up to see how much (or whether) your micrographia is progressing.

- Talk to your occupational therapist (OT) about tips to help you manage this symptom.
- Use an electric typewriter or computer for your written communications.
- Use lined paper that's sold with school supplies (several sizes are available) to help your pen stay in line.

Swallowing: You Can't Take It for Granted

In some PWP, *dysphagia*—swallowing difficulties—becomes a problem as PD progresses. You may try to write the symptoms off to an unrelated condition, but these need to be evaluated by a doctor, speech therapist, or speech pathologist. Don't ignore the onset of swallowing difficulties. Watch for these symptoms:

- Difficulty in eating and the need for a beverage to wash food down

- Episodes of food going down the wrong way or food seeming to get stuck in the throat
- Coughing or throat-clearing during or immediately after consuming food
- Unexplained weight loss
- Refusal of food or drink because swallowing is too difficult and eating has become an unpleasant experience
- Fever due to aspiration in the lung
- An increase in saliva or thickened mucous-like saliva
- Drooling—a little or a lot

Problems you may have with both saliva and drooling are likely due to your lack of regular swallowing. Two tips to prevent drooling and control saliva include the following:

- Keep your head up and your mouth closed when you're not talking or eating.

- Take frequent sips of water throughout the day. Doing this not only reminds you to swallow and keeps you hydrated but also waters down that thicker saliva.

Your doctor or speech professional may perform an X-ray procedure using barium to assess the swallowing muscles in action. You may be asked to eat a sample of various foods and beverages so that the doctor can evaluate how different foods and drinks affect your ability to swallow. And you may be tested at various times in your dosing cycle to determine how your medications may be affecting your swallowing.

After the evaluation, your doctor can recommend ways to ease your swallowing difficulties and make eating and drinking easier. Possible suggestions include:

- Timing your meals during the on cycle of your PD medications
- Cutting food into small bites, chewing thoroughly, and taking a sip of water before the next bite (yup, the old dieter's trick)
- Blending fruits and veggies to create a drink—the popular

smoothie that may be easier to swallow.

These may sound like simple solutions, but don't attempt to self-diagnose a swallowing problem. It could be a condition completely unrelated to your PD.

Your Vision: A Bump in the Road

Another significant problem that can crop up as your PD progresses is the potential for changes in your vision—blurred vision, difficulty focusing (and reading), dry eyes, and such.

Some of these conditions are frequently a part of the aging process and have easy solutions. For example, your doctor may prescribe a special eye drop or suggest an over-the-counter (OTC) product for dry eyes. Blurred vision may also be nothing more than the need for a change in your lens prescription.

On the other hand, your dry eyes may result from the decreased number of times you blink due to your PD. Fortunately the irritation and discomfort respond to the same artificial tears product your doctor recommends for similar problems related to aging.

Other vision problems that can affect PWP are spasm of the eyelid or excessive blinking (blepharospasm) and double vision. Interestingly, the popular cosmetic injection, *Botox,* can treat the problem of excessive blinking. Double vision may be the result of the slowed and uncoordinated movements of your eyes, and it can be controlled by special lenses (prisms). Wearing a patch over one eye can help while you wait to see the eye doctor.

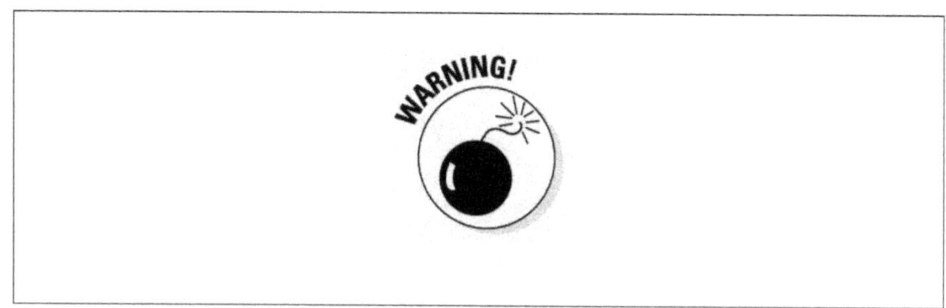

As with any health issue, do not attempt to self-diagnose or treat. See your eye doctor, describe your symptoms, and let the expert prescribe a solution.

To Drive or Not to Drive

Changes from the progression of your PD have the potential to seriously impair your ability to safely operate motorized vehicles, and that can be huge for a PWP. Added to vision problems is the potential for

- Wearing off of your meds at inopportune times
- The possible worsening of your rigidity that impairs the coordination necessary to operate a motor vehicle
- Slowed reaction timing—hazardous for any driver

What to do? How to continue to drive in spite of your PD? How to know when it's no longer an option? Follow these suggestions to assure your safety (not to mention the safety of other people) before you get behind the wheel:

- Be smart about when you drive. Consider limiting (or eliminating) driving after dark. This isn't solely a PD issue; lots of people struggle with night driving as they age.
- Don't drive if another driver's available to take the wheel. This includes public transportation when it's available.
- Don't drive after consuming even the smallest amount of alcohol. You really can't predict the effects of combining a drink with your meds.
- If you (or your partner) question your ability to drive, play it safe by asking your occupational therapist (OT) to refer you to a Driver Rehabilitation Specialist (also an OT but with expertise in this area). Let that person assess your ability and,

if possible, recommend changes (such as not driving at night or for long distances) that permit you to keep driving.

- For legal reasons, if your PD isn't a factor in your driving ability, have your doctor note in your chart that you're capable of driving—day or night. This written verification can protect you if an accident occurs and you're not at fault.

Especially for men, driving is a mark of independence—that macho thing. Get over it. If the end of your driving days isolates and depresses you because you refuse to consider alternatives, that's on you. You have choices, including asking a friend or family member (who just happens to be looking for a concrete way to help) for a lift.

Freezing and Rigidity: When Your Head Says "Go," but Your Body Says "No"

Advanced PD often affects your ability to walk safely. What used to be unconscious, easy maneuvers that you took for granted are now major hurdles, just waiting to trip you up. This section discusses three of the most common problems: freezing, festination, and rigidity. Also, it includes suggestions to minimize the greatest concern—your risk of falling.

Freezing and festination: It's all in the legs

You're walking along fine and then—Bam!—like the cartoon character who steps in glue, you're stuck! *Freezing* is the sudden inability to step forward, and it typically happens in three situations:

- **As you step out:** *Start* hesitation classically occurs when you attempt to take the first step forward. The feet are glued to the floor and you may feel like you're walking in place. While the feet are stuck, the rest of the body may lurch forward, placing you at great risk for falling.
- **In mid-stride:** Even after you get started, freezing often happens in doorways or when you need to take

a step as you perform another action, like turning the doorknob.

- **When stopping or turning:** Freezing and hesitation can really complicate the act of turning around or changing direction—another circumstance that's ripe for a fall.

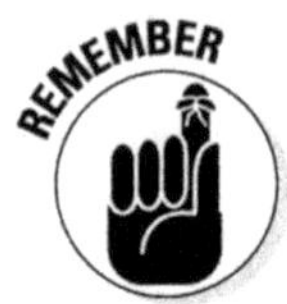

A growing number of products are designed specifically to address the problem of freezing, such as some of the walking aids listed in Appendix B. In addition, exercise videos and booklets offer programs specifically for PWP. Check out Appendix B as well as Chapter 12.

Another typical walking problem in advanced PD is *festination* (from the Latin word *festinato* or *haste*) where you take several short, almost running steps in an effort to regain your balance. This usually occurs as you break out of an episode of freezing.

You can use several tricks to maintain the rhythm of your walking:

- March in place or hum a marching tune.
- Take a step to the side before attempting to move forward. (This change in direction seems to interrupt the freezing sensation and allows you to continue your forward movement.)
- Step over an imaginary line on the ground.
- Visualize your foot moving through space three feet forward.

Rigidity: When your whole body locks up

Rigidity (stiffness in the muscles and limbs) as we discuss in Chapter 2 may first become evident in a reduced arm swing when walking or as the mask, loss of animated facial expression (see

"When Communication Becomes Difficult" earlier in this chapter). As PD progresses or if medication becomes less effective, the severity of rigidity can escalate. Rigidity can also result in muscular pain. In normal movement, activating one muscle (the *agonist*) is offset by relaxing the muscle that performs the opposing action (the *antagonist*). In rigidity, the opposing muscle fails to relax.

Your doctor can determine the degree of rigidity by gently moving the arm, leg, torso, or shoulder while you're standing or sitting in a relaxed position. One classic type of rigidity is known as *cogwheel,* where the arm, for example, can move only in short, jerky, or ratchet-like movements. Cogwheel rigidity is usually associated with resting tremor (tremor is present only in times of inactivity). Another common type of rigidity is *lead pipe,* when the muscles feel heavy and weak and using them causes fatigue.

A program of regular exercise and stretching (see Chapter 12) can be the most effective weapon to fight increasing stiffness and rigidity. Many communities offer special exercise programs through the local YMCA or hospital for people with conditions that cause muscle stiffness, weakness, and rigidity. Talk to your physical therapist (PT) or support group about the availability of such a program in your area (or about getting a program started).

PD and Falling—A Tricky Balancing Act

The greatest risk as PD advances is the danger of falling. By some estimates, two-thirds of all PWP experience falls in the mid-to-later stages. This percentage is significant because falls are the number one cause of hospitalization for the PWP due to fractures or head injuries, and because they're the precipitant factor in worsening of symptoms or even death due to onset of pneumonia.

Your PD symptoms contribute enormously to your possibility of falling. Think about the following scenarios:

- Your shuffling gait practically begs for the opportunity to trip over a rug or uneven pavement.
- Your general stiffness and slowness affect reaction time, so you can't stop yourself from falling by grabbing onto something.
- Your tendency to overcompensate for impaired balance by swaying backward when you turn or stand compromises your balance.

As a PWP, you're at risk to fall from four sources. The following sections cover those sources and the steps you can take to reduce your risk of falling.

Mind those meds

Most medications to manage PD symptoms have side effects, including "may cause dizziness." Medications for other health conditions (such as high blood pressure) can add to the problem. If you experience any change in maintaining your balance (stumbling, dizziness, lightheadedness, overcompensating to stay upright, and so forth), report these changes to your doctor immediately. And if you're experiencing new symptoms of dizziness or imbalance and you've had a recent change in meds, the change may be contributing to the problem. Don't try to guess—call the doctor.

Anything you can do to prevent a fall is worth the effort. The following suggestions may help:

- Ask your doctor to order an assessment of your current status by a PT and OT. (See Chapter 6 for info on these specialists.) Ideally the therapist(s) can compare this assessment to one you had shortly after your diagnosis to evaluate the amount of change.
- The therapist can evaluate your movements and risks for falling and then suggest changes in your home environment to prevent falls. (See Chapter 21 for tips on making this home survey yourself.)
- Ask your doctor whether your meds come in a dissolving tablet (you take them without water) so you can take a dose before you get up. At some point, you may want to ask your doctor to prescribe a hospital bed that you can raise and lower for greater assistance.

Steady as she goes

Training and adaptive devices (including the proper cane or walker) can help you move safely and independently. Please don't just assume that Uncle Dan's old cane is right for you. Ask your therapist to properly fit a device to you.

Falls (and possible injuries that require hospitalization) can lead some people to pull back on activity. If your fear of falling limits your activity, you may be doing more harm than you think because staying active—physically and mentally—goes hand in hand with staving off PD symptoms (and thus preventing more falls). Talk to your doctor about the possibility of a PT or OT assessment and therapy that helps you adapt and get active again.

Make adjustments along the way

Impaired balance can be part of your PD's progression (due to your increasing muscle stiffness, rigidity, a stooped posture, and more frequent episodes of freezing). See the earlier section "Freezing and Rigidity: When Your Head Says 'Go,' but Your Body Says 'No.'" Never is your team of professional care partners more important than now. Your doctor, PT, and OT can assess your needs and make recommendations to help you maintain your balance. In the meantime, this short list of suggestions can help you prevent a fall:

- Use that cane or walker that your doctor or PT ordered and customized for your needs.
- Avoid footwear with rubber soles that may stick to the floor. Ask your PT to suggest the best footwear for you.
- Use a recommended trick for maintaining a rhythm as you walk (see "Freezing and festination: It's

all in the legs" earlier in this chapter).

- Focus on walking rather than distractions. For example, don't try to talk on a portable phone and walk around at the same time.
- Take time to turn (TTT). Walking a few extra steps to make a wide turn is far better than pivoting suddenly and losing your balance.

Overcoming Sleep Disturbances

Anything that causes a disruption of normal sleep on an ongoing basis and prevents you from getting the rest you need is considered a sleep disturbance. Disturbances may have a number of causes: genetic or environmental factors (such as shift work), age, medications, and diet.

PWP are particularly prone to develop sleep disturbances for a wide variety of symptom-related reasons:

- Difficulty turning in bed or medication-induced dyskinesias may disturb the level of muscle relaxation necessary to sleep.

- Urinary urgency and frequency may force you to visit the bathroom several times during the night.
- Medication to treat your PD symptoms, if taken too close to bedtime, may cause vivid dreams or agitation that awakens you.
- Anxiety and depression, which frequently affect PWP (see Chapter 13), can make falling asleep difficult (anxiety) and can cause you to wake early or sleep too much (depression).

In addition, PWP may experience a number of specific sleep disturbances. The most important one is *rapid eye movement (REM) sleep behavior disorder,* a condition that makes you act out your dreams, unknowingly talk out loud, move your limbs, and sometimes even hit your bed partner! All of these actions can create a state of chronic sleep deprivation that leads to fatigue, excessive daytime sleepiness, and visual hallucinations.

However, keep in mind that many sleep disturbances can be improved simply by developing better sleep habits. The American Academy of Neurology offers the following tips:

- Sleep only when drowsy and only in the bedroom.
- Keep lights and noise low when trying to sleep, but keep a night light on to prevent falls if you need to get up in the night.
- Limit your intake of tobacco products, caffeine (chocolate, coffee, non-herbal tea, and such), and alcohol.
- Don't eat a heavy meal or participate in strenuous exercise for four to six hours before bedtime.
- Make use of relaxation and stress relief techniques (see Chapter 11).

Of course, like any new or troublesome symptom, discuss a sleep disturbance with your neurologist. The problem may be a side effect of your medications or a signal of a more serious condition such as sleep apnea syndrome, which requires specialized management.

Those Embarrassing Constipation and Urinary Issues

The good news: Although a nuisance for PWP, urinary and bowel issues are often treatable and manageable even with the progression of PD.

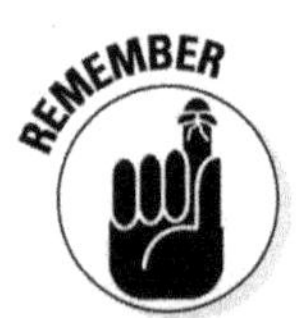

As we note in Chapter 17, never automatically dismiss urinary or bowel problems as unrelated to your PD. If incontinence or constipation becomes a problem as your PD progresses (or you've had issues in the past but they seem to be worsening), tell your doctor. While both conditions are common side effects of many medications (even common OTC meds), simply stopping or changing meds may not relieve symptoms.

In some cases PWP may suffer from an overactive bladder and feel an urgency to get to the bathroom as soon as possible, especially at night. Other PWP may experience an inability to fully empty the bladder, so they need to go again within a short time. Malfunction of the bladder isn't uncommon in PD. If you're experiencing such symptoms, you need to tell your doctor. In males, the problem can be an enlarged prostate gland; in women it may be an infection (called a *urinary tract infection* or *UTI*). In either case, your doctor may recommend that you see a urologist to rule out other causes.

The slowed movement that is a core part of PD can make constipation a relatively common problem for PWP. Because of other issues that can crop up with the progression of PD (swallowing difficulties that lead to a poorer diet, not drinking enough liquids, and infrequent exercise due to increased impairment to movement and balance control), constipation can become a recurrent problem for many PWP.

Let your doctor know of any changes in your normal bowel or urinary habits. In the meantime, you know the routine (your mother probably drummed it into you when you were a kid):

- **Drink plenty of water:** Yes, even if you need to go all the time.
- **Eat your roughage:** Also known as fiber (fruits, veggies, and whole grains). See www.mypyramid.gov.
- **Get daily exercise:** No, reaching for the remote doesn't count!

Dealing with the Big "D"—Dementia

Dementia may be one of the most frightening and unsettling words in the English language. Just to be very clear, the term means

- A person's intellectual function is impaired to the degree that it affects normal and routine activities (such as decision making, balancing a checkbook, and such) and relationships with other people.

- Possible changes occur in behavior and personality. A person with dementia may experience delusions or hallucinations.
- At least two normal functions of the brain (including memory, reasoning, perception, judgment, and such) are affected. Memory loss by itself is not dementia.

Dementia—senile or otherwise—isn't a normal part of aging.

Probably the question uppermost in your mind is: Is dementia part of PD's progression? The answer is: It may be, but it may not necessarily be true for you. In general, dementia seems to more frequently affect patients over the age of 70 and those in the late stages of the disease.

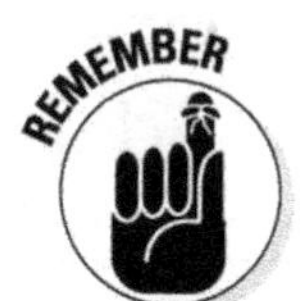

Everyone experiences the progression of PD in a unique way. So learn what you can about dementia and consider how you and your care partner may handle its possible onset. Then get back to living your life.

PD is not Alzheimer's disease

Today Alzheimer's disease (AD) is one of the most commonly recognized conditions associated with dementia. A person with AD faces a progressive loss of intellectual and mental function. Dementia in AD is a *primary* dementia. This means it doesn't result from any other disease or condition.

In contrast, for people with conditions that affect movement or other functions (such as PD), dementia is a secondary dementia. That is, it appears to arise from a separate source. For example, a person with PD may also have high blood pressure or other cardiovascular conditions and may develop symptoms of dementia related to those conditions. This form is then termed *vascular dementia.*

PWP may develop AD in their later years, or they may develop *Lewy body dementia,* a disturbance of their cognition characterized mainly by fluctuations in attention and alertness, executive dysfunction, and recurrent visual hallucinations. (When dementia occurs very early in PD, the term *Lewy body disease* indicates a separate disease in its own right.) But whether the onset of the secondary dementia is *linked* to PD or simply *co-exists* (like PD plus diabetes) is currently unknown. Recent studies of brains at different stages of PD suggest that dementia may be the very last pathological stage of the disease.

The point is this: The onset of dementia in a PWP isn't a foregone conclusion, and it isn't the same as AD. You need to report any sign of cognitive malfunction to your doctor, because your sudden hallucinations or excessive sleepiness and dull mind may have a perfectly logical (and treatable) explanation.

Reviewing those cognitive symptoms

Although Chapter 3 has a full discussion of cognitive symptoms, a quick review is helpful in this chapter's context of PD progression.

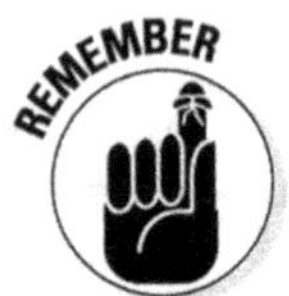

Having some cognitive symptoms doesn't necessarily mean you're headed for full-blown dementia. Don't panic, but do talk to your doctor if you're experiencing any of the following:

- **Anxiety or depression** are part and parcel of PD. Focus on the fact that they're treatable. If you ignore or refuse to acknowledge these symptoms, shame on you. (If you haven't read Chapter 13, do it soon.)
- **Executive dysfunction** can include troubles with balancing your check-book, following directions, making routine decisions, and such. Fortunately, you can strengthen and exercise your mind and possibly keep this problem at bay. (See the

following section "When Medical Treatments Are Limited.")

- **Hallucinations** (seeing objects that really aren't there—perhaps a child or animal passing quickly by your door or simply feeling the presence of a person without actually seeing that person) can be a side effect of your medications. But as your PD advances, these visual (and usually harmless) hallucinations maybe associated with a cognitive disorder. As with everything that seems out of the norm, you (or your care partner) need to let your doctor know. Simple medication changes or adding others medications to block hallucinations may help.

When Medical Treatments Are Limited

Identifying the various symptoms that may worsen or appear as your PD advances is only one piece of the puzzle. Another piece is addressing those changes. What options do you have when medical treatments can't provide the answer?

You have a number of resources—all within your grasp—for fighting back if you have to face the onset of new symptoms or the progression of your present symptoms. The following guidelines can help you stay the course:

- Continue to eat a healthy diet rich in antioxidants (see Chapter 12).
- Continue your daily exercise program (also discussed in Chapter 12).
- Continue to exercise that mind! Mental activities (no, TV doesn't count) can help to keep your mind agile.
- If possible, consider taking a class or starting a new hobby.
- At the very least, remain socially active and engaged in the world and the community around you.

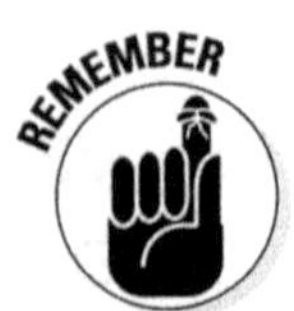

Yes, you may be approaching the point where you rely on other people more. But this doesn't mean you have to surrender all decisions and control.

Your lifestyle and life choices can play an enormous role in your ability to post-pone your PD's progression. Keep fighting! Keep moving! Keep living!

A Word for the PD Care Partner

As your partner's PD progresses, you may face some tough challenges like having to persuade him to give up driving or acknowledge that he's showing more and more signs of cognitive impairment that can impact his safety. Such challenges can seem even more difficult because you've both been living with PD for a number of years. Obvious symptoms that the PD is getting worse can add strain to the relationship. The following tips may help you hold it together as you and your PWP enter this new phase of living with PD:

- Acknowledge changes as they come and seek the advice of the neurologist especially if you notice any unusual progression of symptoms (like sleep disturbances or onset of visual hallucinations) or recurring behavior (excessive eye-blinking or increased urinary urgency).

- Continue to prepare for potential lifestyle changes that may become necessary (such as a change in living accommodations) and check out availability of options in your community.
- Let someone else be the villain when it comes to taking away driving privileges. If you're concerned, let the PWP's doctor know. The doctor can order a driving evaluation and make recommendations based on that.
- If the doctor doesn't respond to your concerns about your partner's driving, contact a representative in your state motor vehicle department and ask her to require a road test as a step in renewing the license.
- If *you* begin to feel overwhelmed with more and more of the responsibilities (financial, physical, emotional), talk to your support group contacts or facilitator, your

clergyperson, or the counselor you found when you and your PWP set up the healthcare team (see Chapter 6); ask for some concrete tips for coping.

- Realize that you're in danger of burning out. Attending to your needs for regular short-term breaks and an occasional long-term respite are keys to keep on keeping on. Plan for these breaks and consider them as vital to living with PD as your partner's timely medications.

If you and your partner have prepared for this day, you've already discussed some difficult decisions. Your partner now needs to accept and appreciate that you're simply carrying out those decisions you made months or years ago. If your partner is incapable of understanding (or appreciating) that fact, remind yourself that he's still in control. But you need to remember: Having made the choices together, you're now simply carrying out his wishes. (For more advice on coping with progressing care, read Chapter 19.)

Chapter 19

When Care Partners Become Caregivers

In This Chapter

- Recognizing the need for change
- Seeing those relationships in a new light
- Making the best of it: Other options
- Leaping the biggest hurdles
- Lining up the secondary team
- Caring words for the caregiver

You're likely to live for many years in spite of your Parkinson's disease (PD). The prognosis is hopeful and every day brings us all closer to a cure. But as your PD progresses, the day may come—most likely following a fall and maybe a fracture that requires hospitalization—when you'll need more hands-on, direct care.

We hope you've had a care *partner* as you've made your PD journey to this point. But that can be good and bad news. The good news is that this person is the most likely candidate to become your primary caregiver, and he or she is probably very familiar with you and the path your PD has taken. The bad news is that you've gotten pretty used to being in charge. Handing off that control will take some adjustment.

As your need for care increases, you'll almost certainly be surrounded by different tiers of care. Your primary caregiver is the person who takes the lead, manages your care day-to-day, and acts as your spokesperson if you can't speak for yourself. But you'll also need secondary caregivers. These people (usually other family members and friends) take on a specific role, like handling your finances or doing the grocery shopping.

In this chapter, we consider that transition from partnering to receiving the care of another person because of your symptoms' progression (see Chapter 18 for more on these). This chapter covers specific changes in your caregiver's new role and how your relationship with that person may adjust. We also offer alternative arrangements that may be necessary over time, give you a heads-up on the biggest challenges of this transition, and suggest ways to develop your secondary caregivers. Finally, we offer straight talk and important suggestions for your care partner.

Understanding Your Primary Caregiver's Role

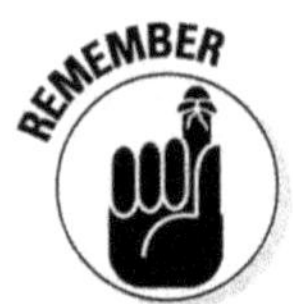

By definition, caregivers provide some type of hands-on assistance to other people. That assistance may be in the area of handling finances, managing legal affairs, providing emotional support, attending to routine chores, administering personal care, or any combination of these categories. According to the Family Caregiver Alliance, as many as 52 million family care-givers in the United States provide care for an adult (age 20 and over) family member or friend.

Most caregivers (75 percent) are women, and about half of all caregivers are employed elsewhere full-time.

Your caregiver is the person who takes primary responsibility in providing more intensive home and personal care assistance. This person is who you trust to abide by your wishes—the ones you made clear in better times—and to speak for you if you're unable to speak for yourself.

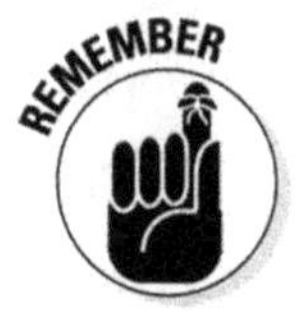

Your caregiver isn't the person with PD. Life will go on for this person after the time for giving care has passed. And he deserves to attend to that life while still attending to your needs. As your relationship adjusts to a new balance of roles, remember that this is the same person who's been right there with you as your *partner*. He's well aware of the emotional and psychological impact these challenging times have on both of you.

Giving care versus partnering in care

Your roles are changing now. More and more it's your care-partner-turned-caregiver who must take charge of decisions and actions that affect your welfare and safety. Decisions that once focused on *your* needs must now increasingly focus on your *caregiver's* needs, abilities, and emotional strength in order to deliver what you need when you need it without sacrificing her normal routine.

Never will it be more tempting to give in to the anger and resentment that this widening chasm can create. Never will your care-partner-turned-caregiver need your love, appreciation, and emotional support more.

And yet an important element of partnering remains. If you and your partner have prepared for this day, discussed the difficult decisions that you knew you might face, and explored options to address your increasing needs, then your partner is simply carrying out the decisions you both made months or even years ago.

Is your care partner a novice or a natural caregiver?

Some people are natural nurturers. Others are not. Some come to the role of caregiver with years of experience already under their belts. Other folks who are new to the role may find themselves entering a strange world that they're not prepared to tackle. But most caregivers have one fact in common: The need to step in sneaks up on them. One day their loved one is managing fairly well, and the next day the caregiver suddenly needs to intervene. The ongoing care becomes not only necessary, but essential.

Keep in mind that not everyone is up to the job. Just because a person is your spouse or adult child and the most obvious candidate, this doesn't mean that he's physically and emotionally prepared to take on increasingly complex care-giving duties. You and your care partner need to keep an open mind and be willing to creatively decide how best to meet your needs as your PD progresses.

It's called the 36-hour day for a reason

Jus how long the need for care will continue is hard to estimate. It can be any-where from a year to decades. But if the caregiver devotes 20 to 40 hours a week (as statistics indicate) to giving care in addition to the other roles she's juggling, then the idea of a 36-hour day fits.

In addition to selecting the best caregiver for the job, you and your care partner need to get real about how much time it's going to take *and* where that time will come from. Two lives are at stake here—yours and your caregiver's. At this stage (as in the earlier stages), each of you has the right to maintain some semblance of a lifestyle that fills your physical, mental, emotional, and spiritual needs. (For more ideas on how to make your priorities a reality, check out Chapters 7 and 15 for your relationships and Chapters 6, 13, and 17 for physical, emotional, and spiritual suggestions.)

Considering How Your Relationships May Change

If you've prepared for this day, you and your significant other (or adult child or other care partner) have discussed the what-will-happen-when questions.

And you've thought about how to address your increasing need to rely on other people. The most likely candidates for caregiver are pretty obvious, but each situation comes with a history that can affect this shift in roles.

When you rely on your spouse or significant other: A balancing act

"Grow old along with me..." the old saying goes.

In a marriage or union between two people, each person settles into a role. She pays the bills and manages the day-to-day budget. He handles their financial and healthcare security. She's the gardener; he's the cook. She's the social butterfly; he prefers staying home with a good book. Through the years, they develop ways of compromising, moving out of their comfort zones, and rein venting themselves individually as they find their way as a couple.

So, what happens if everything shifts? He has advanced PD and can no longer safely prepare the meals. She takes this on. When going out becomes more difficult for him, she adapts by staying home to be with him. He feels guilty that his PD impacts her life so much; she reassures him but can't deny a sense of mourning at how their lives have changed. As the caregiving becomes more intense, perhaps she abandons more and more of those activities that gave her identity.

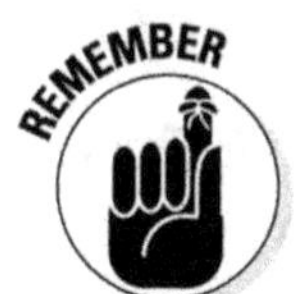

When one partner becomes the caregiver, both partners need to maintain balance as their duties and responsibilities shift. The best way you and your care partner can accomplish this shift is through your willingness to accept the help of other people. This help can free your partner to pursue (in moderation) her life, and (if she accepts this help as your contribution to the relationship) it can relieve her guilt for wanting a life beyond your PD.

When your adult child steps up: You're still the parent

Sometimes the relationship that comes from an adult child caring for a parent has been called *parenting our parents.* Wrong! Roles may shift as you turn to your child for advice on finances or assistance with daily chores, but the relationship between you and your child has a history. There's no reversal here. (See Chapter 15 for more discussion on this relationship.)

If your adult child becomes your primary caregiver, your history influences the relationship you forge. Although the ways you've communicated (or not) through the years may have mellowed, the base of your relationship doesn't change just because you now need help. And this reality may be good, or it may cause some rough moments.

The key for this caregiving relationship is one of mutual respect. As an adult, your child deserves the same trust and respect that you would extend to any person of maturity and experience. At the same time, that child needs to accept that—regardless of your frailties and even childlike dependencies—you're still a grown-up with a history of managing your own life.

When your sibling comes to your aid: Rivalries remain

Family history plays a part with siblings too. Your position within the family order (eldest, middle, youngest) continues to impact the relationship. "Mom always liked you best" isn't forgotten, although someone may mention it in jest these days. Old jealousies, wounds, and slights that you never addressed as adults can still fester. Labels from when you were small can linger. "Mary was the smart one." "Jim was the family comedian."

If a sibling seems the most likely candidate to become your caregiver and spokesperson, the time to mend fences is way before that day arrives. You also need to set ground rules about the way you live your life and interact with other people. If your sibling can't respect your ways and expects you to adapt to his, the relationship may be under stress from day one. And, trust us, the last thing you need in your life is more stress.

When your friends offer to help: Are they in it for the long haul?

If you're single and have no family member close enough (geographically or emotionally) to consider as your caregiver, you may turn increasingly to a long-time friend for help and support. Although this pattern can and does work for many people, take care. A lifelong friendship can be destroyed if both sides aren't absolutely upfront about giving and receiving care.

Identify the specific ways you anticipate needing help. Start with one task—perhaps transportation to and from doctor appointments or a daily call or visit to be sure you're okay. Friends are usually quite willing (even anxious) to step up, but they need direction. Bottom line: If they need to back off, they need to know you'll understand and can find another source for help.

Exploring Alternative Arrangements

If you've been living alone, you may need to look outside your immediate home for the care partner who's willing to take on caregiving as your PD progresses. In fact, you may want to split the job up and enlist more than one caregiver.

When the most obvious caregiver lives far away

In today's world, family members often scatter across a wide area. The most obvious caregiver may be someone living miles away. Short of you or this person making a major move, what are your choices?

Making a long-distance arrangement

One caregiver in Wisconsin managed care for her parents in Virginia over an eight-year period without anyone having to move. When long-distance care-givers take care of loved ones, the keys are knowledge and preparation.

Take these two steps:

1. **Know ahead of time what programs and services your community has for support and care.**
2. **Prepare for the day that your needs increase:**
   - Establish contacts within those community programs.
   - Identify emergency caregivers who can step in for a short time until the long-distance caregiver can arrive.

Establishing an emergency backup

Emergency caregivers are people who are available to step in when something unforeseen arises. Their role is temporary but important.

Your emergency caregiver may be a neighbor who's home during the day (while your primary caregiver works) or a friend who's agreed to assume this key role. It may be your clergyperson who can marshall the forces of the congregation to step in until more permanent help arrives.

Whoever you identify for this role, you—and especially your long-distance caregiver—need to establish a plan for emergency action sooner rather than later. If you fall and your primary caregiver is miles away, who will come to your aid?

When no one applies

In rare cases, no single person can step in and assume the role of primary caregiver. When that happens, don't despair. You have at least two options for preparing for the day when you need more hands-on care.

The first option

Assess how you can remain in your home and get the help you need. Some aspects of this plan are easier than others. For example,

- Many pharmacies and grocery stores offer a delivery service for medications and food.
- You can address safety issues by installing a phone service and wearing a pager. If you don't contact the service within a specified time each day (or even twice a day), then the service contacts someone to come and check on you. Or if you fall and need help, you can activate the pager.

The second option

Other facets of care are more complex. How are you going to manage routine tasks such as showering, shaving, or shampooing? How are you going to manage financial matters if you begin to experience diminished mental capacity?

Consider a change in residence sooner rather than later. At the very least, community services can be a lifeline for you. Or you may consider an actual move. Options such as assisted living facilities and so-called *step* communities are two possibilities. For a full discussion of care and housing options and how to manage the costs, see Chapters 21 and 22.

Making the Transition

When the transition from partnering to caregiving begins in earnest, you and your caregiver need to be ready for the learning curve. Consider these new challenges:

- Moving from independence to the need for assistance
- Rapidly shifting from partner to caregiver, a seemingly full-time job
- Moving from blind stubbornness to acceptance
- Consciously recognizing the emotional roller coaster you've boarded—right when your physical and emotional defenses are down

Your best tactic is to acknowledge the difficult feelings (see Chapter 24) that come with those challenges and deal with them head on. Get professional help to deal with the transition if you need it.

Just make sure that you understand that accepting help from others—regardless of how independent and self-sufficient you've always tried to be—is simply one more tool you and your primary care partner have. Allowing others (friends, extended family, the community) to provide assistance gives you much needed support in preserving your energy to live life as fully as possible for as long as possible.

Learning to accept help

Humans are by nature fiercely independent and perhaps never more so than when that autonomy is threatened by illness or other circumstances beyond their control.

One of the concepts we try to instill throughout this book is that fighting PD is a team effort. If it takes a village to raise a child properly, it takes a contingent of healthcare professionals, family, and friends to maintain a life with PD. You may be the quarterback, but you need every one of those other players to help you run those plays and live on your own terms.

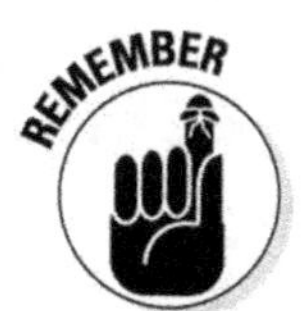

There's no shame in accepting the help of other people. As a matter of fact, *you're* often helping *them!* You empower them by needing them. And you enrich their lives by giving them a way to tangibly demonstrate their love and respect for you.

You know how much you hate this PD being all about you—the glances, the murmured comments when people think you're out of earshot. You have just one way to change that: Take control, and accept the help you need.

Still not convinced the time has come to seek additional help? Think again. Maybe you're reading this chapter because you already suspect you and your care partner can no longer manage totally on your own. But refusing to acknowledge it (and then make the necessary changes and accept help) can result in serious setbacks for both of you. Some of these can be:

- A toll on your relationship
- Financial costs associated with emergencies brought on by your refusal to accept help
- Isolation that comes from managing your PD to the exclusion of everything and everyone else

- Confusion from managing alone, trying to protect your independence
- Ignored warning signs (such as anger, depression, guilt, and other difficult feelings)
- Damaged health (physical, mental, emotional) and financial well-being for you and your care partner

Whether you enlist the help of other people or make a more permanent change (like moving to a different residence where support and care are readily available), don't be stubborn about this. Don't toy with your life and the life of your beloved, devoted care partner. Snap out of it!

Take charge by establishing a routine for daily, weekly, and long-term breaks (be sure you read the section "Dealing with burnout" later in this chapter) and by accepting the help and support that's within your reach.

Remembering that your PD isn't your caregiver's fault

The song says you always hurt the one you love. And it happens fairly innocently. Your care partner knows you aren't always at your best and doesn't expect you to be. You can let go of the brave façade, the "I'm doing great" demeanor, with this person.

But avoid going too far with this. The dark side of being yourself comes out when you start taking out your anger and frustration on that person. This emotion may come in the form of a short temper, snappish comments, or actual physical lashing out. It may also come in more subtle ways, like shutting the person out through silence or isolating the person from his own life by your neediness.

Your care partner has surrendered a piece of his life to continue this journey with you. Just how great that sacrifice turns out to be may be up to you.

Dealing with burnout

If you or your care partner were not dealing with the terrible situation, if both of you were living normal lives, wouldn't you make room for regular breaks from routine? Consider how most jobs include breaks, holidays, vacation time, and personal days. You deserve at least that same consideration!

Review your current situation

Burnout is common in the workplace and even more so among caregivers. However, rarely do you hear about burnout in the person with PD (PWP) or in people with other chronic, progressive conditions that require constant adjustment and adaptation. Ask yourself and your care partner the following questions:

- Is it becoming increasingly difficult for each of you to face the daily challenges of your PD?
- Is your care partner showing signs of health changes—sleeplessness, under-eating or overeating, headaches, or vague complaints of aches and pains?

- Do you or your care partner react to good news or complaints with irritation, cynicism, or sarcasm? (In other words, has your ability to show interest in or concern for other people been compromised?)
- Are the two of you often irritable and impatient with each other?
- Are you seeing signs that you or your care partner is becoming increasingly isolated, sad, lonely, or resentful of others?

Then ask these big questions and be brutally honest in answering:

- Do you or your care partner reject suggestions and offers of help because you believe other people just don't get it? (They haven't been through this, so they can't possibly understand!)
- Do you honestly believe that only your care partner and you can make this work?

If you answered "Yes" to two of the first five questions for yourself or your care partner, think *burnout.* If you answered "Yes" to one or both of the last two questions, you need a break, possibly some counseling, and you need it now.

Ask for additional help

Ideally, sit down with your care partner and consider the following ideas together:

- Identify your personal support network and your care partner's. ***Note:*** They're not necessarily the same people. To do this, list the one or two people that each of you would call if you just needed to vent. Then add the names of three or four people you'd call for specific help or the occasional favor.
- Of these people, have you or your care partner turned down help from one or more of them?
- If you've rejected their support, how can you reopen the door and welcome them back as active partners in care?

If the person accepts your overture and asks what you need, be prepared with specifics. For example, "Can you just stop by for a visit while my care partner goes to the store? It's getting harder for her to take me along, and, frankly, the break does us both good."

Consider counseling to get your head and spirit straight

Depending on how far you've distanced yourselves from other people, professional counseling may be necessary. But you have other choices that carry built-in benefits of community and social interaction. Check out these three possibilities:

- **Support group:** Okay, you may have resisted this option up until now, but get over it—if not for yourself, then for your care partner. Properly facilitated support groups can be a real source of new ideas, local information and updates, and even inspiration for managing your PD more effectively.

You may need to visit more than one group to find a good match, but smaller communities may not have a group specifically for PD. To find support groups in your area, go to the National Parkinson Foundation Web site (www.parkinson.org), or, for more general information, go to the Web site of the National Family Caregivers Association (www.nfcacares.org).

• **Community:** Every community has counseling resources for low or even no cost. For example:

- Religious communities have one or two clergypersons well known for providing comfort and counsel. The clergyperson doesn't need to be yours (or even of your faith).
- Hospitals, your local library, and civic groups may offer community programs with experienced speakers addressing topics of loss, aging, living with chronic illness, and so forth.
- Funeral homes often offer grief counseling by a professional who's trained in helping people work through a loss. Certainly you and your care partner have suffered loss as your PD's progressed.

• **Professional:** At some point you or your care partner may benefit from the guidance of a professional. There's no shame in this. Your physician, hospital or home care social worker, and local Office on Aging are good resources for referrals.

Plan for the healing power of R&R

Good news: You can avoid much of the damage caused by burnout if you build regular respite into your routine—early on. This means planning daily and weekly breaks as well as the occasional (but just as regular) longer hiatus, as we describe in the following:

- **Daily short-term *respite*** means at least two timeouts—separately or together. Perhaps your care partner takes a walk while you watch a sports event on television, or you call a friend while she takes a long, hot bath, or the two of you order takeout from a favorite restaurant, or you watch a favorite movie together. Whatever the respite, be sure you plan it, schedule it, and don't cancel it (okay, short postponements are acceptable).
- **Weekly breaks** may include trips to the beauty salon or manicurist,

card night, choir practice, a movie, or a club meeting. These breaks last a couple of hours, and support group meetings don't count because *respite* means getting away from *everything* to do with PD. Plan the breaks, write them on the calendar in ink, and make them non-negotiable—unless the house is on fire.

- **The longer hiatus** can take many forms but usually lasts several hours to several days. Only you and your care partner can best identify the rest and relaxation you need. It may be a trip to the city for shopping, dining out, and seeing a play. It may be a place without a phone that gives you time to unwind with a book, take a walk in the woods, stroll along a beach, and so on. Such breaks take careful planning but they're doable. And the pay-off can be enormous for you as individuals and for your relationship.

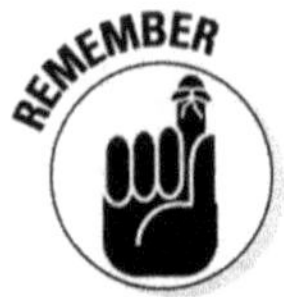

If your care partner receives vacation, holiday, and personal time from work, it's not *respite* if he spends it catching up with a household, a family, and your PD. Respite isn't about labeling time; it's about how time is used. It's taking a break and getting away from everything to do with giving or receiving care.

Recruiting Secondary Caregivers

Okay, your chronic PD has progressed. Little tasks that once were doable are now nearly exhausting—and frankly not always worth the effort. Spending the day in your pj's is easier than the hassle of getting dressed. Brushing or styling your hair is a joke, and shaving or trying to apply make-up? Forget it!

Now you carefully time your appointments or activities to your on-off cycles. Your concentration isn't what it once was, and you're beginning to worry that you may be letting important details (like paying the light bill) slip.

On top of all this, you're seriously worried about your partner—the worry lines around her eyes and mouth, the constant exhaustion, and the lack of attention to personal needs, activities, and grooming. Your partner needs some help—and so do you.

Calling another meeting

We hope you and your family met soon after your diagnosis to talk about the ways PD was likely going to impact your lives (see Chapter 7). Now, as the symptoms worsen and new symptoms seem inevitable, you need to gather the troops once again. This time the agenda is different.

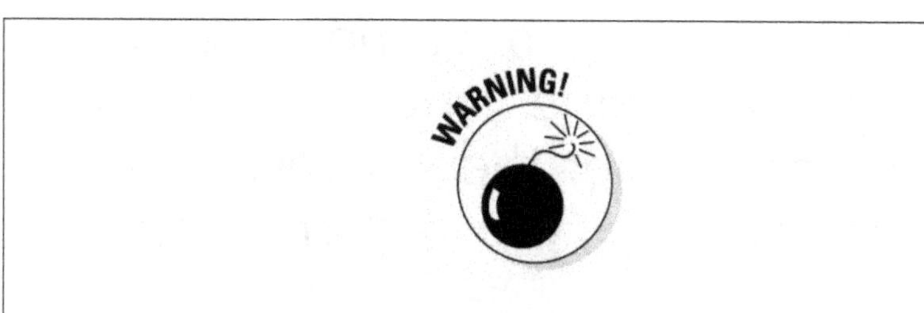

In some cases your adult children may bring everyone together. This family meeting may take on the trappings of an intervention if your family believes that you and your care partner are being overly stubborn about asking for and accepting help. Far better for you to acknowledge early on that you need additional help and take charge of the meeting on your terms.

Extending the invitation

Woody Allen once said that 80 percent of success is simply showing up. And that comment is especially true when you have a family meeting to discuss help and support—you need the family to actually show up. Their good intentions just won't cut it. Although we don't suggest subterfuge for getting family members on board, you need to do what you can to gather the family in one place at one time. If that plan's next to impossible, then choose a family holiday when you plan to be together—Thanksgiving or a major birthday for you or your care partner.

Consider these suggestions to help organize this meeting:

- Make it clear to family members that the day will include a discussion of the future for you and your care partner.
- If the gathering involves young children, make plans to occupy them for two to three hours. Ideally, arrange for them to be at another site so they don't interrupt the meeting.
- If a family member refuses to attend the meeting, assure the other family members that you'll speak with this person privately about a commitment to your care. And if that person clearly isn't on board with this arrangement, then drop it for now. Perhaps down the road (maybe when someone else is burning out) this person may step up.

Preparing the agenda

For this meeting, you have three goals:

- You and your roster of care partners need to face facts. Your PD has advanced, and your spouse, significant other, adult child, or other rock you've been leaning on can't do it all.
- You now need more hands-on and supportive care for you and your primary care partner.
- Everyone needs to understand the situation and figure out how to make some definitive contribution.

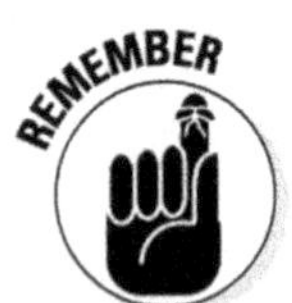

Initially you and your care partner will approach family for this care and support. But in some situations the family is either unwilling or unavailable. In that case you can follow a similar guide for a meeting with friends and neighbors who have expressed a desire to help. Just keep in mind that your friends and neighbors aren't family—they don't owe you anything.

The meeting will outline the following details:

- Help that you need now (chores, bathing, transportation, and so forth)
  - Specifically name the task; quantify how often you need the help and when you need it. (Some tasks are seasonal, like putting up screens and cleaning out gutters; others are regular, like helping you shower or staying with you once a week while your care partner is out.)
  - Indicate community services (and their costs) that can provide the assistance
- Help that you'll likely need within the coming year
  - How often and when
  - Availability and cost of community or paid services

You probably won't need help with everything—at least not all at once. But identify all the areas you may need assistance as your PD progresses. The following is a partial list to get you started:

- **Hygiene:** Bathing or showering, oral hygiene, dressing, personal grooming (hair, nails, and so on), other personal hygiene such as odor due to urinary incontinence
- **Medications:** Organizing and storing, dispensing, refilling prescriptions
- **Transportation:** To and from medical appointments, to and from community or social events, to and from shopping
- **Exercise and recreation:** Prescribed exercise for flexibility and strengthening, personal exercise preference such as yoga or T'ai Chi, pursuit of hobbies and leisure time activities
- **Basic nursing tasks:** Ambulation (walking from room to room), transferring (from bed to chair to car and such), care of medical equipment such as a catheter
- **Emergency care** (prepare every caregiver in basic first aid): Wound

care, falls, fractures, fainting, choking, adverse reactions to medications

- **Household chores:** Exterior home maintenance (regular like grass cutting; seasonal like snow-shoveling), interior home maintenance (regular like weekly cleaning; occasional like changing the furnace filter), errands (like grocery shopping and trips to the post office), meal preparation
- **Financial tasks:** Bill paying (like utilities or medical and household bills), taxes (preparing, filing), money management (like investments and pensions)

As you prepare these lists, don't be too quick to surrender a task (such as grocery shopping) if it gives you or your primary care partner a break from confinement to the house. In this case, the opportunity for socialization and being out in the world may have greater value than the assistance. Perhaps someone can stay with you while your partner shops. Then that secondary caregiver can assist in bringing in the groceries and putting them away.

Turning over the meeting

Surprise! We suggest that you open the meeting, lay out the agenda (see the previous section) ... and then leave. Why should you do this when you and your life are under discussion? Simple. Family members may find it difficult to admit limitations and aversions to giving care; saying this to your face can be even more difficult. When you leave, let your primary care partner take over the facilitation of the meeting, or, better yet, you may want to ask a third party (such as your support group leader or clergyperson) to conduct the meeting. The point is to create an environment where those in attendance feel free to express concerns and limits without hurting your feelings.

Especially in families with a history of discord, asking an objective third party to direct the entire meeting is a good move. A trusted clergyperson, counselors, and the facilitator of your support group are possible candidates. In this case, both you and your primary care partner leave the meeting after the opening.

Getting everyone talking and committing

Open the meeting by stating that you fully intend to manage as much as you can for as long as you can. But you do need their assistance (not control) and patience to accept that tasks may take you longer and require more effort.

Distribute printed copies of the agenda that includes your list of tasks (see the earlier section "Preparing the agenda" for ideas). Then excuse yourself (see the previous section "Turning over the meeting"). Your care partner or third party then facilitates the meeting as follows:

1. **Give everyone time to consider the list and their emotional commitment (10 to 15 minutes should do).**

   Note: Don't try to limit any part of this meeting to a specific schedule. You want to make this meeting an open discussion, not one constrained by time.

2. **Ask everyone to mark tasks that they'll consider taking on.**

   Explain that people won't have to take on every task they mark. You'll use the results of this process to assign specific tasks, establish backup help for a task, and identify gaps that may need outside help.

3. **Open the floor to questions, discussion, and additional suggestions for the list.**

4. **Go through items one by one and identify coverage (or lack thereof).**

5. **Tally the cost of outside help for the apparent gaps. Ask family**

members to indicate (in writing for your care partner's eyes only) what amounts they're willing to contribute to that total each month.

6. Finally, adjourn the meeting with the assurance that you'll plan a follow-up meeting after you and your care partner have gone over the information and made a tentative schedule.

After the meeting, you and your care partner can review the information and get actual commitments for hands-on help and financial contributions.

Accepting aid with appreciation and gratitude

Now that you have the commitment of family members, you and your primary care partner have an important task: You need to accept their willingness to help by making specific assignments.

The division of contributions will not be equal or fair. Everyone needs to face that fact from the outset. The physical and emotional toll for a family member living nearby can be very different from a member who lives at some distance. Similarly, one family member may not be able to accept that you need help with such personal tasks as combing your hair, taking a shower, or going to the bathroom.

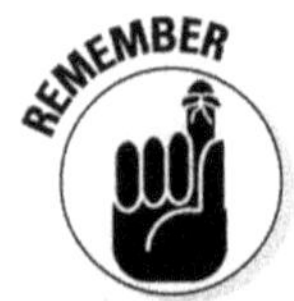

You and your primary care partner must not pass judgment but must try to find ways each personality can contribute. If hands-on care is beyond a person's capacity, assign them to *outside* tasks, such as home maintenance, shopping, finances, taxes, and so on.

Some individuals are just naturally more nurturing. One of your adult children or siblings may mark practically everything on the list. Resist the urge to take him up on that. The last thing you need is for these secondary care-givers to burn out when you need them most.

Teen-aged children, grandchildren, extended family members, close friends, and other people may welcome the opportunity to help you and your care partner in concrete ways. Don't leave them out of the discussion, although you may want to approach them separately. If so, do that shortly after the meeting with adults in your family—perhaps that same afternoon.

You and your care partner probably have a realistic idea of the time and effort each task takes (especially the ones involving personal, hands-on care). You also understand the emotional toll of dealing with PD better than these relative newbies. Keep all these concerns in mind as you consider who may be the best provider for each task.

Whatever the contribution, as long as the provider gives it with love and the best of intentions, accept it and say "Thank you."

A Word for the PD Care Partner

You didn't ask for this, but here you are. Now you need to find a way to attend to the needs of the PWP in addition to other facets of your life. Many of those facets may be (probably are) vital to the situation. For example, your work may be the prime source of income these days. It also may provide the insurance that both you and the PWP need.

Your health is also a factor. You can hardly manage the escalating tasks of a caregiver if your own health is compromised. So, good eating habits, daily physical exercise, and adequate rest are more than good ideas—they make a huge difference in your overall ability to tackle this new challenge.

Get real about the time this is going to take

The Family Caregiver Alliance estimates that the average caregiver spends 18 to 20 hours each week giving care. One-fifth of family caregivers provide 40 or more hours of care per week. Even if you don't work outside the home or work part-time, you have other facets of your life that need your attention. You have you that needs and deserves your attention.

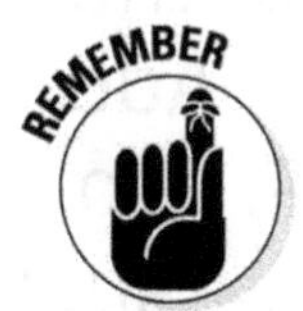

You don't have PD—your partner does. And you won't have PD after your partner moves beyond your ability to provide full-time, hands-on attention. You'll have a life—and we hope it's still filled with the people and activities that have sustained you since before PD became a part of it.

Consider the roles you play now: spouse or significant other, adult child, parent, sibling, employee (or employer), homemaker, civic or community leader (in your town, religious community, or such), volunteer. Add to these official roles a list of the activities you enjoy, such as reading, biking, traveling, gardening, and so on. Finally, add any additional hobbies you enjoy (and don't necessarily share with the PWP), such as needlework, photography, sports, playing cards, and such.

Wow! When you write it all down, chances are good that you have a life that's pretty full. Add one more item: Besides the PWP, do you have other family members, such as an aging parent or in-law, who will likely need your care and support in the next few years?

The big question is: How are you going to fit caregiving into that busy life? Put another way, what will you have to put aside or give up altogether to be an effective caregiver over possibly several years?

Get creative about finding the time

Time management experts advise you to look at time as blocks. Start with your five weekdays—that's five 24-hour blocks. Block out the non-negotiables: work (hours per day) and sleep (at least 7 hours a night). What's left on a normal weekday? Full-time work and sleep account for 15 hours, leaving 9 hours available. Okay, so far.

Now add time to get ready for work, travel to and from work, shopping and errands, laundry and other housework, and meals. Whew! Chances are you just knocked off another two hours a day and you still have to find time for meal preparation, eating those meals, laundry and housework, checking up on other family members, catching up with friends, making time for choir practice or a workout—and oh yes, partnering in care. Where does the time go? Better question: Where will the time come from?

America as a society has gotten very good at multi-tasking, and that practice may save you time in a few places. For example, can you make phone calls while preparing a meal or doing the laundry? Can you work part of your week from home so you can do the actual job in the evening and open up the day for something like a doctor's appointment, grocery shopping, and that workout?

How about taking advantage of available community services such as adult day care (see Chapter 21)? Can they provide the PWP some of the care you currently give (such as a hot meal or hair care) in order to free up time for you?

The options are out there. You and the PWP just have to be willing to accept the help and accept the fact that it may not be done your way or as well as you do it. But if these options can give you back the time you've surrendered to mundane tasks so you can once again enjoy a quiet evening of television or visiting with friends, then they're certainly worth considering.

Be prepared to delegate

The temptation in giving care is to simply do it yourself. Maybe it seems faster and easier than trying to explain what you need. And maybe you get energy from the praise and admiration you receive when you handle everything on your own.

The world has its super-moms. Are you becoming super-caregiver, trapped into believing (and convincing other people) that you and the PWP are managing fine? Are you sending signals that these people can go about their lives with no guilt or concern? *Whoa!*

In the early and mid-stages of PD, you and the PWP managed for some time without relying on others. Then one day you realize that the PD, its physical demands, and its mental and emotional demands are falling squarely on your shoulders.

The point is:

- If you haven't already opened the door (and your mind) to accept the help of other people (see the previous section "Recruiting Secondary Caregivers"), this is the moment.
- If you haven't held a family meeting, do it now.
- If you've had the meeting, call the family together and let them know the need for help and support has reached another level.

Review what else they can do and what they can add to their present financial contributions.

In the process of taking on more care responsibilities, don't make the mistake of ignoring the PWP. Ask yourself these questions:

- Are you (or others) assuming that the PWP can't perform tasks or make decisions that are in fact still possible?
- Are you making sure that the PWP is still part of the discussion and decision-making?
- Are you keeping in mind that, for your loved one, this is another loss in the battle to maintain autonomy and independence?

Bill of Rights for the PD care partner

As the care partner for someone with PD, you perform an incredibly valuable and loving service. Anyone willing to put his life on hold in order to make the life of another better deserves the respect and appreciation of everyone involved. Just in case you have days when you feel as if that respect is not forthcoming (and you will have such days), make a copy of the following Bill of Rights for care partners, carry it with you, and take it out now and then to read through.

I have the right

- To take proper care of myself because doing so will make me a better care partner for the PWP
- To seek the help and support of others and to have the PWP accept that such support is necessary
- To maintain certain facets of my life beyond the PWP, just as I would have if that person didn't have PD
- To occasionally (and humanely) express anger, sadness, and other difficult feelings
- To reject any attempt by others (including the PWP) to manipulate me (either consciously or unconsciously) through guilt
- To receive respect, appreciation, and acceptance for the support and care I provide, knowing that I am giving it my best possible effort
- To take pride in my efforts and to recognize the courage and sacrifice required to provide that support and care
- To protect my individuality and my right to make a life for myself beyond the support and care the PWP needs

• To expect and demand that, even as new strides are made toward the treatment and cure of PD, similar strides be made toward aiding and caring for those of us who partner in care

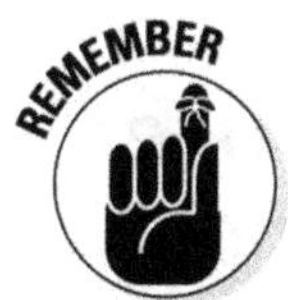

This isn't about you. Presumably you have years ahead of you, but your PWP faces a progressive decline. And you still have choices that the PWP no longer has. On the other hand, no one expects you to martyr yourself in the cause of giving care. That's where respite comes in—for you and your loved one. If you haven't read it yet, be sure you check out the earlier section "Dealing with burnout" for specifics on healthy respites.

Chapter 20

Putting Your Financial and Legal House in Order

In This Chapter

- Organizing: A place for everything
- Checking the pulse of your financial health
- Maneuvering through the insurance maze
- Making your choices known—and legal

Managing long-term illnesses like Parkinson's disease (PD) has more than a physical, mental, and spiritual price tag. The financial cost is also significant. And closely related to financial considerations are the legal issues that need your attention throughout the journey.

As with the rest of this book, in this chapter we preach planning and preparation. Chances are good that before receiving the PD diagnosis, you had made financial plans for your future, so you already have a lot in place. If not, you need to attend to these matters sooner rather than later because PD can progressively affect your capacity for decision-making. The information in this chapter gets you through the financial and legal red tape of protecting your assets and the futures of loved ones.

Gathering Important Information

The first step in managing your financial and legal affairs is to gather all the information and documents in one place. Some people are already terrifically organized; they can put their hands on key documents from three years ago in a flash. But a lot of people don't do as well. Some of these folks think nothing of showing up at the tax auditor's office with shoeboxes stuffed with receipts, cancelled checks, and handwritten notes; they dump it all on the poor auditor's desk and then assume that the auditor can make sense of it.

Whichever group you fall into, set aside some time, get a notebook and pen (or work off your computer if that's preferable), and find a place to work on this important piece of preserving your security.

Inventorying legal and financial documents

You need a clear inventory of key identity information, like Social Security number, insurance numbers, bank account numbers, and so on. Also, if you've appointed a power of attorney for legal or health matters, that document (and copies of it) must be readily available. Your health history is also a vital piece of this inventory. In fact, everything that may be needed—when you're unable to provide it or give its location—needs to be a part of this inventory.

Prepare a document in your computer files or make a list in a notebook with the following information. Then carefully store this information where it's secure from theft or fire (such as in a home safe) and be sure your care partner and others you trust can readily access it.

- **Access to personal information:** For each of the following include pin number and password clue (or actual password); contact name and phone number for technical support; online addresses as appropriate:
  - E-mail account
  - Voicemail
  - Personal and business Web sites
  - Online banking and shopping accounts (such as credit cards, electronic transfer accounts [ETA], or bills paid automatically or online)

- **Personal documents:** Record the location of each of the following:
    - Medical history and records
    - Family history
    - Birth certificate
    - Adoption documents
    - Naturalization papers
    - Marriage license
    - Divorce decree
    - School records
    - Employment history
    - Social Security card (including the number)
    - Driver's license (including number and expiration date)
    - Income tax filings
    - Savings certificates and bonds
    - Stock certificates
    - Safe deposit box (including information about location of the key)
    - Military discharge information (including branch of service and service ID number)
    - Passport (including number and expiration date)
    - Religious papers (including names of preferred place of

worship; clergy person and phone number; important religious records)

• List of memberships (including names of organizations; contact information; membership numbers)

• Organ donor wishes (give a copy to your physicians for your medical records)

• End of life and funeral instructions (including funeral home and cemetery names; contact names and numbers; location of original documents—especially if you prepay)

• Name of your favorite charity (for donations in lieu of flowers)

- **Information for dependents:** List their names, birth dates, and contact information.
- **Inventories:** List all of the following items. In addition to this list, consider taking photos of the items. Store the list and photos in an online file and keep a copy in your safe deposit box. For especially valuable items, get appraisals and keep the appraisals with a photo of the item in your safe deposit box.

- Home inventory including fixtures, furnishings, appliances, equipment, and so on
- Personal valuables including jewelry, artwork, antiques, books, clothes, mementos, and so on
- Business inventory including fixtures, furniture, stock, and so on

- **Personal bank and credit union accounts:** For each of the following entries include name of company or institution; contact name and phone number; account or file identity number(s); name(s) on the account and location of documents.
  - Personal loans
  - Liens against property
  - Paid liens against property
  - Loans paid on installment
  - Business accounts
  - Business loans
  - Pension and retirement accounts
- **Insurance:** For each of the following entries, include name of company or institution; contact name and phone number; policy and any group number; name(s) on

the policy and location of documents:

• Health insurance and Medicare

• Vehicle insurance (including registration number and location of the title)

• Other insurance (life, disability, long-term care, homeowner's, renter's, business, liability, valuables, and so on)

- **Legal papers:** Record the location of the original for each of the following:

  • Will and living will, including name and phone number of attorney and other people with copies

  • Durable power of attorney (finance and healthcare), including name and phone number of the person appointed, the attorney, and other people with copies

- **A list of contents of your safe deposit box:** Be sure to include the following items in your safe deposit box:

  • Copies (possibly photos) of your home, personal, and business inventories (see these categories earlier in this list)

   - Appraisals and photos of especially valuable items
   - Original documents and files
   - Original Social Security card
   - A copy of your driver's license
   - A copy of your health insurance and Medicare cards
   - A copy of other insurance (life, disability, long-term care, home-owner's, renter's, business, liability, valuables, and so on)

- **Miscellaneous:** Record the location of each of the following:
   - Storage units' contracts (including location of unit; name and phone number of company; unit number; location of key or combination)
   - Home and business safe (including key or combination)

Getting the info into the right hands

You aren't finished yet. In addition to completing the inventory, you need to tie up these other loose strings:

- Make sure your care partner and other trusted family or friends are aware of this inventory and how to access it.
- Place all of the documents and files in a safe deposit box (keeping a copy at home) or in a fireproof file container at home.
- Be sure someone other than you and your care partner knows where you store the documents and files. As an alternative, file a copy of key documents with your physician, attorney, or financial advisor as appropriate.
- Make sure that your care partner and one other trusted family member or friend has copies of your medical information (your Social Security number, insurance cards, list of medications, and so on).
- Be sure that your checking and savings accounts are accessible (if you're incapacitated) by putting your care partner's name on the accounts.
- Be sure your safe deposit box is accessible by putting your care

partner's name on the account (especially if you're going to store key documents like your will or living will or the originals of your power of attorney documents there).

- Make sure you give your doctor(s) copies of any advanced directives (like Do Not Resuscitate [DNR] orders); also, have a copy available to hand to the admissions representative any time you check in to the hospital or the emergency room.
- Give your doctor(s) written permission to discuss your health with your care partner.

Assessing Your Financial Health

Your ability to orchestrate your healthcare and solid financial future for you and your family is tied to your ability to understand the complexities of healthcare in America today. In many cases, the decisions that insurance companies and government programs make are based on generalizations, not your specific situation.

So, getting a handle on your specific economic well-being is a wise move. The information you put together in the following sections can provide a better idea of your financial health at this stage of your life, and this understanding can help you and your care partner make the best decisions to protect your futures.

Tracking income and out-go

In addition to an inventory, you need a clear idea of your resources versus your expenses. In your notebook or on your computer, set up a table with two columns, one titled *Resources* and the other *Expenses.* The information you enter under each column is pretty self-explanatory. Under Resources, list:

- Cash on hand (in checking and savings accounts as well as literal cash on hand)
- Annual income (from salary, trusts, royalties, dividends, property rental, and so on)
- Pay-outs due you (from pensions, investments, and so on)

- Property value (home, car, antiques, jewelry, land, and so on)

For Expenses, enter annual data for:

- Standard household expenses (food, utilities, rent or mortgage, insurance payments, payments on loans, and so on)
- Medical expenses (doctor visits, medications, medical equipment, therapy sessions, and so on)
- Occasional but regular expenses (clothing, household items, service for the car, and such)

Projecting costs over the long term

You have a condition that is progressive and will change over time. Predicting how that will translate into dollars and cents is difficult, to say the least. But you do know that costs will increase as your income decreases. What to do?

Yep, you need to make another list. So get out your trusty notebook or open a file on your computer and enter your best estimates for the following additional expenses you can anticipate as your PD progresses. Estimate the cost per month for each item.

- Lost wages
- Lost benefits
- House changes or remodeling
- Transportation expenses
- Medical expenses
    - Medications
    - In-home assistance (aides)
    - Medical equipment (walker, wheelchair, hospital bed)
    - Therapy not covered by insurance (physical, occupational, speech)
    - Medical bills not covered by insurance
- Respite costs (for you and your care partner)
    - Day care
    - Vacation care
    - Weekly in-home relief
    - Counseling

Using your assets to cover medical expenses

A home or other real estate can be a financial asset to cover the escalating costs of medical care. If you're still making payments on your home, you may be able to get a second or a refinanced mortgage. If you own your home out-right, a reverse mortgage may be an option.

With a reverse mortgage, you receive monthly payments from a lender (usually the bank) while you continue to own and live in the property. The amount of cash you receive is based on your equity in the home, your age, current interest rates, the value of the property, and its location. You can receive payments in one of three ways:

- **Term plan:** Fixed monthly payments over a specific time period
- **Tenure plan:** Fixed monthly payments for as long as you continue to live in the house
- **Line-of-credit plan:** Cash advance withdrawals from a fixed total sum

Eligibility requirements for a reverse mortgage don't include income limits but

- You must be at least age 62.
- You must own the home outright.

- The home must be your principal residence based on voter registration information.

Do reverse mortgages have a downside? Yep. Two of the significant downers are the following:

- Up-front fees can be steep for insuring and administering the reverse mortgage.
- If you choose to use part of your cash advances from the reverse mort-gage to pay those fees, those sums plus interest are added to the bottom line of those fees.

How do you repay the loan? After the borrower moves out of the home or dies, the home can be sold to repay the loan, or family members can retain the home and repay the loan in other ways.

The good news? The total of the reverse mortgage loan can never be greater than the value of the home at the time the loan is repaid, even if the loan balance is greater than the home's value at that time.

Deciding to take a second or reverse mortgage isn't as simple as it may appear. Before you take such a step, engage the services of a professional counselor (such as your financial planner, your attorney, the bank's reverse loan officer, or all three).

For more information, check out the U.S. Department of Housing and Urban Development (HUD) Web site at www.hud.gov.

Understanding the Intricacies of Insurance

With the seemingly gazillion insurance products on the market, figuring out which product best meets your needs can be a fulltime job. For people diagnosed with young onset PD (YOPD) or people with PD (PWP) who are still working and receiving employee benefits, check out the section on insurance in Chapter 8.

Before choosing an insurance policy of any type, go online to www.ambest.com, the Web site of A.M. Best, a company that rates insurance companies. You want to see a rating of at least A+, preferably A++. A high rating assures you that this company is financially stable and likely to be around when you actually need the benefits.

You also want to check whether the company has raised premiums on existing policies. When an insurance company's management has to make this move, one or two reasons are behind the raise:

- They didn't do their homework before setting the premium.
- They're planning to raise rates on a regular basis; unfortunately, just when a person needs the benefits, he drops the policy because he can't afford the high premiums any longer.

For most people 60 years and over, the insurance game is a little more straightforward. Although you may have trouble taking out certain types of insurance because of your PD, other options exist. For example, if you're a veteran, you may qualify for veterans' benefits that include insurance. Or your state may offer a special state health insurance plan to cover people with pre-existing conditions that aren't covered by other insurers.

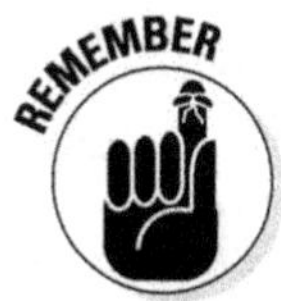

Whatever your options, your goal is pretty clear: You want to work with your insurance advisor to protect you and your family against the ravages of long-term illness on your financial security.

Qualifying for federally funded programs

This is the good news: Federally funded healthcare programs provide health insurance for some Americans; Medicare and its sister program, Medicaid, are the two most prominent. But as the section below explains, all federally funded programs aren't created equal, and although they're certainly a big help, they're simply not going to pay all your healthcare costs.

Be sure your doctors accept Medicare—not every doctor does.

Medicare

Medicare is a federally funded and administered national health insurance program available to any American citizen who is age 65 and older or who is eligible for Social Security disability benefits. Enrollment is automatic regardless of health, income, or political persuasion.

But all is not rosy. The original Medicare program was designed in 1965, when the goal was to provide financial help for seniors due to the rising costs of *acute* (immediate) care. In other words, the program was intended to help pay for care following a catastrophic event such as a heart attack, a fall that results in a hip fracture, and so on. Unfortunately, the program can be confusing in terms of what it covers and what it doesn't cover. (See the sidebar, "Medicare: A primer.")

The Medicare program works on a system of *assignment,* which means the government assigns the number of days you can be hospitalized and the payment levels for each service. So, if your final hospitalization bill reads $75,247.63 and Medicare has assigned only $50,000 to the procedure, a $25,247.63 shortfall exists. Whoa! What happens then? (See "Medigap" in this section for more info on this equation.)

For more information on Medicare coverage, you can call 800-MEDICARE (800-633-4227) or go to www.medicare.gov and request publication #CMS-10050-28, the annual update on Medicare programs and coverage.

Medigap

Medigap is the slang expression for Medicare supplemental insurance policies. You need one of these policies if you're receiving Medicare benefits because—drum roll, please—a gap (sometimes a cavern) exists between the cost of medical care and Medicare's payments. A gap also exists between the services Medicare covers and the services you need.

As a minimum, you need a Medigap policy to cover the 20 percent remainder of charges that Medicare covers at 80 percent. But beyond that, look for a policy that covers what Medicare doesn't cover at all:

- Hospitalization expenses for a year or more past the Medicare allowance
- Coverage for most excess charges not covered by Medicare (such as doctor bills beyond allowable fees)

- Coverage for care received outside the United States or Canada

Fortunately, several policies are available, and these companies must accept anyone who's eligible for Medicare. The concept of pre-existing condition is not part of their vocabulary and you have no wait period. For more information on selecting a policy, call 800-MEDICARE (800-633-4227) and ask for CMS publication #02110, "Choosing a Medigap Policy."

Medicaid

Medicaid is another federal healthcare program with a twist. Although the funding comes from the federal government, each state runs its own programs. And the rules can vary wildly. However, all programs base eligibility on income, and that amount is very close to the federally determined poverty level. Income is the only factor in Medicaid; age doesn't affect eligibility.

When you're at a certain level of income (and remain there), Medicaid covers care costs for the rest of your life. What's the catch? Most states get to decide where, when, and from whom you receive that care.

For more information about your state's requirements for Medicaid eligibility, contact your state Office on Aging.

Looking into long-term care insurance—Not just for old folks

We hope you've already looked into a long-term care (LTC) policy well before being diagnosed with PD (either because you're reaching the age where people consider such issues or because your employer offers a plan). In some cases, pre-existing conditions (such as PD) can disqualify you automatically (or seriously limit your options). If it's too late for you, definitely look into a long-term care policy for your care partner because it may have secondary benefits that help you if your partner becomes unable to provide the care you need.

Although many people can benefit from LTC coverage, two instances where LTC insurance isn't essential are:

- When your income is low (or you're willing to spend down your assets as discussed in the earlier section "Medicaid")
- When you will likely qualify for Medicaid

At the other end of the spectrum, perhaps you're in the Fortune 400 crowd of multimillionaires, in which case your assets are such that you can afford to cover the costs of your care without seriously impacting your lifestyle. Just remember: Some estimates place annual costs of managing healthcare with a chronic progressive condition between $65,000 and $100,000. Did you catch that? That's the per-year cost. If your assets need to stretch to cover 10, 15, or 20 years, you do the math.

Using private health insurance, disability benefits, HIPAA, and COBRA

For many people, health insurance is a benefit offered by their employer, but too many people fail to examine the actual benefits of their coverage until they need it. Don't make that mistake. Take a look at your current coverage and identify where it may be leaving you exposed. For example, does it include coverage for medications? If not, is there a rider or supplemental policy you can add to help cover those costs? Review the following discussion of health insurance basics; then you (or your partner if she has the policy) may want to sit down with someone in Human Resources and review the gaps in your coverage.

- **Private health insurance** comes in two forms:
- *Individual policies* that you purchase on your own give you choices

and coverage that last until age 65. These policies can't be can-celled, and premiums can't increase on the basis of your health condition.

Coverage can be expensive, and at the outset, you can be turned down or denied coverage for treatment for PD or other pre-existing conditions.

• *Group policies* are funded at least in part through your employer. You may have little or no choice on features, but the coverage is usually available with no penalties for pre-existing conditions when you start a job.

• **Long- and short-term disability coverage** is available through many employers or as an individual product. The ground rules are essentially the same as for health coverage:

• For individual policies, you need to be in good health when you apply.

• The group policy may require a period of employment (typically 6 to 12 months) and a waiting period of several months during which the employee has not sought treatment for the condition before being eligible for disability benefits.

Benefits are based on a percentage of base salary, but that salary is still taxable. No adjustments are available for inflation or cost-of-living increases. For more information on disability benefits, see Chapter 8.

• **HIPAA** is a government acronym for the **Health Insurance Portability and Accountability Act,** a relatively new program designed to protect working people.

In a nutshell, HIPAA requires states to make all health insurance portable. This means that if you leave one job for another or to start your own business, you can't be denied coverage regardless of health as long as you're under age 65. Each state decides which carrier provides this portable product, but you can't be denied coverage. For a fact sheet on HIPAA check out www.dol.gov/ebsa/newsroom/fshipaa.html.

• **COBRA,** another federal government alphabet-soup acronym, stands for **Consolidated Omnibus Budget Reconciliation Act.** This program protects and benefits the employee, giving you the option to continue your employer's group insurance for up to 18 months at your expense after leaving your job.

This option guarantees that your coverage isn't interrupted. You pay the group rate (including what your employer was contributing on your behalf), which is usually far less expensive than the same coverage in an individual policy (if you can even get an individual policy).

Relying on other resources to pay for care

As the government continues to wrestle with the issue of affordable health insurance, Congress and many states continue to enact legislation that partially addresses the problem.

For example, a growing number of states have established health insurance co-ops or pools for people who are denied coverage (usually due to a pre-existing condition). ***Note:*** Such programs usually have a residency requirement, and the cost of coverage runs higher than similar coverage if you were completely healthy. To find out whether your state offers such a program, contact your State Insurance Department.

Check that medical bill before you pay up

How many times have you gotten a statement from your insurance provider that shows the name of a doctor you never saw or heard of? How many times has payment by your insurer been denied because the billed service duplicates coverage already paid? How many times have you called the hospital or lab and been told the strange doctor was the one who read the results? Since when is reading the results not part of the lab work? Your insurance carrier is likely to catch such double-billing practices and decline to pay. Not to worry. The purpose is to try and get a higher insurance payment. If that's declined, the provider usually drops the matter rather than bill you out-of-pocket.

According to Medical Billing Advocates of America (an advocacy organization), every hospital Web site and lobby proudly posts a list of patient rights. Included in that list is the right to request an itemized statement or explanation of items on your bill that you don't understand or believe you didn't receive. Unfortunately most patients never take advantage of this right, so medical billing errors go undetected. Either the insurance company pays them (adding to the spiraling costs of health care across America) or the patient pays.

An itemized bill may be overwhelming at first (some can run on for 20 to 30 pages), but every time you catch an error, you put the billing office and the insurance company on notice. For example:

• Administration of oxygen may be a common protocol for the procedure you had, but if you didn't need or didn't received that oxygen, you shouldn't pay for it.

• Maybe your doctor ordered a pain medicine on an as-needed (or as-requested) basis. You know you never requested that medicine, yet it's on the bill.

• A scan through an itemized bill may reveal outlandish charges such as $10 for a cotton swab. Go to the discount store and buy a package of a thousand swabs for a couple of bucks. Take them with you when you go to question the bill. It'll make your point.

Managing your medical costs is one way you can maintain control as your PD progresses. Requesting an itemized statement and questioning services you didn't receive or were overcharged for delivers the message loud and clear: You may have PD, but you're still in charge. By the way, the billing office isn't allowed to charge you for making a copy of the bill even if it runs into a couple hundred of pages.

In 2004, Congress created Health Savings Accounts (HSA) for people who purchase a government-approved, high-deductible health plan (HDHP). The buyer pre-funds a substantial percentage of the deductible each year in a tax-deductible savings account similar to an IRA. Funds deposited in the account can be used to

- Pay the deductible
- Cover the costs of medical and dental services not covered under your policy including alternative medical treatment

Any part of the deposit not used in a given year carries forward. As your PD progresses, you're likely to meet or exceed the deductible in any given year, but this plan may be an option for your care partner.

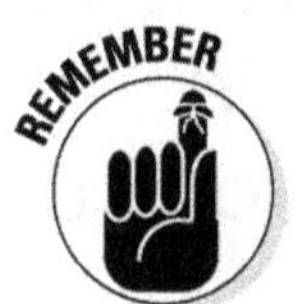

To find additional information about programs and disability coverage, check out Chapter 8 or go online to www.socialsecurity.gov.

Making Sure Your Wishes Are Sacrosanct

One key to good long-term-planning is to put certain documents in place well before you or your care partner needs to access them. These documents include:

- A will, of course
- Trusts in your children's names if you have children to protect
- A durable power of attorney for finances and healthcare if your state has provisions for them
- Your end-of-life wishes
- Advance directives (make sure you've shared those wishes in writing with your doctor[s] and your family)

Durable power of attorney

Appointing someone to act on your behalf is the purpose of a *power of attorney* or simple POA. The standard document allows you to assign someone the right to manage financial and personal matters for you. The catch is that this person's appointment only lasts as long as you remain capable of making those decisions yourself.

For the time when you can't make decisions known, you still need a spokesperson you can trust to move forward as you want. At this point, the *durable* POA comes into play. Two types exist:

- **Durable power of attorney:** You appoint someone to speak on your behalf for financial and other non-healthcare matters when you no longer can.
- **Durable power of attorney for healthcare:** You appoint someone to make medical and healthcare decisions for you when you're unable to make them yourself.

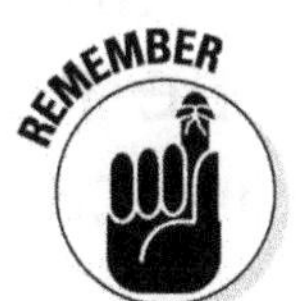

Not all states recognize the same documents. Check with your attorney to understand your state's laws on these issues. If these documents are available, don't put off officially naming your non-healthcare and healthcare representative.

Whether you're living with PD or you're perfectly health, stuff happens and none of us can guarantee that we won't end up unconscious in an emergency room, unable to make our wishes known.

Advance directives and living wills

The trend in medical care today has moved away from the paternalistic model where the doctor made decisions for the patient. Today the patient has the autonomy to state medical and end-of-life choices and to expect that those choices will be honored. But what happens when you can't speak up for yourself?

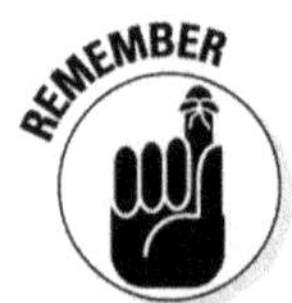

Give advance consent to all your doctors as well as your lawyer to talk with your care partner as needed. The rules and forms for doing this will vary from one state to another, so ask your lawyer to make sure this consent is a part of your legal portfolio.

Advance directives and living wills are tools for stating your desires regarding decisions the doctors and your family are facing when you're unable to participate in the decision. This concept has dual benefits:

- You take the pressure off your doctors and family members from making emotional and tough decisions when they're under enormous stress.
- You can make your exact choices clear in a legally binding document.

For example, the choice of terminal sedation is legal in most states. Terminal sedation isn't considered assisted suicide or euthanasia because the goal is to ease suffering, not to induce death. You (or your healthcare power of attorney) can ask the doctor to order medication at the end of your life to ease pain or difficult breathing.

Another specific to consider is whether you want an autopsy that can help researchers understand more how PD affects the brain. If terminal sedation, autopsy, or a procedure equally specific is part of your decision, you need to state this in your living will and make sure that a copy is on file with each doctor likely to treat you.

Last will and testament

A *will* states your choices regarding the distribution of your property and mementos after you die. This is a legal document, and although you may believe writing down your wishes (or telling them to your care partner) is enough, you can save everyone headaches (and probably a good measure of trauma) after you're gone if you take the time to create a legally witnessed and signed document that makes your wishes binding for your survivors. To help you in that, the Funeral Consumers Alliance offers a packet of materials entitled *Before I Go, You Should Know* available through their Web site at www.funerals.org.

Tough stuff, but even the healthiest of people need to address these seemingly gloomy issues. Getting on top of them early on is just one more way you can take control and move forward with *your* life—on *your* terms.

Chapter 21

It's Just Bricks and Mortar: Housing Options You Can Live With

In This Chapter

- Staying in your home sweet (safe) home
- Expanding your sources of care: Community programs and services
- Taking that first (hardest) step: Deciding to move
- Remaining in control: Choosing the right care community

In times of personal crisis, *home* often becomes a synonym for refuge or safe harbor. It's the one place most people can go and be themselves without feeling the need to keep up appearances or a brave front. It's also the place where people surround themselves with items that bring back memories of good times, successes, and even trials endured through the years.

The day will come when you and your care partner need to reassess your current living situation in terms of its safety and practicality. As time and your Parkinson's disease (PD) progress, you may develop balance problems that result in falls and fractures. In many cases, you can make adjustments to your present home that allow you to remain there in comfort. However, you may eventually need to choose between a building that represents your past and a place where you have the assistance you need for a productive and satisfying future.

And in the spirit of our mantra—prepare, don't project—you can get to work on these housing issues well before the need is imminent. This chapter helps you do just that. We first guide you through the safety issues of your present home and cover the community services that enable you to remain there. Then we take you through the tough steps of deciding to move. Finally the chapter breaks down the variety of residences you can choose from when you've decided the time is right.

Making Your Home PD User-Friendly

Your first step in thinking through this whole nest quest is to take a good look at your current residence. You may be surprised to discover how even small changes can give you additional months, if not years, to enjoy your current home.

Safety first: Assessing your home

Accidents in the home are one of the most common causes of injury and death in America. With your PD and the meds that can make you more prone to falling (see Chapter 18 for more on this), a check of your home is imperative. You may want to schedule one as often as you check the batteries in your smoke detectors—which is at least once a year, right?

Your local fire or police department may offer a home safety assessment at no cost. If so, take advantage of this great community service. There are also home safety assessments offered by trained nurses, and this service is usually covered by Medicare and some insurance companies. If neither of those professional surveys is available for you, you can also go through the following checklist to get started on your own home safety assessment:

- **Oh say, can you see?**
- Make sure lighting is adequate both inside and outside the home.
- Pay special attention to lighting in stairways and hallways.
- Place nightlights in the bathroom and along the path from bedroom to bathroom.
- Check lamps and electrical appliances. Do the cords and wiring show wear and need for repairs?

• Avoid using extension cords if at all possible; when they're absolutely necessary, anchor them to the wall (not the floor) to prevent tripping.

• Bundle and tie up excess footage on computer and other electronics cords; then anchor them safely under the desk or along the baseboard.

• **Underfoot stuff can be dangerous!**

• Get rid of all scatter rugs (even those with rubber backing) and carefully check for worn carpeting or edges that are coming free of their tacking; make necessary repairs.

• Make sure floors (tiled, wood, or uncarpeted flooring) aren't slippery.

Test floors in a pair of socks. If you can do the slide, the floors need to be stripped of the wax or compound that's making them slippery.

• Remove any raised threshold strip that separates one room from another; make the transition smooth.

• Install nonskid runners on uncarpeted stairways. Each stairway needs a sturdy handrail on at least one side and light controls at the top and bottom of the stairway. Use bright neon tape to mark stairs in especially dark places.

• Shop for shoes with nonskid soles and no laces, the kind boaters prefer.

• **Two key spaces are accidents waiting to happen.**

• In the kitchen: Standard safety rules apply. Keep curtains or flammable materials away from the stove and make sure all appliances are in good working order. Assess whether items in the kitchen are convenient for you. For example, are glasses better on a lower shelf? Can you move the skillet from the drawer under the oven to a hook or a higher cabinet?

• In the bathroom: Place nonskid strips in the bathtub and shower; install grab bars wherever they make life easier—bathtub, shower, and toilet. Set the hot water heater at 110 degrees or lower to prevent accidental burning.

• **Don't forget:**

• Place emergency and other medical contact numbers next to every phone.

• Install smoke detectors (or check present ones) in every stairway and in the kitchen; place fire extinguishers in an accessible place on every floor level including the basement; determine an escape route in the event of fire.

• Check for needed repairs to sidewalks and driveways: broken asphalt or concrete, uneven brickwork in paths and sidewalks, and so on. Consider installing ramps for the time when managing even a few stairs becomes difficult.

• Double-check your house's security. Are all locks on windows and doors working properly? Be sure screens, storm windows, and doors are properly and securely installed. Get to know your neighbors and let one or two trusted neighbors know who to contact if they have concerns about your safety or the security of the property.

Got your to-do list ready? Great. Time to get busy!

If possible, make this a family project. List everything that needs attention and then subdivide that list into large and small jobs. Tackle any fairly extensive changes for improving movement (such as removing threshold strips) first. Such structural barriers—usually in multiple places in your home—may put you in the greatest danger for falling.

De-cluttering and hazard-proofing

Take a good, long look at the contents of your residence. Address the clutter that may be hazardous and clean out unnecessary *stuff.* For example, does your son still play that drum set, or could it be moved into the attic or better yet sent to his house for the grandkids to use?

Rearranging to go with the (traffic) flow

You've de-cluttered your living space, so now you're ready to consider repositioning your furnishings. You want to create the best traffic flow, meet your needs for comfort, and still have some design appeal. (Wedging your television in the far corner may offer more space, but not a whole lot more!)

Some people seem to have an eye for positioning furnishings for maximum convenience and visual appeal. The rest of the world needs help—a decorator, a particular family member, a friend, or a friend of a friend who has a real knack.

But you can do a little preliminary evaluating on your own. What suggestions can you incorporate from your assessment (see the previous section, "Safety first: Assessing your home") and from the safety check by the police or fire department? For example, would a simple change in the placement of the sofa make it easier to access the doorway in the event of a fire or other emergency?

How can you put the rooms of your home to better use—not just because you have PD but because they may serve everyone better? Forget those room labels and think outside the box. If you're going to be spending more time on the computer—checking out information and staying in touch with—maybe that little-used guest room could become your headquarters. Even if you didn't have PD, chances are the rooms of your home could be far more user-friendly for the real life you lead. Besides, change and playing around with new ideas can be fun!

Taking Advantage of Community Care Programs

If you choose to remain in your own home for as long as possible, you have some options for extending that timetable even after your PD begins to put you at risk for falls or other traumas. But staying at home and bringing in care services has financial considerations. Most services—even if your insurance or Medicare covers part of them—are for a limited period of time and focus on a higher level of care, such as the services of a nurse or physical therapist. The following sections help you weigh your options.

In-home services

In-home help may be your first line of defense against moving because it can provide two significant services:

- Household help, such as meal preparation, shopping, and home maintenance
- Personal and medical assistance, such as help with personal hygiene, dressing, or medications

Most large communities have agencies that offer in-home care-assessment services at no cost. They can suggest support options for you and your care partner. Smaller communities or rural areas likely have a well-known network of independent contractors—people experienced in offering the elementary services you may need at some stage of your PD.

To find independent contractors and community services, consider the following strategies:

• Talk to neighbors, friends, and the nurse or office manager in your physician's office for references.

• Check with your local librarian or search your telephone directory's business listings for agencies offering services.

• Call the local hospital's social services department or your regional Office on Aging (in the phone book under *state* or *county government offices*).

• Use a computer to check out several sites that may be helpful such as www.eldercare.gov. Search the Internet using key words like *home care* and your community's name.

Expand your search to the county level and surrounding communities if you live in a smaller community.

Even if these people can't offer the answers you need, don't stop there. Ask them for other people to contact. Thank them for their help and follow their suggestions for that next contact.

Consider exploring the types of services in Table 21-1 for your area and file the information for when you may need it down the road.

Table 21-1 Services for In-Home Assistance

Service	*Contact Name and Number*	*Cost*	*Notes*
Errand services			
Home repairs			
Transportation			
Meal programs			
Medical equipment and supplies			
Delivery: Meds			
Delivery: Groceries			
Housekeeping			

Table 12-1

Some programs may involve little or no cost. For example, youth groups may offer snow-shoveling or routine home maintenance. Grocery stores and pharmacies may offer free delivery. Government-funded meal programs for seniors can provide not only a hot, nutritious meal but also the opportunity to get out and interact socially with other people.

On the other hand, some services may come with sticker shock that has you reeling and saying, "Are you kidding? I'll do it myself," or "If I can't, my care partner will!" But take care not to burn those bridges too quickly. What happens when you can't manage some tasks on your own? What happens when your care partner is ill, needs to go away, or has to work overtime and can't be there when you need the help? What about your escalating need for care? Are you really prepared to ask your care partner to assume all the household and personal care tasks that the two of you may have shared up to now?

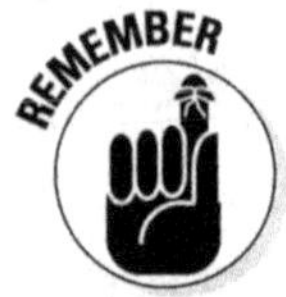

Don't be stubborn about accepting care from other people—even when you have to pay for it. If the service provides help for you *and* extra time for your enjoyable activities (not to mention independence!), it may seem downright priceless.

Home healthcare services

Home healthcare is a higher level of medical assistance that isn't part of the normal services offered through either your doctor's office or the hospital. At the same time it includes services that your doctor or the hospital's social worker and discharge planner might *prescribe* for you (such as a visiting nurse to come to your home and check up on you after you've had a fall).

The good news: If your physician orders or prescribes professional in-home care, your insurance or Medicare pays most, if not all, of the bill. After the professional (a nurse or physical therapist, for example) is approved, you may also become eligible for personal-hygiene care and housekeeping services you've needed.

The not-so-great news: Such home health-services are finite—they continue for as long as medically necessary. After the need for professional service is over, the personal care also ends. Likewise, when you can reasonably travel to the site of the professional services (like physical therapy), the home delivery ends.

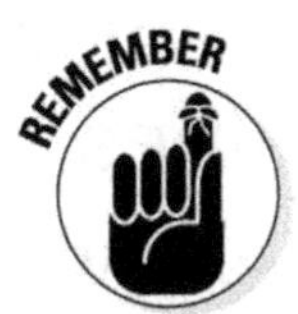

The most common situation for home healthcare is following a hospitalization, often because of a fall that causes a hip fracture or other broken bones. Check out Chapter 6 for a full discussion on what to expect (and do) if you've been discharged from the hospital and still need extra care. Such services—whether they follow a hospitalization or another scenario—are finite and short-term, but they are available. ***Note:*** The downside is that you have to demonstrate your knowledge of them and then ask for them.

Adult day care

Adult day care is relatively new in the United States and therefore not as geo-graphically widespread as the need is. Day care programs for adults can offer an array of services in a variety of settings—from community rooms in religious or senior centers to free-standing facilities.

In most cases, day care programs focus on socialization rather than health-care services. Still, they offer more health support than traditional senior centers because day care programs have staff trained to provide nursing assistance and routine medical support (such as overseeing medication dosages, assistance with transferring from one position to another, and, in some instances, personal care services such as bathing and barber or beautician services).

Day care can bridge an important gap in the continuum of care services. When your PD symptoms keep you from safely getting out and about on your own or when your care partner needs to work, day care offers an opportunity for you to be with other people and remain active.

Keep the following facts in mind:

- Not all states license or certify day care centers for adults. This means safety, cleanliness, and regular reviews of staffing and program standards aren't regulated.
- Because programs can vary greatly, be sure you understand what services are included in the fee and what services you pay for on an as-needed basis.

- Some centers may offer a free trial day; if they don't, then visit the center (if possible, more than once) before making your decision.

Adult day care isn't for everyone and may not be right for you if you're still an active participant in other social and community circles. But it's an option to consider as your PD progresses. Adult day care can lengthen the time you're able to remain in your own home, and it can provide occasional respite for your care partner.

Respite care

The concept of respite isn't just for your care partner. (Review Chapter 19 for this discussion.) When you have a chronic, progressive condition like PD, you too need time off. Trying to keep up that brave and optimistic demeanor can be enormously exhausting. Managing symptoms and fighting for every bit of function and independence can sap the energy of even the strongest PWP.

You deserve a break—a regular timeout from thinking about PD at least once a week. (Although we cover this more completely in Chapter 19, the routine's important enough to reinforce here.) You also need (and deserve) the occasional longer R&R to

- Take a deep breath and be cared for without feeling as if you're imposing on your family or under their watchful eye
- Come to terms with the progression of your PD

Believe it or not, such places exist. In the early stages of your PD when your symptoms are well managed by your treatment plan, consider traveling to:

- A retreat center that offers rejuvenation, often at a reasonable cost.
- A cabin or lodge in a state park where you can spend a few days or a week for a reasonable cost in settings that inspire introspection.
- A major city if you really can't deal with all that quiet time. Treat yourself to a stay in a hotel, tickets to a play or sporting event, shopping, dining (as opposed to

simply *eating*), and letting strangers pamper you.

As your PD progresses, options for respite are available in an environment of safety and care appropriate to your needs. For example,

- Adult day care programs (see the earlier section "Adult day care") can give you and your care partner a few hours of respite.
- Hospitals, step-care communities (see the section "Communities of care" later in this chapter), rehabilitation centers, and dedicated Parkinson's centers on medical-center campuses may offer overnight, weekend, or vacation *respite care.*

Even if you're not ready to make use of such programs right now, gather information about the ones in your area. You may find that such a service is handy when an emergency arises (such as your care partner's mother needs help in another state) and your care partner worries about leaving you.

Deciding When It's Time to Move

One day in the future, your current residence may simply not work for you. (Frankly that day comes for a lot of folks who aren't even dealing with PD!) Certainly you've had other life passages when change wasn't necessarily welcomed, but required. You managed then—and perhaps you even thrived in the new setting. You can certainly do it again—especially if the move simplifies your care and frees you to enjoy other activities.

Bidding your abode adieu

The truth is that you're going to know in your heart of hearts when your home is no longer practical. You can't climb the stairs. Your bathroom—in spite of its maze of grab bars and safety features—is too small or difficult to use. Your wheelchair doesn't fit through the doorways or roll easily across the carpeted floors. You and your care partner are becoming isolated from friends, family, and the community activities you love.

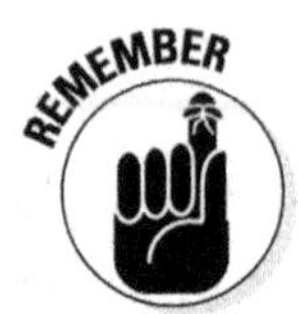

The only problem is if you refuse to admit that the time is right. If you've prepared for this day (as we've been known to preach), the struggle can be far less distressing. The decision won't be easy, but you can skip the panic and anxiety of not knowing where to turn because you already know your options. You're ready to pick one and get on with your life.

Weighing the pros and cons of moving

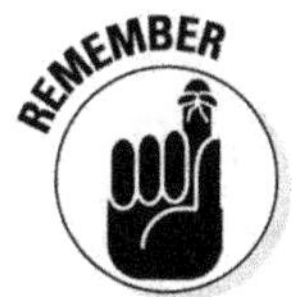

Certainly you don't want to move before you're ready, but you do need to let go of any fantasies about the future and face reality. Is it practical and safe to continue living in your home? More to the point, can your life, routine, and ease of functioning improve if you move?

One person with Parkinson's (PWP) didn't leave his home without a fight. Before he was willing to admit it was time, he tried everything—an alert necklace so he could call for help if he fell (which he did frequently), a hospital bed for his living room so he didn't have to go to the upstairs bedrooms, a portable commode next to the bed so he didn't have go to the bathroom during the night, and a private-duty aide at night so his wife could get her rest.

One day he looked around the house and realized that it wasn't the refuge he had loved for so many years. The memories it held had been pushed aside to make room for the trappings of his illness—his home had become one giant sick-room. And he didn't want that for himself or his wife.

Moving is 90 percent attitude

However you come to the decision—willingly or kicking and screaming—moving day is tough. It's tough on you and on the people who love you and share the memories that made your house a home.

Further, this is a major step in the progression of your PD—the admission that you need to (rather than *choose to*) move. This is the time to talk about your feelings with a counselor or trusted friend—one who has no stake in the emotional real estate of the home itself. In short, you need to take the time to grieve this passage the same way you mourn any major passage in your life. Talking about your sadness and regrets eventually leads to acceptance and even (perhaps) anticipation of the next step.

Redefining Your Castle

Leaving the old homestead is the end of the world only if you say it is. Remember the discussion of your coping style—the old fight or flight scenario? (Check out Chapter 7 for a refresher if you need one.) Well, in this case, flight is turning your back on the positive possibilities of housing opportunities. Fight, on the other hand, is taking charge of this new challenge by considering the options you've researched and by choosing the best one with your care partner.

Weighing your options

You may be surprised at the possibilities after you begin to consider solutions for moving to a place that will permit you to continue to have as much independence and control over your routine as possible. The following sections describe some of the more common choices.

Moving in with a family member

Okay, stop shuddering. Moving in with a family member can work as long as both parties work through the details of the living arrangements and routines *before* making the decision to share living space. In every household there are routine chores and schedules. What's yours and what's the schedule for the rest of the household? If you're moving in with an adult child, are there also grandchildren in the house? Then their schedules (and rights to privacy and socializing with friends) must also be taken into consideration. Ideally you will have a specific space of your own in the house—your room (hopefully furnished with your things) and possible (hopefully) your own bathroom. And the rules for you? Keep in mind that this is your relative's home—not yours. By all means, state your needs at the outset, but then settle in and do your part to become a welcomed member of the household.

Considering a more practical apartment, condo, or house

Some options aren't as drastic as moving to a care facility. If you're having mobility problems in your current residence, what can make that easier? Perhaps your home is multi-level, or the doorways are too narrow, or the rooms are too small to accommodate a wheelchair or the safe use of your walker. In such cases, consider a house, condominium, or apartment that's on one level and constructed for an aging population. Much new construction today offers wider doorways, smooth thresholds, and safety features in bathrooms as standard fare. Several other options are also available:

- **Accessory dwelling units (ADUs):** ADUs are living spaces within an existing home or on the same property. (Remember the concept of the mother-in-law apartment?) Can you remodel your present (and beloved) home to include a small apartment where you can live comfortably and safely while your adult child moves into the main house? Can you use the ADU as a residence for a live-in caregiver who, in exchange for room and board, provides care services for you?

An alternative is to move into an ADU within the home or on the property of your son or daughter whose been encouraging you to move in. An ADU gives you (and your child) privacy and autonomy while relieving the stress of living some distance apart.

Check local zoning ordinances and assess the practicality of constructing an ADU. If you're determined to stay in your home for as long as possible, the ADU can help lengthen that stay.

- **Subsidized senior housing:** In many communities, apartment or housing complexes use state and federal funding to accommodate middle- or low-income senior citizens. In such facilities, rents reflect a percentage of income.

• **Board-and-care homes:** If you have no live-in care partner, a board-and-care home may be an option. Also referred to as *group homes,* these facilities are usually large homes that have been converted to serve people who can no longer manage on their own but who don't need a higher level of care. These homes are in residential neighborhoods, and residents have their own bedrooms and share common areas of the house. Sometimes the makeup of the residents revolves around a common factor such as age, gender, or disability. A paid staff prepares meals, assists with some care, and may engage residents in group activities. ***Note:*** Such facilities aren't eligible for public funding such as Medicare or Medicaid.

Communities of care

In response to the aging of America (and the rest of the world), the options for long-term care have grown in the last several decades. Today the most common types of services are grouped according to client-ability: independent, needs some assistance, needs major assistance, and end-of-life. The facilities may have different names in different states, and the services and costs vary widely.

To locate services in your area (or in another community closer to adult children or a preferred climate), consider the following:

- Call the local Area Agency on Aging (look under state- or federal-government listings in your phone directory).
- Call the Eldercare Locator at 800-677-1116.
- Go online to www.eldercare.gov.

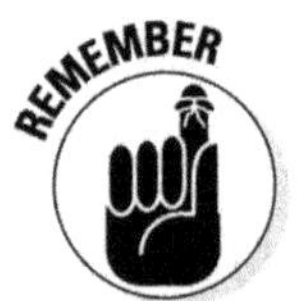

Medicare covers costs on the same basis as medically necessary services in a resident's private home (for example, if the doctor orders physical therapy for you, Medicare might cover such *skilled* home-care with some possibility of personal care as long as such services aren't already provided by the facility).

This section breaks out five basic types of long-term care facilities along with their specific features, pros, and cons.

Continuing care retirement centers (CCRCs or step-care communities)

These facilities offer levels of care from independent through nursing care. The primary advantage is that you don't have to research new facilities, make a major move, or leave behind friends and staff as your needs change. You and your significant other can live together; if one partner needs a higher level of care, the other can remain nearby.

Services, levels of care, and admission procedures and requirements can vary widely in such facilities. Get all the rules up front before you choose. Also, remember that should the time come when you need a higher level of care, you want to be sure that the nursing part of any step community is certified as a *skilled-care* facility (meaning they're qualified to accept Medicare payment for skilled rehabilitative services). The facility should also be certified for Medicaid (see Chapter 20 for more on this federal program). To be thorough, you may want to check their state inspection record. For more information, check out www.carf.org/aging.

Some communities may not include a nursing care facility. If this is the case, ask whether they have an association with a nursing facility in the community and whether residents of the CCRC get preferential consideration if the nursing facility has a waiting list. The same words of caution apply: Be sure this facility is certified to ensure you receive the best possible care.

Independent apartment with services

Many step-community residents begin by residing in an apartment or cottage with their personal belongings. Such units may tie into the overall community through safety features (such as call bells in bathrooms), activities (such as field trips or book discussion groups), and meals in a common dining room. ***Note:*** This level is similar to traditional freestanding apartment or condominium complexes. Residents come and go as they please, manage their own healthcare, and maintain roles of choice in the larger community.

Assisted living

These facilities can vary greatly in terms of standard services and those services offered at an extra cost. Be sure you ask for the specifics regarding both of them. In general, such facilities include assistance with activities of daily living (ADLs), such as bathing, dressing, and transferring from chair to bed and back.

Standard services may also include the management and administration of medicines, transportation to and from doctor appointments, and most meals. Residents usually live in their own efficiency or one-bedroom apartment within a building or complex of buildings that also houses common areas such as a dining room, chapel, activity room, and library. Most assisted living facilities have a standard monthly fee and then additional services that you can purchase on an as-needed or as-wanted basis.

On the downside, if the facility isn't part of a step community with its on-campus skilled nursing facility and you fall and need extended rehabilitation, that will mean another move (plus having to pay for two places if you intend to return to the assisted living facility).

Skilled nursing facility (SNF) or rehabilitation center

Skilled nursing facilities or rehab centers are facilities that provide *skilled* care and must be specifically licensed to provide these professional rehabilitative services. Nursing facilities that aren't licensed for skilled care (as well as those that are) also offer what is called *non-skilled, custodial, or maintenance care.* These non-skilled wings of the facility serve people in the advanced stages of illness or life with a wide range of support, personal care, routine health services, and social opportunities.

SNFs can serve a variety of populations—people of all ages who may reside there for varying lengths of time, including:

- People recovering from surgery may spend several weeks in a nursing home or rehabilitation center before returning to more independent living.
- People who suffer from dementia, such as Alzheimer's, often live in nursing home care centers when the community or their family can no longer manage the person's care. Often the care centers have special units that maintain the safety and dignity of people suffering from dementia.
- People whose care needs exceed the family's or community's ability to meet those needs may live in this type of facility. Many facilities have special units where people who are frail but alert and relatively active can be safe and secure while taking part in the facility's activities and social opportunities.

- People in need of care occasionally stay here on a short-term basis to give the caregiver a much-needed break.

The best nursing homes have full occupancy, so visit early on and get your name on the wait list if this is the place you want to be for any future rehab or residency services. ***Note:*** When your name comes to the top of the list, the administrator calls you. If you're not ready to move to the nursing home, you can request that your name stay on the list.

Hospice

Hospice care is becoming an increasingly preferred option for patients who are clearly coming to the end of life. Hospice programs provide personal care for the patient and also offer counseling for the families and friends. The program may be in a special facility, a hospital, or a nursing home, but in many cases hospice services are also available in your own home. After the pro-gram accepts you, a team of doctors, nurses, home health aides, social workers, counselors, and even trained volunteers help you and your family cope with the final days of your illness.

To find a program in your area, ask your hospital social worker, and remember that while Medicare may cover some costs, it won't cover round-the-clock care at home.

Assessing for a perfect fit

Only you and your care partner can describe in detail the needs you have as individuals and as a care team. But as you make that list together and use it to evaluate various housing options, keep these key factors in mind:

- Be realistic about your possible future needs and the ability of you and your care partners to meet those needs every day over what could be several years.

- List residential care options in your area and in the area of an adult child, friend, or close relative where you may consider moving. Then assess and compare similar facilities for quality and consistency of care.
- Visit those facilities (at all levels) that meet your criteria and assess them using the checklist at the end of this chapter.
- Talk to people—staff and clients at the facility, people in the community, neighbors, and friends. Ask what they've heard, what they know, and what their Aunt Millie's experience was.
- Always choose on the basis of which facility best meets *your* needs.

Making a list, checking it twice: Evaluating the facilities

When you visit a facility, focus on the people in the program and note their interactions with staff. Two words of caution:

- Don't let the *window dressing* (beautiful furnishings, plantings, free lattes, treats for prospective clients, and other such details) sway you.
- Don't be taken in by an unusually warm welcome or excesses of flattery and interest by your tour guide.

These folks are in business to sell a product and a service. And you, dear reader, are their target audience.

Following is a checklist for your tours of various facilities. In a notebook, record the number of each item and then any notes you have about that service (use a separate page for each facility). Consider placing a numeric value next to each service to reflect your overall observation (for example a 5 is *excellent* and a 1 is *very poor*). Not all items apply to every location, and services offered by one facility and not others may influence your final decision depending on your current idea of what you will need and the reality of what might be needed down the road.

- Entrance is user-friendly and attractive.

- Staff welcomed and was prepared for appointment or tour.
- Light, doorways, and hallways adequate to accommodate people with wheel chair or walker.
- Facility is free of any noxious or unpleasant odor; clean and attractively furnished.
- Grab bars are in bathrooms and handrails in hallways.
- Temperature is comfortable for clients.
- Smoking is either not permitted or allowed only in clearly marked, designated areas.
- Exits are clearly marked; smoke detectors and sprinklers are throughout the facility.
- Furnishings are sturdy and appropriate for people with movement disorders.
- If meals are served, clients have choices and special diets are available.
- Staff interacts with clients and treats every client as an adult and with respect.
- Staff members are certified (where appropriate) or receive ongoing

training; hiring includes background checks.

- Tour guide calls residents by name and is clearly known to them.
- If appropriate, a registered nurse is on staff in addition to the facility administrator.
- The ratio of staff to client is reasonable.
- Staff takes a team approach with the client and family in developing a plan of care.
- The administrative team has been in place at least one year.
- Ownership of the facility has not changed more than once in five years.
- In a residential facility, residents may bring personal furnishings.
- Resident living spaces have adequate and personal closet and dresser space even if room is shared.
- If rooms are shared, residents have a voice in choosing a roommate.
- Tour guide offers copies of resident-rights documents and any reports of state or facility inspections for review.

- Activities are age-appropriate and conducted with respect to the experience and history of the clients.
- The facility has an outdoor area for client use; staff is available to assist the residents in accessing that area.
- Facility has an emergency evacuation plan that includes plans for unusual events such as tornadoes, hurricanes, and so on if appropriate.
- Services alluded to in promotional materials are indeed included in the base cost; extra services and their cost are clearly spelled out.

Certification and licensing isn't a requirement in all states or for all types of care facilities, but facilities that must meet such regulations (either state or federal or both) undergo regular (and unannounced) inspections to ensure compliance.

Certainly any facility that accepts Medicare or Medicaid or both must be licensed and inspected. The results of such inspections are a matter of public record. If you're considering a setting that provides full residential care and is licensed for payment through Medicare or Medicaid, you can view the results of the most recent inspection results online at www.medicare.gov/NH Compare.

A Few Words for You and Your Care Partner

The day may come (or it may never come) when your PD progresses to the point where you need constant round-the-clock care that is beyond the limits of what can be provided to you at home or in a semi-independent setting (such as an assisted living facility). Should that day come and you decide to move to a full-care facility, you and your care partner need to be prepared for some changes.

For example, the PWP must be prepared to accept help from strangers for even his most basic needs including dressing, bathing, getting to and from the bathroom, and such, and he may need to rely on someone else to speak for him and make his wishes known. And the care partner will need to down-shift her role from caregiver back to care partner (Chapter 19 explains the difference), which will involve monitoring the way care is provided by others instead of providing that care herself. The care partner also will need to advocate for the PWP, making sure that the PWP's final wishes are followed.

If the facility isn't used to caring for PWP, the care partner may also need to be firm about the importance of timing in the delivery of medications—even if that means the care partner must lobby for the staff to deliver meds outside of their normal routine rounds. Care partners, be prepared to have these tough conversations and stand your ground.

For both of you, this doesn't have to be a time of sadness. Instead it can be a time to let go of the stresses of the last many years and look back instead to the triumphs of having maintained a full life in spite of having PD.

Part VI

The Part of Tens

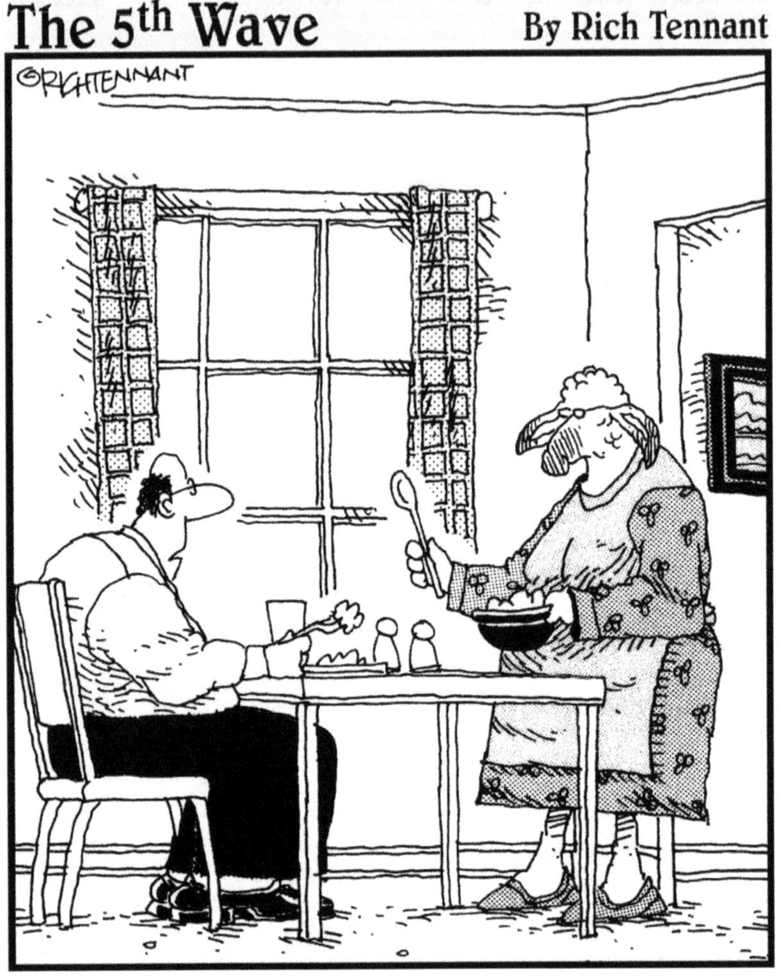

"Tell me again what the goal of the clinical trail is?"

In this part...

Every *For Dummies* book ends with a few top-ten lists. This one is no exception. We use this part to offer tips for handling the difficult feelings of living with a progressive and incurable condition. We also have a list that gently reminds you that your care partner is living with PD every day too. And finally we reissue our plea for you to get involved in the extraordinary community of people living with Parkinson's around the world. You'll be richer for the experience—we promise!

Chapter 22

Ten Ways to Deal with Difficult Feelings

In This Chapter

- Recognizing feelings that can do real damage
- Coping with difficult times and moving on

Coping with feelings has no hard and fast rules. Just like the wild elation of falling in love may seem impossible to control, the bouts of intensely negative feelings that can accompany Parkinson's disease (PD) may also appear beyond your control. Because of the depression, anxiety, and other symptoms of your PD, you may find these feelings more of a challenge over time. To top it off, other people don't easily recognize when you're upset, which only requires more of your limited patience at these troublesome times. Here are ten ideas that may help you begin coping with these feelings.

Banishing the Concept of "Bad"

Placing some sort of value system on feelings is a no-win situation, yet people do it all the time. "I feel bad" doesn't mean that someone's physically ill but rather that he's wrestling with one or more emotions that make him feel out of sorts. By taking the time to examine and name this feeling, a person's more likely to find relief—and minimize the guilt. So, whenever you recognize you're in a funk, consider these two tips:

- Name the feeling (do not judge it as good or bad) by completing this statement: "I am (angry/jealous/sad) because______."
- Do not resort to artificial comforts and cover-ups for the pain (like binge-eating, popping a pill, or drowning the feeling in a stiff drink).

Halting the Isolation

Any chronic, progressive illness carries a measure of isolation—for you and your care partner. You get so tired of having to admit that you can't go here or do that. As your illness progresses and you truly have more trouble getting out and about, that sense of isolation can become overwhelming. Heal the feeling by:

- Meeting regularly with other persons with Parkinson's (PWP).
- Encouraging (and accepting) the offers of people to come to you to share an hour, a meal, or an entire evening.
- Connecting through e-mail and phone calls.
- Exercising—take a walk or take part in a sport like golf.
- Tapping into whatever spiritual therapies work for you.

Corralling the Anger

Anger at your PD is one issue, but anger at those who love you and are attempting to meet your needs is quite another. On its own, anger is a completely normal response to living with a condition like PD that hampers your control and freedom. And getting really ticked off once in awhile can even be healthy. But generalized and unidentified anger that festers can do some real damage. So get a handle on your anger from the outset by:

- Recognizing that your mask-like facial expression may compromise your efforts to convey your frustrations and anger.
- Naming the cause and then seizing the moment—rant and rage for a couple of minutes, punch a pillow, or count to ten.
- Putting your anger in perspective—talk it over with someone to look for the actual underlying causes for the outburst.

Taming the Guilt

Guilt is sneaky. It creeps up on you after a jealous, frustrated, or angry reaction. It chafes as you perceive people putting their lives on hold for you. Like anger, guilt can build on other difficult feelings. But, just as you do with anger, you need to name the guilt and nip it in the bud by:

- Asking yourself whether you're being fair to people around you by accepting and appreciating their efforts.
- Taking stock and reassuring yourself that you're doing all you can to maintain your function in the face of your PD.

Subduing Your Fears

Face it. We live in a pretty scary world, mostly because of the uncertainties that surround us—planes flying into buildings, pandemic threats of famine and contagious disease, and then some. As a PWP, your fears may be far more specific than these world events. You're concerned that you may have passed this disease on to your children; you worry that your PD will incapacitate you before you can achieve certain milestones, such as seeing your daughter married or holding your first grandchild. Face your fears by:

- Reviewing the information on anxiety and depression in Chapter 13.

- Accepting that life is uncertain. The best anyone can do is to live each day to its fullest and *not* wait to celebrate and appreciate.

Venting Your Frustration

Frustration can arise from many situations. You may get frustrated with your inability to hold a comb or toothbrush. Or you may grit your teeth when you perceive your care partner's taking over tasks you can do for yourself. Or maybe you gag with the lack of straight answers to your questions about PD and its progression. And on and on. Here's an excellent solution: Call or e-mail one of the people in your support group (or go to an online group such as brain.hastypas try.net/forums) and vent! Then get back to life.

Cooling the Jealousy

Jealousy is such a normal human reaction. You've dealt with it your entire life—when a friend got a bigger house or a better car; when a co-worker got the pro-motion you wanted; when your sister lost 30 pounds without trying (or so she said!). As a PWP, odds are good that your green monster rears its jealous head when your family and friends are free to go and do as they please without even thinking about it. You, on the other hand, have to plan and time activities. Life is not fair. You know this one. Face it by:

- Reminding yourself of *your* successes. Could that co-worker handle the challenge of PD with the kind of grace and humor you do (most of the time)?
- Expressing (in a kind and gentle way) your feelings of jealousy to the person. Chances are good that you'll discover the person is equally jealous of you.

Stopping the Spirals of Sadness

There's a *little* sad and then there's a *lot* sad. A little sad is when you feel sorry for yourself but the feeling passes quickly—usually within a few hours. A lot sad is when sadness spirals into full-blown mourning or grieving, the way you'd feel if you suffered some life-changing event such as the death of a loved one or the break-up of a relationship.

For PWP, intense sadness may be connected to the life they had planned before they heard they had PD. Left to its own devices, sadness of this magnitude can spiral into full-blown depression. You need to nip it in the bud by first acknowledging your right to mourn the life that will no longer be and then by embracing the possibilities that are before you now.

If working your way through the sadness becomes overwhelming, seek professional support by talking to your clergyperson or the counselor you put on your care team to help you through tough times (see Chapter 6).

Caring About Apathy

"I just don't care anymore." "Nothing's going to change." Answers? You care or you wouldn't have made it this far. So start by discussing these feelings with your doctor. If you're not already engaged in some form of talk therapy with a counselor, this is a good time to consider that option.

Dumping Depression

Short spurts of sadness can be healthy reactions as you adapt to life with a chronic and progressive condition. But when such feelings last weeks with no let-up, you may be facing depression. You need to treat it the way you'd treat any physical symptoms that don't go away after a short time. If feelings of helplessness, hopelessness, escalating apathy, or spiraling sadness persist beyond a few days, get help. Start by reading Chapter 13; then talk to your neurologist about treatments for handling depression in PD.

Chapter 23

Ten Ways to Care for Your Care Partner

In This Chapter

- Understanding your care partner's life
- Making life a little easier for your care partner
- Recognizing the simple pleasures

Life turned an unexpected corner the day you were diagnosed with Parkinson's disease (PD) for at least two people—you and your primary care partner.

Your care partner is your champion—speaking up when you can't, making sure that the medical community focuses on you as an individual and not just as another *case,* and performing the thousand and one tasks that keep life running for both of you. Your care partner deserves not only your empathy and understanding but also your support and attention.

This chapter gives you ten ways to acknowledge the sacrifice and encourage a healthy form of selfishness for your care partner.

Honor the Partnership

A partnership is a two-way street. It's not all about you and your needs. You and your partner honor your partnership by recognizing it as a mutual exchange of ideas as you find your way together through this change in lifestyle. Initially the focus is on you, and that's only right. But eventually you need to get a grip on your own reaction to PD and take a long, hard look at its effect on people around you, especially the person next to you, your partner in care. These are some ideas for doing just that:

- In any discussion about adapting to your needs, be sure you address (via words and actions) how those needs will impact your partner's routine.
- Be open to the idea of getting support and assistance from someone other than your care

partner. For that matter, suggest calling in reinforcements yourself. Perhaps your sister (who's offered to help in the past) can drive you to the hairdresser so your care partner has an after-noon to himself.

- Listen to what your partner is really saying. For example, in a discussion about your care partner doing tasks that you can still manage (although it may take you longer), maybe she admits that doing the tasks herself is just easier instead of waiting because of all she has to do. That answer may be a good clue that she's feeling overwhelmed, and you need to discuss ways to get her some help.

Acknowledge Life beyond PD

When every waking moment seems to focus on doctor's appointments, medications, maintaining function, and fighting depression, you need to stop and take a moment to really consider how much of your (healthy) care partner's life has been given over to your PD. How many of your conversations begin and end with PD? How much of your day and your care partner's focus on managing symptoms and maintaining your independence? What facets of your relationship before PD are beginning to slip through the cracks? Address that imbalance right now before it's too late. Talk through just how you can work together to make sure PD doesn't become your and your care partner's life.

One way to remind each other that there's more to life than your PD is to declare certain times of day *no-PD zones.* For example, agree to talk about topics other than your PD during and after dinner. You'll both sleep better if you spend the evening discussing lighter topics and catching up in general.

Accentuate the Positive

Care partners may actually resist talking about pleasurable experiences in their lives. For example, because you can't ride any longer, she may avoid discussing the amazing bike ride she just completed. Or she may feel uncomfortable talking about some political infighting at work because she fears that the details seem so petty and silly to you. Or she may worry that if she talks about a friend's impending vacation, it may just remind you that you'll probably never make that trip to Paris you dreamed of. You have a responsibility to encourage such sharing by making it clear that your partner is in some ways your extended eyes and ears, bringing you news and funny stories that have always entertained you.

Strike a Balance in Caregiving

Surely one of the most exhausting tasks for any care partner is trying to guess how much care is enough and how much is too much. How is your care partner supposed to know whether you're too exhausted to do something for yourself or you're determined to complete a task, even if you take all day? Care partners have many talents and they develop new ones over time, but mind-reading will never be on that list. If your care partner seems to be *doing* rather than *helping,* let that imbalance go for the moment, but find a time later to talk through the problems it may be causing.

Ask, Don't Demand

Listen to yourself. When you need help, do you begin the request with a verb? "Get me the remote." "Come here." "Button this."

Your care partner is not a private in your war against PD. Your care partner is right there in the trenches with you. Show some respect. This advice is not a request—it's a demand!

Use the Magic Words Often

Surely you learned them as kids: *please* and *thank you.* Never have they had more power. In the grown-up version, you need to move beyond simple statements—you need to show as well as tell. The smile, the touch of the hand, the small surprise that focuses just on your care partner are all magic in their own way. And the true magic is that you feel a little more like your old self if you can take care of your partner now and then.

Get Over Yourself

Yes, you've been dealt a really bad hand, but you're still here. For now you have a life that includes this person who has put his life on hold to take this journey with you. You also have a choice: live each day thinking about all the problems you may face as your PD progresses, or *live each day!*

Accept Services as a Gift for Your Care Partner

Asking other people to take care of needs that you once managed is depressing, especially if that person's a stranger who's paid to deliver a service.

(And especially if that service is so personal and private that you find it difficult to accept, such as bathing you or helping you to the bathroom.) Try to accept this help as one way of caring for your partner. Does this service free your partner to attend to some other task or simply enjoy a break? Does the help save time that both of you can put to better use?

Find Joy in Life

Caring for someone whose outlook is positive and hopeful—in spite of set-backs—is far less stressful than trying to bolster the spirit of someone constantly seeing the dark side. Your care partner has gone through all of the emotions you have: anger, fear, depression, the gamut. True, PD isn't attacking your care partner's ability to function, but PD is attacking both your lives. Remember, you set the tone for how people respond to your PD. If you've shivered in the shadows for a while, try crossing over to that sunnier side of the street, and take your care partner with you.

Encourage Laughter and Dreams

Your care partner deserves a life beyond your PD, a life as full of pleasure and promise as possible under the circumstances, a life that keeps dreams alive. You can encourage and nurture that life for your partner. Start by flipping to the "Bill of Rights for the PD Care Partner" in Chapter 19. Post the list where you and your care partner see it every day. And when your care partner resists nurturing and caring for herself, ask her to read the list aloud. Then talk about issues that can and must change so you can help care for your partner—physically, mentally, and spiritually.

Chapter 24

Michael J. Fox, Muhammad Ali, and YOU: Ten Ways to Make a Real Difference

In This Chapter

- Using your power of one
- Getting out and speaking up

The Parkinson's community is unique in that most PD organizations at the national level are super-organized, well-connected, and have earned the respect of the powerbrokers who can affect change. Think of the benefits people with PD (PWP) have gained from the efforts of Michael J. Fox and Muhammad Ali, for example, and then multiply that by 1.5 million—the number of PWP in the United States alone. Wow! There's power in those numbers!

But you don't have to be a celebrity to make a huge difference. Here are ten ideas to get you started.

Read More About It

Start by making yourself a local expert on PD. Check out the resources in Appendix B—especially those that offer information to share with other people. Get them on board for a specific issue that needs attention. (See "Get to Know Your Local Officials" a little later in this chapter.)

Vote Early and Often

The shocking fact is that Americans are becoming increasingly apathetic about voting. How often have you heard someone say, "It doesn't matter—politicians are all the same"? Well, if you as a PWP don't care, who *is* going to care? Your elected officials' support for dollars for research and adequate care options is vital for the future of treating and curing PD.

Absentee voting is always an option if getting to the polls is too difficult.

Get to Know Your Local Officials

Local elected officials work for you and often live in your community. Don't hesitate to talk directly to them about key issues that could impact you or others with a chronic progressive condition like PD. For example, if a zoning law is preventing a rehabilitation clinic from locating in your community, let your elected officials know why this clinic is important for you and other people with chronic conditions.

If the issue is a state or national matter, consider making contact (by phone, e-mail, or letter) with an official's senior staff person. Locally or nationally, build relationships with your elected officials—not one of checking up but one of informing that can lead to a difference for many people in the community (and votes for re-election).

Never underestimate the power of a single note or phone call. And don't forget to follow up! If you've written or called an elected official and been told someone will get back to you, but no one has, call again.

Don't Just Be Informed—Pass It On

Okay, you don't want to overdo this but *carpe diem*—seize the day! Say you're at dinner with friends and the conversation has settled on politics. You know a key bill's coming up for a vote that can really impact PD research. Talk about it! Relate its importance to facts that will stick in people's minds and perhaps lead them to contact their congressperson to cast a key vote.

A less in-your-face way to inform people as you go about your daily routine is to stay involved and talk about projects and interests you're involved in even if they're not PD related. Why? Because this is your opportunity to show that PWP can be contributing members to society in spite of PD.

Support Your Local Support Group

Attend meetings and consider getting more involved in the group's effort to influence community leaders (or even national politicians). Even if the support group isn't specifically for PWP, you can find power in numbers. Signing a petition, participating in a charity event, or raising money for research are all ways you can help build a better future for PWP.

Rally Local Support

Consider ways you can build awareness through your local library, employer, and community organizations. For example, encourage your librarian to invest in informative books, videos, and CDs for people with chronic, progressive conditions and their care partners. Ask your employer and community organization leaders to offer literature and seminars that help people with these conditions and their families to manage their time and caregiving. Employers benefit from less absenteeism and a more focused and productive work force, and community groups become more engaged in the needs of the community. (Get things started by ordering a set of the excellent booklets from the National Parkinson Foundation listed in Appendix B.)

Pitch Your Story to Local Media Outlets

People who put together the local news (print, radio, and television) are eager to hear from you. Can you imagine how they would delight in a story about a 60-something doctor with PD performing his first piano recital with a group of kids? What about the young onset Parkinson's disease (YOPD) person's care partner who also works fulltime, cares for their school-aged children, and volunteers?

Before you call your local news desk, check with the person whose story you plan to offer (even if that's your care partner). In telling the story, include:

- A local angle—the story is about a person in your community
- The key that makes it unique and not just another health story—as in the piano-playing doctor mentioned earlier
- The visuals (for print and television; for example, is there a photo op at the recital so a photographer can attend along with the journalist?)

Never forget that your story could help others struggling with chronic illness.

Join the Parkinson's Action Network

Advocacy requires conviction and passion for a cause. The national PD community has banded together (for the most part) and named the Parkinson's Action Network (PAN) to speak in Washington DC for the entire PD community. You can be a part of that national call to action by logging on to the PAN Web site at www.parkinsonsaction.org or calling 800-850-4726 to find a local or area chapter or to get on their mailing list for updates.

Raise Money for Research

Of course, if politics isn't your gig, you can raise awareness as well as dollars for research several other ways. For example, some events (such as a marathon or walkathon) require quite a bit of organization and teamwork. Sign up to volunteer and get your friends and family on board as well.

You also can be effective on your own. How many times have you read of someone biking or walking across

America and collecting donations along the way to raise awareness of some cause? Personally taking action doesn't mean you need to plan a trek across America, but what else can you do on your own to raise awareness and financial support? Try holding a yard sale with all the money going to PD research or ask family and friends to make a monetary contribution in your name to a PD organization in lieu of gifts on holidays, birthdays, and other gift occasions. (After all, do you really need another book, t-shirt, or CD?)

Celebrate National PD Month in April

PD gets its own month for national awareness—April (think springtime, renewal, and hope). How appropriate! How can you and your care partner mark this special month? The following are some easy ideas:

- Donate a copy of this book (or another on PD) to your local library.
- Plan to schedule one of the events suggested earlier in this chapter during the month of April.

- Go to New York City and take part in the annual Parkinson's Unity Walk. (Check out www.unitywalk.org for full information.)
- Buy a couple dozen red tulips (a floral symbol of the fight against PD) and pass them out to your friends, family, and everyone on your health-care team to thank them for making the journey with you.

Part VII

Appendixes

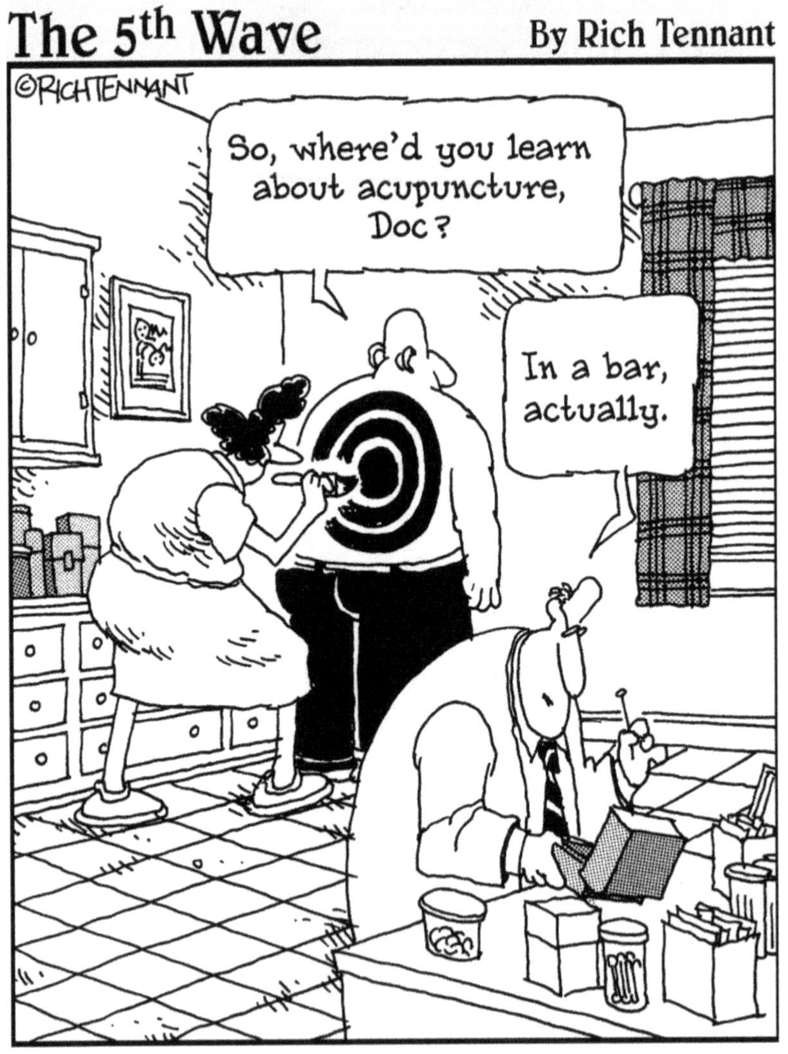
The 5th Wave
By Rich Tennant
©RICHTENNANT
So, where'd you learn about acupuncture, Doc?
In a bar, actually.

In this part...

In Appendix A you find a glossary that defines terms frequently tossed around in the world of Parkinson's disease. These are terms you should get to know because your doctors, other people with PD, and even the journalists who report the latest PD news use them.

Appendix B is a collection of resources that we introduce throughout this guide. The list includes national PD organizations with Web sites that can help in everything, from locating a neurologist or support group to updating you on the latest advances in medicines and treatments. We also include a list of programs and assistive devices that can make your life easier. Even if you don't have access to a computer (or don't know how to use one), get your child, grandchild, or the local librarian to help you discover these resources for enhancing your life.

Appendix A

Glossary

action tremor: An *involuntary,* rhythmic movement of the hand, arm, foot, or leg when a person performs a *voluntary* action such as lifting a fork, writing, or stepping onto a ladder. See *resting tremor.*

activities of daily living (ADLs): Routine activities that are part of a person's normal day (such as dressing, bathing, eating, toileting, transferring from bed to chair, walking from one room to another, participating in social and leisure activities).

advocacy: The process of influencing people via education, group actions, and publicity for a cause.

agonist: A muscle that contracts so the body can perform a specific movement; also a chemical or drug that stimulates a specific receptor to signal a desired action. *See dopamine agonist.*

akinesia: Also called *freezing;* temporary inability to initiate a desired movement.

antioxidants: Body chemicals that neutralize *free radicals.*

antiparkinsonian drugs: Drugs or medicines for the management and control of Parkinson's disease and its symptoms.

apraxia: The inability to execute a voluntary movement despite normal function and mental understanding of the desired action.

ataxia: Loss of balance and coordination.

athetosis: *Involuntary,* repetitive movements, especially with the hands, fingers, and (sometimes) feet.

basal ganglia: Groups of cells deep in the base of the brain that help the cortex in controlling *voluntary* movement and coordination.

bilateral: Occurring on or affecting both sides of the body or organ.

bradykinesia: The gradual slowing or loss of spontaneous movement that results in impaired abilities to perform a task or change positions.

bradyphrenia: The gradual slowing or loss of ability to process information.

carbidopa: A drug that, when combined with *levodopa,* reduces the side effects of levodopa yet improves overall effectiveness of levodopa by allowing more of it to enter the brain.

care partner/caregiver: Usually a family member (spouse, parent, sibling) who provides the emotional (and eventually physical) support and care for a person diagnosed with a chronic, progressive condition.

central nervous system (CNS): The network responsible for cueing the human body's mental and physical actions; consists of the brain and the spinal cord.

clinical trial: The research and testing required by the Food and Drug Administration (FDA) to determine whether new medicines, medical devices, and treatments are safe and effective before approving them for patients.

cognition: Those mental skills necessary to process information (such as perception, memory, reasoning, judgment, intellect, and creativity).

cogwheeling: The slow, jerky, or ratcheting sensation the doctor perceives when moving a patient's rigid limb at the joint.

computerized axial tomography (CAT or CT scan): A diagnostic computer procedure that uses a series of X-rays to produce a two-dimensional image of the body or specific body part.

Catechol O-methyltransferase (COMT) inhibitors: Drugs that block an enzyme that breaks down *levodopa* before the levodopa can convert into *dopamine,* thereby increasing the therapeutic supply of levodopa to the brain.

deep brain stimulation (DBS): A surgical procedure that helps control symptoms of advanced PD; electrodes are implanted in the brain and controlled through a battery-operated device known as an implanted pulse generator (IPG) or pacemaker.

delusion: A fixed belief that is false, not proven by objective evidence.

dementia: The neurological condition or sign of progressive decline in intellectual ability (such as impaired judgment, memory loss, confusion, personality changes, and disorientation) caused by one or a combination of underlying conditions, such as Alzheimer's disease and strokes.

depression: Sustained, prolonged feelings of hopelessness, helplessness, and sadness.

diagnosis: A doctor's conclusions based on a patient's medical history and symptoms as well as the doctor's observations and tests.

dopamine: The natural chemical substance present in areas of the brain that regulate movement, motivation, and feelings of pleasure. See *neurotransmitter.*

dopamine agonist (DA): *Antiparkinsonian drugs* that imitate and supplement the brain's naturally produced *dopamine.*

dysarthria: Difficulties with speech caused by impaired movement of muscles; results in slurred or muffled words or the inability to project one's voice or speak at a normal volume.

dyskinesia: Abnormal *involuntary movements* (examples are sudden muscle contractions; rapid, jerky or lurching movements; fidgeting or restless movements of upper body, arms, legs, or head); may be a response to long-term use of *antiparkinsonian meds* and may worsen with stress.

dysphagia: The impaired ability to swallow.

dystonia: A movement disorder that causes significant and unexpected muscle contractions or spasms that result in abnormal and *involuntary* movement and posture. Can be a symptom of Parkinson's disease.

essential tremor (ET): More common than *primary PD,* this movement disorder causes an uncontrolled *tremor* of the hands, neck, head or voice; most apparent when performing a *voluntary* action, such as lifting a cup. See *action tremor.*

executive function: The intellectual ability to set goals, make decisions, and perform multi-stepped processes such as balancing a checkbook.

festination: A series of progressively quicker, shuffling, almost-running small steps after walking is initiated; sensation of the upper body wanting to move forward but the legs are unable to follow appropriately.

Food and Drug Administration (FDA): The federal body charged with monitoring clinical trials and assuring the safety and effectiveness of a medicine or therapy before it's available to the public.

free radicals: Potentially toxic substances produced by the normal metabolism in all human cells; left uncontrolled, they can damage or destroy vital brain cells.

freezing: The sudden and temporary inability of a *PWP* to initiate a movement such as going through a doorway or exiting a car. See *akinesia.*

gait: Medical term for walking; includes the individual style of walking.

gene: The building block of inheritance contained in every human cell; a change in the gene can predispose the individual to a disease.

genetic: Anything related to genes or inherited characteristics, including diseases.

globus pallidus: One of the areas of the *basal ganglia* most affected by the lack of *dopamine* in Parkinson's disease.

hallucination: Unreal perceptions that a person may experience while awake; hearing or seeing objects or people that are not present. Visual hallucinations may be a side effect of *antiparkinsonian meds.*

hypokinesia: Decreased or reduced movement.

hypomimia: The lack of facial expression and absence of eye-blinking caused by Parkinson's disease. Also called *mask* or "facial mask."

hypophonic: Reduced vocal volume and clarity.

idiopathic: A diagnostic term meaning "of unknown origin or without apparent cause."

involuntary movement: Movement that happens without the person's intention or control.

levodopa (L-dopa): The most commonly used drug for treatment of PD; restores levels of *dopamine* in the brain.

Lewy bodies: Abnormal, round clumps of protein in damaged and dying *dopamine*-producing brain cells.

magnetic resonance imaging (MRI): A noninvasive, diagnostic imaging tool that uses an electromagnetic field to create cross-sectional illustrations of particular organs and systems in the human body.

mask: See *hypomimia.*

micrographia: The small, cramped handwriting due to impaired fine motor skills in some *PWP.*

motor fluctuations: Daily variations of the benefits from *antiparkinsonian drugs.* Usually occur as PD progresses. Also called *on-off phenomenon, wearing off,* and *dyskinesia.*

movement disorders: A category of neurological conditions that impair normal control of movements; includes *Parkinson's disease* and similar disorders (*parkinsonism* disorders), *essential tremor, dystonia,* tics, chorea, and other less common diseases.

multiple system atrophy: A neurological disorder characterized by *parkinsonism* that is poorly responsive to *levodopa;* typically associated early in its progression with other signs of neurological dysfunction including low blood pressure when standing (orthostatic hypotension), impotence, urinary incontinence, severe *gait* imbalance, slurred speech, incoordination, loss of cognitive function, and *dementia.*

National Institutes of Health (NIH): The primary federal agency charged with conducting and supporting medical research.

National Institute of Neurological Disorders and Stroke (NINDS): The branch of *NIH* that focuses on diseases and conditions that affect the brain and *central nervous system.*

neurodegenerative: A neurological disease (such as Alzheimer's and Parkinson's) marked by the progressive loss of *neurons.*

neurologist: A specialist in the diagnosis and treatment of neurological disorders of the brain, spinal cord, nerves, and muscles (such as PD, stroke, Alzheimer, and multiple sclerosis).

neuron: A type of cell (mainly in the nervous system) that processes and transmits information for specific functions.

neuroprotective therapy: Any treatment with the ability to prevent or slow the loss of vital *neurons* affected by a *neurodegenerative* disease.

neurosurgeon: A surgeon specializing in the treatment of neurological disorders.

neurotransmitter: The body's natural chemicals (such as *dopamine*) that send messages from one nerve cell to another or from nerve cells to muscles.

occupational therapy: Skilled rehabilitation techniques that help people with neurological conditions perform routine daily tasks at home; maximizes physical potential through lifestyle adaptations and possible use of assistive devices.

on-off phenomenon: Severe *motor fluctuations* that are particularly frequent, sudden, and unpredictable; also called "yo-yo" syndrome.

pallidotomy: A surgical procedure that lesions (burns) parts of the *globus pallidus* to lessen PD symptoms; now largely replaced by *deep brain stimulation* (DBS).

palsy: Also called "paralysis;" loss of the ability to move a body part. Parkinson's disease was originally called "shaking palsy."

parkinsonism: A group of movement disorders characterized by a variable combination of *tremor, rigidity, bradykenesia,* and *postural instability.*

Parkinson's disease (PD): A slowly progressing neurological disease resulting in the loss of *dopamine*-producing brain cells in the *substantia nigra.* The disease normally responds to the medication *levodopa.*

person (or persons) with Parkinson's disease: See *PWP.*

physical therapy: The use of stretching and strengthening exercises and machines to help *PWP* maintain (or regain) strength, balance, coordination, flexibility, endurance, and function for as long as possible.

pill-rolling: A characteristic finger *tremor* in which the thumb and index finger slowly rub against each other as if rolling something into a small ball. Typically (almost exclusively) seen in patients with *Parkinson's disease.*

placebo effect: A change or improvement (physical or emotional) in a patient who has been given a medication with no therapeutic benefits (as in clinical trials); there is no medical explanation for the change.

positron emission tomography (PET scan): A diagnostic imaging tool that uses an injected radioactive form of various compounds (such as glucose *levodopa*) to produce color maps of the sections of the brain and assist in the diagnosis of Parkinson's disease.

postural instability: A person's lack of balance or coordination when walking; usually results in awkward forward- or backward-leaning that may result in a fall as the person attempts to compensate for lack of balance.

postural tremor: *Tremor* or shaking that occurs when a person's arms are stretched outright to the front.

prognosis: A doctor's prediction of a condition's progression based on the patient's medical history and response to treatment as well as the doctor's knowledge of the disease.

propulsive gait: Also called *parkinsonian gait;* walking that is characterized by a stooped, rigid posture with head and neck bent forward; shorter and faster steps propel the person forward, placing him at risk for falling. See *festination* and *retropulsive gait.*

PWP: Abbreviation for "person (people) with Parkinson's disease;" sometimes appears as "PLWP" for "person (people) living with Parkinson's."

range of motion (ROM): The measurement of a person's ability to fully straighten or bend a joint (knee, elbow, hip, ankle, shoulder, or spine).

receptor: The part of a nerve cell that receives a message from a *neurotransmitter* (*dopamine,* for example).

resting tremor: A *tremor* or shaking that occurs when a body part is relaxed and supported (hand resting on the arm of a chair) but not engaged in activity; typically tremor ceases or lessens if the limb is engaged in activity.

retropulsive gait: A movement characterized by a person propelling herself backward in an attempt to maintain balance, thereby placing herself at risk for falling. See *propulsive gait.*

rigidity: The abnormal stiffness of a joint or limb.

seborrhea: Increased volume of oily perspiration.

sialorrhea: Drooling.

side effects: Undesirable problems a patient experiences when taking a certain medication; prescription meds list major side effects in their printed information and over-the-counter products list them on the packaging.

Sinemet: The brand name for *levodopa/carbidopa,* the most common medication for treating PD symptoms.

speech therapy: Rehabilitative techniques that help restore or strengthen speech and swallowing muscles affected by PD.

stem cell: Undeveloped or undifferentiated cells that can duplicate themselves or become cells of various body tissues; may originate from an adult tissue or an undeveloped embryo. Current studies consider these cells as potential cures for *neurodegenerative* diseases.

striatum: Part of the *basal ganglia* affected by the lack of *dopamine.* See *globus pallidus* and *subthalamic nucleus.*

substantia nigra: The small area of the brain that houses cells that produce the *neurotransmitter dopamine;* specifically affected by Parkinson's disease.

subthalamic nucleus: One of the small groups of cells in the *basal ganglia* primarily affected by PD; the most frequent surgical target for *DBS.* See *deep brain stimulation.*

support group: A gathering of people with a common connection (such as PWP or PD *care partners*) who meet regularly to share information, receive education, and sustain one another.

thalamotomy: A surgical procedure intended to relieve *tremor;* now largely replaced by *DBS.* See *deep brain stimulation.*

transcranial magnetic stimulation (TMS): A procedure in which an electromagnetic coil briefly stimulates specific areas of the brain in order to modulate their activity; used experimentally to treat depression and PD.

tremor: A repetitive and involuntary movement such as trembling or shaking; usually in the hands but possible in feet, legs, arms, head, or voice.

trigger event: An event (a fall or head trauma), exposure (to toxins or other environmental materials), or unusual stress (loss of job or death of a loved one) that exposes a condition's previously unrecognized symptoms.

unilateral: Occurring on one side of the body.

voluntary movement: Movement performed with full intention and control.

wearing off: Reappearance of PD symptoms before the next dose of *levodopa* is due. See *motor fluctuations.*

young onset PD: PD diagnosed in people under the age of 50.

Appendix B

Additional Resources

Even though this handy guide covers Parkinson's disease (PD) from A to Z and offers a world of suggestions in dealing with it, we realize you may not be satisfied with reading just one book. You may want to know everything you can, or you may want more information about a specific topic within this huge subject. So, to round out this all-purpose guide, our appendix highlights other valuable sources for credible information and practical tools. This is by no means an exhaustive list—but it does include some truly valuable *stuff* to broaden your understanding of PD.

Requesting Free Print Materials

The National Parkinson Foundation (www.parkinson.org or 800-327-4545) has a terrific series of booklets about living with PD. Each booklet touches on a specific topic, and the foundation is always coming up with new topics (or revising the current ones). The best news is that these booklets are free. A sampling of the current titles includes:

- ***Parkinson's Disease: What You and Your Family Should Know***
- ***Parkinson's Disease: Nutrition Matters***
- ***Activities of Daily Living: Practical Pointers for Parkinson's Disease***
- ***Parkinson's Disease: Caring and Coping***

Gathering Free Info Online

As soon as possible, bookmark the following Web sites on your computer. Visit them regularly for updates on the latest treatments, tips on managing symptoms, and suggestions for your care partner. You can even use the Web to locate a neurologist, a local support group, or a medical center that specializes in the treatment of PD.

Don't have a computer? Talk to your local librarian. Better yet, put a child or grandchild on the case. They're the experts at searching the Internet, and when you research a question or topic together, it can be great quality time.

Making national PD organizations your first stop

The PD community is well organized. Each of the following Web sites provides a full range of information from medical updates to tips for coping.

• **American Parkinson Disease Association Inc.:** www.apdaparkinson.org

Click on *Young Parkinson's* for The Arlette Johnson Young Parkinson Information and Referral Center; also click on *Local Information and Referral*

Center on the home page to locate a support group or chapter.

Also: 135 Parkinson Avenue Staten Island, NY 10305; Phone 800-223-2732 or 718-981-8001

• **The Bachmann-Strauss Dystonia & Parkinson Foundation:** www.dystonia-parkinsons.org

This foundation focuses on research updates for dystonia and PD.

Also: One Gustave L. Levy Place, Box 1490, New York, NY 10029; Phone 212-241-5614

• **The Michael J. Fox Foundation:** www.michaeljfox.org

Click on *Sign up for e-mail* on the home page to receive the newsletter plus regular e-mail updates on research and other advances toward a cure.

Also: 20 Grand Central Station, P.O. Box 4777, New York, NY 10163; Phone 800-708-7644

• **The Muhammad Ali Parkinson Center:** www.maprc.com

Click on *Register* to help the center gather data on PD prevalence in the United States.

Also: 500 W. Thomas Road, Suite 720, Phoenix, Arizona 85013; Phone 602-406-4931

• **National Parkinson Foundation:** www.parkinson.org

Click on *Library/Publications* for a complete list and order form for the free publications mentioned at the beginning of this appendix; also click on *Support Groups* to locate a group in your area.

Also: 1501 N.W. 9th Avenue/Bob Hope Road, Miami FL 33136; Phone 800-327-4545

• **Parkinson's Action Network:** w ww.parkinsonsaction.org

Click on *Become an Advocate* and get involved in the fight for a cure.

Also: 1025 Vermont Ave. NW, Suite 1120, Washington, DC 20005; Phone 800-850-4726

• **Parkinson's Disease Foundation:** www.pdf.org

Click on *Ask an Expert* to submit a question or to link to expert information.

Also: 1359 Broadway, Suite 1509, New York, NY 10018; Phone 212-923-4700

• **Young Onset Parkinson's Association:** www.yopa.org

Click on *YOPA Support* to locate a support group for YOPD in your area.

Also: 22136 Westheimer Parkway #343, Katy, TX 77450; Phone 1-888-WE-R-YOPA (1-888-937-9672)

Locating a neurologist near you

These sites help you find a neurologist or interpret the medical jargon:

• **American Academy of Neurology:** www.aan.com

Click on *Contact Us* to ask about a neurologist in your area.

• **Cleveland Clinic Foundation:** www.clevelandclinic.org

In the *Search* box, type *Parkinson's* for links to the Center on PD.

• **Medline Plus:** www.nia.nih.gov/HealthInformation/Publications

This site provides federal government info on PD, caregiving, and aging.

• **Medscape:** www.medscape.com

Click on *Neurology and Neurosurgery* link; then on the *Resource Center* list, click on *Parkinson's disease.*

• **NeurologyChannel:** www.neurologychannel.com

Click on *MD Locator* to locate a neurologist in your area.

Connecting with a rehab therapist

Physical, occupational, and speech therapy may be part of your care plan for managing PD symptoms. These national associations can help you locate the appropriate therapist in your area if you doctor hasn't already done so.

- **American Physical Therapy Association:** www.apta.org or by phone at 800-999-2782
- **American Occupational Therapy Association, Inc.:** www.aota.org or by phone at 800-377-8555
- **American Speech-Language-Hearing Association:** www.asha.org or by phone at 800-638-8255

Seeking assistance with your meds

Check out the Pharmaceutical Research and Manufacturers of America (PhRMA) at www.phrma.org. Click on *Patient Assistance Programs* to find out more about financial assistance for meds. Click on *About PhRma* and then *Member List* to locate the manufacturer of any medicine you're taking.

Finding tools that make your life easier

A number of devices are available to make life easier and to prolong independence for people with PD. The following resources offer places to check out as the need arises.

Exercise and speech tools

These resources offer exercise and speech programs you can use at home. They come in a variety of formats from printed booklet with illustrations to videos and audio tapes.

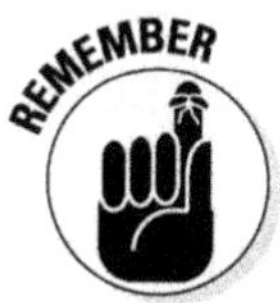

Be sure you show the program to your neurologist or rehab therapist before using any program on your own.

- ***Aquatic Exercises for Parkinson's Disease:*** From The American Parkinson Disease Association, Inc.: www.apdaparkinson.org/user/PublicationOrder.asp
- ***Exercise: A Guide from the National Institute on Aging:*** www.nia.nih.gov/HealthInformation/Publications/ExerciseGuide
- ***The LSVT (Lee Silverman Voice Treatment):*** www.lsvt.org
- ***Motivating Moves for People with Parkinson's:*** www.motivatingmoves.com
- ***The PDF Exercise Program:*** www.pdf.org/publications/brochures
- ***SIT AND BE FIT:*** www.sitandbefit.com

- Additional related Web sites at http ://parkinsonexercise.com

Clothing, medical alert systems, and other helpful aids

The following sites provide a range of aids from clothing with easy closures to canes that may help avoid *freezing* (legs locked, unable to step forward) to medic alert gear. New products come on the market every year.

- **Clothing Solutions:** www.clothings olutions.com
- **Exerstrider:** www.exerstrider.com
- **Fashion Ease:** www.fashionease.co m
- **Liberty Cane:** www.libertycane.co m
- **Philips Lifeline:** www.lifelinesys.co m
- **Luminaud, Inc.:** www.luminaud.co m
- **Med-Alert:** www.1800medalert.com
- **MedicAlert:** www.medicalert.org
- **Sears Health and Wellness:** ww w.searshealthandwellness.com
- **U-Step Walking Stabilizer:** www. ustep.com

Complementary and alternative therapies

If you and your neurologist decide that some form of alternative therapy may prove helpful, these three resources can help.

- **American Massage Therapy Association:** www.amtamassage.org
- **National Center for Complementary and Alternative Medicine:** www.nccam.nih.gov
- **Yoga Journal:** www.yogajournal.com

Looking into financial and legal matters

Finances and legal matters are nothing to play around with. You need the help of (or at least a consultation with) an expert. These resources can help:

- **American Institute of Certified Public Accountants:** www.aicpa.org
- **American Association of Daily Money Managers:** www.aadmm.com

- **American Association of Retired Persons:** www.aarp.org
- **Financial Planning Association:** www.fpanet.org
- **Medicare:** www.medicare.gov
- **Medicare Rights Center:** www.medicarerights.org

Sharing sites with your care partner

Bookmark these sites for your care partner:

- **CARE:** www.pdcaregiver.org
- **Eldercare Locator:** www.eldercare.gov
- **National Alliance for Caregiving:** www.caregiving.org
- **National Family Caregivers Association:** www.nfcacares.org
- **Parkinson Foundation of the Heartland:** www.parkinsonheartland.org
- **Parkinson's Training for Caregivers:** www.parkinsonseducator.com
- **The Parkinson's Web:** http://pdweb.mgh.harvard.edu

- **National Parkinson's Foundation *(Caregiver Resources):*** www.parkinson.org/site

Other Books Worth the $$

New books on living with PD are published every year and your local library may have these recent works. If it doesn't, suggest the librarian add it to the library's wish list, or consider donating a copy yourself.

- ***100 Questions and Answers about Parkinson Disease*** by Abraham Lieberman, MD with Marcia McCall (Jones and Barlett Publishing)
- ***A Life Shaken: My Encounter with Parkinson's Disease*** by Joel Havermann (Johns Hopkins University Press)
- ***Lucky Man: A Memoir*** by Michael J. Fox (Hyperion)
- ***Parkinson's Disease: A Guide for Patient and Family*** (Fifth Edition) by Roger C. Duvosin and Jacob Sage (Lippincott Williams & Wilkins)
- ***Parkinson's Disease and the Family: A New Guide*** by Nutan

Sharma and Elaine Richman (Harvard University Press)

Figure I

SPORTS, FITNESS, PARENTING, RELIGION & SPIRITUALITY

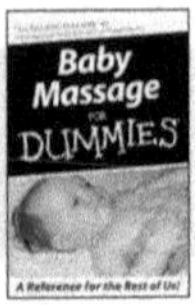

Also available:

- Catholicism For Dummies
- Exercise Balls For Dummies
- Fitness For Dummies
- Football For Dummies
- Judaism For Dummies
- Potty Training For Dummies
- Buddhism For Dummies
- Pregnancy For Dummies
- Ten Minute Tone-Ups For Dummies
- NASCAR For Dummies
- Religion For Dummies
- Soccer For Dummies
- Women in the Bible For Dummies

TRAVEL

Also available:

- Alaska For Dummies
- Cruise Vacations For Dummies
- England For Dummies
- Europe For Dummies
- Germany For Dummies
- Hawaii For Dummies
- Italy For Dummies
- Las Vegas For Dummies
- London For Dummies
- Paris For Dummies
- RV Vacations For Dummies
- Walt Disney World & Orlando For Dummies

GRAPHICS, DESIGN & WEB DEVELOPMENT

Also available:

- 3D Game Animation For Dummies
- AutoCAD 2006 For Dummies
- Building a Web Site For Dummies
- Creating Web Pages For Dummies
- Creating Web Pages All-in-One Desk Reference For Dummies
- Dreamweaver 8 For Dummies
- InDesign CS2 For Dummies
- Macromedia Flash 8 For Dummies
- Photoshop CS2 and Digital Photography For Dummies
- Photoshop Elements 4 For Dummies
- Syndicating Web Sites with RSS Feeds For Dummies
- Yahoo! SiteBuilder For Dummies

NETWORKING, SECURITY, PROGRAMMING & DATABASES

Also available:

- Access 2007 For Dummies
- ASP.NET 2 For Dummies
- C# 2005 For Dummies
- Hacking For Dummies
- Hacking Wireless Networks For Dummies
- Java For Dummies
- Microsoft SQL Server 2005 For Dummies
- Networking All-in-One Desk Reference For Dummies
- Preventing Identity Theft For Dummies
- Telecom For Dummies
- Visual Studio 2005 All-in-One Desk Reference For Dummies
- XML For Dummies

Figure II

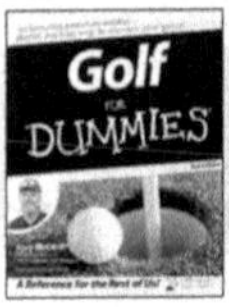

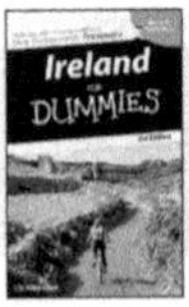

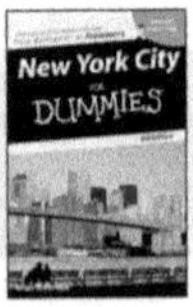

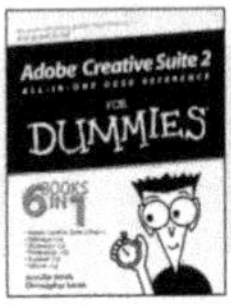

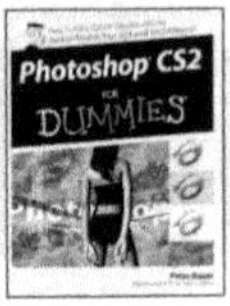

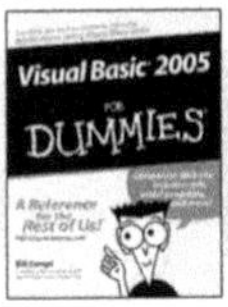

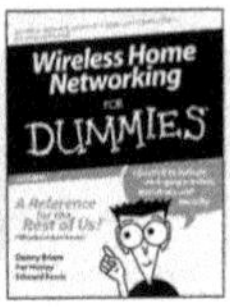

Parkinson's Disease For Dummies®—Cheat Sheet

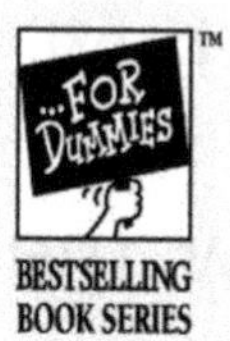

Managing Your Medication Routine

- Carry a complete list of current prescription (Rx) and over-the-counter (OTC) medications. Give a copy to your care partner as well.
- Tell all doctors of allergies or other problems.
- Ask the doctor:
    - Name of medicine
    - Purpose
    - Dosing schedule (how much, how often)
    - How to take and how long to take
    - Side effects

- Ask the pharmacist to:
    - Check new Rx with your current Rx and OTC meds for possible interaction
    - Print label in large print
    - Provide easy-to-open cap
    - Explain how to take med
- At home:
    - Add new med to list of meds you carry with you
    - Read and file information print-out
    - Take med exactly as prescribed

Words and Acronyms to Know

- akinesia: Inability to move spontaneously
- ataxia: Impaired balance and coordination
- bradykinesia: Slowed movement
- carbidopa/levodopa: Medication to relieve PD symptoms
- dopamine: Acts as one of the brain's messengers to signal movement and maintain balance and coordination

- dyskinesia: Abnormal involuntary movements
- PD: Parkinson's disease
- PWP: Person (or people) with Parkinson's disease
- T.R.A.P.: Acronym for 4 primary PD symptoms:
  - Tremor: Shaking of limb (usually hand) while at rest
  - Rigidity: Muscle stiffness and resistance to movement
  - Akinesia/bradykinesia: See above
  - Postural instability: See *ataxia* above

Bookmark These Web Sites

American Parkinson Disease Association, Inc.: www.apdaparkinson.org

- The Michael J. Fox Foundation: www.michaeljfox.org
- National Parkinson Foundation: www.parkinson.org
- Parkinson Action Network: www.parkinsonsaction.org
- Parkinson's Disease Foundation: www.pdf.org

- National Institute of Neurological Disorders and Stroke: www.ninds.nih.gov

Red-Flag Medications

The following classes of medications may be incompatible with routine PD meds. Provide the following list to all medical professionals before they prescribe any new medicine (Rx or OTC), and review any new medications with your neurologist before you begin taking them:

- Antinausea dopamine agonists
- Gastrointestinal anticholinergics
- Antipsychotics
- Postoperative pain-management drugs (Demerol in particular)

Contact the National Parkinson Foundation (www.parkinson.org or 800-327-4545) for a wallet-sized card that lists drugs that may be contraindicated.

Your Daily CHECK-IN

Here's a quick and easy way to remind yourself that living *well* with PD is possible. Read this list once a day – twice if it's a rough day.

- ***C***hallenge—acknowledge and face the facts
- ***H***umor—find and revel in the absurd
- ***E***mpowerment—refuse to surrender your life and relationships to PD
- ***C***ollaboration—team with your family, friends, and healthcare providers
- ***K***nowledge—know the difference between myth and fact and keep up with the latest developments
- ***I***ntegration—treat the body, mind, and spirit
- ***N***ever—give up!

When You Go to the Hospital or ER

- Have copies of the following information ready; give them to the Admissions office, the doctors, and ER or floor staff:
  - Your neurologist's contact information – phone, pager, e-mail, and fax info
  - Your doctor's written instructions for stopping and starting

your PD meds during ER or hospital treatment

- A list of all Rx and OTC medications you currently take
- A list of the red-flag medications (see previous page)

- Examine meds you are given in the hospital. If you don't recognize a med, ask what it is, who prescribed it, and why you're taking it.
- Make sure your care partner has copies of all personal info (as noted in Chapter 9) including insurance info and copies of your advance directive and living will.
- Have your care partner monitor all ER- or hospital-administered meds.
- Before leaving the hospital, get a list of medications you're now taking.
- After you're home, contact your neurologist to review the list of new meds.

Emergency Contacts

Fill in these blanks to keep important phone numbers close at hand:

Primary care partner:_____ (h)_____ (w)_____ (cell)_____

Secondary care partner: _____ (h)_____ (w)_____ (cell)_____

Neighbor: _____ (h)_____ (w)_____ (cell)_____

Support group member/leader_____ (h)_____ (w)_____ (cell)_____

Primary doctor: _____ (h)_____ (w)_____ (cell)_____

Neurologist: _____ (h)_____ (w)_____ (cell)_____

Pharmacist:_____ (w)_____

For more information about Wiley Publishing, call 1-800-762-2974.

For Dummies: Bestselling Book Series for Beginners

A

D

E

H

I

M

N

O

P

Q

R

S

T

U

V

W

Y

CPSIA information can be obtained
at www.ICGtesting.com
Printed in the USA
BVHW010049220922
647492BV00024B/376

Web Coding & Development

ALL-IN-ONE

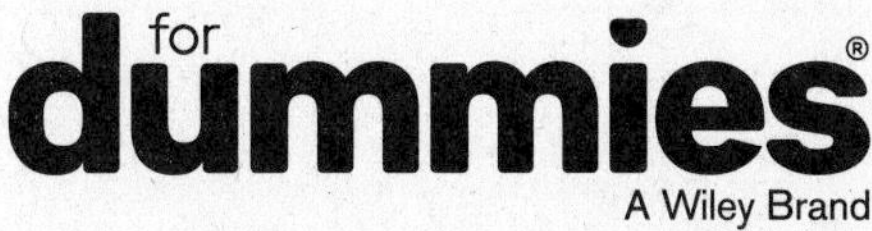

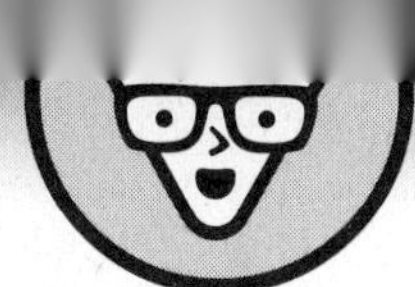

Web Coding & Development

ALL-IN-ONE

by Paul McFedries

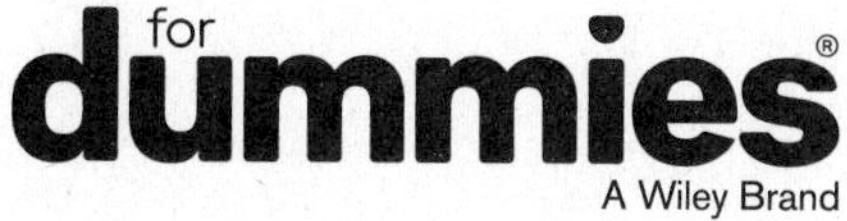

2/19
$40

Web Coding & Development All-in-One For Dummies®

Published by: **John Wiley & Sons, Inc.,** 111 River Street, Hoboken, NJ 07030-5774, www.wiley.com

For general information on our other products and services, please contact our Customer Care Department within the U.S. at 877-762-2974, outside the U.S. at 317-572-3993, or fax 317-572-4002. For technical support, please visit https://hub.wiley.com/community/support/dummies.

Wiley publishes in a variety of print and electronic formats and by print-on-demand. Some material included with standard print versions of this book may not be included in e-books or in print-on-demand. If this book refers to media such as a CD or DVD that is not included in the version you purchased, you may download this material at http://booksupport.wiley.com. For more information about Wiley products, visit www.wiley.com.

Library of Congress Control Number: 2018935649

ISBN: 978-1-119-47392-3; ISBN: 978-1-119-47383-1 (ePDF); ISBN: 978-1-119-47379-4 (ePub)

Manufactured in the United States of America

C10004238_091018

Contents at a Glance

Table of Contents

Introduction

When the web first came to the attention of the world's non-geeks back in the mid-1990s, the vastness and variety of its treasures were a wonder to behold. However, it didn't take long before a few courageous and intrepid souls dug a little deeper into this phenomenon and discovered something truly phenomenal: *They* could make web pages, too!

Why was that so amazing? Well, think back to those old days and think, in particular, of what it meant to create what we now call *content*. Think about television shows, radio programs, magazines, newspapers, books, and the other media of the time. The one thing they all had in common was that their creation was a decidedly *un*common thing. It required a *team* of professionals, a *massive* distribution system, and a *lot* of money. In short, it wasn't something that your average Okie from Muskogee would have any hope of duplicating.

The web appeared to change all of that because learning HTML was within the grasp of anybody who could feed himself, it had a built-in massive distribution system (the Internet, natch), and it required little or no money. For the first time in history, content was democratized and was no longer defined as the sole province of governments and mega-corporations.

Then reality set in.

People soon realized that merely building a website wasn't enough to attract "eyeballs," as the marketers say. A site had to have interesting, useful, or fun content, or people would stay away in droves. Not only that, but this good content had to be combined with a solid site design, which meant that web designers needed a thorough knowledge of HTML and CSS.

But, alas, eventually even all of that was not enough. To make their websites dynamic and interesting, to make their sites easy to navigate, and to give their sites those extra bells and whistles that surfers had come to expect, something more than content, HTML, and CSS was needed.

That missing link was *code*.

What we've all learned the hard way over the past few years is that you simply can't put together a world-class website unless you have some coding prowess in your site design toolkit. You need to know how to program your way out of the basic problems that afflict most sites; how to use scripting to go beyond the inherent limitations of HTML and CSS; and how to use code to send and receive data from a web server. And it isn't enough just to copy the generic scripts that are available on the web and paste them into your pages. First of all, most of those scripts are very poorly written, and second of all, they invariably need some customization to work properly on your site.

About This Book

My goal in this book is to give you a complete education on web coding and development. You learn how to set up the tools you need, how to use HTML and CSS to design and build your site, how to use JavaScript and jQuery to program your pages, and how to use PHP and MySQL to program your web server. My aim is to show you that these technologies aren't hard to learn, and that even the greenest rookie programmers can learn how to put together web pages that will amaze their family and friends (and themselves).

If you're looking for lots of programming history, computer science theory, and long-winded explanations of concepts, I'm sorry but you won't find it here. My philosophy throughout this book comes from Linus Torvalds, the creator of the Linux operating system: "Talk is cheap. Show me the code." I explain what needs to be explained and then I move on without further ado (or, most of the time, without any ado at all) to examples and scripts that do more to illuminate a concept that any verbose explanations I could muster (and believe me, I can muster verbosity with the best of them).

How you approach this book depends on your current level of web coding expertise (or lack thereof):

- If you're just starting out, begin at the beginning with Book 1 and work at your own pace sequentially through to Books 2 and 3. This will give you all the knowledge you need to pick and choose what you want to learn throughout the rest of the book.
- If you know HTML and CSS, you can probably get away with taking a fast look at Book 2, then settle in with Book 3 and beyond.
- If you've done some JavaScript coding already, I suggest working quickly through the material in Book 3, then dig into Book 4 a little slower if you don't already know jQuery. You'll then be ready to branch out and explore the rest of the book as you see fit.
- If you're a relatively experienced JavaScript programmer, use Books 3 and 4 as a refresher, then tackle Book 5 to learn how to code the back end. I've got a few tricks in there that you might find interesting. After that, feel free to

consider the rest of the book a kind of coding smorgasbord that you can sample as your web development taste buds dictate.

Foolish Assumptions

This book is not a primer on the Internet or on using the World Wide Web. This is a coding and development book, pure and simple. This means I assume the following:

- You know how to operate a basic text editor, and how to get around the operating system and file system on your computer.
- You have an Internet connection.
- You know how to use your web browser.

Yep, that's it.

"I've never coded before!"

If you've never done a stitch of computer programming before, even if you're not quite sure what programming really is, don't worry about it for a second because I had you in mind when I wrote this book. For too many years programming has been the property of "hackers" and other technowizards. That made some sense because the programming languages they were using — with bizarre names such as C++ and Perl — were exceedingly difficult to learn, and even harder to master.

This book's main coding technologies — HTML, CSS, JavaScript, jQuery, PHP, and MySQL — are different. They're nowhere near as hard to learn as those for-nerds-only languages. I honestly believe that *anyone* can become a savvy and successful web coder, and this book is, I hope, the proof of that assertion. Just follow along, examine my code carefully (particularly in the first few chapters), and practice what you learn, and you *will* master web coding and development.

"I have coded before!"

What if you've done some programming in the past? For example, you might have dipped a toe or two in the JavaScript waters already, or you might have dabbled with HTML and CSS. Will this book be too basic for you? No, not at all. My other main goal in this book is to provide you with a ton of truly *useful* examples that you can customize and incorporate into your own site. The book's first few chapters start slowly to avoid scaring off those new to this programming business. But once you get past the basics, I introduce you to lots of great techniques and tricks that will take your web coding skills to a higher level.

Icons Used in This Book

This icon points out juicy tidbits that are likely to be repeatedly useful to you — so please don't forget them.

Think of these icons as the fodder of advice columns. They offer (hopefully) wise advice or a bit more information about a topic under discussion.

Look out! In this book, you see this icon when I'm trying to help you avoid mistakes that can cost you time, money, or embarrassment.

When you see this icon, you've come across material that isn't critical to understand but will satisfy the curious. Think "inquiring minds want to know" when you see this icon.

Beyond the Book

Some extra content for this book is available on the web. Go online to find the following:

- **The examples used in the book:** You can find these here:

  ```
  mcfedries.com/webcodingfordummies
  ```

  The examples are organized by book and then by chapter within each book. For each example, you can view the code, copy it to your computer's clipboard, and run the code in the browser.

- **The WebDev Workshop:** To edit the book's examples and try your own code and see instant results, fire up the following site:

  ```
  webdev.mcfedries.com
  ```

  You won't break anything, so feel free to use the site run some experiments and play around with HTML, CSS, JavaScript, and jQuery.

1

Getting Ready to Code for the Web

Contents at a Glance

» **Understanding the front-end technologies of HTML and CSS**

» **Understanding the back-end technologies of MySQL and PHP**

» **Figuring out how JavaScript fits into all of this**

» **Learning about dynamic web pages, web apps, and mobile web apps**

Chapter 1

How Web Coding and Development Work

More than mere consumers of technology, we are makers, adapting technology to our needs and integrating it into our lives.

— DALE DOUGHERTY

The 1950s were a hobbyist's paradise with magazines such as *Mechanix Illustrated* and *Popular Science* showing the do-it-yourselfer how to build a go-kart for the kids and how to soup up a lawnmower with an actual motor! Sixty years later, we're now firmly entrenched in the age of do-it-yourself tech, where folks indulge their inner geek to engage in various forms of digital tinkering and hacking. The personification of this high-tech hobbyist renaissance is the *maker*, a modern artisan who lives to create things, rather than merely consume them. Today's makers exhibit a wide range of talents, but the skill most sought-after not only by would-be makers themselves, but by the people who hire them, is web coding and development.

Have you ever visited a website and thought, "Hey, I can do better than that!"? Have you found yourself growing tired of merely reading text and viewing images that someone else has put on the web? Is there something creative in you — stories, images, expertise, opinions — that you want to share with the world? If you answered a resounding "Yes!" to any of these questions, then congratulations: You have everything you need to get started with web coding and development. You have, in short, the makings of a maker.

The Nuts and Bolts of Web Coding and Development

If, as the King said very gravely in Lewis Carroll's *Alice in Wonderland,* it's best to "begin at the beginning," then you've come to the right place. My goal here is to get you off on the right foot by showing you what web coding and web development are.

How the web works

Before you can understand web coding and development, you need to take a step back and understand a bit about how the web itself works. In particular, you need to know what happens behind the scenes when you click a link or type a web page address into your browser. Fortunately, you don't need to be a network engineer to understand this stuff, because I can explain the basics without much in the way of jargon. Here's a high-level blow-by-blow of what happens:

1. **You tell the web browser the web page you want to visit.**

   You do that either by clicking a link to the page or by typing the location — known as the *uniform resource locator* or *URL* (usually pronounced "you-are-ell," but also sometimes "earl") — into the browser's address bar (see Figure 1-1).

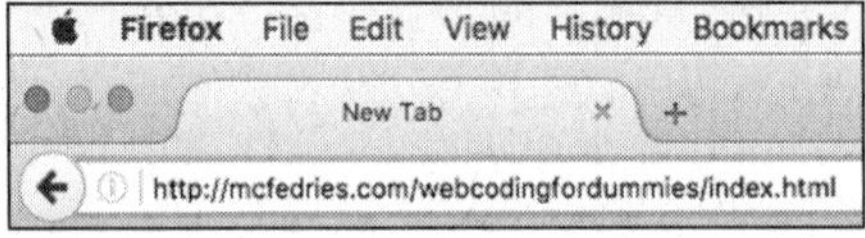

FIGURE 1-1: One way to get to a web page is to type the URL in the browser's address bar.

2. **The browser decodes the URL.**

   Decoding the URL means two things: First, it checks the prefix of the URL to see what type of resource you're requesting; this is usually `http://` or `https://`, both of which indicate that the resource is a web page. Second, it gets the

URL's domain name — the `something.com` or `whatever.org` part — and asks the *domain name system* (DNS) to translate this into a unique location — called the IP (Internet Protocol) address — for the web server that hosts the page (see Figure 1-2).

FIGURE 1-2: The browser extracts the prefix, domain, and the server address from the URL.

Decoding http://mcfedries.com/webcodingfordummies/index.html...

Results:

Prefix: `http://`
Domain name: `mcfedries.com`
Web server IP address: `162.144.120.37`

3. **The browser contacts the web server and requests the web page.**

With the web server's unique IP address in hand, the web browser sets up a communications channel with the server and then uses that channel to send along a request for the web page (see Figure 1-3).

Dear 162.144.120.37:

At your earliest convenience, please send me the mcfedries.com web page located at webcodingfordummies/index.html.

Sincerely,
W. Browser

FIGURE 1-3: The browser asks the web server for the web page.

4. **The web server decodes the page request.**

Decoding the page request involves a number of steps. First, if the web server is shared between multiple user accounts, the server begins by locating the user account that owns the requested page. The server then uses the page address to find the directory that holds the page and the file in which the page code is stored (see Figure 1-4).

FIGURE 1-4: The server uses the page request to get the account, directory, and filename.

Decoding mcfedries.com/webcodingfordummies/index.html...

Results:

User account: `paulmcfedries`
Directory: `webcodingfordummies`
Filename: `index.html`

5. **The web server sends the web page file to the web browser (see Figure 1-5).**

Dear W. Browser:

Thank you for contacting us. Here is the file you requested. Let us know if you need anything else.

Best,
mcfedries.com Web Server

FIGURE 1-5: The web server sends the requested web page file to the browser.

6. **The web browser decodes the web page file.**

   Decoding the page file means looking for text to display, instructions on how to display that text, and other resources required by the page, such as images and fonts (see Figure 1-6).

Decoding index.html…

Results:

Text: Received
Formatting: Request `styles.css`
Images: Request `logo.png`, `cover.jpg`
Audio: None
Video: None
Data: Request book examples

FIGURE 1-6: The web browser scours the page file to see if it needs anything else from the server.

7. **If the web page requires more resources, the web browser asks the server to pass along those resources (see Figure 1-7).**

Dear 162.144.120.37:

Thank you for the page file. If it's not too much trouble, could you please also send along the following:

styles.css
logo.png
cover.jpg
Book examples from the database

FIGURE 1-7: The web browser goes back to the server to ask for the other data needed to display the web page.

8. **For each of the requested resources, the web server locates the associated file and sends it to the browser (see Figure 1-8).**

> *Dear W. Browser:*
>
> *You're very welcome. We're here to serve! We're gathering your order and will send along the extra data you requested shortly.*
>
> *Best,*
> *mcfedries.com Web Server*

FIGURE 1-8: The web server sends the browser the rest of the requested files.

9. **The web browser gathers up all the text, images, and other resources and displays the page in all its digital splendor in the browser's content window (see Figure 1-9).**

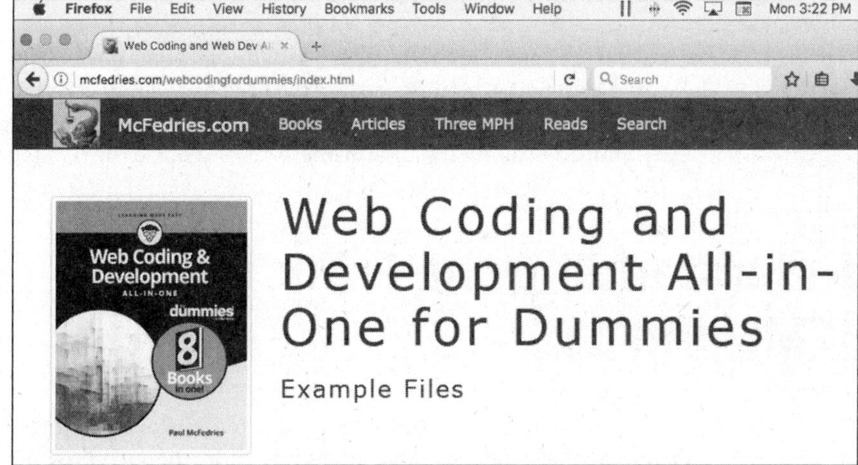

FIGURE 1-9: At long last, the web browser displays the web page.

How the web works, take two

Another way to look at this process is to think of the web as a giant mall or shopping center, where each website is a storefront in that mall. When you request a web page from a particular site, the browser takes you into that site's store and asks the clerk for the web page. The clerk goes into the back of the store, locates the page, and hands it to the browser. The browser checks the page and asks for any other needed files, which the clerk retrieves from the back. This process is repeated until the browser has everything it needs, and it then puts all the page pieces together for you, right there in the front of the store.

This metaphor might seem a bit silly, but it serves to introduce yet another metaphor, which itself illustrates one of the most important concepts in web development. In the same way that our website store has a front and a back, so, too, is web development separated into a front end and a back end:

- **Front end:** That part of the web page that the web browser displays in the browser window. That is, it's the page stuff you see and interact with.
- **Back end:** That part of the web page that resides on the web server. That is, it's the page stuff that the server gathers based on the requests it receives from the browser.

As a consumer of web pages, you only ever deal with the front end, and even then you only passively engage with the page by reading its content, looking at its images, or clicking its links or buttons.

However, as a maker of web pages — that is, as a web developer — your job entails dealing with both the front end and the back end. Moreover, that job includes coding what others see on the front end, coding how the server gathers its data on the back end, and coding the intermediate tasks that tie the two together.

Understanding the Front End: HTML and CSS

As I mention in the previous section, the *front end* of the web development process involves what users see and interact with in the web browser window. It's the job of the web developer to take a page design — which you might come up with yourself, but is more often something cooked up by a creative type who specializes in web design — and make it web-ready. Getting a design ready for the web means translating the design into the code required for the browser to display the page somewhat faithfully. (I added the hedge word "somewhat" there because it's not always easy to take a design that looks great in Photoshop or Illustrator and make it look just as good on the web. However, with the techniques you learn in this book, you'll almost always be able to come pretty close.)

You need code to create the front end of a web page because without it your page will be quite dull. For example, consider the following text:

```
COPENHAGEN—Researchers from Aalborg University announced today
   that they have finally discovered the long sought-after
   Soup-Nuts Continuum. Scientists around the world have been
```

```
   searching for this elusive item ever since Albert Einstein's
   mother-in-law proposed its existence in 1922.

"Today is an incredible day for the physics community and for
   humanity as a whole," said senior researcher Lars Grüntwerk.
   "Today, for the first time in history, we are on the verge of
   knowing everything from soup to, well, you know, nuts."
```

If you plop that text onto the web, you get the result shown in Figure 1-10. As you can see, the text is very plain, and the browser didn't even bother to include the paragraph break.

COPENHAGEN—Researchers from Aalborg University announced today that they have finally discovered the long sought-after Soup-Nuts Continuum. Scientists around the world have been searching for this elusive item ever since Albert Einstein's mother-in-law proposed its existence in 1922. "Today is an incredible day for the physics community and for humanity as a whole," said senior researcher Lars Grüntwerk. "Today, for the first time in history, we are on the verge of knowing everything from soup to, well, you know, nuts."

FIGURE 1-10: Text-only web pages are dishwater-dull.

So, if you can't just throw naked text onto the web, what's a would-be web developer to do? Ah, that's where you start earning your web scout merit badges by adding code that tells the browser how you want the text displayed. That code comes in two flavors: structure and formatting.

Adding structure: HTML

The first thing you usually do to code a web page is give it some structure. This means breaking up the text into paragraphs, adding special sections such as a header and footer, organizing text into bulleted or numbered lists, dividing the page into columns, and much more. The web coding technology that governs these and other web page structures is called (deep breath) *Hypertext Markup Language,* or *HTML,* for short.

HTML consists of a few dozen special symbols called *tags* that you sprinkle strategically throughout the page. For example, if you want to tell the web browser that a particular chunk of text is a separate paragraph, you place the `<p>` tag (the `p` here is short for paragraph) before the text and the `</p>` tag after the text.

In the code that follows, I've added these paragraph tags to the plain text that I show earlier. As you can see in Figure 1-11, the web browser displays the text as two separate paragraphs, no questions asked.

```
<p>
COPENHAGEN—Researchers from Aalborg University announced today
   that they have finally discovered the long sought-after
```

```
  Soup-Nuts Continuum. Scientists around the world have been
  searching for this elusive item ever since Albert Einstein's
  mother-in-law proposed its existence in 1922.
</p>
<p>
"Today is an incredible day for the physics community and for
  humanity as a whole," said senior researcher Lars Grüntwerk.
  "Today, for the first time in history, we are on the verge of
  knowing everything from soup to, well, you know, nuts."
</p>
```

COPENHAGEN—Researchers from Aalborg University announced today that they have finally discovered the long sought-after Soup-Nuts Continuum. Scientists around the world have been searching for this elusive item ever since Albert Einstein's mother-in-law proposed its existence in 1922.

"Today is an incredible day for the physics community and for humanity as a whole," said senior researcher Lars Grüntwerk. "Today, for the first time in history, we are on the verge of knowing everything from soup to, well, you know, nuts."

FIGURE 1-11: Adding paragraph tags to the text separates the text into two paragraphs.

REMEMBER

HTML is one of the fundamental topics of web development, and you learn all about it in Book 2, Chapter 1.

Adding style: CSS

HTML takes care of the structure of the page, but if you want to change the formatting of the page, then you need to turn to a second front-end technology: *cascading style sheets*, known almost universally as just *CSS*. With CSS in hand, you can play around with the page colors and fonts, you can add margins and borders around things, and you can mess with the position and dimensions of page elements.

CSS consists of a large number of *properties* that enable you to customize many aspects of the page to make it look the way you want. For example, the `width` property lets you specify how wide a page element should be; the `font-family` property enables you to specify a typeface for an element; and the `font-size` property lets you dictate the type size of an element. Here's some CSS code that applies all three of these properties to every `p` element (that is, every `<p>` tag) that appears in a page (note that `px` is short for pixels):

```
p {
    width: 700px;
    font-family: sans-serif;
    font-size: 24px;
}
```

When used with the sample text from the previous two sections, you get the much nicer-looking text shown in Figure 1-12.

COPENHAGEN—Researchers from Aalborg University announced today that they have finally discovered the long sought-after Soup-Nuts Continuum. Scientists around the world have been searching for this elusive item ever since Albert Einstein's mother-in-law proposed its existence in 1922.

"Today is an incredible day for the physics community and for humanity as a whole," said senior researcher Lars Grüntwerk. "Today, for the first time in history, we are on the verge of knowing everything from soup to, well, you know, nuts."

FIGURE 1-12: With the judicious use of a few CSS properties, you can greatly improve the look of a page.

REMEMBER

CSS is a cornerstone of web development. You learn much more about it in Book 2, Chapters 2, 3, and 4.

Understanding the Back End: PHP and MySQL

Many web pages are all about the front end. That is, they consist of nothing but text that has been structured by HTML tags and styled by CSS properties, plus a few extra files such as images and fonts. Sure, all these files are transferred from the web server to the browser, but that's the extent of the back end's involvement.

These simple pages are ideal when you have content that doesn't change very often, if ever. With these so-called *static* pages, you plop in your text, add some HTML and CSS, perhaps point to an image or two, and you're done.

But there's another class of page that has content that changes frequently. It could be posts added once or twice a day, or sports or weather updates added once or twice an hour. With these so-called *dynamic* pages, you might have some text, HTML, CSS, and other content that's static, but you almost certainly don't want to be updating the changing content by hand.

Rather than making constant manual changes to such pages, you can convince the back end to do it for you. You do that by taking advantage of two popular back-end technologies: MySQL and PHP.

Storing data on the server: MySQL

MySQL is a relational database management system that runs on the server. You use it to store the data you want to use as the source for some (or perhaps even all) of the data you want to display on your web page. Using a tool called Structured Query Language (SQL, pronounced "ess-kew-ell," or sometimes "sequel"), you can specify which subset of your data you want to use.

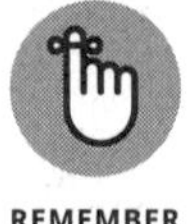
REMEMBER

If phrases such as "relational database management system" and "Structured Query Language" have you furrowing your brow, don't sweat it: I explain all in Book 5, Chapter 2.

Accessing data on the server: PHP

PHP is a programming language used on the server. It's a very powerful and full-featured language, but for the purposes of this book, you use PHP mostly to interact with MySQL databases. You can use PHP to extract from MySQL the subset of data you want to display, manipulate that data into a form that's readable by the front end, and then send the data to the browser.

REMEMBER

You learn about the PHP language in Book 5, Chapter 1, and you learn how to use PHP to access MySQL data in Book 5, Chapter 3.

How It All Fits Together: JavaScript and jQuery

Okay, so now you have a front end consisting of HTML structure and CSS styling, and a back end consisting of MySQL data and PHP code. How do these two seemingly disparate worlds meet to create a full web page experience?

In the website-as-store metaphor that I introduce earlier in this chapter, I use the image of a store clerk taking an order from the web browser and then going into the back of the store to fulfill that order. That clerk is the obvious link between the front end and the back end, so what technology does that clerk represent? She actually represents two technologies that I use in this book: JavaScript and jQuery.

Front end, meet back end: JavaScript

The secret sauce that brings the front end and the back end together to create the vast majority of the web pages you see today, is JavaScript. JavaScript is a programming language and is the default language used for coding websites today. JavaScript is, first and foremost, a front-end web development language. That is, JavaScript runs inside the web browser and it has access to everything on the page: the text, the images, the HTML tags, the CSS properties, and more. Having access to all the page stuff means that you can use code to manipulate, modify, even add and delete web page elements.

But although JavaScript runs in the browser, it's also capable of reaching out to the server to access back-end stuff. For example, with JavaScript you can send data to the server to store that data in a MySQL database. Similarly, with JavaScript you can request data from the server and then use code to display that data on the web page.

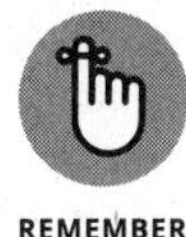

REMEMBER

JavaScript is very powerful, very useful, and very cool, so Book 3 takes nine full chapters to help you learn it well. Also, you learn how JavaScript acts as a bridge between the front end and the back end in Book 6, Chapter 1.

Making your web coding life easier: jQuery

JavaScript is extremely powerful, but sometimes using certain JavaScript statements and structures can be a bit unwieldly. For example, here's a bit of JavaScript code:

```
var subheads = document.getElementsByClassName('subheadings');
```

This will no doubt look like gibberish to you now, but my purpose here is only to have you remark the length of that statement. Now compare the following:

```
var subheads = $('.subheadings');
```

Believe it or not, these statements do exactly the same thing, except the second one is written using a JavaScript package called jQuery. jQuery is a collection — called a *library* — of JavaScript code that makes it easier and faster to code for the web. Not only does jQuery give you shorter ways to reference web page elements, but it also incorporates routines that make it easier for you to manipulate HTML tags and CSS properties, navigate and manipulate web page elements, add animation effects, and much more.

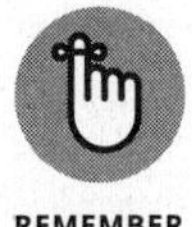

REMEMBER

jQuery is extremely powerful and useful stuff, and you'll be thankful you've got it in your web development toolkit. You learn just enough jQuery to be dangerous in Book 4.

How Dynamic Web Pages Work

It's one thing to know about HTML and CSS and PHP and all the rest, but it's quite another to actually do something useful with these technologies. That, really, is the goal of this book, and to that end the book spends several chapters later covering how to create wonderful things called *dynamic web pages*. A dynamic web page is one that includes content that, rather than being hard-wired into the page, is generated on-the-fly from the web server. This means the page content can change based on a request by the user, by data being added to or modified on the server, or in response to some event, such as the clicking of a button or link.

It likely sounds a bit like voodoo to you now, so perhaps a bit more detail is in order. For example, suppose you want to use a web page to display some data that resides on the server. Here's a general look at the steps involved in that process:

1. **JavaScript determines the data that it needs from the server.**

   JavaScript has various ways it can do this, such as extracting the information from the URL, reading an item the user has selected from a list, or responding to a click from the user.

2. **JavaScript sends a request for that data to the server.**

   In most cases, and certainly in every case you see in this book, JavaScript sends this request by calling a PHP script on the server.

3. **The PHP script receives the request and passes it along to MySQL.**

   The PHP script uses the information obtained from JavaScript to create an SQL command that MySQL can understand.

4. **MySQL uses the SQL command to extract the required information from the database and then return that data to the PHP script.**

5. **The PHP script manipulates the returned MySQL data into a form that JavaScript can use.**

   JavaScript can't read raw MySQL data, so one of PHP's most important tasks is to convert that data into a format called JavaScript Object Notation (JSON, for short, and pronounced like the name Jason) that JavaScript is on friendly terms with (see Book 6, Chapter 1 for more about this process).

6. **PHP sends the JSON data back to JavaScript.**

7. **JavaScript displays the data on the web page.**

   One of the joys of JavaScript is that you get tremendous control over how you display the data to the user. Through existing HTML and CSS, and by manipulating these and other web page elements using JavaScript, you can show your data in the best possible light.

REMEMBER

To expand on these steps and learn how to create your own dynamic web pages, check out the three chapters in Book 6.

What Is a Web App?

You no doubt have a bunch of apps residing on your smartphone. If you use Windows 10 on your PC, then you have not only the pre-installed apps such as Mail and Calendar, but you might also have one or more apps downloaded from the Windows Store. If the Mac is more your style, then you're probably quite familiar with apps such as Music and Messages, and you might have installed a few others from the App Store. We live, in other words, in a world full of apps which, in the context of your phone or computer, are software programs dedicated to a single topic or task.

So what then is a *web app?* It's actually something very similar to an app on a device or PC. That is, it's a website, built using web technologies such as HTML, CSS, and JavaScript, that has two main characteristics:

- The web app is focused on a single topic or task.
- The web app offers some sort of interface that enables the user to operate the app in one or more ways.

In short, a web app is a website that looks and acts like an app on a device or computer. This is opposed to a regular website, which usually tackles several topics or tasks and has an interface that for the most part only enables users to navigate the site.

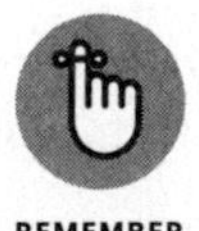

REMEMBER

To get the scoop on building your very own web apps, head on over to the four chapters in Book 7.

What Is a Mobile Web App?

In late 2016, the world reached a milestone of sorts when the percentage of people accessing the web via mobile devices such as smartphones and tablets surpassed the percentage of people doing the web thing using desktops and notebooks. The gap between mobile web users and everyone else has only widened since then, so it's safe to say that we live in a mobile web world now.

What does that mean for you as a web developer? It means you can't afford to ignore mobile users when you build your web pages. It means you can't code your web pages using a gigantic desktop monitor and assume that everything will look great on a relatively tiny smartphone screen. It means that you'd do well to embrace the mobile web in a big old bear hug by creating not just web apps, but *mobile web apps*. What's the difference? A mobile web app is the same as a web app — that is, it has content and an interface dedicated to a single topic or task — but with a design built from the ground up to look good and work well in a mobile device. This is known as the *mobile-first* approach to web development, and it's one of the hottest topics in the web coding world.

REMEMBER

To learn how to create your own mobile web apps, look no farther than the two chapters in Book 8.

What's the Difference between Web Coding and Web Development?

After all this talk of HTML, CSS, MySQL, JavaScript, and jQuery, after the bird's-eye view of dynamic sites, web apps, and mobile web apps, you might be wondering when the heck I'm going to answer the most pressing question of the all: What in the name of Sir Tim Berners-Lee (inventor of the web) is the difference between web coding and web development?

I'm glad you asked! Some people would probably answer that question by saying that there's no real difference at all, because "web coding" and "web development" are two ways of referring to the same thing: Creating web pages using programming tools.

Hey, it's a free country, but to my mind I think there's a useful distinction to be made between web coding and web development:

- *Web coding* is the pure programming part of creating a web page, particularly using JavaScript/jQuery on the front end and PHP on the back end.
- *Web development* is the complete web page creation package, from building a page with HTML tags, to formatting the page with CSS, to storing data on the back end with MySQL, to accessing that data with PHP, to bridging the front and back ends using JavaScript and jQuery.

However you look at it, this book teaches you everything you need to know to become both a web coder and a web developer.

» Gathering the tools you need for a local development setup

» Installing a local web development environment on a Windows PC

» Installing a local web development environment on a Mac

» Learning what to look for in a good text editor

Chapter 2
Setting Up Your Web Development Home

He is happiest, be he king or peasant, who finds peace in his home.

— JOHANN WOLFGANG VON GOETHE

One of the truly amazing things about web development is that, with the exception of the databases on the server, all you ever work with are basic text files. But surely all the structure you add with HTML tags requires some obscure and complex file type? No way, José: It's text all the way down. What about all that formatting stuff associated with CSS? Nope: nothing but text. PHP? Text. JavaScript and jQuery? Text and, again, text.

What this text-only landscape means is that you don't need any highfalutin, high-priced software to develop for the web. A humble text editor is all you require to dip a toe or two in the web coding waters.

But what if you want to get more than your feet wet in web coding? What if you want to dive in, swim around, perhaps do a little snorkeling? Ah, then you need to take things up a notch or three and set up a proper web development environment on your computer. This will give you everything you need to build, test, and refine your web development projects. In this chapter, you get your web coding adventure off to a rousing start by exploring how to set up a complete web development environment on your Windows PC or Mac.

What Is a Local Web Development Environment?

In programming circles, an *integrated development environment* (IDE) is a collection of software programs that make it easy and efficient to write code. Most development environments are tailored to a particular programming language and come with tools for editing, testing, and compiling code (that is, converting the code to its final form as an application).

In the web coding game, we don't have IDEs, per se, but we do have a similar beast called a *local web development environment*, which is also a collection of software. It usually includes the following:

- A web server
- A relational database management system (RDBMS) to run on the web server
- A server-side programming language
- An interface for controlling (starting, stopping, and so on) the web server
- An interface for accessing and manipulating the RDBMS

The key point to grok here is that this is a "local" web development environment, which means that it gets installed on your PC or Mac. This enables you to build and test your web development projects right on your computer. You don't need a web hosting service or even an Internet connection, for that matter. Everything runs conveniently on your computer, so you can concentrate on coding and leave the deployment of the site until you're ready.

Do You Need a Local Web Development Environment?

Okay, if it's possible to use a simple text editor to develop web pages, why not do just that? After all, every Windows PC and Mac in existence comes with a pre-installed text editor, and there are lots of free third-party text editors ripe for downloading, so why bother installing the software for a local web development environment?

To be perfectly honest, I'm not going to stand here and tell you that a local web development setup is a must. Certainly if all you're doing for now is getting started with a few static web pages built using HTML, CSS, and JavaScript, then you don't yet need access to the back end. Similarly, if you're building websites and web apps for your own use and you already have a web host that gives you access to MySQL and PHP, then you can definitely get away with using just your trusty text editor.

However, there are two major exceptions that pretty much require you to build your web stuff locally:

- If you're building a website or app for someone else and you don't have access to their web server.
- If you're building a new version of an existing website or app, which means that you don't want to mess with the production code while tinkering (and therefore making mistakes) with the new code.

That said, there's also something undeniably cool about having a big-time web server purring away in the background of your computer. So, even if you don't think you'll need a full-blown web development environment in the short term, think about installing one anyway, if only so you can say you're "running Apache 2.4 locally" at your next cocktail party.

Setting Up the XAMPP for Windows Development Environment

If you're running Windows, then I highly recommend the web development environment XAMPP for Windows, which in its most recent version (at least as I write this in early 2018) requires Windows Vista or later. XAMPP for Windows is loaded with dozens of features, but for our needs the following are the most important:

- **Apache:** This is an open-source web server that runs about half of all the websites on Earth.
- **MariaDB:** This is an open-source server database that is fully compatible with MySQL (discussed in Book 1, Chapter 1).

» **PHP:** This is the server-side programming language that I talk about briefly in Book 1, Chapter 1.

» **phpMyAdmin:** This is an interface that enables you to access and manipulate MariaDB databases.

So all of this requires big bucks, right? Nope. XAMPP for Windows is completely free.

To get started, head for the Apache Friends website at `www.apachefriends.org`, and then download XAMPP for Windows. Be sure to get the most recent version.

Installing XAMPP for Windows

Once the download is complete, follow these steps to install XAMPP for Windows:

1. **Open the installation file that you downloaded.**

   The download is an executable file, so you can double-click it to get the installation off the ground.

2. **Enter your User Account Control (UAC) credentials to allow the install.**

   If you're the administrator of your PC, click Yes. Otherwise, you need to enter the username and password of the PC's administrator account.

3. **When XAMPP displays a warning about installing with UAC activated, click OK.**

   This oddly worded warning means that if you install XAMPP in the default folder (usually `C:\Program Files`), then it might have problems running normally because UAC imposes restrictions on that folder. You can ignore this because later (see Step 6) I show you how to install XAMPP in a different folder that doesn't suffer from this problem.

4. **When the XAMPP Setup Wizard appears, click Next.**

5. **In the Select Components dialog box (see Figure 2-1), deselect the check box beside any component you don't want installed, and then click Next.**

   For a basic install, you only need Apache, MySQL, PHP, and phpMyAdmin. If your PC is running low on disk space, consider not installing the other components. If you're rich in disk space, go ahead and install everything because, hey, after all of this you might be inspired to learn Perl (which is another server-side programming language).

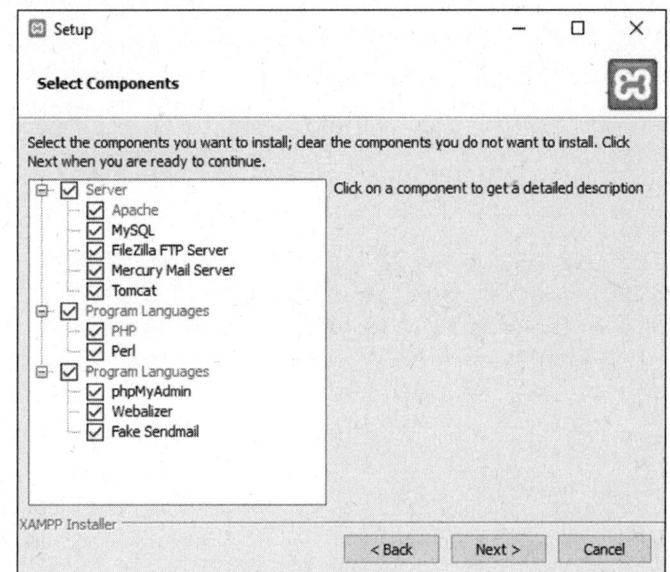

FIGURE 2-1: Use this Setup Wizard dialog box to deselect the check box beside any component you don't want installed.

6. **In the Installation Folder dialog box, type the location where you want XAMPP installed, then click Next.**

   Be sure to avoid the folders `C:\Program Files` and `C:\Program Files (x86)`, for the reason I described back in Step 3. Most folks create a `xampp` folder in C:\ and install everything there (see Figure 2-2).

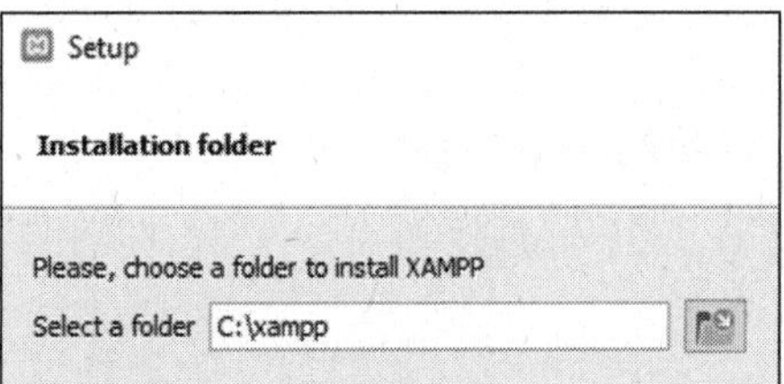

FIGURE 2-2: To install XAMPP, use a subfolder in the main C:\ folder (such as `C:\xampp`).

7. **The Setup Wizard lets you know that Bitnami for XAMPP can install content management systems such as WordPress and Drupal. Click OK.**

   If you don't care about any of this, be sure to deselect the Learn More About Bitnami for XAMPP check box before you click OK.

8. **Click Next to begin the installation.**
9. **If you see a Windows Security Alert similar to the one shown in Figure 2-3, select the Private Networks check box, deselect the Public Networks check box, and then click Allow Access.**

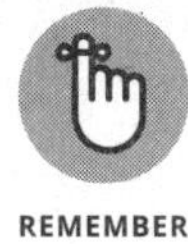
REMEMBER

However, just because you select the Private Networks check box, it doesn't mean that people on your network can access (much less mess with) your local web server. XAMPP for Windows is configured out of the box to be accessible only from the computer on which it's installed.

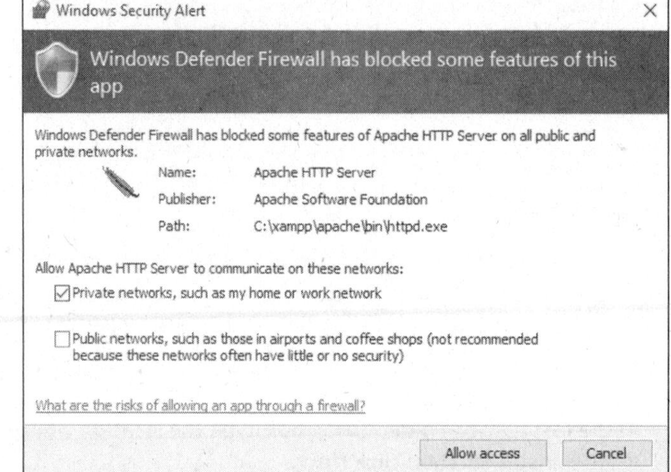

FIGURE 2-3: If the Windows Security Alert dialog box shows up, be sure to allow Apache to communicate on your private network, but not on any public networks.

10. **When the install is complete, click Finish.**

    Be sure to deselect the Do You Want to Start the Control Panel Now check box. I talk about the correct way to start the Control Panel in the next section.

Running the XAMPP for Windows Control Panel

The XAMPP Control Panel enables you to start, stop, and configure the XAMPP apps, particularly the Apache web server and the MySQL database system. For best results, you should start the program with administrator privileges, which you can do by following these steps:

1. **Click Start.**
2. **Find and open the XAMPP folder in the All Apps list.**

   Depending on your version of Windows, you might have to click All Apps to get to the All Apps list.
3. **Right-click XAMPP Control Panel, click More, and then click Run as Administrator.**

Depending on your version of Windows, you might not have to click More to get to the Run as Administrator command.

4. **If you're the administrator of your PC, click Yes. Otherwise, you need to enter the username and password of the PC's administrator account.**
5. **The first time you run the Control Panel, you're asked to choose a language. Select the radio button for the language you prefer, then click Save.**

The XAMPP Control Panel appears, as shown in Figure 2-4.

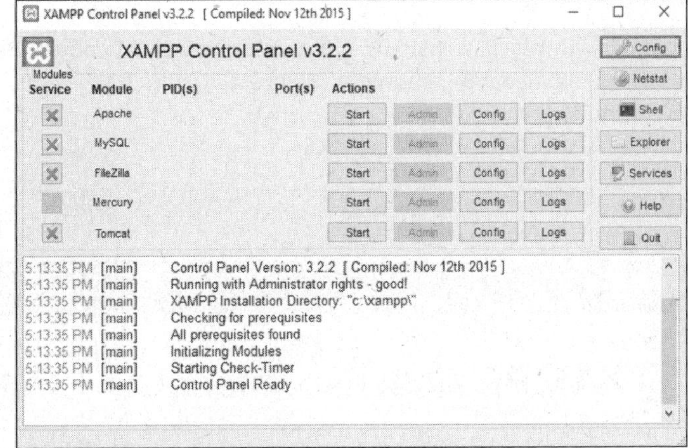

FIGURE 2-4: You use the XAMPP Control Panel to control and configure apps such as Apache and MySQL.

To start an app, click the corresponding Start button. That button name changes to Stop, meaning you can later stop the service by clicking its Stop button.

TIP

You'll always want the Apache and MySQL apps running, so you can save a bit of time by having the XAMPP Control Panel launch these two apps automatically when you open the program. Click Config, select the Apache and MySQL check boxes, and then click Save.

REMEMBER

If when you start an app you see a Windows Security Alert dialog box similar to the one shown earlier in Figure 2-3. Select the Private Networks check box, deselect the Public Networks check box, and then click Allow Access.

Accessing your local web server

With XAMPP for Windows installed and Apache up and running, congratulations are in order: You've got a web server running on your PC! That's great, but how do you access your shiny, new web server? There are two ways, depending on what you're doing:

» **Adding files and folders to the web server:** Place the files and folders in the `htdocs` subfolder of your main XAMPP install folder. For example, if you installed XAMPP to `C:\xampp`, then your web server's root folder will be `C:\xampp\htdocs`.

» **Viewing the files and folders on the server:** Open your favorite web browser and navigate to the `localhost` address (or to `127.0.0.1`, which gets you to the same place). If you have the XAMPP Control Panel open, you can also click the Apache app's Admin button.

By default, your local website is configured to automatically redirect `localhost` to `localhost/dashboard/`, shown in Figure 2-5, which gives you access to several XAMPP tools.

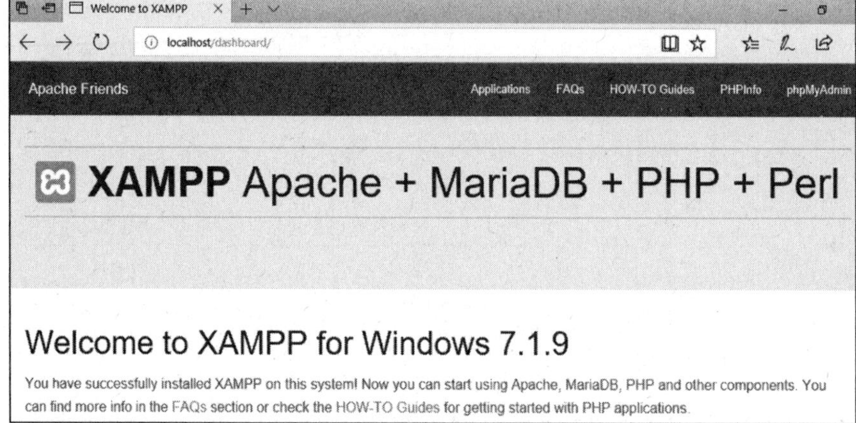

FIGURE 2-5: The `localhost/dashboard/` address gives you access to a few XAMPP tools.

In the page header, you can use the following links:

» **Apache Friends:** Returns you to the main Dashboard page.

» **Applications:** Provides information about installing Bitnami applications on the server.

» **FAQs:** Displays a list of XAMPP frequently asked questions.

» **How-To Guides:** Displays a list of links to step-by-step guides for a number of XAMPP for Windows tasks.

» **PHPInfo:** Displays a for-geeks-only page of information about the version of PHP that you have installed.

- **phpMyAdmin:** Opens the phpMyAdmin tool, which lets you create and manipulate MariaDB/MySQL databases. You can also open phpMyAdmin by navigating directly to `localhost/phpmyadmin/`, or in the XAMPP Control Panel, by clicking the MySQL app's Admin button. However you get there, just be sure to have the MySQL app running before you open phpMyAdmin.

Setting Up the XAMPP for OS X Development Environment

If you'll be doing your web work on a Mac, then I recommend the web development environment XAMPP for OS X, which in its most recent version (at least as I write this in early 2018) requires OS X Snow Leopard (10.6) or later. XAMPP for OS X is packed with programs and features, but you'll probably only concern yourself with the following:

- **Apache:** This is an open-source web server that runs about half of all the websites on Earth.
- **MariaDB:** This is an open-source server database that is fully compatible with MySQL (discussed in Book 1, Chapter 1).
- **PHP:** This is the server-side programming language that I mention in Book 1, Chapter 1.
- **phpMyAdmin:** This is an interface that enables you to access and work with MariaDB databases.

The best news of all is XAMPP for OS X is completely, utterly, and forever free. Nice! To get the show on the road, surf to the Apache Friends website at `www.apachefriends.org`, and then download the most recent version of XAMPP for OS X.

Installing XAMPP for OS X

Once the download is done, follow these steps to install XAMPP for OS X:

1. **Double-click the installation file that you downloaded.**
2. **Double-click the XAMPP icon.**
3. **If macOS warns you about opening an application downloaded from the Internet, say "It's cool, bro" and click Open.**
4. **Enter your macOS administrator password and then click OK.**

5. **When the XAMPP Setup Wizard appears, click Next.**
6. **In the Select Components dialog, deselect the XAMPP Developer Files check box, as shown in Figure 2-6, and then click Next.**

   The developer files might sound like they're right up your alley, but they're actually for people who want to add to or modify the code for XAMPP itself.

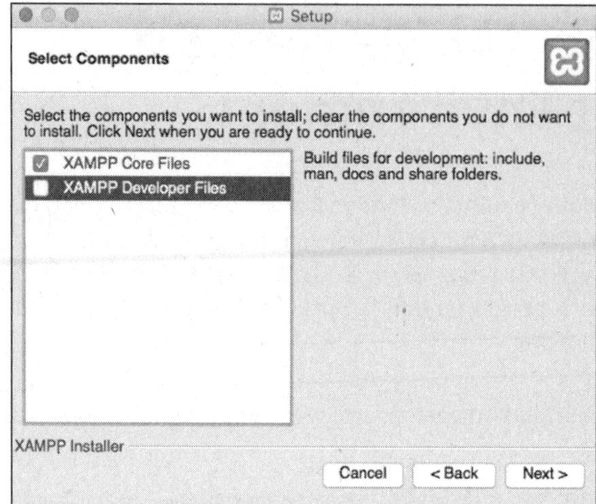

FIGURE 2-6: Use this Setup Wizard dialog to deselect the check box beside XAMPP Developer Files.

7. **In the Installation Directory dialog, click Next.**
8. **The Setup Wizard lets you know that Bitnami for XAMPP can install content management systems such as WordPress and Drupal. Click Next.**

   If you don't care about any of this, be sure to deselect the Learn More About Bitnami for XAMPP check box before you click Next.
9. **Click Next to launch the installation.**
10. **When the install is complete, click Finish.**

    If you want to head right into the XAMPP Manager, leave the Launch XAMPP check box selected.

REMEMBER

What about the security of your local web server? Fortunately, that's not an issue because people on your network can't access your web server. XAMPP is configured by default to be accessible only from the Mac on which it's installed.

Running the XAMPP Application Manager

The XAMPP Application Manager enables you to start, stop, and configure the XAMPP servers, particularly the Apache web server and the MySQL database system. To launch the XAMPP Application Manager, you have two choices:

- If you still have the final Setup Wizard dialog onscreen, leave the Launch XAMPP check box selected and click Finish.
- In Finder, open the Applications folder, open the XAMPP folder, and then double-click Manager-OSX.

The XAMPP Application Manager appears. To work with the XAMPP servers, click the Manage Servers tab, shown in Figure 2-7.

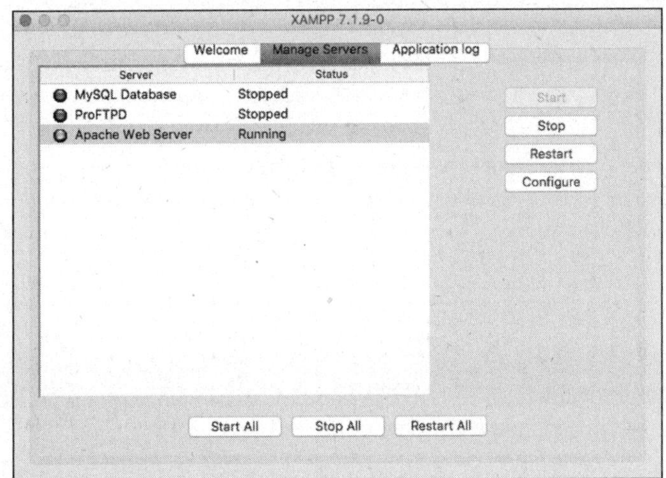

FIGURE 2-7: You use the XAMPP Control Panel to control and configure services such as Apache and MySQL.

In the Manage Servers tab, you can perform the following actions:

- **Start a server.** Click the server and then click Start.
- **Start all the servers.** Click Start All.
- **Restart a server.** Click the server and then click Restart.
- **Restart all the servers.** Click Restart All.
- **Stop a server.** Click the server and then click Stop.
- **Stop all the servers.** Click Stop All.

Accessing your local web server

With XAMPP for OS X installed and Apache up and running, it's time for high-fives all around because you've got a web server running on your Mac! That's awesome, but how do you access your web server? There are two ways, depending on what you're doing:

- **Adding files and folders to the web server:** Place the files and folders in the `htdocs` subfolder of your main XAMPP install folder. To get there, open Applications, then XAMPP, then double-click htdocs. If you have the XAMPP Application Manager open, click the Welcome tab, click Open Application Folder, then open htdocs.
- **Viewing the files and folders on the server:** Open your favorite web browser and navigate to the `localhost` address (or to `127.0.0.1`, which gets you to the same place). If you have the XAMPP Application Manager running, click the Welcome tab and then click Go To Application.

By default, your local website is configured to automatically redirect `localhost` to `localhost/dashboard/`, shown in Figure 2-8, which gives you access to several XAMPP tools.

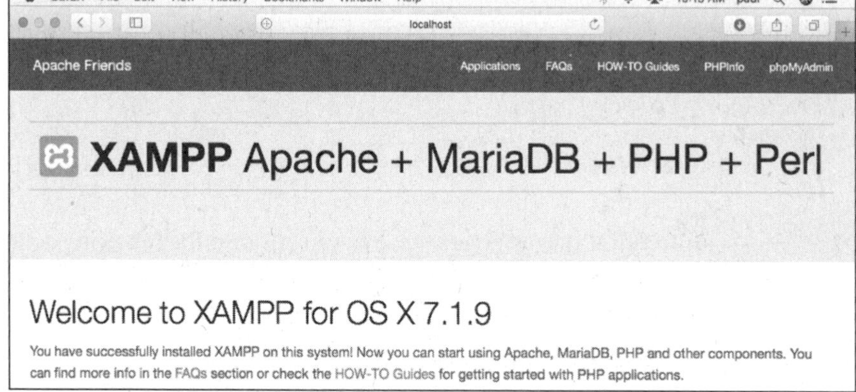

FIGURE 2-8: The `localhost/dashboard/` address gives you access to a few XAMPP for OS X features.

In the page header, you can use the following links:

- **Apache Friends:** Returns you to the main Dashboard page.
- **Applications:** Provides information about installing Bitnami applications on the server.
- **FAQs:** Displays a list of XAMPP frequently asked questions.
- **How-To Guides:** Displays a list of links to step-by-step guides for a number of XAMPP for OS X tasks.

- **PHPInfo:** Displays a for-geeks-only page of information about the version of PHP that you have installed.
- **phpMyAdmin:** Opens the phpMyAdmin tool, which lets you create and manipulate MariaDB/MySQL databases. You can also open phpMyAdmin by navigating directly to `localhost/phpmyadmin/`. Either way, make sure you have the MySQL Database server running before you open phpMyAdmin.

Choosing Your Text Editor

I mention at the beginning of this chapter that all you need to develop web pages is a text editor. However, saying that all you need to code is a text editor is like saying that all you need to live is food: It's certainly true, but more than a little short on specifics. After all, to a large extent the quality of your life depends on the food you eat. If you survive on nothing but bread and water, well "surviving" is all you're doing. What you really need is a balanced diet that supplies all the nutrients your body needs. And pie.

The bread-and-water version of a text editor is the barebones program that came with your computer: Notepad if you run Windows, or TextEdit if you have a Mac. You can survive as a web developer using these programs, but that's not living, if you ask me. You need the editing equivalent of vitamins and minerals (and, yes, pie) if you want to flourish as a web coder. These nutrients are the features and tools that are crucial to being an efficient and organized developer:

- **Syntax highlighting:** *Syntax* refers to the arrangement of characters and symbols that create correct programming code, and *syntax highlighting* is an editing feature that color-codes certain syntax elements for easier reading. For example, while regular text might appear black, all the HTML tags might be shown in blue and the CSS properties might appear red. The best text editors let you choose the syntax colors, either by offering prefab themes, or by letting you apply custom colors.
- **Line numbers:** It might seem like a small thing, but having a text editor that numbers each line, as shown in Figure 2-9, can be a major timesaver. When the web browser alerts you to an error in your code (see Book 3, Chapter 9), it gives you an error message and, crucially, the line number of the error. This enables you to quickly locate the culprit and (fingers crossed) fix the problem pronto.
- **Code previews:** A good text editor will let you see a preview of how your code will look in a web browser. The preview might appear in the same window as your code, or in a separate window, and it should update automatically as you modify and save your code.

```
<!DOCTYPE html>
<html lang="en">
    <head>
        <meta charset="utf-8">
        <title>Web Coding and Web Dev AIO for Dummies</title>
        <meta name="author" content="Paul McFedries">
        <meta name="viewport" content="width=device-width, initial-scale=1.0">
        <link rel="stylesheet" href="/css/styles.css">
        <script src="/js/jquery-1.11.1.min.js"></script>
        <script src="/js/clipboard.min.js"></script>
        <script src="/js/my-js.js"></script>
        <script>
            $(document).ready(function () {
                // Load the nav bar
                $("#navbar-code").load("/includes/navbar-code.txt");

                // Load the footer
                $("#footer-code").load("/php/write-footer.php");

                // Get the example files
                $.getJSON('get-examples.php', function(data) {
                    var str = '';
                    var strCode = '';
                    var strExample = '';
                    var currBook = data[0].Book;
                    var currChapter = data[0].Chapter;

                    // Write the initial item
                    str += '<div class="wcd-book" id="book' + currBook + '">';
                    str += '    Book ' + data[0].Book + ': ' + data[0].BookTitle;
                    str += '    <div class="wcd-chapters" id="book' + currBook + '-chapters">';
                    str += '        <div class="wcd-chapter" id="book' + currBook + '-chapter' + currChapter + '">';
                    str += '            Chapter ' + data[0].Chapter + ': ' + data[0].ChapterTitle;
```

FIGURE 2-9: Line numbers, as seen here down the left side of the window, are a crucial text editor feature.

- **Code completion:** This is a handy feature that, when you start typing something, displays a list of possible code items that complete your typing. You can then select the one you want and press Tab or Enter to add it to your code without having to type the whole thing.
- **Text processing:** The best text editors offer a selection of text processing features, such as automatic indentation of code blocks, converting tabs to spaces and vice versa, shifting chunks of code right or left, removing unneeded spaces at the end of lines, hiding blocks of code, and more.

The good news is that there's no shortage of text editors that support all these features and many more. That's also the bad news, because it means you have a huge range of programs to choose from. To help you get started, here, in alphabetical order, are a few editors to take for test drives:

- **Atom:** Available for Windows and Mac. Free! `http://atom.io`
- **Brackets:** Available for Windows and Mac. Also free! `http://brackets.io/`
- **Coda:** Available for Mac only. $99, but a free trial is available. `www.panic.com/coda`
- **Notepad++:** Available for Windows only. Another freebie. `https://notepad-plus-plus.org/`
- **Sublime Text:** Available for both Windows and Mac. $80, but a free trial is available. `www.sublimetext.com`
- **TextMate:** Available for Mac only. $60, but a free trial is available. `http://macromates.com/`

» Examining the various choices for hosting your site

» Choosing the host that's right for you

» Looking around your new web home

» Getting your site files to your web host

Chapter 3

Finding and Setting Up a Web Host

You will end up with better software by releasing as early as practically possible, and then spending the rest of your time iterating rapidly based on real-world feedback. So trust me on this one: Even if version 1 sucks, ship it anyway.

— JEFF ATTWOOD

You build your web pages from the comfort of your Mac or PC, and if you've chosen your text editor well (as I describe in Book 1, Chapter 2), then you can even use your computer to preview how your web pages will look in a browser.

That's fine and dandy, but I think you'll agree that the whole point of building a web page is to, you know, put it on the web! First, you need to subject your code to the wilds of the wider web to make sure it works out there. Even if it seems to be running like a champ on your local server, you can't give it the seal of approval until you've proven that it runs champlike on a remote server. Second, once your code is ready, then the only way the public can appreciate your handiwork is to get it out where they can see it.

Whether you're testing or shipping your code, you need somewhere to put it, and that's what this chapter is about. Here you explore the wide and sometimes wacky world of web hosts. You delve into what they offer, investigate ways to choose a good one, and then take a tour of your web home away from home.

Understanding Web Hosting Providers

A common question posed by web development newcomers is "Where the heck do I put my web page when it's done?" If you've asked that question, you're doing okay because it means you're clued in to something crucial: Just because you've created a web page and you have an Internet connection doesn't mean your site is automatically a part of the web.

After all, people on the web have no way of getting to your computer. Even if you're working with a local web development environment (which I discuss in Book 1, Chapter 2), you're working in splendid isolation because no one either on your network or on the Internet can access that environment.

In other words, your computer isn't set up to hand out documents (such as web pages) to remote visitors who ask for them. Computers that can do this are called *servers* (because they "serve" stuff out to the web), and computers that specialize in distributing web pages are called *web servers.* So your web page isn't on the web until you store it on a remote web server. Because this computer is, in effect, playing "host" to your pages, such machines are also called *web hosts.* Companies that run these web hosts are called *web hosting providers.*

Now, just how do you go about finding a web host? Well, the answer to that depends on a bunch of factors, including the type of site you have, how you get connected to the Internet in the first place, and how much money (if any) you're willing to fork out for the privilege. In the end, you have three choices:

- Your existing Internet provider
- A free hosting provider
- A commercial hosting provider

Using your existing Internet provider

If you access the Internet via a corporate or educational network, your institution might have its own web server you can use. If you get online via an Internet service provider (ISP), phone or email its customer service department to ask whether the company has a web server available. Almost all ISPs provide space so their customers can put up personal pages free of charge.

Finding a free hosting provider

If cash is in short supply, a few hosting providers will bring your website in from the cold out of the goodness of their hearts. In some cases, these services are open only to specific groups such as students, artists, nonprofit organizations, and so on. However, plenty of providers put up personal sites free of charge.

What's the catch? Well, there are almost always restrictions both on how much data you can store and on the type of data you can store (no ads, no dirty pictures, and so on). You might also be required to display some kind of "banner" advertisement for the hosting provider on your pages.

Signing up with a commercial hosting provider

For personal and business-related websites, many web artisans end up renting a chunk of a web server from a commercial hosting provider. You normally hand over a setup fee to get your account going and then you're looking at a monthly fee.

Why shell out all that dough when there are so many free sites lying around? Because, as with most things in life, you get what you pay for. By paying for your host, you generally get more features, better service, and fewer annoyances (such as the ads that some free sites have to display).

A Buyer's Guide to Web Hosting

Unfortunately, choosing a web host isn't as straightforward as you might like it to be. For one thing, hundreds of hosts are out there clamoring for your business; for another, the pitches and come-ons your average web host employs are strewn with jargon and technical terms. I can't help reduce the number of web hosts, but I can help you understand what those hosts are yammering on about. Here's a list of the terms you're most likely to come across when researching web hosts:

- **Storage space:** Refers to the amount of room allotted to you on the host's web server to store your files. The amount of acreage you get determines the amount of data you can store. For example, if you get a 1MB (1 megabyte) limit, you can't store more than 1MB worth of files on the server. HTML files don't take up much real estate, but large graphics sure do, so you need to watch your limit. For example, you could probably store about 200 pages in 1MB of storage (assuming about 5KB per page), but only about 20 images (assuming about 50KB per image). Generally speaking, the more you pay for a host, the more storage space you get.

» **Bandwidth:** A measure of how much of your data the server serves. For example, suppose the HTML file for your page is 1KB (1 kilobyte) and the graphics associated with the page consume 9KB. If someone accesses your page, the server ships out a total of 10KB; if ten people access the page (either at the same time or over a period of time), the total bandwidth is 100KB. Most hosts give you a bandwidth limit (or "cap"), which is most often a certain number of megabytes or gigabytes per month. (A gigabyte is equal to about 1,000 megabytes.) Again, the more you pay, the greater the bandwidth you get.

WARNING

If you exceed your bandwidth limit, users will usually still be able to get to your pages (although some hosts shut down access to an offending site). However, almost all web hosts charge you an extra fee for exceeding your bandwidth, so check this out before signing up. The usual penalty is a set fee per every megabyte or gigabyte over your cap.

» **Domain name:** A general Internet address, such as wiley.com or whitehouse.gov. They tend to be easier to remember than the long-winded addresses most web hosts supply you by default, so they're a popular feature. Two types of domain names are available:

- A regular domain name (such as *yourdomain*.com or *yourdomain*.org)
- A subdomain name (such as *yourdomain.webhostdomain*.com)

To get a regular domain, you either need to use one of the many domain registration services such as GoDaddy or `Register.com`. A more convenient route is to choose a web hosting provider that will do this for you. Either way, it will usually cost you $35 per year (although some hosts offer cheap domains as a "loss leader" and recoup their costs with hosting fees; also, discount domain registrars such as GoDaddy offer domains for as little as $9.99 per year). If you go the direct route, almost all web hosts will host your domain, which means that people who use your domain name will get directed to your website on the host's web server. For this to work, you must tweak the domain settings on the registrar. This usually involves changing the DNS servers associated with the domain so that they point at the web host's domain name servers. Your web host will give you instructions on how to do this.

With a subdomain name, "webhostdomain.com" is the domain name of the web hosting company, and it simply tacks on whatever name you want to the beginning. Many web hosts will provide you with this type of domain, often for free.

- **Email addresses:** Most hosts offer you one or more email addresses along with your web space. The more you pay, the more mailboxes you get. Some hosts offer *email forwarding,* which enables you to have messages that are sent to your web host address rerouted to some other email address.
- **Shared server:** If the host offers a *shared server* (or *virtual server*), it means that you'll be sharing the server with other websites — dozens or even hundreds of them. The web host takes care of all the highly technical server management chores, so all you have to do is maintain your site. This is by far the best (and cheapest) choice for individuals or small business types.
- **Dedicated server:** You get your very own server computer on the host. That may sound like a good thing, but it's usually up to you to manage the server, which can be a dauntingly technical task. Also, dedicated servers are much more expensive than shared servers.
- **Operating system:** The operating system on the web server. You usually have two choices: Unix (or Linux) and Windows Server. Unix systems have the reputation of being very reliable and fast, even under heavy traffic loads, so they're usually the best choice for a shared server. Windows systems are a better choice for dedicated servers because they're easier to administer than their Unix brethren. Note, too, that Unix servers are case sensitive in terms of file and directory names, while Windows servers are not.
- **Databases:** The number of databases you get to create with your account. Unix systems usually offer MySQL databases, whereas Windows servers offer SQL Server databases.
- **Administration interface:** This is the host app that you use to perform tasks on the server, such as uploading files or creating users. Many hosts offer the excellent cPanel interface, and most Unix-based systems offer the phpMyAdmin app for managing your MySQL data.
- **Ad requirements:** A few free web hosts require you to display some type of advertising on your pages. This could be a banner ad across the top of the page, a "pop-up" ad that appears each time a person accesses your pages, or a "watermark" ad, usually a semitransparent logo that hovers over your page. Fortunately, free hosts that insist on ads are rare these days.
- **Uptime:** The percentage of time the host's server is up and serving. There's no such thing as 100 percent uptime because all servers require maintenance and upgrades at some point. However, the best hosts have uptime numbers over 99 percent. (If a host doesn't advertise its uptime, it's probably because it's very low. Be sure to ask before committing yourself.)
- **Tech support:** If you have problems setting up or accessing your site, you want to know that help — in the form of *tech support* — is just around the corner. The best hosts offer 24/7 tech support, which means you can contact the company — either by phone or email — 24 hours a day, 7 days a week.

- **FTP support:** You usually use the Internet's *FTP* service to transfer your files from your computer to the web host. If a host offers *FTP access* (some hosts have their own method for transferring files), be sure you can use it any time you want and there are no restrictions on the amount of data you can transfer at one time.
- **Website statistics:** Tell you things such as how many people have visited your site, which pages are the most popular, how much bandwidth you're consuming, which browsers and browser versions surfers are using, and more. Most decent hosts offer a ready-made stats package, but the best ones also give you access to the "raw" log files so you can play with the data yourself.
- **Ecommerce:** Some hosts offer a service that lets you set up a web "store" so you can sell stuff on your site. That service usually includes a "shopping script," access to credit card authorization and other payment systems, and the ability to set up a secure connection. You usually get this only in the more expensive hosting packages, and you'll most often have to pay a setup fee to get your store built.
- **Scalability:** The host is able to modify your site's features as required. For example, if your site becomes very popular, you might need to increase your bandwidth limit. If the host is scalable, it can easily change your limit (or any other feature of your site).

Finding a Web Host

Okay, you're ready to start researching the hosts to find one that suits your web style. As I mention earlier, there are hundreds, perhaps even thousands, of hosts, so how is a body supposed to whittle them down to some kind of short list? Here are some ideas:

- **Ask your friends and colleagues.** The best way to find a good host is that old standby, word of mouth. If someone you trust says a host is good, chances are you won't be disappointed. This is assuming you and your pal have similar hosting needs. If you want a full-blown ecommerce site, don't solicit recommendations from someone who has only a humble home page.
- **Solicit host reviews from experts.** Ask existing webmasters and other people "in the know" about which hosts they recommend or have heard good things about. A good place to find such experts is Web Hosting Talk (`www.webhostingtalk.com`), a collection of forums related to web hosting.

- **Contact web host customers.** Visit sites that use a particular web host, and send an email message to the webmaster asking what she thinks of the host's service.
- **Peruse the lists of web hosts.** A number of sites track and compare web hosts, so they're an easy way to get in a lot of research. Careful, though, because there are a lot of sketchy lists out there that are only trying to make a buck by getting you to click ads. Here are some reputable places to start:
  - **CNET Web Hosting Solutions:** `www.cnet.com/web-hosting`
  - **PC Magazine Web Site Hosting Services Reviews:** `www.pcmag.com/reviews/web-hosting-services`
  - **Review Hell:** `www.reviewhell.com`
  - **Review Signal Web Hosting Reviews:** `http://reviewsignal.com/webhosting`

Finding Your Way around Your New Web Home

After you sign up with a web hosting provider and your account is established, the web administrator creates two things for you: a directory on the server you can use to store your website files, and your very own web address. (This is also true if you're using a web server associated with your corporate or school network.) The directory — which is known in the biz as your *root directory* — usually takes one of the following forms:

```
/yourname/
/home/yourname/
/yourname/public_html/
```

In each case, *yourname* is the login name (or username) the provider assigns to you, or it may be your domain name (with or without the .com part). Remember, your root directory is a slice of the host's web server, and this slice is yours to monkey around with as you see fit. This usually means you can do all or most of the following to the root:

- Add files to the directory.
- Add subdirectories to the directory.
- Move or copy files from one directory to another.

» Rename files or directories.

» Delete files from the directory.

Your web address normally takes one of the following shapes:

```
http://provider/yourname/
http://yourname.provider/
http://www.yourname.com/
```

Here, *provider* is the host name of your provider (for example, www.hostcompany.com or just hostcompany.com), and *yourname* is your login name or domain name. Here are some examples:

```
http://www.hostcompany.com/mywebsite/
http://mywebsite.hostcompany.com/
http://www.mywebsite.com/
```

Your directory and your web address

There's a direct and important relationship between your server directory and your address. That is, your address actually "points to" your directory and enables other people to view the files you store in that directory. For example, suppose I decide to store a file named `thingamajig.html` in my directory and my main address is `http://mywebsite.hostcompany.com/`. This means someone else can view that page by typing the following URL into a web browser:

```
http://mywebsite.hostcompany.com/thingamajig.html
```

Similarly, suppose I create a subdirectory named `stuff` and use it to store a file named `index.html`. A surfer can view that file by convincing a web browser to head for the following URL:

```
http://mywebsite.hostcompany.com/stuff/index.html
```

In other words, folks can surf to your files and directories by strategically tacking on the appropriate filenames and directory names after your main web address.

Making your hard disk mirror your web home

As a web developer, one of the key ways to keep your projects organized is to set up your directories on your computer, and then mirror those directories on your web host. Believe me, this will make your uploading duties immeasurably easier.

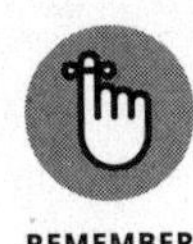

REMEMBER

Moving a file from your computer to a remote location (such as your web host's server) is known in the file transfer trade as *uploading.*

This process begins at the root. On the web host, you already have a root directory assigned to you by the hosting provider, so now you need to designate a folder on your computer to be the root mirror. If you're using the XAMPP web development environment (see Book 1, Chapter 2), then the XAMPP installation's `htdocs` subfolder is perfect as your local root. Otherwise, choose or create a folder on your computer to use as the local root.

What you do from here depends on the number of web development projects you're going to build, and the number of files in each project:

- **A single web development project consisting of just a few files:** In this case, just put all the files into the root directory.
- **A single web development project consisting of many files:** The more likely scenario for a typical web development project is to have multiple HTML, CSS, JavaScript, and PHP files, plus lots of ancillary files such as images and fonts. Although it's okay to place all your HTML files in the root directory, do yourself a favor and organize all your other files into subfolders by file type: a `css` subfolder for CSS files, a `js` subfolder for JavaScript files, and so on.
- **Multiple web development projects:** As a web developer, you'll almost certainly create tons of web projects, so it's crucial to organize them. The ideal way to do that is to create a separate root subdirectory for each project. Then within each of these subdirectories, you can create sub-subdirectories for file types such as CSS, JavaScript, images, and so on.

To help you see why mirroring your local and remote directory structures is so useful, suppose you set up a subfolder on your computer named `graphics` that you use to store your image files. To insert into your page a file named `mydog.jpg` from that folder, you'd use the following reference:

```
graphics/mydog.jpg
```

When you send your HTML file to the server and you then display the file in a browser, it looks for `mydog.jpg` in the `graphics` subdirectory. If you don't have such a subdirectory — either you didn't create it or you used a different name, such as `images` — the browser won't find `mydog.jpg` and your image won't show. In other words, if you match the subdirectories on your web server with the subfolders on your computer, your page will work properly without modifications both at home and on the web.

WARNING

One common faux pas beginning web developers make is to include the local drive and all the folder names when referencing a file. Here's an example:

```
C:\xampp\htdocs\graphics\mydog.jpg
```

This image will show up just fine when it's viewed from your computer, but it will fail miserably when you upload it to the server and view it on the web. That's because the `C:\xampp\htdocs\` part exists only on your computer.

WARNING

The Unix (or Linux) computers that play host to the vast majority of web servers are downright finicky when it comes to the uppercase and lowercase letters used in file and directory names. It's crucial that you check the file references in your code to be sure the file and directory names you use match the combination of uppercase and lowercase letters used on your server. For example, suppose you have a CSS file on your server that's named `styles.css`. If your HTML references that file as, say, `STYLES.CSS`, the server won't find the file and your styles won't get applied.

Uploading your site files

Once your web page or site is ready for its debut, it's time to get your files to your host's web server. If the server is on your company or school network, you send the files over the network to the directory set up by your system administrator. Otherwise, you upload the files to the root directory created for you on the hosting provider's web server.

How you go about uploading your site files depends on the web host, but here are the four most common scenarios:

- **Use an FTP program.** It's a rare web host that doesn't offer support for the File Transfer Protocol (FTP, for short), which is the Internet's most popular method for transfer files from here to there. To use FTP, you usually need to get a piece of software called an *FTP client,* which enables you to connect to your web host's FTP server (your host can provide you with instructions for this) and offers an interface for standard file tasks, such as navigating and creating folders, uploading the files, deleting and renaming files, and so on. Popular Windows clients are CuteFTP (`www.globalscape.com/cuteftp`) and Cyberduck (`https://cyberduck.io`). For the Mac, try Transmit (`https://panic.com/transmit`) or FileZilla (`https://filezilla-project.org`).
- **Use your text editor's file upload feature.** Some text editors come with an FTP client built-in, so you can edit a file and then immediately upload it with a single command. The Coda text editor (`https://panic.com/coda`) supports this too-handy-for-words feature.

» **Use the File Manager feature of cPanel.** I mention earlier that lots of web hosts offer an administration tool called cPanel that offers an interface for hosting tasks such as email and domain management. cPanel also offers a File Manager feature that you can use to upload files and perform other file management chores.

» **Use the web host's proprietary upload tool.** For some reason, a few web hosts only offer their own proprietary interface for uploading and messing around with files and directories. See your host's Help or Support page for instructions.

Making changes to your web files

What happens if you send a web development file to your web host and then realize you've made a typing gaffe or you spy a coding mistake? Or what if you have more information to add to one of your web pages? How do you make changes to the files you've already sent?

Well, here's the short answer: You don't. That's right, after you've sent your files, you never have to bother with them again. That doesn't mean you can never update your site, however. Instead, you make your changes to the files that reside on your computer and then send these revised files to your web host. These files replace the old files, and your site is updated just like that.

WARNING

Be sure you send the updated file to the correct directory on the server. Otherwise, you may overwrite a file that happens to have the same name in some other directory.

2 Coding the Front End, Part 1: HTML & CSS

Contents at a Glance

- » Figuring out HTML tags and attributes
- » Understanding the basic blueprint for all web pages
- » Adding text, images, and links to your page
- » Building bulleted and numbered lists

Chapter 1
Structuring the Page with HTML

I am always fascinated by the structure of things; why do things work this way and not that way.

— URSUS WEHRLI

When it comes to web development, it's no exaggeration to say that the one indispensable thing, the *sine qua non* for those of you who studied Latin in school, is HTML. That's because absolutely everything else you make as a web developer — your CSS rules, your JavaScript code, even your PHP scripts — can't hang its hat anywhere but on some HTML. These other web development technologies don't even make sense outside of an HTML context.

So, in a sense, this chapter is the most important for you as a web coder because all the rest of the book depends to a greater or lesser degree on the HTML know-how found in the following pages. If that sounds intimidating, not to worry: One of the great things about HTML is that it's not a huge topic, so you can get up to full HTML speed without a massive investment of time and effort.

Because HTML is so important, you'll be happy to know that I don't rush things. You'll get a thorough grounding in all things HTML, and when you're done you'll be more than ready to tackle the rest of your web development education.

Getting the Hang of HTML

Building a web page from scratch using your bare hands may seem like a daunting task. It doesn't help that the codes you use to set up, configure, and format a web page are called the Hypertext Markup Language (HTML for short), a name that could only warm the cockles of a geek's heart. I take a mercifully brief look at each term:

- **Hypertext:** In prehistoric times — that is, the 1980s — tall-forehead types referred to any text that, when selected, takes you to a different document, as *hypertext*. So this is just an oblique reference to the links that are the defining characteristic of web pages.
- **Markup:** Instructions that specify how the content of a web page should be displayed in the web browser.
- **Language:** The set of codes that comprise all the markup possibilities for a page.

But even though the name HTML is intimidating, the codes used by HTML aren't even close to being hard to learn. There are only a few of them, and in many cases they even make sense!

At its most basic, HTML is nothing more than a collection of markup codes — called *tags* — that specify the structure of your web page. In HTML, "structure" is a rubbery concept that can refer to anything from the overall layout of the page all the way down to a single word or even just a character or two.

You can think of a tag as a kind of container. What types of things can it contain? Mostly text, although lots of tags contain things like chunks of the web page and even other tags.

Most tags use the following generic format:

```
<tag>content</tag>
```

What you have here are a couple codes that define a container. Most of these codes are one- or two-letter abbreviations, but sometimes they're entire words. You always surround these codes with angle brackets <>; the brackets tell the web browser that it's dealing with a chunk of HTML and not just some random text.

The first of these codes — `<tag>` — is called the *start tag* and it marks the opening of the container; the second of the codes — `</tag>` — is called the *end tag* and it marks the closing of the container. (Note the extra slash (/) that appears in the end tag.)

In between you have the *content*, which refers to whatever is contained in the tag. For example, I start with a simple sentence that might appear in a web page:

```
Okay, listen up people because this is important!
```

Figure 1-1 shows how this might look in a web browser.

FIGURE 1-1: The sample sentence as it appears in a web browser.

Okay, listen up people because this is important!

Ho hum, right? Suppose you want to punch this up a bit by emphasizing "important." In HTML, the tag for emphasis is `<em>`, so you'd modify your sentence like so:

```
Okay, listen up people because this is <em>important</em>!
```

See how I've surrounded the word `important` with `<em>` and `</em>`? The first `<em>` is the start tag and it says to the browser, "Yo, Browser Boy! You know the text that comes after this? Be a good fellow and treat it as emphasized text." This continues until the browser reaches the end tag `</em>`, which lets the browser know it's supposed to stop what it's doing. So the `</em>` tells the browser, "Okay, okay, that's enough with the emphasis already!"

All web browsers display emphasized text in italics, so that's how the word now appears, as you can eyeball in Figure 1-2.

FIGURE 1-2: The sentence revised to italicize the word `important`.

Okay, listen up people because this is *important*!

There are tags for lots of other structures, including important text, paragraphs, headings, page titles, links, and lists. HTML is just the sum total of all these tags.

WARNING

One of the most common mistakes rookie web weavers make is to forget the slash (/) that identifies an end tag. If your page looks wrong when you view it in a browser, look for a missing slash. Also look for a backslash (\) instead of a slash, which is another common error.

Understanding Tag Attributes

You'll often use tags straight up, but all tags are capable of being modified in various ways. This might be as simple as supplying a unique identifier to the tag for use in a script or a style, or it might be a way to change how the tag operates. Either way, you modify a tag by adding one or more *attributes* to the start tag. Most attributes use the following generic syntax:

```
<tag attribute="value">
```

Here, you replace `attribute` with the name of the attribute you want to apply to the tag, and you replace `value` with the value you want to assign the attribute.

For example, the `<hr>` tag adds a horizontal line across the web page (`hr` stands for *horizontal rule*). You use only the start tag in this case (as a simple line, it can't "contain" anything, so no end tag is needed), as demonstrated in the following example:

```
Okay, listen up people because this is <em>important</em>!
<hr>
```

As you can see in Figure 1-3, the web browser draws a line right across the page.

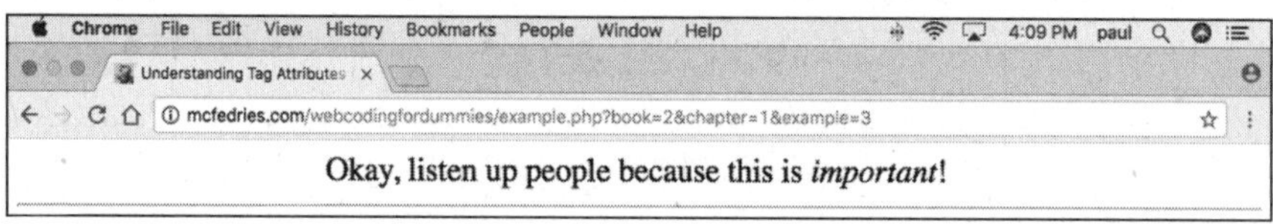

FIGURE 1-3: When you add the `<hr>` tag, a horizontal line appears across the page.

You can also add the `width` attribute to the `<hr>` tag and specify the width you prefer. For example, if you only want the line to traverse half the page width, set the `width` attribute to `"50%"`, as shown here:

```
Okay, listen up people because this is <em>important</em>!
<hr width="50%">
```

As Figure 1-4 shows, the web browser obeys your command and draws a line that takes up only half the width of the page.

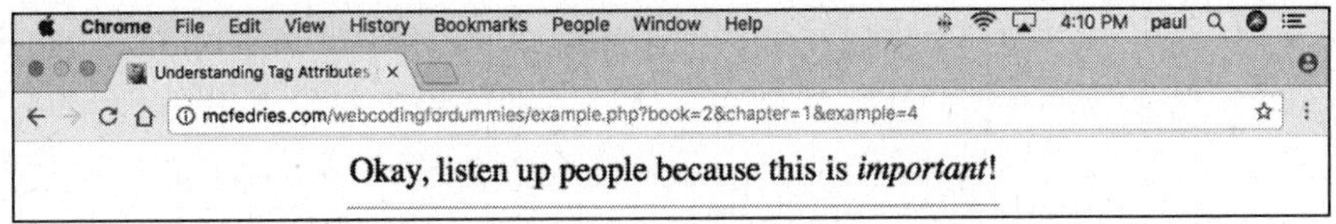

FIGURE 1-4: The `<hr width="50%">` tag creates a horizontal line across half the page.

Learning the Fundamental Structure of an HTML5 Web Page

In this section, I show you the tags that serve as the basic blueprint you'll use for all your web pages.

Your HTML files will always lead off with the following tag:

```
<!DOCTYPE html>
```

This tag (it has no end tag) is the so-called *Doctype declaration*, and it lets the web browser know what type of document it's about to process (an HTML document, in this case).

Next up you add the `<html lang="en">` tag. This tag doesn't do a whole lot except tell any web browser that tries to read the file that it's dealing with a file that contains HTML doodads. It also uses the `lang` attribute to specify the document's language, which in this case is English.

Similarly, the last line in your document will always be the corresponding end tag: `</html>`. You can think of this tag as the HTML equivalent for "The End." So, each of your web pages will include this on the second line:

```
<html lang="en">
```

and this on the last line:

```
</html>
```

The next items serve to divide the page into two sections: the head and the body. The head section is like an introduction to the page. Web browsers use the head to glean various types of information about the page. A number of items can appear in the head section, but the only one that makes any real sense at this early stage is the title of the page, which I talk about in the next section.

To define the head, add <head> and </head> tags immediately below the <html> tag you typed in earlier. So your web page should now look like this:

```
<!DOCTYPE html>
<html lang="en">
<head>
</head>
</html>
```

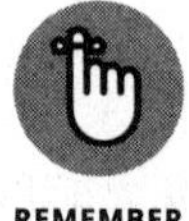

REMEMBER

Although technically it makes no difference if you enter your tag names in uppercase or lowercase letters, the HTML powers-that-be prefer to see HTML tags in lowercase letters, so that's the style I use in this book, and I encourage you to do the same.

While you're in the head section, let's add a head-scratcher:

```
<meta charset="utf-8">
```

You place this between the <head> and </head> tags (indented four spaces for easier reading). It tells the web browser that your web page uses the UTF-8 character set, which you can mostly ignore except to know that UTF-8 contains almost every character (domestic and foreign), punctuation mark, and symbol known to humankind.

The body section is where you enter the text and other fun stuff that the browser will actually display. To define the body, place <body> and </body> tags after the head section (that is, below the </head> tag):

```
<!DOCTYPE html>
<html lang="en">
<head>
    <meta charset="utf-8">
</head>
<body>
</body>
</html>
```

WARNING

A common page error is to include two or more copies of these basic tags, particularly the <body> tag. For best results, be sure you use each of these seven basic structural tags only one time on each page.

Giving your page a title

When you surf the web, you've probably noticed that your browser displays some text in the current tab. That tab text is the web page title, which is a short (or sometimes long) phrase that gives the page a name. You can give your own web page a name by adding the `<title>` tag to the page's head section.

To define a title, surround the title text with the `<title>` and `</title>` tags. For example, if you want the title of your page to be "My Home Sweet Home Page," enter it as follows:

```
<title>My Home Sweet Home Page</title>
```

Note that you always place the title inside the head section, so your basic HTML document now looks like this:

```
<!DOCTYPE html>
<html lang="en">
<head>
    <meta charset="utf-8">
    <title>My Home Sweet Home Page</title>
</head>
<body>
</body>
</html>
```

Figure 1-5 shows this HTML file loaded into a web browser. Notice how the title appears in the browser's tab bar.

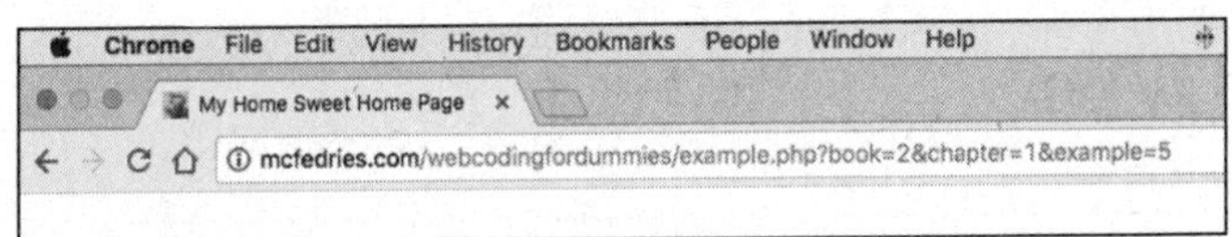

FIGURE 1-5: The text you insert into the `<title>` tag shows up in the browser tab.

Here are a few things to keep in mind when thinking of a title for your page:

- Be sure your title describes what the page is all about.
- Don't make your title too long. If you do, the browser might chop it off because there's not enough room to display it in the tab. Fifty or 60 characters are usually the max.
- Use titles that make sense when someone views them out of context. For example, if someone really likes your page, that person might add it to his or her list of favorites or bookmarks. The browser displays the page title in the favorites list, so it's important that the title makes sense when she looks at the bookmarks later on.

» Don't use cryptic or vague titles. Titling a page "Link #42" or "My Web Page" might make sense to you, but your readers will almost certainly be scratching their heads.

Adding some text

Now it's time to put some flesh on your web page's bones by entering the text you want to appear in the body of the page. For the most part, you can type the text between the `<body>` and `</body>` tags, like this:

```
<!DOCTYPE html>
<html lang="en">
<head>
    <meta charset="utf-8">
    <title>My Home Sweet Home Page</title>
</head>
<body>
Hello HTML World!
</body>
</html>
```

Figure 1-6 shows how a web browser displays this HTML.

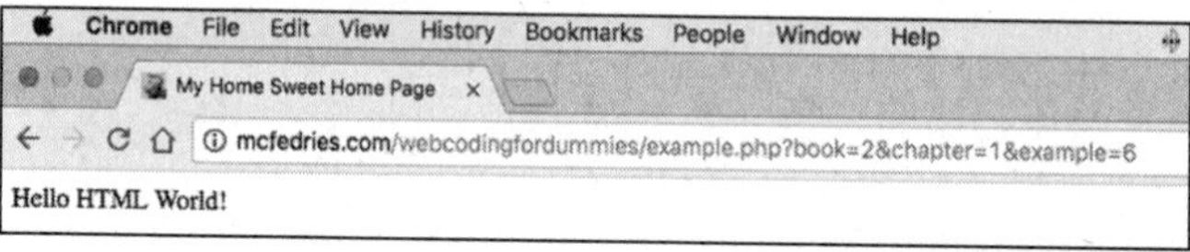

FIGURE 1-6: Text you add to the page body appears in the browser's content window.

Before you start typing willy-nilly, however, there are a few things you should know:

» You might think you can line things up and create some interesting effects by stringing together two or more spaces. Ha! Web browsers chew up all those extra spaces and spit them out into the nether regions of cyberspace. Why? Well, the philosophy of the web is that you can use only HTML tags to lay out a document. So a run of multiple spaces (or *white space,* as it's called) is ignored.

» Tabs also fall under the rubric of white space. You can enter tabs all day long, but the browser ignores them completely.

- Browsers also like to ignore the carriage return. It might sound reasonable to the likes of you and me that pressing Enter (or Return on a Mac) starts a new paragraph, but that's not so in the HTML world.
- If you want to separate two chunks of text, you have multiple ways to go, but here are the two easiest:
  - **If you want no space between the texts:** Place a `<br>` (for line break) tag between the two bits of text.
  - **If you want some breathing room between the texts:** Surround each chunk of text with the `<p>` and `</p>` (for paragraph) tags.
- If HTML documents are just plain text, does that mean you're out of luck if you need to use characters such as © and €? Luckily, no. For the most part, you can just add these characters to your file. However, HTML also has special codes for these kinds of characters. I talk about them a bit later in this chapter.
- If, for some reason, you're using a word processor instead of a text editor, know that it won't help to format your text using the program's built-in commands. The browser cheerfully ignores even the most elaborate formatting jobs because browsers understand only HTML (and CSS and JavaScript). And besides, a document with formatting is, by definition, not a pure text file, so a browser might bite the dust trying to load it.

Some Notes on Structure versus Style

One of the key points of front-end web development is to separate the structure of the web page from its styling. This makes the page faster to build, easier to maintain, and more predictable across a range of browsers and operating systems. HTML provides the structure side, while CSS handles the styling.

That's fine as far as it goes, but HTML performs its structural duties with a couple of quirks you need to understand:

- **This isn't your father's idea of structure.** That is, when you think of the structure of a document, you probably think of larger chunks such as articles, sections, and paragraphs. HTML does all that, but it also deals with structure at the level of sentences, words, and even characters.
- **HTML's structures often come with some styling attached.** Or, I should say, all web browsers come with predefined styling that they use when they render some HTML tags. Yes, I know I just said that it's best to separate

structure and style, so this can be a tad confusing. Think of it this way: When you build a new deck using cedar, your completed deck has a natural "cedar" look to it, but you're free to apply a coat of varnish or paint. HTML is the cedar, whereas CSS is the paint.

I mention these quirks because they can help to answer some questions that might arise as you work with HTML tags.

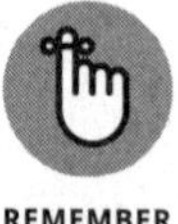
REMEMBER

Another key to understanding why HTML does what it does, is that much of HTML — especially its most recent incarnation, HTML5 — has been set up so that a web page is "understandable" to an extent by software that analyzes the page. One important example is a screen reader used by some visually impaired surfers. If a screen reader can easily figure out the entire structure of the page from its HTML tags, then it can present the page properly to the user. Similarly, software that seeks to index, read, or otherwise analyze the page will only be able to do this successfully if the page's HTML tags are a faithful representation of the page's intended structure.

Applying the Basic Text Tags

HTML has a few tags that enable you to add structure to text. Many web developers use these tags only for the built-in browser formatting that comes with them, but you really should try and use the tags *semantically,* as the geeks say, which means to use them based on the meaning you want the text to convey.

Emphasizing text

One of the most common meanings you can attach to text is emphasis. By putting a little extra oomph on a word or phrase, you tell the reader to add stress to that text, which can subtly alter the meaning of your words. For example, consider the following sentence:

```
You'll never fit in there with that ridiculous thing on your
   head!
```

Now consider the same sentence with emphasis added to one word:

```
You'll never fit in there with that ridiculous thing on your
   head!
```

You emphasize text on a web page by surrounding that text with the `<em>` and `</em>` tags:

```
You'll <em>never</em> fit in there with that ridiculous thing on
   your head!
```

All web browsers render the emphasized text in italics, as shown in Figure 1-7.

FIGURE 1-7: The web browser renders emphasized text using italics.

You'll *never* fit in there with that ridiculous thing on your head!

I should also mention that HTML has a closely related tag: `<i>`. The `<i>` tag's job is to mark up *alternative text*, which refers to any text that you want treated with a different mood or role than regular text. Common examples include book titles, technical terms, foreign words, or a person's thoughts. All web browsers render text between `<i>` and `</i>` in italics.

Marking important text

One common meaning that you'll often want your text to convey is importance. It might be some significant step in a procedure, a vital prerequisite or condition for something, or a crucial passage within a longer text block. In each case, you're dealing with text that you don't want your readers to miss, so it needs to stand out from the regular prose that surrounds it.

In HTML, you mark text as important by surrounding it with the `<strong>` and `</strong>` tags, as in this example:

```
Dear reader: Do you see the red button in the upper-right
corner of this page? <strong>Never click the red
button!</strong> You have been warned.
```

All web browsers render text marked up with the `<strong>` tag in bold, as shown in Figure 1-8.

FIGURE 1-8: The browser renders important text using bold.

Dear reader: Do you see the red button in the upper-right corner of this page?
Never click the red button! You have been warned.

Just to keep us all on our web development toes, HTML also offers a close cousin of the `<strong>` tag: the `<b>` tag. You use the `<b>` tag to mark up keywords in the text. A *keyword* is a term that you want to draw attention to because it plays a different role than the regular text. It could be a company name or a person's name (think of those famous "bold-faced names" that are the staple of celebrity gossip columns). The browser renders text between the `<b>` and `</b>` tags in a bold font.

Nesting tags

It's perfectly legal — and often necessary — to combine multiple tag types by nesting one inside the other. For example, check out this code:

```
Dear reader: Do you see the red button in the upper-right
corner of this page? <strong>Never, I repeat <em>never</em>,
click the red button!</strong> You have been warned.
```

See what I did there? In the text between the `<strong>` and `</strong>` tags, I marked up a word with the `<em>` and `</em>` tags. The result? You got it: bold, italic text, as shown in Figure 1-9.

FIGURE 1-9: The browser usually combines nested tags, such as the bold, italic text shown here.

Dear reader: Do you see the red button in the upper-right corner of this page?
Never, I repeat *never*, click the red button! You have been warned.

Adding headings

Earlier you saw that you can give your web page a title using the aptly named `<title>` tag. However, that title only appears in the browser's title bar and tab. What if you want to add a title that appears in the body of the page? That's almost easier done than said because HTML comes with a few tags that enable you to define *headings*, which are bits of text that appear in a separate paragraph and usually stick out from the surrounding text by being bigger, appearing in a bold typeface, and so on.

There are six heading tags in all, ranging from `<h1>`, which uses the largest type size, down to `<h6>`, which uses the smallest size. Here's some web page code that demonstrates the six heading tags, and Figure 1-10 shows how they look in a web browser:

```
<h1>This is Heading 1</h1>
<h2>This is Heading 2</h2>
```

```
<h3>This is Heading 3</h3>
<h4>This is Heading 4</h4>
<h5>This is Heading 5</h5>
<h6>This is Heading 6</h6>
```


FIGURE 1-10: The six HTML heading tags.

What's up with all the different headings? The idea is that you use them to create a kind of outline for your web page. How you do this depends on the page, but here's one possibility:

- Use `<h1>` for the overall page title.
- Use `<h2>` for the page subtitle.
- Use `<h3>` for the titles of the main sections of your page.
- Use `<h4>` for the titles of the subsections of your page.

Adding quotations

You might have noticed that each chapter of this book begins with a short, apt quotation because, hey, who doesn't love a good quote, right? The readers of your web pages will be quote-appreciators, too, I'm sure, so why not sprinkle your text with a few words from the wise?

In HTML, you designate a passage of text as a quotation by using the `<blockquote>` tag. Here's an example:

```
Here's what the great jurist Oliver Wendell Holmes, Sr. had to
   say about puns:
```

```
<blockquote>
A pun does not commonly justify a blow in return.
But if a blow were given for such cause, and death
ensued, the jury would be judges both of the facts
and of the pun, and might, if the latter were of an
aggravated character, return a verdict of justifiable
homicide.
</blockquote>
Clearly, the dude was not a pun fan.
```

The web browser renders the text between `<blockquote>` and `</blockquote>` in its own paragraph that it also indents slightly from the left margin, as shown in Figure 1-11.

FIGURE 1-11: The web browser renders `<blockquote>` text indented slighted from the left.

Here's what the great jurist Oliver Wendell Holmes, Sr. had to say about puns:

> A pun does not commonly justify a blow in return. But if a blow were given for such cause, and death ensued, the jury would be judges both of the facts and of the pun, and might, if the latter were of an aggravated character, return a verdict of justifiable homicide.

Clearly, the dude was not a pun fan.

Creating Links

When all is said and done (actually, long before that), your website will consist of anywhere from 2 to 102 pages (or even more, if you've got lots to say). Here's the thing, though: If you manage to cajole someone onto your home page, how do you get that person to your other pages? That really is what the web is all about, isn't it, getting folks from one page to another? And of course, you already know the answer to the question. You get visitors from your home page to your other pages by creating links that take people from here to there. In this section, you learn how to build your own links and how to finally put the "hypertext" into HTML.

Linking basics

The HTML tags that do the link thing are `<a>` and `</a>`. Here's how the `<a>` tag works:

```
<a href="address">
```

Here, `href` stands for *hypertext reference,* which is just a fancy-schmancy way of saying "address" or "URL." Your job is to replace *address* with the actual address of the web page you want to use for the link. And yes, you have to enclose the address in quotation marks. Here's an example:

```
<a href="http://webcodingplayground.io">
```

You're not done yet, though, not by a long shot (insert groan of disappointment here). What are you missing? Right: You have to give the reader some descriptive link text to click. That's pretty straightforward because all you do is insert the text between the `<a>` and `</a>` tags, like this:

```
<a href="address">Link text</a>
```

Need an example? You got it:

```
For web coding fun, check out the
<a href="http://webcodingplayground.io">
Web Coding Playground</a>!
```

Figure 1-12 shows how it looks in a web browser. Notice how the browser colors and underlines the link text, and when I point my mouse at the link, the address I specified in the `<a>` tag (albeit without the `http://` prefix) appears in the browser's status area.

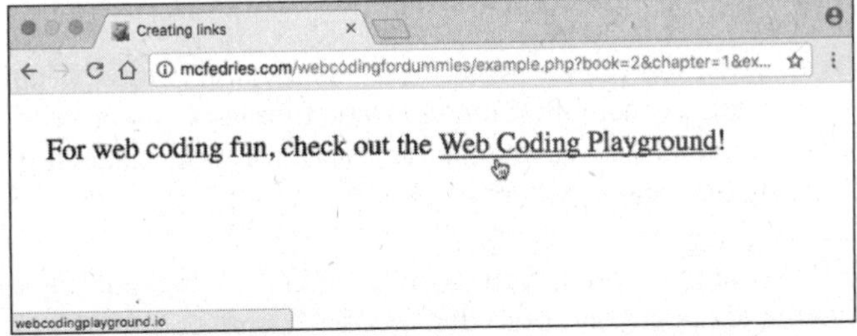

FIGURE 1-12: How the link appears in the web browser.

Anchors aweigh: Internal links

When a surfer clicks a standard link, the page loads and the browser displays the top part of the page. However, it's possible to set up a special kind of link that will force the browser to initially display some other part of the page, such as a section in the middle of the page. For these special links, I use the term *internal links,* because they take the reader directly to some inner part of the page.

When would you ever use an internal link? Most of your HTML pages will probably be short and sweet, and the web surfers who drop by will have no trouble navigating their way around. But if, like me, you suffer from a bad case of terminal verbosity combined with bouts of extreme long windedness, you'll end up with web pages that are lengthy, to say the least. Rather than force your readers to scroll through your tomelike creations, you can set up links to various sections of the document. You could then assemble these links at the top of the page to form a sort of "hypertable of contents," as an example.

Internal links actually link to a specially marked section — called an *anchor* — that you've inserted somewhere in the same page. To understand how anchors work, think of how you might mark a spot in a book you're reading. You might dog-ear the page, attach a note, or place something between the pages, such as a bookmark or your cat's tail.

An anchor performs the same function: It "marks" a particular spot in a web page, and you can then use a regular `<a>` tag to link to that spot. Here's the general format for an anchor tag:

```
<element id="name">
```

As you can see, an anchor tag looks a lot like a regular tag, except that it also includes the `id` attribute, which is set to the name you want to give the anchor. Here's an example:

```
<section id="section1">
```

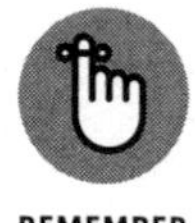

REMEMBER

You can use whatever you want for the name, but it must begin with a letter and it can include any combination of letters, numbers, underscores (_), and hyphens (-). Also, `id` values are case-sensitive, so the browser treats the `id` value `section1` differently than the `id` value `Section1`.

To set up the anchor link, you create a regular `<a>` tag, but the `href` value becomes the name of the anchor, preceded by a hash symbol (#):

```
<a href="#name">
```

Here's an example that links to the anchor I showed earlier:

```
<a href="#section1">
```

Although you'll mostly use anchors to link to sections of the same web page, there's no law against using them to link to specific sections of other pages. What you do is add the appropriate anchor to the other page and then link to it by adding the anchor's name (preceded, as usual, by #) to the end of the page's filename. Here's an example:

```
<a href="chapter57.html#section1">
```

Building Bulleted and Numbered Lists

For some reason, people love lists: Best (and Worst) Dressed lists, Top Ten lists, My All-Time Favorite *X* lists, where *X* is whatever you want it to be: movies, songs, books, *I Love Lucy* episodes — you name it. People like lists, for whatever reasons.

Okay, so let's make some lists. Easy, right? Well, sure, any website jockey can just plop a Best Tootsie Roll Flavors Ever list on a page by typing each item, one after the other. Perhaps our list maker even gets a bit clever and inserts the `<br>` tag between each item, which displays them on separate lines. Ooooh.

Yes, you can make a list that way, and it works well enough, I suppose, but there's a better way. HTML has a few tags that are specially designed to give you much more control over your list-building chores. For example, you can create a bulleted list that actually has those little bullets out front of each item. Nice! Want a Top Ten list, instead? HTML has your back by offering special tags for numbered lists, too.

Making your point with bulleted lists

A no-frills, `<br>`-separated list isn't very useful or readable because it doesn't come with any type of eye candy that helps differentiate one item from the next. An official, HTML-approved bulleted list solves that problem by leading off each item with a bullet — a cute little black dot.

Bulleted lists use two types of tags:

- The entire list is surrounded by the `<ul>` and `</ul>` tags. Why "ul"? Well, what the rest of the world calls a bulleted list, the HTML poohbahs call an *unordered list.*
- Each item in the list is preceded by the `<li>` (list item) tag and is closed with the `</li>` end tag.

The general setup looks like this:

```
<ul>
    <li>Bullet text goes here</li>
    <li>And here<li>
    <li>And here</li>
    <li>You get the idea...</li>
</ul>
```

Notice that I've indented the list items by four spaces, which makes it easier to see that they're part of a <ul></ul> container. Here's an example to chew on:

```
<h3>My All-Time Favorite Oxymorons</h3>
<ul>
    <li>Pretty ugly</li>
    <li>Military intelligence</li>
    <li>Jumbo shrimp</li>
    <li>Original copy</li>
    <li>Random order</li>
    <li>Act naturally</li>
    <li>Tight slacks</li>
    <li>Freezer burn</li>
    <li>Sight unseen</li>
    <li>Microsoft Works</li>
</ul>
```

Figure 1-13 shows how the web browser renders this code, cute little bullets and all.

My All-Time Favorite Oxymorons

- Pretty ugly
- Military intelligence
- Jumbo shrimp
- Original copy
- Random order
- Act naturally
- Tight slacks
- Freezer burn
- Sight unseen
- Microsoft Works

FIGURE 1-13: A typical bulleted list.

Numbered lists: Easy as one, two, three

If you want to include a numbered list of items — it could be a Top Ten list, bowling league standings, steps to follow, or any kind of ranking — don't bother adding in the numbers yourself. Instead, you can use a *numbered list* to make the web browser generate the numbers for you.

Like bulleted lists, numbered lists use two types of tags:

- The entire list is surrounded by the `<ol>` and `</ol>` tags. The "ol" here is short for *ordered list,* because those HTML nerds just have to be different, don't they?
- Each item in the list is surrounded by `<li>` and `</li>`.

Here's the general structure to use:

```
<ol>
    <li>First item</li>
    <li>Second item</li>
    <li>Third item</li>
    <li>You got this...</li>
</ol>
```

I've indented the list items by four spaces to make it easier to see that they're inside an `<ol></ol>` container. Here's an example:

```
<h3>My Ten Favorite U.S. College Nicknames</h3>
<ol>
    <li>U.C. Santa Cruz Banana Slugs</li>
    <li>Delta State Fighting Okra</li>
    <li>Kent State Golden Flashes</li>
    <li>Evergreen State College Geoducks</li>
    <li>New Mexico Tech Pygmies</li>
    <li>South Carolina Fighting Gamecocks</li>
    <li>Southern Illinois Salukis</li>
    <li>Whittier Poets</li>
    <li>Western Illinois Leathernecks</li>
    <li>Delaware Fightin' Blue Hens</li>
</ol>
```

Notice that I didn't include any numbers before each list item. However, when I display this document in a browser (see Figure 1-14), the numbers are automatically inserted. Pretty slick, huh?

My Ten Favorite U.S. College Nicknames

1. U.C. Santa Cruz Banana Slugs
2. Delta State Fighting Okra
3. Kent State Golden Flashes
4. Evergreen State College Geoducks
5. New Mexico Tech Pygmies
6. South Carolina Fighting Gamecocks
7. Southern Illinois Salukis
8. Whittier Poets
9. Western Illinois Leathernecks
10. Delaware Fightin' Blue Hens

FIGURE 1-14: When the web browser renders the ordered list, it's kind enough to add the numbers for you automatically.

Inserting Special Characters

Earlier in this chapter, I talk briefly about a special `<meta>` tag that goes into the head section:

```
<meta charset="utf-8">
```

It might not look like it, but that tag adds a bit of magic to your web page. The voodoo is that now you can add special characters such as © and ™ directly to your web page text and the web browser will display them without complaint.

The trick is how you add these characters directly to your text, and that depends on your operating system. First, if you're using Windows, you have two choices:

- Hold down the Alt key and then press the character's four-digit ASCII code using your keyboard's numeric keypad. For example, you type an em dash (—) by pressing Alt+0151.
- Paste the character from the Character Map application that comes with Windows.

If you're a Mac user, you also have two choices:

- Type the character's special keyboard shortcut. For example, you type an em dash (—) by pressing Option+Shift+- (hyphen).
- Paste the character from the Symbols Viewer that comes with macOS.

Having said all of that, I should point out that there's another way to add special characters to a page. The web wizards who created HTML came up with special codes called *character entities* (which is surely a name only a true geek would love) that represent these oddball symbols.

These codes come in two flavors: a *character reference* and an *entity name*. Character references are basically just numbers, and the entity names are friendlier symbols that describe the character you're trying to display. For example, you can display the registered trademark symbol (™) by using either the ® character reference or the ® entity name, as shown here:

```
Print-On-Non-Demand&#174;
```

or

```
Print-On-Non-Demand&reg;
```

Note that both character references and entity names begin with an ampersand (&) and end with a semicolon (;). Don't forget either character when using special characters in your own pages.

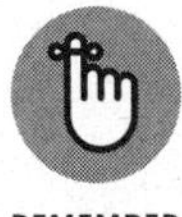
REMEMBER

One very common use of character references is for displaying HTML tags without the web browser rendering them as tags. To do this, replace the tag's less-than sign (<) with < (or <) and the tag's greater-than sign (>) with > (or >).

Inserting Images

Whether you want to tell stories, give instructions, pontificate, or just plain rant about something, you can do all of that and more by adding text to your page. But to make it more interesting for your readers, add a bit of eye candy every now and then. To that end, there's an HTML tag you can use to add one or more images to your page.

However, before we get too far into this picture business, I should tell you that, unfortunately, you can't use just any old image on a web page. Browsers are limited in the types of images they can display. There are, in fact, three main types of image formats you can use:

- **GIF:** The original web graphics format (it's short for Graphics Interchange Format). GIF (it's pronounced "giff" or "jiff") is limited to 256 colors, so it's best for simple images like line art, clip art, text, and so on. GIFs are also useful for creating simple animations.
- **JPEG:** Gets its name from the Joint Photographic Experts Group that invented it. JPEG (it's pronounced "jay-peg") supports complex images that have many millions of colors. The main advantage of JPEG files is that, given the same image, they're smaller than GIFs, so they take less time to download. Careful,

though: JPEG uses *lossy* compression, which means that it makes the image smaller by discarding redundant pixels. The greater the compression, the more pixels that are discarded, and the less sharp the image will appear. That said, if you have a photo or similarly complex image, JPEG is almost always the best choice because it gives the smallest file size.

- **PNG:** The Portable Network Graphics format supports millions of colors. PNG (and it's pronounced "p-n-g" or "ping") is a compressed format, but unlike JPEGs, PNGs use *lossless* compression. This means images retain sharpness, but the file sizes can get quite big. If you have an illustration or icon that uses solid colors, or a photo that contains large areas of near-solid color, PNG is a good choice. PNG also supports transparency.

Okay, enough of all that. Time to start squeezing some images onto your web page. As I mention earlier, there's an HTML code that tells a browser to display an image. It's the `<img>` tag, and here's how it works:

```
<img src="filename" alt="description">
```

Here, `src` is short for source, *`filename`* is the name of the graphics file you want to display, and *`description`* is a short description of the image (which is read by screen readers and seen by browsers who aren't displaying images). Note that there's no end tag to add here.

Look at an example. Suppose you have an image named `logo.png`. To add it to your page, you use the following line:

```
<img src="logo.png" alt="The Logophilia Ltd. company logo">
```

In effect, this tag says to the browser, "Excuse me? Would you be so kind as to go out and grab the image file named `logo.png` and insert it in the page right here where the `<img>` tag is?" Dutifully, the browser loads the image and displays it in the page.

For this simple example to work, bear in mind that your HTML file and your graphics file need to be sitting in the same directory. Many webmasters create a subdirectory just for images, which keeps things neat and tidy. If you plan on doing this, be sure you study my instructions for using directories and subdirectories in Book 1, Chapter 3.

Here's an example and Figure 1-15 shows how things appear in a web browser:

```
To see a World in a Grain of Sand<br>
And a Heaven in a Wild Flower
<img src="/images/macro-flower-and-ant.jpg" alt="Macro photo
  showing an ant exploring a flower">
```

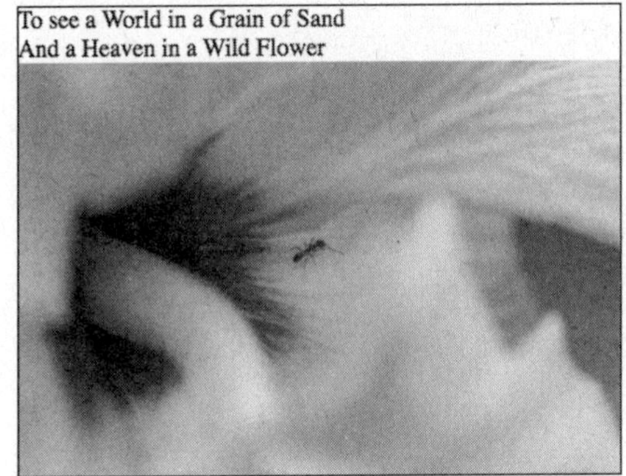

FIGURE 1-15: A web page with an image thrown in.

Carving Up the Page

Adding a bit of text, some links, and maybe a list or three to the body of the page is a good start, but any web page worth posting will require much more than that. For starters, all your web pages will require a high-level structure. Why? Well, think about the high-level structure of this book, which includes the front and back covers, the table of contents, an index, and eight mini-books, each of which contains several chapters, which, in turn consist of many sections and paragraphs within those sections. It's all nice and neat and well-organized, if I do say so myself.

Now imagine, instead, that this entire book was just page after page of undifferentiated text: no mini-books, no chapters, no sections, no paragraphs, plus no table of contents or index. I've just described a book-reader's worst nightmare, and I'm sure I couldn't even pay you to read such a thing.

Your web pages will suffer from the same fate unless you add some structure to the body section, and for that you need to turn to HTML's high-level structure tags.

The first thing to understand about these tags is that they're designed to infuse meaning — that is, semantics — into your page structures. You'll see what this means as I introduce each tag, but for now get a load of the abstract page shown in Figure 1-16.

I next discuss each of the tags shown in Figure 1-16.

The <header> tag

You use the `<header>` tag to create a *page header,* which is usually a strip across the top of the page that includes elements such as the site or page title and a logo. (Don't confuse this with the page's head section that appears between the `<head>` and `</head>` tags.)

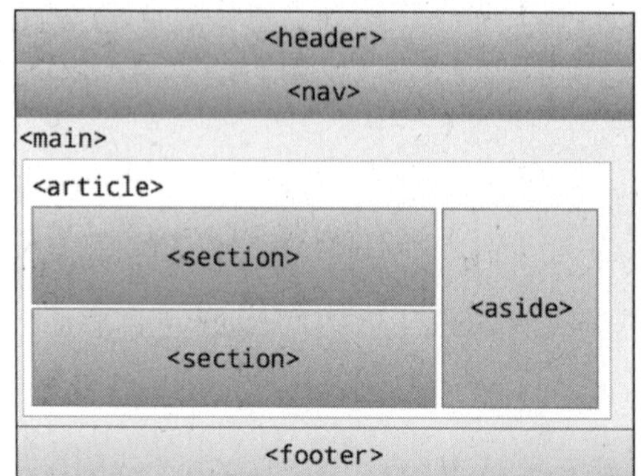

FIGURE 1-16: An abstract view of HTML5's semantic page structure tags.

Since the header almost always appears at the top of the page, the `<header>` tag is usually seen right after the `<body>` tag, as shown in the following example (and Figure 1-17):

```
<body>
    <header>
        <img src="iis-logo.png" alt="Isn't it Semantic? company
    logo">
        <h1>Welcome to "Isn't it Semantic?"</h1>
        <hr>
    </header>
    ...
</body>
```

FIGURE 1-17: A page header with a logo, title, and horizontal rule.

The <nav> tag

The `<nav>` tag defines a page section that includes a few elements that help visitors navigate your site. These elements could be links to the main sections of the site, links to recently posted content, or a search feature. The `<nav>` section typically appears after the header, as shown here (and in Figure 1-18):

```
<body>
    <header>
        <img src="iis-logo.png" alt="Isn't it Semantic?
    company logo">
```

```
        <h1>Welcome to "Isn't it Semantic?"</h1>
        <hr>
    </header>
    <nav>
        <a href="/">Home</a>
        <a href="semantics.html">Semantics</a>
        <a href="contact.html">Contact</a>
        <a href="about.html">About</a>
    </nav>
    ...
</body>
```

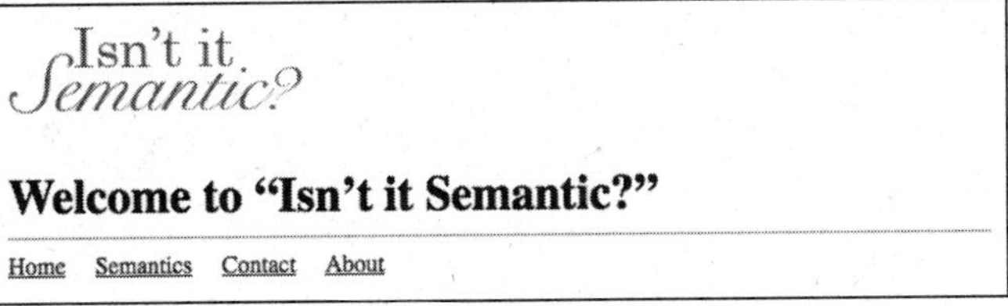

FIGURE 1-18: The <nav> section usually appears just after the <header> section.

The <main> tag

The `<main>` tag sets up a section to hold the content that is, in a sense, the point of the page. For example, if you're creating the page to tell everyone all that you know about Siamese Fighting Fish, then your Siamese Fighting Fish text, images, links, and so on would go into the `<main>` section.

The `<main>` section usually comes right after the `<head>` and `<nav>` sections:

```
<body>
    <header>
        ...
    </header>
    <nav>
        ...
    </nav>
    <main>
        Main content goes here
    </main>
    ...
</body>
```

Structuring the Page with HTML

The <article> tag

You use the `<article>` tag to create a page section that contains a complete composition of some sort: a blog post, an essay, a poem, a review, a diatribe, or a jeremiad.

In most cases, you'll have a single `<article>` tag nested inside your page's `<main>` section:

```
<body>
    <header>
        ...
    </header>
    <nav>
        ...
    </nav>
    <main>
        <article>
            Article content goes here
        </article>
    </main>
    ...
</body>
```

However, it isn't a hard and fast rule that your page can have only one `<article>` tag. In fact, it isn't a rule at all. If you want to have two compositions in your page — and thus two `<article>` sections within your `<main>` tag — be my guest.

The <section> tag

The `<section>` tag indicates a major part of page: usually a heading tag followed by some text. How do you know whether a chunk of the page is "major" or not? The easiest way is to imagine if your page had a table of contents. If you'd want a particular part of your page to be included in that table of contents, then it's major enough to merit the `<section>` tag.

Most of the time, your `<section>` tags will appear within an `<article>` tag:

```
<main>
    <article>

        <section>
            Section 1 heading goes here
            Section 1 text goes here
        </section>
```

```
        <section>
            Section 2 heading goes here
            Section 2 text goes here
        </section>
        ...
    </article>
</main>
```

The <aside> tag

You use the `<aside>` tag to cordon off a bit of the page for content that, although important or relevant for the site as a whole, is at best tangentially related to the page's `<main>` content. The `<aside>` is often a sidebar that includes site news or links to recent content, but it might also include links to other site pages that are related to current page.

The `<aside>` element most often appears within the `<main>` area, but after the `<article>` content.

```
<body>
    <header>
        ...
    </header>
    <nav>
        ...
    </nav>
    <main>
        <article>
            ...
        </article>
        <aside>
            ...
        </aside>
    </main>
    ...
</body>
```

The <footer> tag

You use the `<footer>` tag to create a *page footer,* which is typically a strip across the bottom of the page that includes elements such as a copyright notice, contact info, and social media links.

Since the footer almost always appears at the bottom of the page, the `<footer>` tag is usually seen right before the `</body>` tag, as shown here:

```
<body>
    <header>
        ...
    </header>
    <nav>
        ...
    </nav>
    <main>
        <article>
            ...
        </article>
        <aside>
            ...
        </aside>
    </main>
    <footer>
        ...
    </footer>
</body>
```

Handling non-semantic content with <div>

The `<header>`, `<nav>`, `<main>`, `<article>`, `<section>`, `<aside>`, and `<footer>` elements create meaningful structures within your page, which is why HTML nerds call these *semantic* elements. Even the humble `<p>` tag that I introduced earlier in this chapter is semantic in that it represents a single paragraph, usually within a `<section>` element.

But what's a would-be web weaver to do when she wants to add a chunk of content that just doesn't fit any of the standard semantic tags? That happens a lot, and the solution is to slap that content inside a `<div>` (for "division") element. The `<div>` tag is a generic container that doesn't represent anything meaningful, so it's the perfect place for any non-semantic stuff that needs a home:

```
<div>
    Non-semantic content goes right here
</div>
```

Here's an example:

```
<div>
    Requisite social media links:
</div>
<div>
    <a href="https://facebook.com/">Facebook</a>
    <a href="https://twitter.com/">Twitter</a>
    <a href="https://instagram.com/">Instagram</a>
    <a href="http://www.hbo.com/silicon-valley">Hooli</a>
</div>
```

Notice in Figure 1-19 that the browser renders the two `<div>` elements on separate lines.

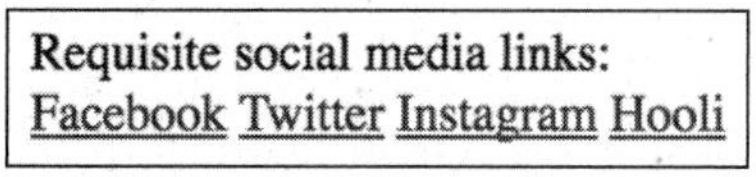

FIGURE 1-19: The browser renders each <div> section on a new line.

Requisite social media links:
Facebook Twitter Instagram Hooli

Handling words and characters with <span>

If you might want to do something with a small chunk of a larger piece of text, such as a phrase, a word, or even a character or three, then you need to turn to a so-called *inline element,* which creates a container that exists within some larger element and flows along with the rest of the content in that larger element.

The most common inline element to use is `<span>`, which creates a container around a bit of text:

```
<p>
Notice how an <span style="font-variant: small-caps">
inline element</span> flows right along with the
rest of the text.
</p>
```

What's happening here is that the <span> tag is applying a style called *small caps* to the text between <span> and </span> (`inline element`). As you can see in Figure 1-20, the <span> text flows along with the rest of the paragraph.

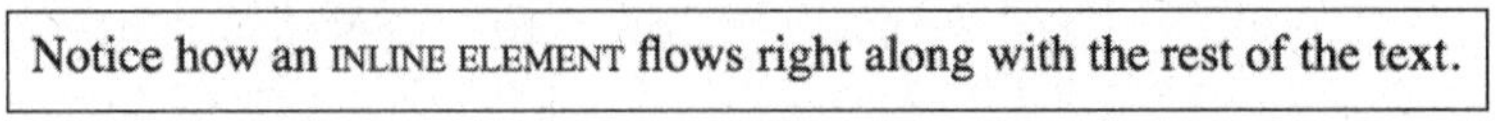

FIGURE 1-20: Using <span> makes the container flow with the surrounding text.

Notice how an INLINE ELEMENT flows right along with the rest of the text.

IN THIS CHAPTER

» Understanding cascading style sheets

» Learning the three methods you can use to add a style sheet

» Applying styles to web page elements

» Working with fonts and colors

» Taking advantage of classes and other style sheet timesavers

Chapter 2
Styling the Page with CSS

HTML elements enable Web-page designers to mark up a document's structure, but beyond trust and hope, you don't have any control over your text's appearance. CSS changes that. CSS puts the designer in the driver's seat.

— HÅKON WIUM LIE, THE "FATHER" OF CSS

One of the things that makes web coding with HTML so addictive is that you can slap up a page using a few basic tags and when you look at the result in the browser, it usually works pretty good. A work of art it's not, but it won't make your eyes sore. That basic functionality and appearance are baked in courtesy of the default formatting that all web browsers apply to various HTML elements. For example, `<strong>` text appears in a bold font, there's a bit of vertical space between `<p>` elements, and `<h1>` text shows up quite a bit larger than regular text.

The browsers' default formatting means that even a basic page looks reasonable, but I'm betting you're reading this book because you want to shoot for something more than reasonable. In this chapter, you discover that the secret to creating great-looking pages is to override the default browser formatting with your own. You explore custom styling and dig into specific styles for essentials such as fonts, alignment, and colors.

Figuring Out Cascading Style Sheets

If you want to control the look of your web pages, then the royal road to that goal is a web coding technology called *cascading style sheets*, or *CSS*. As I mention in Book 2, Chapter 1, your design goal should always be to separate structure and formatting when you build any web project. HTML's job is to take care of the structure part, but to handle the formatting of the page you must turn to CSS. Before getting to the specifics, I answer three simple questions: What's a style? What's a sheet? What's a cascade?

Styles: Bundles of formatting options

If you've ever used a fancy-schmancy word processor such as Microsoft Word, Google Docs, or Apple Pages, you've probably stumbled over a style or two in your travels. In a nutshell, a *style* is a combination of two or more formatting options rolled into one nice, neat package. For example, you might have a "Title" style that combines four formatting options: bold, centered, 24-point type size, and a Verdana typeface. You can then "apply" this style to any text and the program dutifully formats the text with all four options. If you change your mind later and decide your titles should use an 18-point font, all you have to do is redefine the Title style. The program then automatically trudges through the entire document and updates each bit of text that uses the Title style.

In a web page, a style performs a similar function. That is, it enables you to define a series of formatting options for a given page element, such as a tag like `<div>` or `<h1>`. Like word processor styles, web page styles offer two main advantages:

- They save time because you create the definition of the style's formatting once, and the browser applies that formatting each time you use the corresponding page element.
- They make your pages easier to modify because all you need to do is edit the style definition and all the places where the style is used within the page get updated automatically.

For example, Figure 2-1 shows some `<h1>` text as it appears with the web browser's default formatting. Figure 2-2 shows the same `<h1>` text, but now I've souped up the text with several styles, including a border, a font size of 72 pixels, the Verdana typeface, and page centering.

Sheets: Collections of styles

So far so good, but what the heck is a sheet? The term *style sheet* harkens back to the days of yore when old-timey publishing firms would keep track of their preferences for things like typefaces, type sizes, margins, and so on. All these so-called "house styles" were stored in a manual known as a *style sheet*. On the web, a style sheet is similar: It's a collection styles that you can apply to a web page.

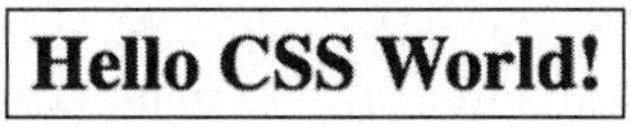

FIGURE 2-1: An <h1> heading that appears with the web browser's default formatting.

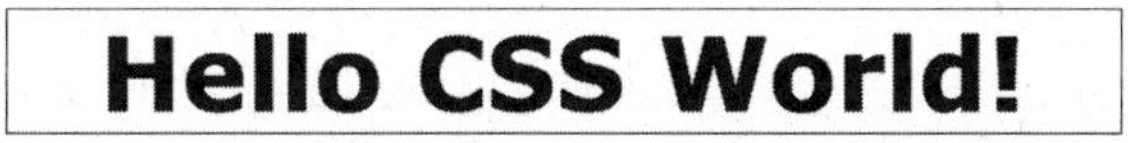

Hello CSS World!

FIGURE 2-2: The same text from Figure 2-1, except now with added styles.

Hello CSS World!

Cascading: How styles propagate

The "cascading" part of the name *cascading style sheets* is a bit technical, but it refers to a mechanism that's built into CSS for propagating styles between elements. For example, suppose you want all your page text to be blue instead of the default black. Does that mean you have to create a "display as blue" CSS instruction for every single text-related tag on your page? No, thank goodness! Instead, you apply it just once, to, say, the <body> tag, and CSS makes sure that every text tag in the <body> tag gets displayed as blue. This is called *cascading* a style.

Getting the Hang of CSS Rules and Declarations

Before I show you how to actually use CSS in your web pages, let's take a second to get a grip on just what a style looks like.

The simplest case is where a single formatting option is applied to an element. Here's the general syntax for this:

```
element {
    property: value;
}
```

Here, *element* is a reference to the web page doodad to which you want the style applied. This reference is often a tag name (such as h1 or div), but CSS has a powerful toolbox of ways you can reference things, which I discuss later in this chapter.

The *property* part is the name of the CSS property you want to apply. CSS offers a large collection of properties, each of which is a short, alphabetic keyword, such as font-family for the typeface, color for the text color, and border-width for the thickness of a border. The property name is followed by a colon (:), a space for readability, the *value* you want to assign to the property, and then a semicolon (;). This is known in the trade as a *CSS declaration* (although the description *property-value pair* is quite common, as well).

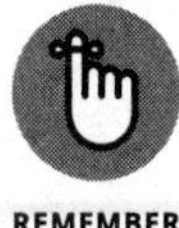
REMEMBER

Always enter the *property* name using lowercase letters. If the *value* includes any characters other than letters or a hyphen, then you need to surround the value with quotation marks.

Notice, too, that the declaration is surrounded by braces ({ and }). All the previous code — from the element name down to the closing brace (}) is called a *style rule*.

For example, the following rule applies a 72-pixel (indicated by the px unit) font size to the <h1> tag:

```
h1 {
    font-size: 72px;
}
```

Your style rules aren't restricted to just a single declaration: You're free to add as many as you need. The following example shows the rule I used to style the h1 element as shown earlier in Figure 2-2:

```
h1 {
    border-width: 1px;
    border-style: solid;
    border-color: black;
    font-size: 72px;
    font-family: Verdana;
    text-align: center;
}
```

REMEMBER

Note that the *declaration block* — that is, the part of the rule within the braces ({ and }) — is most easily read if you indent the declarations with a tab or with either two or four spaces. The order of the declarations isn't crucial; some developers use alphabetical order, whereas others group related properties together.

Besides applying multiple styles to a single element, it's also possible to apply a single style to multiple elements. You set up the style in the usual way, but instead of a single element at the beginning of the rule, you list all the elements that you want to style, separated by commas. In the following example, a yellow background color is applied to the `<header>`, `<aside>`, and `<footer>` tags:

```
header,
aside,
footer {
    background-color: yellow;
}
```

Adding Styles to a Page

With HTML tags, you just plop the tag where you want it to appear on the page, but styles aren't quite so straightforward. In fact, there are three main ways to get your web page styled: inline styles, internal style sheets, and external style sheets.

Inserting inline styles

An *inline style* is a style rule that you insert directly into whatever tag you want to format. Here's the general syntax to use:

```
<element style="property1: value1; property2: value2; ...">
```

That is, you add the `style` attribute to your tag, and then set it equal to one or more declarations, separated by semicolons.

For example, to apply 72-pixel type to an `<h1>` heading, you'd add an inline style that uses the `font-size` CSS property:

```
<h1 style="font-size: 72px;">
```

REMEMBER

Note that an inline style gets applied only to the tag within which it appears. Consider the following code:

```
<h1 style="font-size: 72px;">The Big Kahuna</h1>
<h1>Kahunas: Always Big?</h1>
<h1>Wait, What the Heck Is a Kahuna?</h1>
```

As you can see in Figure 2-3, the larger type size only gets applied to the first `<h1>` tag, whereas the other two `h1` elements appear in the browser's default size.

FIGURE 2-3: Only the top <h1> tag has the inline style, so only its text is styled at 72 pixels.

The Big Kahuna

Kahunas: Always Big?

Wait, What the Heck Is a Kahuna?

Embedding an internal style sheet

Inline styles are a useful tool, but because they get shoehorned inside tags, they tend to be difficult to maintain because they end up scattered all over the page's HTML code. You're also more likely to want a particular style rule applied to multiple page elements.

For easier maintenance of your styles, and to take advantage of the many ways that CSS offers to apply a single style rule to multiple page elements, you need to turn to style sheets, which can be either internal (as I discuss here) or external (as I discuss in the next section).

An *internal style sheet* is a style sheet that resides within the same file as the page's HTML code. Specifically, the style sheet is embedded between the `<style>` and `</style>` tags in the page's head section, like so:

```
<!DOCTYPE html>
<html lang="en">
    <head>
        <style>
            Your style rules go here
        </style>
    </head>
    <body>
...
```

Here's the general syntax to use:

```
<style>
    elementA {
        propertyA1: valueA1;
        propertyA2: valueA2;
        ...
    }
```

```
    elementB {
        propertyB1: valueB1;
        propertyB2: valueB2;
        ...
    }
    ...
</style>
```

As you can see, an internal style sheet consists of one or more style rules embedded within a <style> tag, which is why an internal style sheet is also sometimes called an *embedded style sheet.*

In the following code, I apply border styles to the h1 and h2 elements: solid and dotted, respectively. Figure 2-4 shows the result.

CSS:

```
<style>
    h1 {
        border-width: 2px;
        border-style: solid;
        border-color: black;
    }
    h2 {
        border-width: 2px;
        border-style: dotted;
        border-color: black;
    }
</style>
```

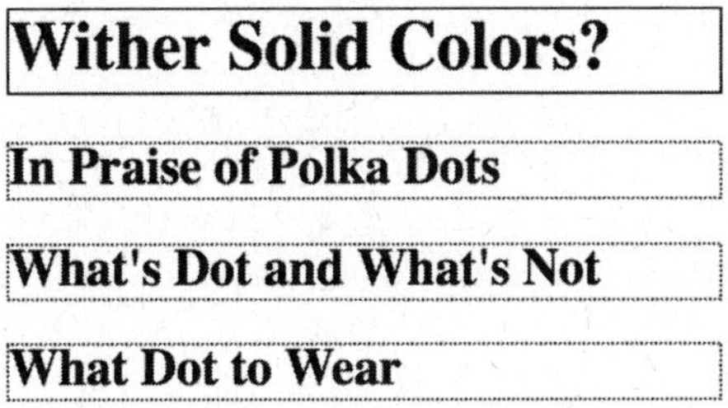

FIGURE 2-4: An internal style sheet that applies different border styles to the h1 (top) and h2 elements.

HTML:

```
<h1>Wither Solid Colors?</h1>
<h2>In Praise of Polka Dots</h2>
```

```
<h2>What's Dot and What's Not</h2>
<h2>What Dot to Wear</h2>
```

Note, in particular, that my single style rule for the h2 element gets applied to all the <h2> tags in the web page. That's the power of an internal style sheet: You only need a single rule to apply one or more styles to every instance of a particular element.

The internal style sheet method is best when you want to apply a particular set of style rules to just a single web page. If you have rules that you want applied to multiple pages, then you need to go the external style sheet route.

Linking to an external style sheet

Style sheets get insanely powerful when you use an *external style sheet*, which is a separate file that contains your style rules. To use these rules within any web page, you add a special <link> tag inside the page head. This tag specifies the name of the external style sheet file, and the browser then uses that file to grab the style rules.

Here are the steps you need to follow to set up an external style sheet:

1. **Use your favorite text editor to create a shiny new text file.**
2. **Add your style rules to this file.**

   Note that you don't need the <style> tag or any other HTML tags.
3. **Save the file.**

   It's traditional to save external style sheet files using a .css extension (for example, styles.css), which helps you remember down the road that this is a style sheet file. You can either save the file in the same folder as your HTML file, or you can create a subfolder (named, say, css or styles).
4. **For every page in which you want to use the styles, add a <link> tag inside the page's head section.**

   Here's the general format to use (where *filename*.css is the name of your external style sheet file):

   ```
   <link rel="stylesheet" href="filename.css">
   ```

   If you created a subfolder for your CSS files, be sure to add the subfolder to the href value (for example, href="styles/*filename*.css").

For example, suppose you create a style sheet file named styles.css, and that file includes the following style rules:

```
h1 {
    color: red;
}
p {
    font-size: 16px;
}
```

You then refer to that file by using the `<link>` tag, as shown here:

```
<!DOCTYPE html>
<html lang="en">
    <head>
        <link rel="stylesheet" href="styles.css">
    </head>
    <body>
        <h1>This Heading Will Appear Red</h1>
        <p>This text will be displayed in a 16-pixel font</p>
    </body>
</html>
```

Why is this so powerful? You can add the same `<link>` tag to any number of web pages and they'll all use the same style rules. This makes it a breeze to create a consistent look and feel for your site. And if you decide that your `<h1>` text should be green instead, all you have to do is edit the style sheet file (`styles.css`). Automatically, every single one of your pages that link to this file will be updated with the new style!

Styling Page Text

You'll spend the bulk of your CSS development time applying styles to your web page text. CSS offers a huge number of text properties, but those I show in Table 2-1 are the most common. I discuss each of these properties in more detail in the sections that follow.

Setting the type size

When it comes to the size of your page text, the CSS tool to pull out of the box is `font-size`:

```
font-size: value;
```

TABLE 2-1 Some Common CSS Text Properties

Property	Example	Description
`font-size`	`font-size: 16px;`	Sets the size of the text
`font-family`	`font-family: serif;`	Sets the typeface of the text
`font-weight`	`font-weight: bold;`	Sets whether the text uses a bold font
`font-style`	`font-style: italic;`	Sets whether the text uses an italic font
`text-decoration`	`text-decoration: underline;`	Applies (or removes) underline or strikethrough styles
`text-align`	`text-align: center;`	Aligns paragraph text horizontally
`text-indent`	`text-indent: 8px;`	Sets the size of the indent for the first line of a paragraph

Here, *`value`* is the size you want to apply to your element, which means a number followed by the unit you want to use. I discuss the units you can use in the next section, but for now we can stick with one of the most common units: pixels. The pixels unit is represented by the letters `px`, and a single pixel is equivalent to 1/96 of an inch. All browsers set a default size for regular text, and that default is usually `16px`. However, if you prefer that, say, all your paragraph (`<p>`) text get displayed at the `20px` size, then you'd include the following rule in your style sheet:

```
p {
    font-size: 20px;
}
```

Getting comfy with CSS measurement units

CSS offers a few measurement units that you need to know. You use these not only for setting type sizes, but also for setting the sizes of padding, borders, margins, shadows, and many other CSS properties. Table 2-2 lists the most common CSS measurement units.

Here are some notes about these units that I hope will decrease that furrow in your brow:

- An *absolute* measurement unit is one that has a fixed size: either 1/96 of an inch in the case of a pixel, or 1/72 of an inch in the case of a point.

TABLE 2-2 Some CSS Measurement Units

Unit	Name	Type	Equals
`px`	pixel	Absolute	1/96 of an inch
`pt`	point	Absolute	1/72 of an inch
`em`	em	Relative	The element's default, inherited, or defined font size
`rem`	root em	Relative	The font size of the root element of the web page
`vw`	viewport width	Relative	1/100 of the current width of the browser's content area
`vh`	viewport height	Relative	1/100 of the current height of the browser's content area

- A *relative* unit is one that doesn't have a fixed size. Instead, the size depends on whatever size is supplied to the element. For example, suppose the browser's default text size is `16px`, which is equivalent then to `1em`. If your page consists of a single `<article>` tag and you set the `article` element's `font-size` property to `1.5em`, then the browser will display text within the `<article>` tag at `24px` (since 16 times 1.5 equals 24). If, however, the browser user has configured her default text size to `20px`, then she'll see your `article` text displayed at `30px` (20 times 1.5 equals 30).
- The `em` unit can sometimes be a head-scratcher because it takes its value from whatever element it's contained within. For example, if your page has an `<article>` tag and you set the `article` element's `font-size` property to `1.5em`, then the browser will display text within the `<article>` tag at `24px` (assuming a `16px` default size). However, if within the `<article>` tag you have a `<section>` tag and you set the `section` element's `font-size` property to `1.25em`, then the browser will display text within the `<section>` tag at `30px` (since 24 times 1.25 equals 30).
- If you want more consistency in your text sizes, use `rem` instead of `em`, since `rem` is always based on the default font size defined by either the web browser or the user. For example, if your page uses a `16px` default size and it has an `<article>` tag with the `font-size` property set to `1.5rem`, then the browser will display text within the `<article>` tag at `24px`. If within the `<article>` tag you have a `<section>` tag and you set the `section` element's `font-size` property to `1.25rem`, then the browser will display text within the `<section>` tag at `20px` (since 16 times 1.25 equals 20).

Applying a font family

You can make a huge difference in the overall look and appeal of your web pages by paying attention to the typefaces you apply to your headings and body text.

A *typeface* is a particular design applied to all letters, numbers, symbols, and other characters. CSS types prefer the term *font family*, hence the property you use to set text in a specific typeface is named `font-family`:

```
font-family: value;
```

Here, `value` is the name of the typeface, which needs to be surrounded by quotation marks if the name contains spaces, numbers, or punctuation marks other than a hyphen (-). Feel free to list multiple typefaces, as long as you separate each with a comma. When you list two or more font families, the browser reads the list from left to right, and uses the first font that's available either on the user's system or in the browser itself.

When it comes to specifying font families, you have three choices:

- **Use a generic font.** This is a font that's implemented by the browser itself and set by using one of the following five keywords: `serif` (offers small cross strokes at the ends of each character), `sans-serif` (doesn't use the cross strokes), `cursive` (looks like handwriting), `fantasy` (a decorative font), or `monospace` (gives equal space to each character). Figure 2-5 shows each of these generic fonts in action.

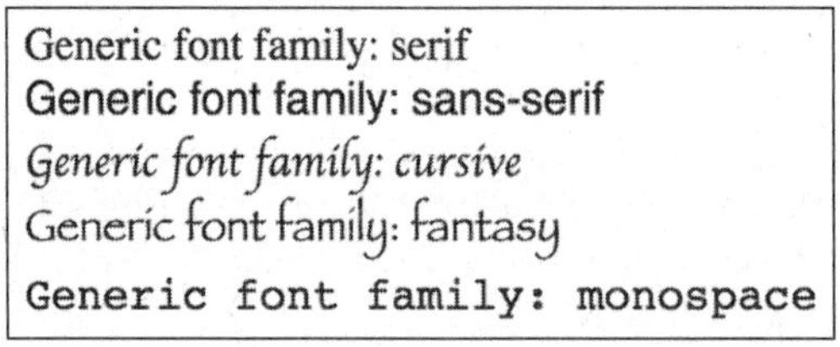

Generic font family: serif
Generic font family: sans-serif
Generic font family: cursive
Generic font family: fantasy
Generic font family: monospace

FIGURE 2-5: Generic fonts are implemented by all web browsers and come in five flavors: `serif`, `sans-serif`, `cursive`, `fantasy`, and `monospace`.

- **Use a system font.** This is a typeface that's installed on the user's computer. How can you possibly know that? You don't. Instead, you have two choices. One possibility is to use a system font that's installed universally. Examples include Georgia and Times New Roman (serifs), Verdana and Tahoma (sans serifs), and Courier New (monospace). The other way to go is to list several system fonts, knowing that the browser will use the first one that's implemented on the user's PC. Here's a sans-serif example:

  ```
  font-family: "Gill Sans", Calibri, Verdana, sans-serif;
  ```

» **Use a Google font.** Google Fonts offers access to hundreds of free and well-crafted fonts that you can use on your site. Go to `https://fonts.google.com`, find a font you like, then click the plus sign (+) beside it. Click "1 Family Selected" and then use the Customize tab to add styles such as bold and italic. In the Embed tab, copy the `<link>` tag and then paste it in your HTML file, somewhere in the <head> section (before your `<style>` tag, if you're using an internal style sheet, or before your CSS `<link>` tag, if you're using an external style sheet). Go back to the Embed tab, copy the `font-family` rule, and then paste that rule into your CSS.

Making text bold

In Book 2, Chapter 1, I talk about how the `<strong>` and `<b>` tags have semantic definitions (important text and keywords, respectively), but you'll often come across situations where you want text to appear bold, but that text isn't important or a keyword. In that case, you can style the text the CSS way with the `font-weight` property:

```
font-weight: value;
```

Here, *`value`* is either the word `bold`, or one of the numbers `100`, `200`, `300`, `400`, `500`, `600`, `700` (this is the same as using `bold`), `800`, and `900`, where the higher numbers give bolder text and the lower numbers give lighter text; `400` is regular text, which you can also specify using the word `normal`. Note, however, that depending on the typeface you're using, not all of these values will give you bolder or lighter text.

Styling text with italics

In Book 2, Chapter 1, I mention that the `<em>` and `<i>` tags have semantic significance (emphasis and alternative text, respectively), but you might have text that should get rendered in italics, but not with emphasis or as alternative text. No problem: Get CSS on the job by adding the `font-style` property to your rule:

```
font-style: italic;
```

Styling links

When you add a link to the page, the web browser displays the link text in a different color (usually blue) and underlined. This might not fit at all with the rest of your page design, so go ahead and adjust the link styling as needed.

You can apply any text style to a link, including changing the font size, the typeface, adding bold or italics, and changing the color (which I discuss later in this chapter).

One common question web coders ask is "Links: underline or not?" Not everyone is a fan of underlined text, and if you fall into that camp, then you can use the following rule to remove the underline from your links:

```
a {
    text-decoration: none;
}
```

WARNING

Creating a custom style for links is standard operating procedure for web developers, but a bit of caution is in order because a mistake made by many new web designers it to style links too much like regular text (particularly when they've removed underlining from their links). Your site visitors should be able to recognize a link from ten paces, so be sure to make your links stick out from the regular text in some way.

Aligning paragraph text

By default, your web page paragraphs line up nice and neat along the left margin of the page. Nothing wrong with that, but what if you want things to align along the right margin, instead? Or perhaps you want to center something on the page. Wouldn't that be nice? You can do all that and more by pulling out the `text-align` property:

```
text-align: left|right|center|justify;
```

In case you're wondering, the `justify` value tells the web browser to align the element's text on both the left and right margin.

Indenting a paragraph's first line

You can signal the reader that a new paragraph is being launched by indenting the first line a bit from the left margin. This is easier done than said with CSS by applying the `text-indent` property:

```
text-indent: value;
```

Here, *value* is a number followed by any of the CSS measurement units I mention earlier in this chapter. For example, a common indent value is 1em, which here I've applied to the p element:

```
p {
    text-indent: 1em;
}
```

Working with Colors

When rendering the page using their default styles, browsers don't do much with colors, other than showing link text a default and familiar blue. But CSS offers some powerful color tools, so there's no reason not to show the world your true colors.

Specifying a color

I begin by showing you the three main ways that CSS provides for specifying the color you want:

- **Use a color keyword.** CSS defines a bit more than 140 color keywords. Some of these are straightforward, such as red, yellow, and purple, while others are, well, a bit whimsical (and hunger-inducing): lemonchiffon, papayawhip, and peachpuff. The Web Coding Playground (wcpg.io/dummies/2-2-14) lists them all, as shown in Figure 2-6.

Color	Keyword	RGB Value
	lightpink	#ffb6c1
	pink	#ffc0cb
	crimson	#dc143c
	lavenderblush	#fff0f5
	palevioletred	#db7093
	hotpink	#ff69b4
	deeppink	#ff1493
	mediumvioletred	#c71585
	orchid	#da70d6

FIGURE 2-6: Go to the Web Coding Playground to see a full list of the CSS color keywords.

- **Use the `rgb()` function.** `rgb()` is a built-in CSS function that takes three values: one for red, one for green, and one for blue (separated by commas). Each of these can be a value between 0 and 255, and these combinations can produce any of the 16 million or so colors on the spectrum. For example, the following function produces a nice red:

  ```
  rgb(255, 99, 71)
  ```

- **Use an RGB code.** An *RGB code* is a six-digit value that takes the form `#rrggbb`, where `rr` is a two-digit value that specifies the red component of the color, *gg* is a two-digit value that specifies the green component, and *bb* is a two-digit value that specifies the blue component. Alas, these two-digit values are hexadecimal — base 16 — numbers, which run from 0 to 9 and then a to f. As two-digit values, the decimal values 0 through 255 are represented as 00 through ff in hexadecimal. For example, the following RGB code produces the same red as in the previous example:

  ```
  #ff6347
  ```

Coloring text

To apply a CSS color to some text, you use the `color` property:

```
color: value;
```

Here, *`value`* can be a color keyword, an `rgb()` function, or an RGB code. The following three rules produce the same color text:

```
color: tomato;
color: rgb(255, 99, 71);
color: #ff6347;
```

Coloring the background

For some extra page pizazz, try adding a color to the background of either the entire page or a particular element. You do this in CSS by using the `background-color` property:

```
background-color: value;
```

Here, *`value`* can be a color keyword, an `rgb()` function, or an RGB code. The following example displays the page with white text on a black background:

```
body {
    color: rgb(255,255,255);
    background-color: rgb(0,0,0);
}
```

WARNING

When you're messing around with text and background colors, make sure you leave enough contrast between the text and background to ensure that your page visitors can still read the text without shaking their fists at you. But I should also warn you that too much contrast isn't conducive to easy reading, either. For example, using pure white for text and pure black for a background (as I did in the preceding code, tsk, tsk) isn't great because there's too much contrast. Darkening the text a shade and lightening the background a notch makes all the difference:

```
body {
    color: rgb(222,222,222);
    background-color: rgb(32,32,32);
}
```

Getting to Know the Web Page Family

One of the prerequisites for becoming a web developer is understanding both the structure of a typical web page and the odd (at least at first) lingo associated with that structure. As an example, I'm going to refer to the semantic HTML elements that I demonstrate in Book 2, Chapter 1 (in Figure 1-16, in particular). Figure 2-7 shows that semantic structure as a tree diagram:

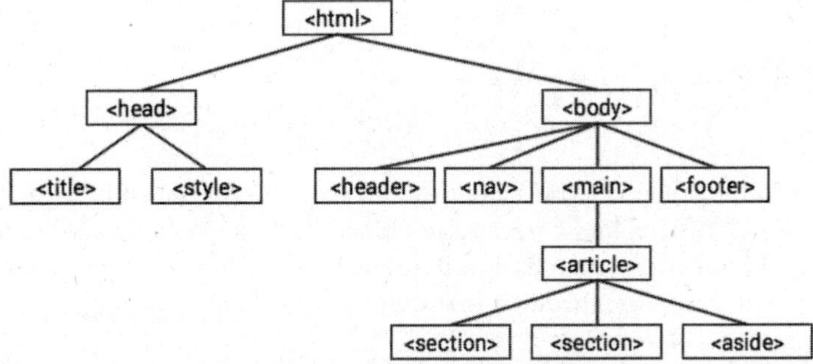

FIGURE 2-7: The structure of a semantic HTML web page.

As you can see, the tree has the `<html>` tag at the top. The second level consists of the `<head>` tag and the `<body>` tag, and the `<head>` tag leads to a third level that consists of the `<title>` and `<style>` tags. For the `<body>` tag, the third level contains four tags: <header>, <nav>, <main>, and <footer>. The <main> tag leads to the <article> tag, which contains two <section> tags and an <aside> tag.

Okay, I can see the "So what?" thought bubble over your head, so I'll get to the heart of the matter. With this structure in mind, you can now identify and define four useful members of the web page family tree:

- **Parent:** An element that contains one or more other elements in the level below it. For example, in Figure 2-7, the <html> tag is the parent of the <head> and <body> tags, whereas the <head> tag is the parent of the <title> and <style> tags.
- **Child:** An element that is contained within another element that sits one level above it in the tree. (Which is another way of saying that the element has a parent.) In Figure 2-7, the <header>, <nav>, <main>, and <footer> tags are children of the <body> tag, whereas the two <section> tags and the <aside> tag are children of the <article> tag.
- **Ancestor:** An element that contains one or more levels of elements. In Figure 2-7, the <body> tag is an ancestor of the <aside> tag, whereas the <html> tag is an ancestor of everything in the page.
- **Descendant:** An element that is contained within another element that sits one or more levels above it in the tree. In Figure 2-7, the <section> tags are descendants of the <main> tag, whereas the <article> tag is a descendant of the <body> tag.

This no doubt seems far removed from web development, but these ideas play a crucial role not only in CSS, but also JavaScript (see Book 3) and jQuery (see Book 4).

Using CSS Selectors

When you add a CSS rule to an internal or external style sheet, you assemble your declarations into a declaration block (that is, you surround them with the { and } thingies) and then assign that block to an element of the page. For example, the following rule throws a few styles at the page's <h1> tags:

```
h1 {
    font-size: 72px;
    font-family: Verdana;
    text-align: center;
}
```

But the element you assign to the declaration block doesn't have to be an HTML tag name. In fact, CSS has a huge number of ways to define what parts of the page you want to style. These methods for defining what to style are called *selectors* (because you use them to "select" those parts of the page you want styled). When you use a tag name, you're specifying a *type selector*. However, there are many more — a few dozen, in fact — but lucky for you, only four should cover most of your web development needs:

- The class selector
- The id selector
- The descendant selector
- The child selector

The class selector

If you master just one CSS selector, make it the class selector, because you'll use it time and again in your web projects. A *class selector* is one that targets its styles at a particular web page class. So, what's a class? I'm glad you asked. A *class* is an attribute assigned to one or more page tags that enables you to create a kind of grouping for those tags. Here's the syntax for adding a class to an element:

```
<element class="class-name">
```

Replace `element` with the tag and replace `class-name` with the name you want to assign. The name must begin with a letter and the rest can be any combination of letters, numbers, hyphens (`-`), and underscores (`_`). Here's an example:

```
<div class="caption">
```

With your classes assigned to your tags as needed, you're ready to start selecting those classes using CSS. You do that by preceding the class name with a dot (`.`) in your style rule:

```
.class-name {
    property1: value1;
    property2: value2;
    ...
}
```

For example, here's a rule for the `caption` class:

```
.caption {
    font-size: .75rem;
    font-style: italic;
}
```

The advantage here is that you can assign the `caption` class to any tag on the page, and CSS will apply the same style rule to each of those elements.

The id selector

In Book 2, Chapter 1, I talk about creating an anchor by adding a unique `id` attribute to a tag, which enabled you to create a link that targeted the anchor:

```
<element id="id-name">
```

Here's an example:

```
<h2 id="subtitle">
```

You can also use the `id` attribute as a CSS selector, which enables you to target a particular element with extreme precision. You set this up by preceding the `id` value with a hashtag symbol (#) in your CSS rule:

```
#id-name {
    property1: value1;
    property2: value2;
    ...
}
```

For example, here's a rule for the `subtitle` id:

```
#subtitle {
    font-size: 2rem;
    font-style: italic;
    color: blue;
}
```

This isn't as useful as the class selector because it can only target a single element, which is why web developers use id selectors only rarely.

The descendant selector

Rather than targeting specific tags, classes, or ids, you might need to target every instance of a particular element that is contained within another element. Those contained elements are called *descendants*, and CSS offers the *descendant selector* for applying styles to them. To set up a descendant selector, you include in your rule the ancestor and the descendant type you want to style, separated by a space:

```
ancestor descendant {
    property1: value1;
    property2: value2;
    ...
}
```

For example, here's a rule that applies a few styles to every `<a>` tag that's contained with an `<aside>` tag:

```
aside a {
    color: red;
    font-style: italic;
    text-decoration: none;
}
```

The child selector

The descendant selector that I discuss in the previous section is one of the most powerful in the CSS kingdom because it targets all the descendants of a particular type that reside within an ancestor, no matter how many levels down the page hierarchy those descendants live. However, it's often more suitable and more manageable to target only those descendants that reside one level down: in short, the children of some parent element.

To aim some styles at the child elements of a parent, you use the CSS *child selector*, where you separate the parent and child elements with a greater-than sign (`>`):

```
parent > child {
    property1: value1;
    property2: value2;
    ...
}
```

For example, here's a rule that targets the links that are the immediate children of an `<aside>` tag:

```
aside > a {
    color: green;
    font-style: bold;
    text-decoration: none;
}
```

Revisiting the Cascade

I close this first CSS chapter with a quick look at three important concepts that you need to drill into your brain if you want to write good CSS and troubleshoot the inevitable CSS problems that will crop up in your web development career:

- **Inheritance:** If a parent element is styled with a property, in many cases its child and descendant elements will also be styled with the same property. This is known in the CSS game as *inheritance*: Parents "pass along" some of their properties to their children and descendants. Notice, however, that I said "some" properties are inherited. Lots of properties — such as the padding, borders, and margins I cover in Book 2, Chapter 3 — don't get inherited, so you need to watch out for inheritance (or its lack) as you code your pages.
- **Weight:** The different ways that you can specify styles for a page have a built-in hierarchy of importance, or *weight* in CSS-speak. Here's that style source hierarchy in ascending order of weight:

  1. Browser styles — The list of default styles that the web browser applies to certain HTML tags. This is known officially as the *user agent style sheet*.
  2. User-specified styles — The styles that the web browser user has configured, such as a new default type size. This is known to CSS pros as a *user style sheet*.
  3. External style sheets.
  4. Internal style sheets.
  5. Inline styles.

  What this means is that if a web browser comes across the same style property in two or more style sources, it uses the property value from the source that has the greater weight. For example, if you set `font-size: 1.5rem` in an external style sheet and then set `font-size: 2rem` with an inline style, the inline style "wins" because it has a greater weight than the external style sheet.

» **Specificity:** What happens when two or more style rules from the same source target the same element? You can't go by weight since they all reside in the same style source, so you have to turn to a concept called *specificity*, instead. This is a score given to each style rule, where the browser implements the rule that garners the highest specificity value. Here's how the browser determines the specificity for a rule:

1. Add one point for each element (such as `div` or span) in the rule's selector.
2. Add 10 points for each class in the selector.
3. Add 100 points for each ID in the selector.
4. If the selector is part of an inline style, add 1,000 points.

In practice, you can use specificity to figure out why a particular element has styles that don't seem right. Quite often, the problem turns out to be that the browser is applying some other style rule that has a higher specificity.

» Setting the sizes of page elements

» Encrusting elements with padding, borders, and margins

» Letting elements float where they may

» Positioning elements exactly where you want them

Chapter 3
Sizing and Positioning Page Elements

Every element in web design is a rectangular box. This was my ah-ha moment that helped me really start to understand CSS-based web design and accomplish the layouts I wanted to accomplish.

— CHRIS COYIER

I'm not going to lie to you: When you're just getting started with CSS, the elements on the page will sometimes seem to defy your every command. Like surly teenagers, they ignore your best advice and refuse to understand that you are — or you are supposed to be — the boss of them. Okay, I did lie to you a little: That can happen to even the most experienced web coders. Why the attitude? Because although web browsers are fine pieces of software for getting around the web, by default they're not very adept at laying out a web page. Like overly permissive grandparents, they just let the page elements do whatever they like. Your job as a parent, er, I mean, a web developer, is to introduce some discipline to the page.

Fortunately, CSS comes with a huge number of tools and techniques that you can wield to make stubborn page elements behave themselves. In this chapter, you discover many of these tools and you explore how best to use them to gain mastery of anything you care to add to a web page. You delve into styles that cover properties such as dimensions (the height and width of things), padding and margins (the amount of space around things), borders (lines around things), and position (where things appear on the page).

Learning about the CSS Box Model

Everything in this chapter is based on something called the CSS *box model*. So I begin by discussing what this box model thing is all about and why it's important.

Every web page consists of a series of HTML tags, and each of those tags represents an element on the page. In the strange and geeky world known as Style Sheet Land, each of these elements is considered to have an invisible box around it (okay, it's a very strange world). You might be tempted to think that this invisible box only surrounds block-level elements, which are those elements that start new sections of text: `<p>`, `<blockquote>`, `<h1>` through `<h6>`, `<div>`, all the page layout semantic tags, such as `<header>`, `<article>`, and `<section>`, and so on. That makes sense, but in fact every single tag, even inline elements such as `<a>` and `<span>`, have a box around them.

This box has the following components:

- **Content:** The stuff inside the box (the text, the images, and so on)
- **Padding:** The space around the content
- **Border:** A line that surrounds the box padding
- **Margin:** The space outside of the border separating the box from other boxes to the left and right, as well as above and below
- **Dimensions:** The height and width of the box
- **Position:** The location of the box within the page

Of these, the first four — the content, padding, border, and margin — comprise the box model, and they're illustrated in Figure 3-1.

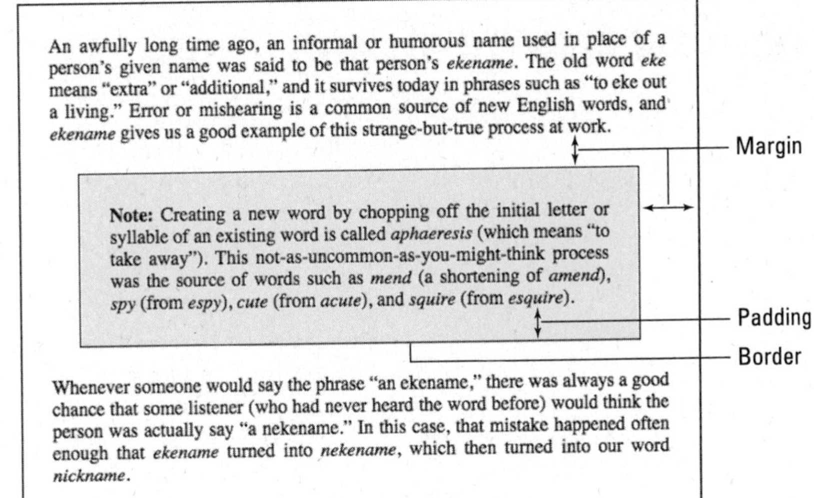

FIGURE 3-1: The components of the CSS box model.

Styling Sizes

When the web browser renders a page, it examines each element and sets the dimensions of that element. For block-level elements such as `<header>` and `<div>`, the browser sets the dimensions as follows:

- **Width:** Set to the width of the element's parent. Because by default the width of the <body> element is set to the width of the browser's content area, in practice all block-level elements have their widths set to the width of the content area.
- **Height:** Set just high enough to hold all the element's content.

You can (and should) run roughshod over these defaults by styling the element's width and height properties:

```
width: value;
height: value;
```

In both cases, you replace *`value`* with a number and one of the CSS measurement units I talk about in Book 2, Chapter 2: `px`, `em`, `rem`, `vw`, or `vh`. For example, if you want your page to take up only half the width of the browser's content area, you'd use the following rule:

```
body {
    width: 50vw;
}
```

TECHNICAL STUFF

MAKING WIDTH AND HEIGHT MAKE SENSE

Width and height seem like such straightforward concepts, but you might as well learn now that CSS has a knack for turning the straightforward into the crooked-sideways. A block element's dimensions are a case in point, because you'd think the "size" of a block element would be the size of its box out to the border: that is, the content, plus the padding, plus the border itself. Nope. By default, the size of a block element's box is just the content part of the box.

That may not sound like a cause for alarm, but it does mean that when you're working with an element's dimensions, you have to take into account its padding widths and border sizes if you want to get things right. Believe me, that is no picnic. Fortunately, help is just around the corner. You can avoid all those extra calculations by forcing the web browser to be sensible and define an element's size to include not just the content, but the padding and border, as well. A CSS property called `box-sizing` is the superhero here:

```
element {
    box-sizing: border-box;
}
```

The declaration `box-sizing: border-box` tells the browser to set the element's height and width to include the content, padding, and border. You could add this declaration to all your block-level element rules, but that's way too much work. Instead, you can use a trick where you use an asterisk (`*`) "element," which is a shorthand way of referencing every element on the page:

```
* {
    box-sizing: border-box;
}
```

Put this at the top of your style sheet, and then you never have to worry about it again.

Most of the time you'll only mess with an element's width, because getting the height right is notoriously difficult because it depends on too many factors: the content, the browser's window size, the user's default font size, and more.

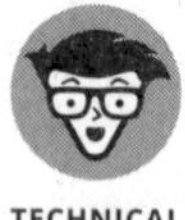

TECHNICAL STUFF

Height and width apply only to block-level elements such as `<article>`, `<div>`, and `<p>`, and not to inline elements such as `<span>` and `<a>`. However, it's possible to convert inline elements into blocks. CSS offers two methods for this inline-to-block makeover:

» **Make it an inline block.** If you want to set an inline element's width, height, or other block-related properties, but still allow the element to flow along with the surrounding text, add the following to the element's CSS rule:

```
display: inline-block;
```

» **Make it a true block.** If you want to set an inline element's block-related properties and you no longer want the element to flow with the surrounding text, turn it into an honest-to-goodness block-level element by adding the following to the element's CSS rule:

```
display: block;
```


Adding Padding

In the CSS box model, the *padding* is the space that surrounds the content out to the border, if the box has one. Your web pages should always have lots of whitespace (that is, blank, content-free chunks of the page), and one way to do that is to give each element generous padding to ensure the element's content isn't crowded either by its border or by surrounding elements.

There are four sections to the padding — above, to the right of, below, and to the left of the content — so CSS offers four corresponding properties for adding padding to an element:

```
element {
    padding-top: top-value;
    padding-right: right-value;
    padding-bottom: bottom-value;
    padding-left: left-value;
}
```

Each value is a number followed by a CSS measurement unit: `px`, `em`, `rem`, `vw`, or `vh`. Here's an example:

```
.margin-note {
    padding-top: 1rem;
    padding-right: 1.5rem;
    padding-bottom: .5rem;
    padding-left: 1.25rem;
}
```

CSS also offers a shorthand syntax that uses the `padding` property. There are four different syntaxes you can use with the `padding` property, and they're all listed in Table 3-1.

TABLE 3-1 **The `padding` Shorthand Property**

Syntax	Description
`padding:` *`value1`*`;`	Applies *value1* to all four sides
`padding:` *`value1 value2`*`;`	Applies *value1* to the top and bottom and *value2* to the right and left
`padding:` *`value1 value2 value3`*`;`	Applies *value1* to the top, *value2* to the right and left, and *value3* to the bottom
`padding:` *`value1 value2 value3 value4`*`;`	Applies *value1* to the top, *value2* to the right, *value3* to the bottom, and *value4* to the left

Here's how you'd rewrite the previous example using the `padding` shorthand:

```
.margin-note {
    padding: 1rem 1.5rem .5rem 1.25rem;
}
```

To illustrate what a difference padding can make in your page designs, take a peek at Figure 3-2. Here you see two <aside> elements, where the one on top looks cramped and uninviting, whereas the one on the bottom offers ample room for reading. These two elements are styled identically, except the one on the bottom has its padding set with the following declaration:

```
padding: 1rem;
```

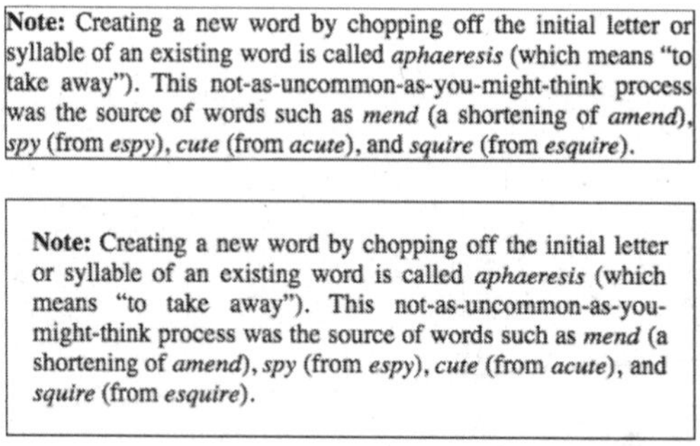

Note: Creating a new word by chopping off the initial letter or syllable of an existing word is called *aphaeresis* (which means "to take away"). This not-as-uncommon-as-you-might-think process was the source of words such as *mend* (a shortening of *amend*), *spy* (from *espy*), *cute* (from *acute*), and *squire* (from *esquire*).

Note: Creating a new word by chopping off the initial letter or syllable of an existing word is called *aphaeresis* (which means "to take away"). This not-as-uncommon-as-you-might-think process was the source of words such as *mend* (a shortening of *amend*), *spy* (from *espy*), *cute* (from *acute*), and *squire* (from *esquire*).

FIGURE 3-2: Without padding (top), your text can look uncomfortably crowded by its surroundings, but when you add padding (bottom), the same text has room to breathe.

Building Borders

Modern web design eschews vertical and horizontal lines as a means of separating content, preferring, instead, to let copious amounts of whitespace do the job. However, that doesn't mean you should never use lines in your designs, particularly borders. An element's *border* is the notional set of lines that enclose the element's content and padding. Borders are an often useful way to make it clear that an element is separate from the surrounding elements in the page.

There are four lines associated with an element's border — above, to the right of, below, and to the left of the padding — so CSS offers four properties for adding borders to an element:

```
element {
    border-top: top-width top-style top-color;
    border-right: right-width right-style right-color;
    border-bottom: bottom-width bottom-style bottom-color;
    border-left: left-width left-style left-color;
}
```

As you can see, each border requires three values:

- **Width:** The thickness of the border line, which you specify using a number followed by a CSS measurement unit: `px`, `em`, `rem`, `vw`, or `vh`. Note, however, that most border widths are measured in pixels, usually `1px`. You can also specify one of the following keywords: `thin`, `medium`, or `thick`.
- **Style:** The type of border line, which must be one of the following keywords: `dotted`, `dashed`, `solid`, `double`, `groove`, `ridge`, `inset`, or `outset`.
- **Color:** The color of the border line. You can use a color keyword, an `rgb()` function, or an RGB code, as I describe in Book 2, Chapter 2.

Here's an example that adds a 1-pixel, dashed, red bottom border to the `header` element:

```
header {
    border-bottom: 1px dashed red;
}
```

If you want to add a full border around an element and you want all four sides to use the same width, style, and color, CSS mercifully offers a shorthand version that uses the `border` property:

```
border: width style color;
```

Here's the declaration I used to add the borders around the elements you see in Figure 3-2:

```
border: 1px solid black;
```

Making Margins

The final component of the CSS box model is the *margin*, which is the space around the border of the box. Margins are an important detail in web design because they prevent elements from rubbing up against the edges of the browser content area, ensure two elements don't overlap each other, and create separation between elements.

As with padding, there are four sections to the margin — above, to the right of, below, and to the left of the border — so CSS offers four corresponding properties for adding margins to an element:

```
element {
    margin-top: top-value;
    margin-right: right-value;
    margin-bottom: bottom-value;
    margin-left: left-value;
}
```

Each value is a number followed by one of the standard CSS measurement units: `px`, `em`, `rem`, `vw`, or `vh`. Here's an example:

```
aside {
    margin-top: 1rem;
    margin-right: .5rem;
    margin-bottom: 2rem;
    margin-left: 1.5rem;
}
```

Like padding, CSS also offers a shorthand syntax that uses the `margin` property. Table 3-2 lists the four syntaxes you can use with the `margin` property.

Here's the shorthand version of the previous example:

```
aside {
    margin: 1rem .5rem 2rem 1.5rem;
}
```

TABLE 3-2 The `margin` Shorthand Property

Syntax	Description
`margin: value1;`	Applies *value1* to all four sides
`margin: value1 value2;`	Applies *value1* to the top and bottom and *value2* to the right and left
`margin: value1 value2 value3;`	Applies *value1* to the top, *value2* to the right and left, and *value3* to the bottom
`margin: value1 value2 value3 value4;`	Applies *value1* to the top, *value2* to the right, *value3* to the bottom, and *value4* to the left

Resetting the padding and margin

If you see a web developer pulling her hair or gnashing her teeth, it's a good bet that she's battling the web browser's default styles for padding and margins. These defaults are one of the biggest sources of frustration for web coders because they force you to relinquish control over one of the most important aspects of web design: the whitespace on the page.

Most modern web developers have learned not to fight against these defaults, but to eliminate them entirely by resetting everything to zero by adding the following rule to the top of every style sheet they build:

```
* {
    margin: 0;
    padding: 0;
}
```

The downside is that you must now specify the margins and padding for all your page elements yourself, but that extra work is really a blessing in disguise because now you have complete control over the whitespace in your page.

Collapsing margins ahead!

CSS has no shortage of eccentricities, and you'll come across most of them in your web development career. Here's a look at one of the odder things that CSS does. First, here's some HTML and CSS code to chew over:

CSS:

```
nav {
    margin-top: .5rem;
```

```
    padding: .75rem;
    border: 1px solid black;
}
```

HTML:

```
<header>
    <img src="/images/notw.png" alt="News of the Word logo">
    <h1>News of the Word</h1>
    <h3>Language news you won't find anywhere else (for good
  reason!)</h3>
</header>
<nav>
    <a href="#">Home</a>
    <a href="#">What's New</a>
    <a href="#">What's Old</a>
    <a href="#">What's What</a>
</nav>
```

I'd like to draw your attention in particular to the `margin-top: .5rem` declaration in the `nav` element's CSS rule. In Figure 3-3, you can see that, sure enough, the browser has rendered a small margin above the `nav` element.

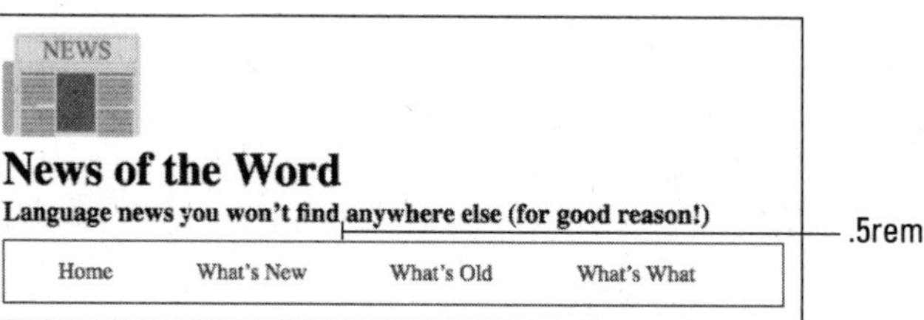

FIGURE 3-3: The nav element (with the border) has a .5rem top border.

Suppose now I decide that I want a bit more space between the `header` and the `nav` elements, so I add a bottom margin to the `header`:

```
header {
    margin-bottom: .5rem;
}
```

Figure 3-4 shows the result.

No, you're not hallucinating: The space between the `header` and `nav` elements didn't change one iota! Welcome to the wacky world of CSS! In this case, the wackiness comes courtesy of a CSS "feature" called *collapsing margins*. When one element's bottom margin butts up against another element's top margin, common sense would dictate that the web browser would add the two margin values together. Hah, you wish! Instead, the browser uses the larger of the two margin values and it throws out the smaller value. That is, it "collapses" the two margin values into a single value.

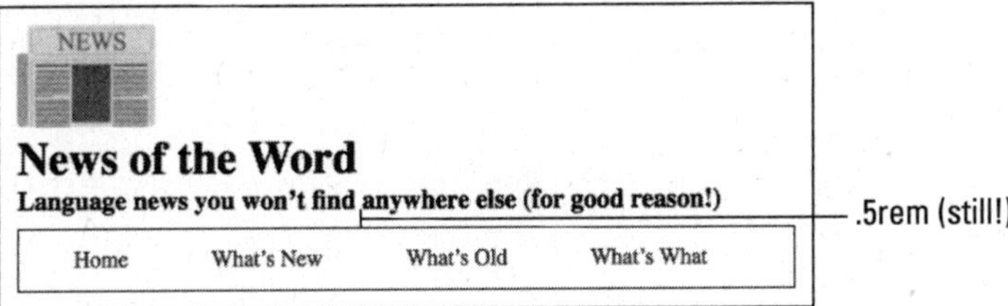

FIGURE 3-4: The header element with a bottom margin added (with the border) has a .5rem top border.

Sizing and Positioning Page Elements

So, does that mean you're stuck? Not at all. To get some extra vertical space between two elements, you have four choices:

- Increase the `margin-top` value of the bottom element.
- Increase the `margin-bottom` value of the top element.
- If you already have `margin-top` defined on the bottom element, and the top element doesn't use a border, add a `padding-bottom` value to the top element.
- If you already have `margin-bottom` defined on the top element, and the bottom element doesn't use a border, add a `padding-top` value to the bottom element.

In the last two bullets, combining a top or bottom margin on one element with a bottom or top padding on the other element works because the browser doesn't collapse a margin/padding combo.

Getting a Grip on Page Flow

When a web browser renders a web page, one of the really boring things it does is lay out the tags by applying the following rules to each element type:

- **Inline elements:** Rendered from left to right within each element's parent container
- **Block-level elements:** Stacked on top of each other, with the first element at the top of the page, the second element below the first, and so on

This is called the *page flow*. For example, consider the following HTML code:

```
<header>
    The page header goes here.
</header>
<nav>
    The navigation doodads go here.
</nav>
<section>
    This is the first section of the page.
</section>
<section>
    This is—you got it—the second section of the page.
</section>
<aside>
    This is the witty or oh-so-interesting aside.
</aside>
<footer>
    The page footer goes here.
</footer>
```

This code is a collection of six block-level elements — a `header`, a `nav`, two `section` tags, an `aside`, and a `footer` — and Figure 3-5 shows how the web browser renders them as a stack of boxes.

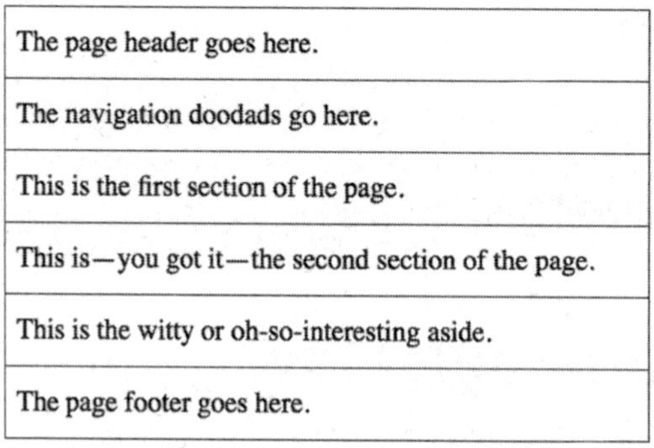

The page header goes here.
The navigation doodads go here.
This is the first section of the page.
This is—you got it—the second section of the page.
This is the witty or oh-so-interesting aside.
The page footer goes here.

FIGURE 3-5: The web browser renders the block-level elements as a stack of boxes.

There's nothing inherently wrong with the default page flow, but having your web page render as a stack of boxes lacks a certain flair. Fortunately for your creative spirit, you're not married to the default, one-box-piled-on-another flow. CSS gives you two useful methods for breaking out of the normal page flow and giving your pages some pizzazz: floating and positioning.

Floating Elements

When you *float* an element, the web browser takes the element out of the default page flow. Where the element ends up on the page depends on whether you float it to the left or to the right:

- **Float left:** The browser places the element as far to the left and as high as possible within the element's parent container.
- **Float right:** The browser places the element as far to the right and as high as possible within the element's parent container.

In both cases, the non-floated elements flow around the floated element.

You convince the web browser to float an element by adding the `float` property:

```
element {
    float: left|right|none;
}
```

For example, consider the following code and its rendering in Figure 3-6.

```
<header>
    <img src="/images/notw.png" alt="News of the Word logo">
    <h1>News of the Word</h1>
    <h3>Language news you won't find anywhere else (for good
  reason!)</h3>
</header>
<nav>
    <a href="#">Home</a>
    <a href="#">What's New</a>
    <a href="#">What's Old</a>
    <a href="#">What's What</a>
</nav>
```

In Figure 3-6, you can see that the web browser is up to its usual page flow tricks: stacking all the block-level elements on top of each other. However, I think this page would look better if the title (the `<h1>` tag) appeared to the right of the logo. To do that, I can float the `<img>` to the left:

```
header img {
    float: left;
    margin-right: 2em;
}
```

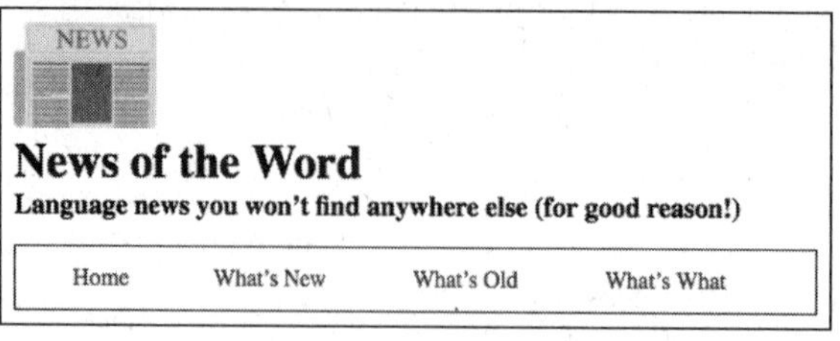

FIGURE 3-6: As usual, the browser displays the block-level elements as a stack of boxes.

Figure 3-7 shows the results. With the logo floated to the left, the rest of the content — the <h1> , <h3>, and <nav> tags — now flows around the <img> tag.

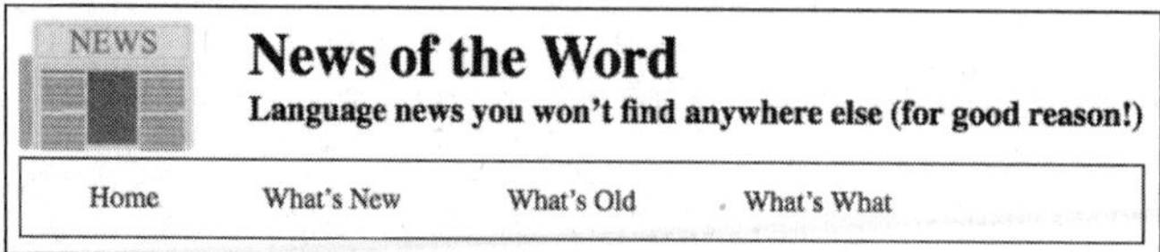

FIGURE 3-7: When the logo gets floated left, the rest of the content flows around it.

Clearing your floats

The default behavior for non-floated stuff is to wrap around anything that's floated, which is often exactly what you want. However, there will be times when you want to avoid having an element wrap around your floats. For example, consider the following code and how it gets rendered, as shown in Figure 3-8.

```
<header>
    <h1>Can't You Read the Sign?</h1>
</header>
<nav>
    <a href="/">Home</a>
    <a href="semantics.html">Signs</a>
    <a href="contact.html">Contact Us</a>
    <a href="about.html">Suggest a Sign</a>
</nav>
<article>
    <img src="/images/keep-off-the-grass.jpg">
</article>
<footer>
    &copy; Can't You Read?, Inc.
</footer>
```

With the <img> tag floated to the left, the rest of the content flows around it, including the content of the <footer> tag, which now appears by the top of the image.

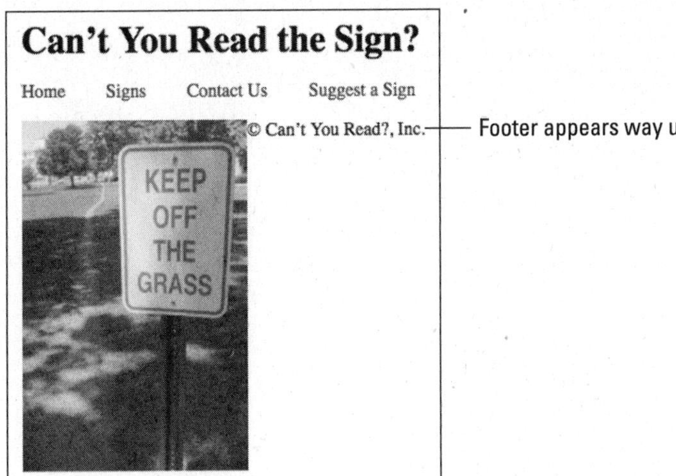

FIGURE 3-8: When the image is floated left, the footer wraps around it and ends up in a weird place.

You want your footer to appear at the bottom of the page, naturally, so how can you fix this? By telling the web browser to position the `footer` element so that it *clears* the floated image, which means that it appears after the image in the page flow. You clear an element by adding the `clear` property:

```
element {
    clear: left|right|both|none;
}
```

Use `clear: left` to clear all left-floated elements, `clear: right` to clear all right-floated elements, or `clear: both` to clear everything. When I add `clear: left` to the footer element, you can see in Figure 3-9 that the footer content now appears at the bottom of the page.

```
footer {
    clear: left;
}
```

Collapsing containers ahead!

The odd behavior of CSS is apparently limitless, and floats offer yet another example. Consider the following HTML and its result in Figure 3-10:

```
<article>

    <section>
        An awfully long time ago...
    </section>
```

```
    <aside>
        <b>Note:</b> Creating a new word by...
    </aside>
</article>
```

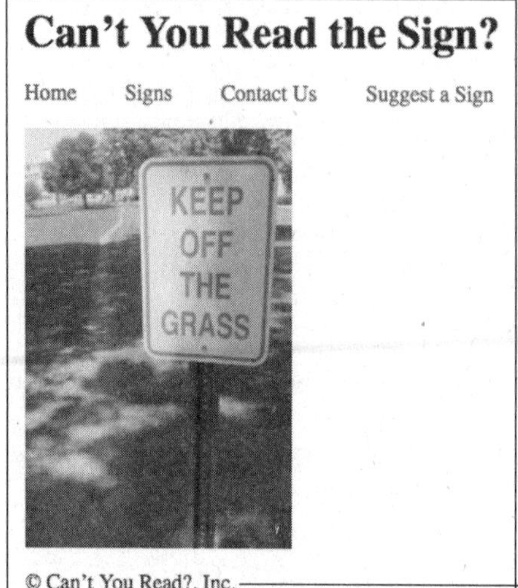

Now the footer's where it should be.

FIGURE 3-9: Adding `clear: left` to the `footer` element causes the footer to clear the left-floated image and appear at the bottom of the page.

An awfully long time ago, an informal or humorous name used in place of a person's given name was said to be that person's *ekename*. The old word *eke* means "extra" or "additional," and it survives today in phrases such as "to eke out a living." Error or mishearing is a common source of new English words, and *ekename* gives us a good example of this strange-but-true process at work. Whenever someone would say the phrase "an ekename," there was always a good chance that some listener (who had never heard the word before) would think the person was actually say "a nekename." In this case, that mistake happened often enough that *ekename* turned into *nekename*, which then turned into our word *nickname*.

Note: Creating a new word by chopping off the initial letter or syllable of an existing word is called *aphaeresis* (which means "to take away"). This not-as-uncommon-as-you-might-think process was the source of words such as *mend* (a shortening of *amend*), *spy* (from *espy*), *cute* (from *acute*), and *squire* (from *esquire*).

FIGURE 3-10: An `<article>` tag containing a `<section>` tag and an `<aside>` tag, rendered using the default page flow.

Note, in particular, that I've styled the `article` element with a border.

Rather than the stack of blocks shown in Figure 3-10, you might prefer to have the `section` and the `aside` elements side-by-side. Great idea! So you add `width` properties to each, and float the `section` element to the left and the `aside` element to the right. Here are the rules and Figure 3-11 shows the result.

```
section {
    float: left;
    width: 25rem;
}
aside {
    float: right;
    width: 15rem;
}
```

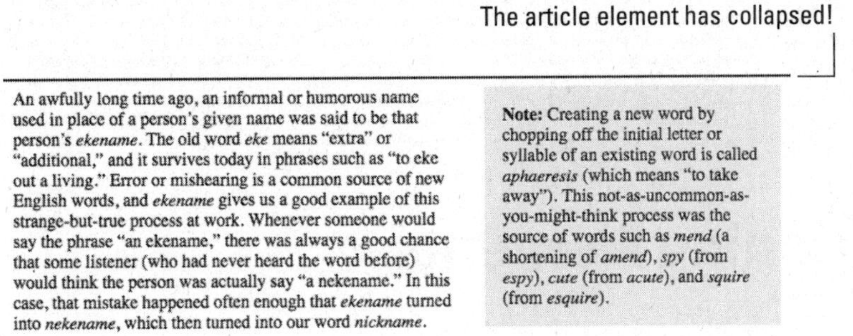

The article element has collapsed!

An awfully long time ago, an informal or humorous name used in place of a person's given name was said to be that person's ***ekename***. The old word ***eke*** means "extra" or "additional," and it survives today in phrases such as "to eke out a living." Error or mishearing is a common source of new English words, and ***ekename*** gives us a good example of this strange-but-true process at work. Whenever someone would say the phrase "an ekename," there was always a good chance that some listener (who had never heard the word before) would think the person was actually say "a nekename." In this case, that mistake happened often enough that ***ekename*** turned into ***nekename***, which then turned into our word ***nickname***.

Note: Creating a new word by chopping off the initial letter or syllable of an existing word is called *aphaeresis* (which means "to take away"). This not-as-uncommon-as-you-might-think process was the source of words such as *mend* (a shortening of *amend*), *spy* (from *espy*), *cute* (from *acute*), and *squire* (from *esquire*).

FIGURE 3-11: With its content floated, the `<article>` element collapses down to just its border.

Well, that's weird! The line across the top is what's left of the `article` element. What happened? Because I floated both the `section` and the `aside` elements, the browser removed them from the page flow, which made the `article` element behave as though it had no content at all. The result? A CSS bugaboo known as *container collapse*.

To fix this, you have to force the parent container to clear its own children.

CSS:

```
.self-clear::after {
    content: "";
    display: block;
    clear: both;
}
```

HTML:

```
<article class="self-clear">
```

First, `::after` is a so called *pseudo-element* that, in this case, tells the browser to create an element and add it to the page flow after whatever element gets the class. What's being added here is an empty string (since you don't want to add anything substantial to the page), and that empty string is displayed as a block that uses `clear: both` to clear the container's children. It's weird, but it works, as you can see in Figure 3-12.

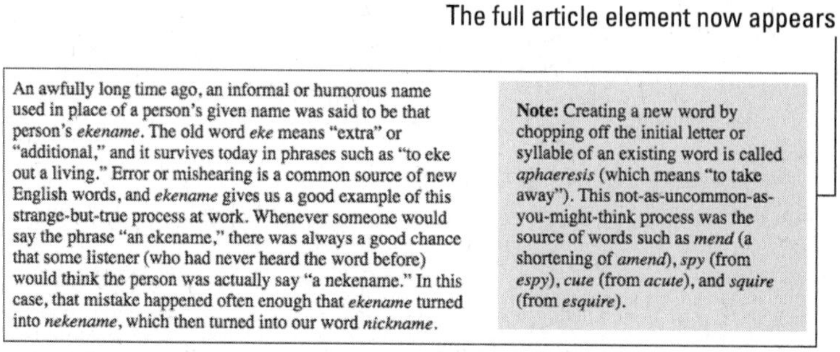

The full article element now appears

An awfully long time ago, an informal or humorous name used in place of a person's given name was said to be that person's ***ekename***. The old word ***eke*** means "extra" or "additional," and it survives today in phrases such as "to eke out a living." Error or mishearing is a common source of new English words, and ***ekename*** gives us a good example of this strange-but-true process at work. Whenever someone would say the phrase "an ekename," there was always a good chance that some listener (who had never heard the word before) would think the person was actually say "a nekename." In this case, that mistake happened often enough that ***ekename*** turned into ***nekename***, which then turned into our word ***nickname***.

Note: Creating a new word by chopping off the initial letter or syllable of an existing word is called *aphaeresis* (which means "to take away"). This not-as-uncommon-as-you-might-think process was the source of words such as ***mend*** (a shortening of ***amend***), ***spy*** (from ***espy***), ***cute*** (from ***acute***), and ***squire*** (from ***esquire***).

FIGURE 3-12: With the `self-clear` class added to the `<article>` tag, the `article` element now clears its own children and is no longer collapsed.

Positioning Elements

The second major method for breaking out of the web browser's default "stacked boxes" page flow is to position an element yourself using CSS properties. For example, you could tell the browser to place an image in the top left corner of the window, no matter where that element's `<img>` tag appears in the page's HTML code. This is known as *positioning* in the CSS world, and it's a very powerful tool, so much so that most web developers use positioning only sparingly.

The first bit of positioning wizardry you need to know is, appropriately, the `position` property:

```
element {
    position: static|relative|absolute|fixed;
}
```

- » `static`: Places the element in its default position in the page flow
- » `relative`: Offsets the element from its default position with respect to its parent container while keeping the element in the page flow
- » `absolute`: Offsets the element from its default position with respect to its parent (or sometimes an earlier ancestor) container while removing the element from the page flow
- » `fixed`: Offsets the element from its default position with respect to the browser window while removing the element from the page flow

Because static positioning is what the browser does by default, I won't say anything more about it. For the other three positioning values — relative, absolute, and fixed — notice that each one offsets the element. Where do these offsets come from? From the following CSS properties:

```
element {
    top: top-value;
    right: right-value;
    bottom: bottom-value;
    left: left-value;
}
```

- top: Shifts the element down
- right: Shifts the element from the right
- bottom: Shifts the element up
- left: Shifts the element from the left

In each case, the value you supply is either a number followed by one of the CSS measurement units (px, em, rem, vw, or vh) or a percentage.

Using relative positioning

Relative positioning is a bit weird because not only does it offset an element relative to its parent container, but it still keeps the element's default space in the page flow intact.

Here's an example:

CSS:

```
.offset-image {
    position: relative;
    left: 200px;
}
```

HTML:

```
<h1>
    holloway
</h1>
```

```
<div>
    <i>n.</i> A sunken footpath or road; a path that is enclosed
  by high embankments on both sides.
</div>
<img src="/images/holloway1.jpg">
<img src="/images/holloway2.jpg" class="offset-image">
<img src="/images/holloway3.jpg">
```

The CSS defines a rule for a class named `offset-image`, which applies relative positioning and offsets the element from the left by `200px`. In the HTML, the `offset-image` class is applied to the middle image. As you can see in Figure 3-13, not only is the middle image shifted from the left, but the space in the page flow where it would have appeared by default remains intact, so the third image's place in the page flow doesn't change. As far as that third image is concerned, the middle image is still right above it.

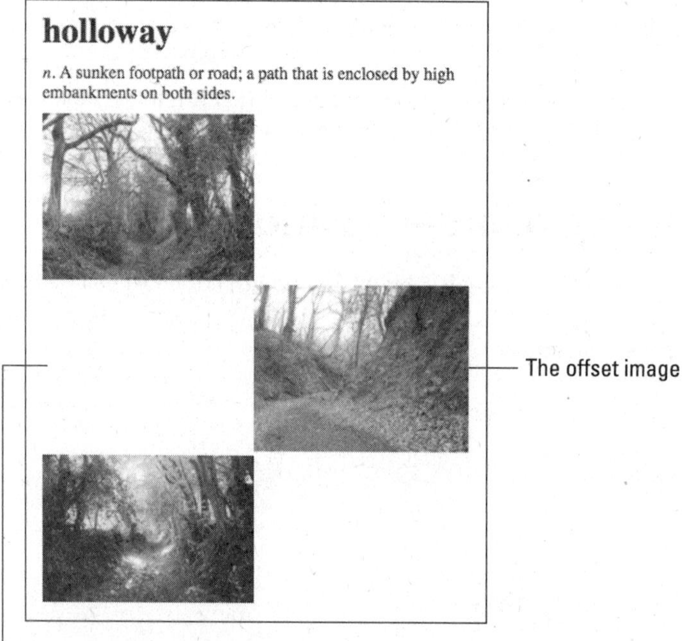

FIGURE 3-13: The middle image uses relative positioning to shift from the left, but its place in the page flow remains.

Giving absolute positioning a whirl

Absolute positioning not only offsets the element from its default position, but it also removes the element from the page flow. Sounds useful, but if the element is no longer part of the page flow, from what element is it offset? Good question, and here's the short answer: the closest ancestor element that uses non-static positioning.

If that has you furrowing your brow, I have a longer answer that should help. To determine which ancestor element is used for the offset of the absolutely positioned element, the browser goes through a procedure similar to this:

1. Move one level up the page hierarchy to the previous ancestor.
2. Check the `position` property of that ancestor element.
3. If the `position` value of the ancestor is `static`, go back to Step 1 and repeat the process for the next level up the hierarchy; otherwise (that is, if the `position` value of the parent is anything other than `static`), then offset the original element with respect to the ancestor.
4. If, after going through Steps 1 to 3 repeatedly, you end up at the top of the page hierarchy — that is, at the `<html>` tag — then use that to offset the element, which means in practice that the element is offset with respect to the browser's content area.

I mention in the previous section that relative positioning is weird because it keeps the element's default position in the page flow intact. However, now that weirdness turns to goodness because if you want a child element to use absolute positioning, then you add `position: relative` to the parent element's style rule. Because you don't also supply an offset to the parent, it stays put in the page flow, but now you have what CSS nerds called a *positioning context* for the child element.

I think an example would be welcome right about now.

CSS:

```
section {
    position: relative;
    border: 1px double black;
}
img {
    position: absolute;
    top: 0;
    right: 0;
}
```

HTML:

```
<section>
    <img src="/images/new.png">
    <h1>
        holloway
    </h1>
    <div>
        <i>n.</i> A sunken footpath or road; a path that is
  enclosed by high embankments on both sides.
    </div>
    <div>
        There are two main methods that create holloways: By
  years (decades, centuries) of constant foot traffic that wears
  down the path (a process usually accelerated somewhat by water
  erosion); or by digging out a path between two properties and
  piling up the dirt on either side.
    </div>
</section>
```

In the CSS, the `section` element is styled with the `position: relative` declaration, and the `img` element is styled with `position: absolute` and `top` and `right` offsets set to `0`. In the HTML, you can see that the `<section>` tag is the parent of the `<img>`, so the latter's absolute positioning will be with respect to the former. With top and right offsets set to `0`, the image will now appear in the top right corner of the section element and, indeed, it does, as you can see in Figure 3-14.

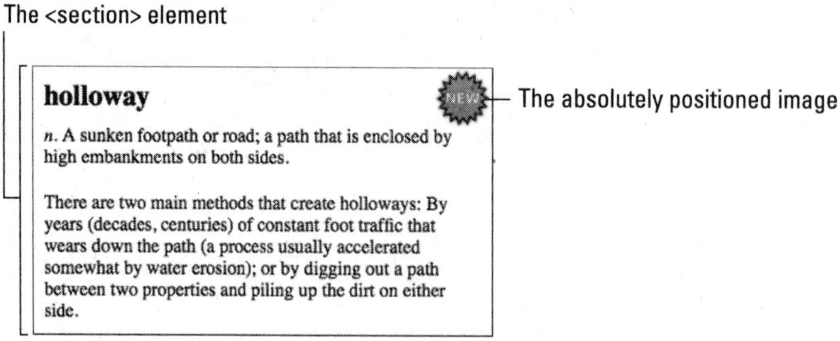

FIGURE 3-14: The `img` element uses absolute positioning to send it to the top right corner of the `section` element.

Trying out fixed positioning

With *fixed positioning,* the element is taken out of the normal page flow and is then offset with respect to the browser's content area, which means the element doesn't move, not even a little, when you scroll the page (that is, the element is "fixed" in its new position).

One of the most common uses of fixed positioning is to plop a header at the top of the page and make it stay there while the user scrolls the rest of the content. Here's an example that shows you how to create such a header:

CSS:

```
header {
    position: fixed;
    top: 0;
    left: 0;
    width: 100%;
    height: 64px;
    border: 1px double black;
    background-color: rgb(147, 196, 125);
}
main {
    margin-top: 64px;
}
```

HTML:

```
<header>
    <img src="/images/holloway3.jpg">
    <h1>
        holloway
    </h1>
</header>
<main>
...
</main>
```

The HTML includes a `header` element with an image and a heading, followed by a longish `main` section that I don't include here for simplicity's sake. In the CSS code, the `header` element is styled with `position: fixed`, and the offsets `top` and `left` set to `0`. These offsets fix the header to the top left of the browser's content area. I also added `width: 100%` to give the header the entire width of the window. Note, too, that I set the header `height` to `64px`. To make sure the `main` section begins below the header, I styled the `main` element with `margin-top: 64px`. Figure 3-15 shows the results.

holloway

n. A sunken footpath or road; a path that is enclosed by high embankments on both sides.

Notes:

There are two main methods that create holloways: By years (decades, centuries) of constant foot traffic that wears down the path (a process usually accelerated somewhat by water erosion); or by digging out a path between two properties and piling up the dirt on either side.

Examples:

> Down in the depths of the holloway, you could see neither metalled roads nor telegraph poles, nor even the most distant glimpses of the outsized golf balls of the early warning radar up on Fylingdales.
> —William Dalrymple, "Holloway by Robert Macfarlane, Stanley Donwood, Dan Richards – review," *The Guardian*, July 19, 2013

FIGURE 3-15: A page with the `header` element fixed to the top of the screen. When you scroll the rest of the page, the header remains where it is.

» Using floated elements for page layout

» Using inline blocks for page layout

» Learning the fundamentals of Flexbox layouts

» Getting a grip on Grid layouts

Chapter 4
Creating the Page Layout

Flexbox is essentially for laying out items in a single dimension — in a row OR a column. Grid is for layout of items in two dimensions — rows AND columns.

— RACHEL ANDREWS

Why are some web pages immediately appealing, while others put the "Ugh" in "ugly"? There are lots of possible reasons: colors, typography, image quality, the density of exclamation points. For my money, however, the number one reason why some pages soar while others are eyesores, is the overall look and feel of the page. We've all visited enough websites in our lives to have developed a kind of sixth sense that tells us immediately whether a page is worth checking out. Sure, colors and fonts play a part in that intuition, but we all respond viscerally to the "big picture" that a page presents.

That big picture refers to the overall layout of the page, and that's the subject you explore in this chapter. Here you discover what page layout is all about, and you investigate several CSS-based methods for making your web pages behave the way you want them to. By the time you're done mastering the nitty-gritty of page layout, you'll be in a position to design and build beautiful and functional pages that'll have them screaming for more.

What Is Page Layout?

The *page layout* is the arrangement of the page elements within the browser's content area, including not only what you see when you first open the page, but also the rest of the page that comes into view as you scroll down. The page layout acts as a kind of blueprint for the page, and like any good blueprint, the page layout details how a page looks at two levels:

- **The macro level:** Refers to the overall layout of the page, which determines how the major sections of the page — `header`, `nav`, `main`, `footer`, and so on — fit together as a whole.
- **The micro level:** Refers to the layout within a section or subsection of the page. For example, the page's `header` element might have one layout, whereas the page's `article` section might have another.

CSS offers four main layout techniques, each of which you can apply at either the macro level or the micro level:

- **Floats:** Arranges elements by floating them.
- **Inline blocks:** Arranges elements by styling them as inline blocks.
- **CSS Flexible Box (flexbox):** Arranges elements either vertically or horizontally within flexible boxes.
- **CSS Grid:** Arranges the elements in a row-and-column structure.

The rest of this chapter discusses each of these techniques, with a special emphasis on the newer technologies of flexbox and Grid.

Laying Out Page Elements with Floats

I discuss floating elements in detail in Book 2, Chapter 3, so I won't repeat myself here. From a page layout standpoint, you generally use floats as needed when you want two or more items to appear side-by-side rather than stacked on top of each other in the default page flow.

The general procedure you follow goes something like this:

1. Work your way down the page, allowing the page elements to lay out using the default page flow.

2. When you come to two or more elements that you want to appear side-by-side, float them to the left (usually) or to the right.
3. When you come to the next element that should follow the default page flow, clear the floats for that element.
4. Repeat Steps 1 to 3 until you reach the end of the page.

For example, say you're following the above procedure and you come to the nav element, which consists of several links. Because the <a> tag is an inline element, you could just toss a bunch of <a> tags inside the nav element and they'd line up alongside each other. That's fine, but you don't get to control the horizontal spacing since an <a> tag isn't a true block.

A common way to work around that problem is to add the links as an unordered list, but with two special additions:

- The `ul` element's `list-style-type` property set to none to hide the bullets.
- The `li` elements (that is, the list items) are styled with `float: left` so they display side-by-side instead of vertically.

Here's the code, and Figure 4-1 shows the result:

CSS:

```
nav {
    height: 2.5rem;
    padding-top: .6rem;
    background-color: #ccc;
}
nav ul {
    list-style-type: none;
    padding-left: 1.75rem;
}
nav li {
    float: left;
    padding-right: 1.75rem;
}
main {
    clear: left;
    margin-top: 1rem;
}
```

HTML:

```
<nav>
    <ul>
        <li><a href="#">Home</a></li>
        <li><a href="#">Blog</a></li>
        <li><a href="#">Store</a></li>
        <li><a href="#">About</a></li>
        <li><a href="#">Contact</a></li>
    </ul>
</nav>
<main>
    Main content goes here...
</main>
```

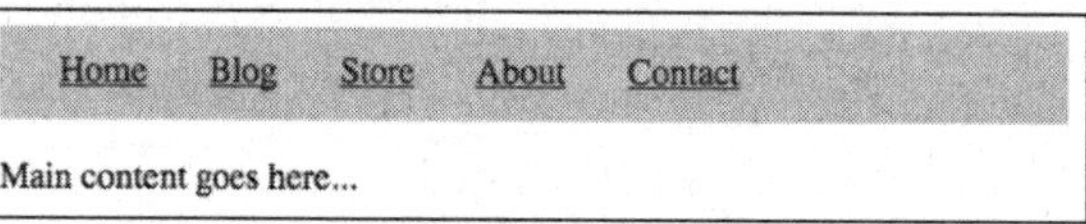

FIGURE 4-1: These links are unordered list items and floated left to appear side-by-side.

You can also use floats to make larger page layout decisions. For example, one common page layout is to have a header at the top of the page, a navigation area below the header, and a footer at the bottom of the page, where all three span the width of the page. Between the navigation area and the header, you have the main content of the page, which is split horizontally between an article on one side and a sidebar on the other.

Here's some barebones code that creates such a page layout:

CSS:

```
body {
    margin: 2rem;
    width: 30rem;
}
header {
    height: 2.5rem;
    border: 1px solid black;
}
```

```
nav {
    height: 2.5rem;
    margin-top: 1rem;
    border: 1px solid black;
}
main {
    margin-top: 1rem;
    height: 10rem;
}
article {
    float: left;
    margin-right: 1rem;
    width: 20rem;
    height: 100%;
    border: 1px solid black;
}
aside {
    float: right;
    width: 9rem;
    height: 100%;
    border: 1px solid black;
}
footer {
    clear: both;
    height: 2.5rem;
    margin-top: 1rem;
    border: 1px solid black;
}
```


HTML:

```
<header>
    Header
</header>
<nav>
    Navigation
</nav>
<main>
    <article>
        Article
    </article>
    <aside>
        Aside
    </aside>
```

```
</main>
<footer>
    Footer
</footer>
```

The key elements to notice here are that the `<article>` and `<aside>` tags are both children of the `<main>` tag, and in the CSS the `article` element is styled with `float: left`, whereas the `aside` element is styled with `float: right`. Figure 4-2 shows the resulting page layout.

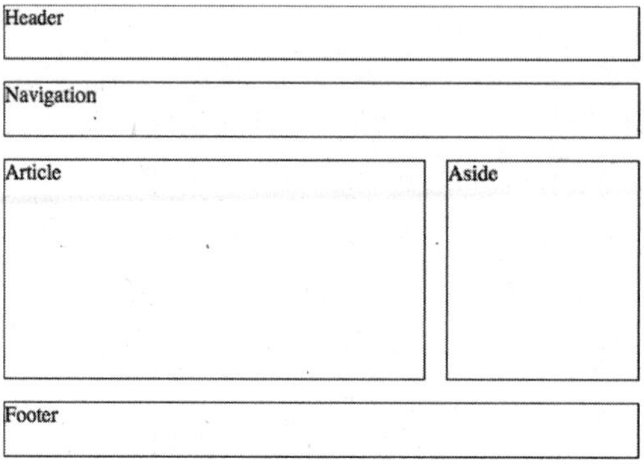

Header

Navigation

Article

Aside

Footer

FIGURE 4-2: A classic web page layout, created by floating the `article` element to the left and the `aside` element to the right.

Laying Out Page Elements with Inline Blocks

When you turn an element into an inline block (by adding `display: inline-block` to the element's style rule), one of two things happens:

- » If you're working with an inline element, that element becomes a block, but it still flows horizontally with the rest of the surrounding inline content.
- » If you're working with a block-level element, that element is removed from the default vertical page flow and now flows horizontally with the rest of the surrounding inline content.

It's the second of these — that is, the removal of a block-level element from the default page flow so that it now flows inline — that interests us from a page layout point of view. That is, you can use inline blocks as needed when you want two or more items to appear side-by-side rather than stacked.

Here's the general procedure to follow:

1. Work your way down the page, allowing the page elements to lay out using the default page flow.
2. When you come to two or more elements that you want to appear side-by-side, convert them to inline blocks.
3. Repeat Steps 1 and 2 until you reach the end of the page.

This procedure is very similar to the float steps I outline in the previous section, with one notable exception: When you use inline blocks, you don't need to clear the following elements because the browser does that for you automatically.

Here's the inline-block version of the `nav` element layout that I went through in the previous section, and Figure 4-3 shows the result:

CSS:

```
nav {
    height: 2.5rem;
    padding-top: .6rem;
    background-color: #ccc;
}
nav ul {
    list-style-type: none;
    padding-left: 1.75rem;
}
nav li {
    display: inline-block;
    padding-right: 1.75rem;
}
main {
    margin-top: 1rem;
}
```

HTML:

```
<nav>
    <ul>
        <li><a href="#">Home</a></li>
        <li><a href="#">Blog</a></li>
        <li><a href="#">Store</a></li>
        <li><a href="#">About</a></li>
        <li><a href="#">Contact</a></li>
    </ul>
```

Creating the Page Layout

```
</nav>
<main>
    Main content goes here...
</main>
```

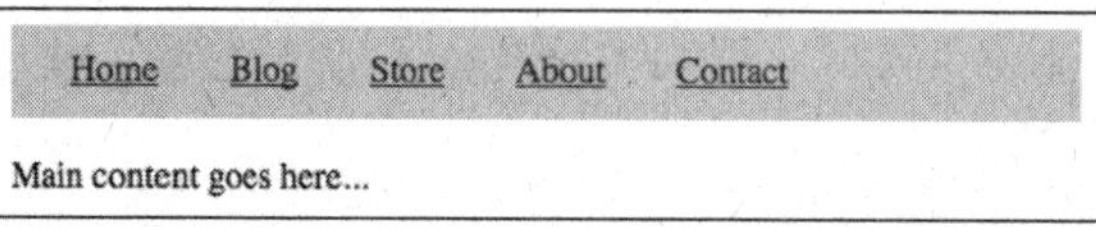

FIGURE 4-3: These links are list items styled as inline blocks to appear side-by-side.

You can also use inline blocks for macro page layouts. For example, to re-create the layout shown earlier in Figure 4-2 using inline blocks, you'd use the following code:

CSS:

```
body {
    margin: 2rem;
    width: 30rem;
}
header {
    height: 2.5rem;
    border: 1px solid black;
}
nav {
    height: 2.5rem;
    margin-top: 1rem;
    border: 1px solid black;
}
main {
    margin-top: 1rem;
    height: 10rem;
}
article {
    display: inline-block;
    margin-right: 1rem;
    width: 20rem;
    height: 100%;
    border: 1px solid black;
}
```

```
aside {
    display: inline-block;
    width: 9rem;
    height: 100%;
    border: 1px solid black;
}
footer {
    height: 2.5rem;
    margin-top: 1rem;
    border: 1px solid black;
}
```

HTML:

```
<header>
    Header
</header>
<nav>
    Navigation
</nav>
<main>
    <article>
        Article
    </article><aside>
        Aside
    </aside>
</main>
<footer>
    Footer
</footer>
```

Notice, first, that in the CSS both the `article` element and the `aside` element are styled with `display: inline-block`. More mysteriously, in the HTML, notice that I jammed together the `</article>` and `<aside>` tags. What's up with that? It's an eccentric feature of using inline blocks in this way that there shouldn't be any whitespace between one inline block and another. It's weird, I know, but it works, as you can see in Figure 4-4.

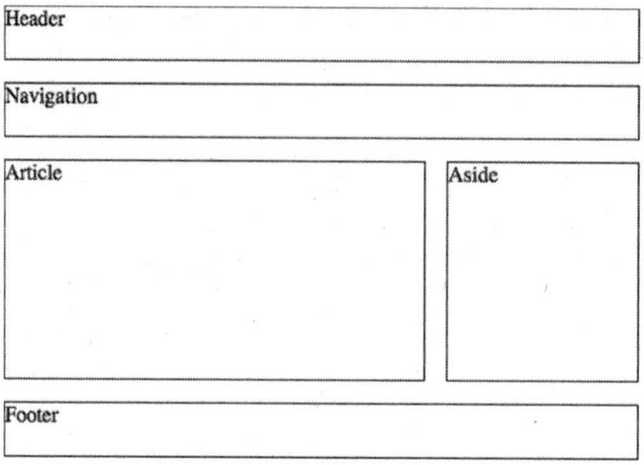

Header

Navigation

Article

Aside

Footer

FIGURE 4-4: The classic web page layout, created by displaying the `article` and `aside` elements as inline blocks.

Making Flexible Layouts with Flexbox

When you use either floats or inline blocks for page layout, there are some banana peels in the path that can trip you up, including forgetting to clear your floats and forgetting to ensure there is no whitespace between two inline blocks.

However, beyond these mere annoyances, there are also a few things that float- or inline-block-based layouts have trouble with:

- It's very hard to get an element's content centered vertically within the element's container.
- It's very hard to get elements evenly spaced horizontally across the full width (or vertically across the full height) of their parent container.
- It's very hard to get a footer element to appear at the bottom of the browser's content area.

Fortunately, these troubles vanish if you use a CSS technology called Flexible Box Layout Module, or *flexbox*, for short. The key here is the "flex" part of the name. As opposed to the default page flow and layouts that use floats and inline blocks, all of which render content using rigid blocks, flexbox renders content using containers that can grow and shrink — I'm talking both width and height here — in response to changing content or browser window size. But flexbox also offers powerful properties that make it a breeze to lay out, align, distribute, and size the child elements of a parent container.

The first thing you need to know is that flexbox divides its world into two categories:

- **Flex container:** This is a block-level element that acts as a parent to the flexible elements inside it.
- **Flex items:** These are the elements that reside within the flex container.

Setting up the flex container

To designate an element as a flex container, you set its `display` property to `flex`:

```
container {
    display: flex;
}
```

With that done, the element's children automatically become flex items.

Flexbox is a one-dimensional layout tool, which means the flex items are arranged within their flex container either horizontally — that is, in a row — or vertically — that is, in a column. This direction is called the *primary axis* and you specify it using the `flex-direction` property:

```
element {
    display: flex;
    flex-direction: row|row-reverse|column|column-reverse;
}
```

- `row`: The primary axis is horizontal and the flex items are arranged from left to right. This is the default value.
- `row-reverse`: The primary axis is horizontal and the flex items are arranged from right to left.
- `column`: The primary axis is vertical and the flex items are arranged from top to bottom.
- `column-reverse`: The primary axis is vertical and the flex items are arranged from bottom to top.

The axis that is perpendicular to the primary axis is called the *secondary axis.*

As an example, here's some CSS and HTML code, and Figure 4-5 shows how it looks if you let the browser lay it out:

CSS:

```
.container {
    border: 5px double black;
}
.item {
    border: 1px solid black;
    padding: .1rem;
    font-family: "Verdana", sans-serif;
    font-size: 5rem;
    text-align: center;
}
.item1 {
    background-color: rgb(240, 240, 240);
}
.item2 {
    background-color: rgb(224, 224, 224);
}
.item3 {
    background-color: rgb(208, 208, 208);
}
.item4 {
    background-color: rgb(192, 192, 192);
}
.item5 {
    background-color: rgb(176, 176, 176);
}
```

HTML:

```
<div class="container">
    <div class="item item1">1</div>
    <div class="item item2">2</div>
    <div class="item item3">3</div>
    <div class="item item4">4</div>
    <div class="item item5">5</div>
</div>
```

The browser does its default thing where it stacks the `div` blocks on top of each other and makes each one take up the full width of its parent `div` (the one with the `container` class), which, in Figure 4-5, has its boundaries marked by the double border.

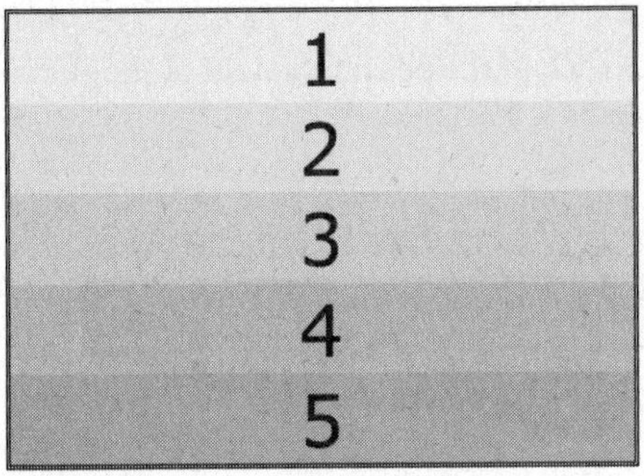

FIGURE 4-5: If you let the browser lay out the elements, you get the default stack of blocks.

Now configure the parent `div` — again, the one with the `container` class — as a flex container with a horizontal primary axis:

```
.container {
    display: flex;
    flex-direction: row;
    border: 5px double black;
}
```

This automatically configures the child `div` elements — the ones with the `item` class — as flex items. As you can see in Figure 4-6, the flex items are now aligned horizontally and only take up as much horizontal space as their content requires.

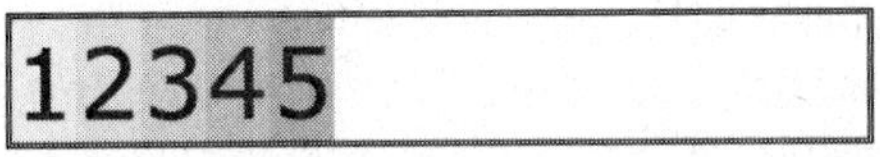

FIGURE 4-6: With their parent as a flex container, the child elements become flex items.

Aligning flex items along the primary axis

Notice in Figure 4-6 that the flex items are bunched together on the left side of the flex container (which has its boundaries shown by the double border). This is the default alignment along the primary axis, but you can change that by modifying the value of the `justify-content` property:

```
container {
    display: flex;
    justify-content: flex-start|flex-end|center|space-
   between|space-around;
}
```

Table 4-1 demonstrates each of the possible values of the `justify-content` property when the primary axis is horizontal.

TABLE 4-1 **Aligning Flex Items along the Primary Axis**

justify-content	Example
flex-start	12345
flex-end	12345
center	12345
space-between	1 2 3 4 5
space-around	1 2 3 4 5

REMEMBER

Here are a few notes about Table 4-1 to recite to yourself before going to bed:

- The `flex-start` alignment is the default, so you can leave out the `justify-content` property if `flex-start` is the alignment you want.
- The space-between alignment works by placing the first flex item at the start of the flex container, the last flex item at the end of the flex container, and then distributing the rest of the flex items evenly in between.
- The space-around alignment works by assigning equal amounts of space before and after each flex item, where the amount of space is calculated to get the flex items distributed evenly along the primary axis. Actually, the distribution isn't quite even, because the inner flex items (2, 3, and 4 in Table 4-1) have two units of space between them, whereas the starting and ending flex items (1 and 5, respectively, in Table 4-1) have only one unit of space to the outside (that is, to the left of item 1 and to the right of item 5).

Aligning flex items along the secondary axis

Besides aligning the flex items along the primary axis, you can also align them along the secondary axis. For example, if you've set `flex-direction` to `row`, which gives you a horizontal primary axis, then the secondary axis is vertical, which means you can also align the flex items vertically. By default, the flex items always take up the entire height of the flex container, but you can get a different secondary axis alignment by changing the value of the `align-items` property:

```
container {
    display: flex;
    align-items: stretch|flex-start|flex-end|center|baseline;
}
```

Table 4-2 demonstrates each of the possible values of the `align-items` property when the secondary axis is vertical.

TABLE 4-2 **Aligning Flex Items along the Secondary Axis**

align-items	Example
stretch	12345
flex-start	12345
flex-end	12345
center	12345
baseline	12345

REMEMBER

Some notes about Table 4-2:

- To make the examples useful, I added some height to the flex container (the edges of which are designated by a double border) and I added random amounts of top and bottom padding to each flex item.
- The `stretch` alignment is the default, so you can leave out the `align-items` property if `stretch` is the alignment you want.
- The `baseline` value aligns the flex items along the bottom edges of the item text. (Technically, given a line of text, the *baseline* is the invisible line upon which lowercase characters such as o and x appear to sit.)

Centering an element horizontally and vertically

In the olden days of CSS, centering an element both horizontally and vertically within its parent was notoriously difficult. Style wizards stayed up until late at night coming up with ways to achieve this feat. They succeeded, but their techniques were obscure and convoluted. Then flexbox came along and changed everything by making it almost ridiculously easy to plop something smack dab in the middle of the page:

```
container {
    display: flex;
    justify-content: center;
    align-items: center;
}
```

Yes, that's all there is to it. Here's an example:

CSS:

```
.container {
    display: flex;
    justify-content: center;
    align-items: center;
    height: 25vh;
    border: 5px double black;
}
.item {
    font-family: "Georgia", serif;
    font-size: 2rem;
}
```

HTML:

```
<div class="container">
    <div class="item">Look, ma, I'm centered!</div>
</div>
```

As you can see in Figure 4-7, the flex item sits right in the middle of its flex container.

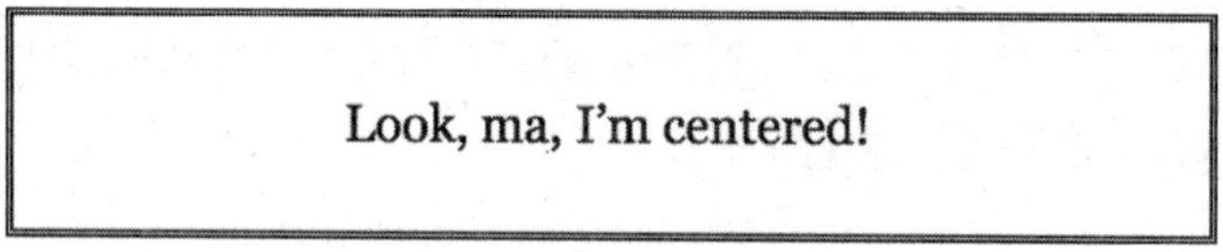

FIGURE 4-7: To center an item, set the container's `justify-content` and `align-items` properties to `center`.

Look, ma, I'm centered!

Laying out a navigation bar with flexbox

Earlier in this chapter, I show some HTML and CSS code for a horizontal layout of a navigation bar. One example uses floats and the other uses inline blocks, but in both cases I had to resort to finicky finagling of vertical and horizontal padding to get the links nicely positioned within the `nav` element.

With flexbox, however, you don't need to resort to such time-consuming tweaking to gets things lined up nice and neat. Here's the flexbox version of the navigation bar, and Figure 4-8 shows how it looks in the browser:

CSS:

```
nav {
    background-color: #ccc;
}
nav ul {
    display: flex;
    justify-content: space-around;
    align-items: center;
    height: 2.5rem;
    list-style-type: none;
}
main {
    margin-top: 1rem;
}
```

HTML:

```
<nav>
    <ul>
        <li><a href="#">Home</a></li>
        <li><a href="#">Blog</a></li>
        <li><a href="#">Store</a></li>
        <li><a href="#">About</a></li>
        <li><a href="#">Contact</a></li>
    </ul>
</nav>
<main>
    Main content goes here...
</main>
```

FIGURE 4-8: Using flexbox, you can modify flex container properties for nicely spaced links.

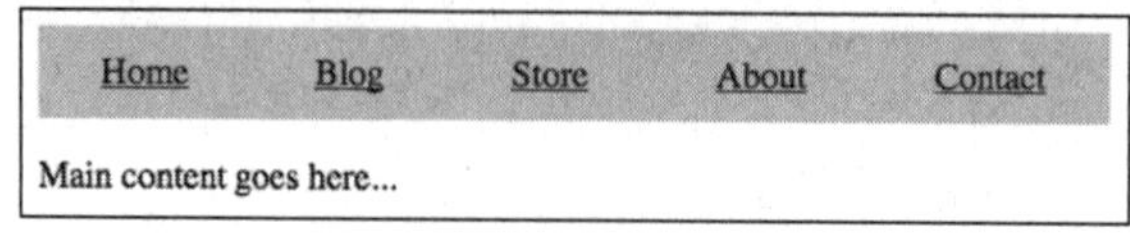

Notice that I made the `ul` element the flex container. By setting `justify-content` to `space-around` and `align-items` to `center`, you get the flex items — that is, the navigation links — perfectly spaced within the navigation bar.

Allowing flex items to grow

By default, when you set the `justify-content` property to `flex-start`, `flex-end`, or `center`, the flex items take up only as much room along the primary axis as they need for their content, as shown earlier in Figure 4-6 and Table 4-1. This is admirably egalitarian, but it does often leave a bunch of empty space in the flex container. Interestingly, one of the meanings behind the "flex" in flexbox is that you can make one or more flex items grow to fill that empty space.

You configure a flex item to grow by setting the `flex-grow` property on the item:

```
item {
    flex-grow: value;
}
```

Here, *`value`* is a number greater than or equal to `0`. The default value is `0`, which tells the browser not to grow the flex items. That usually results in empty space in the flex container, as shown in Figure 4-9.

FIGURE 4-9: By default, all flex items have a `flex-grow` value of `0`, resulting in empty space.

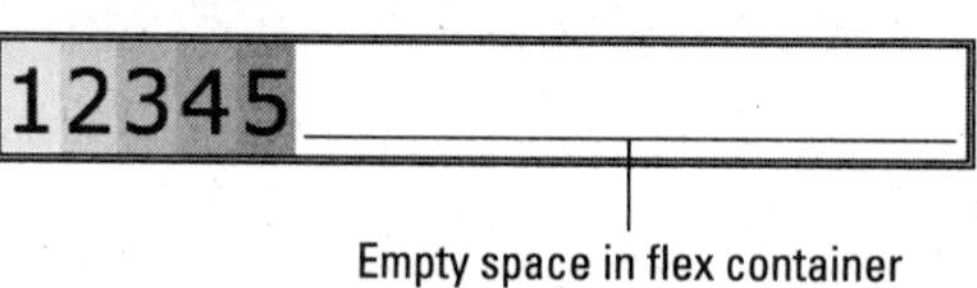

For positive values of `flex-grow`, there are three scenarios to consider:

» **You assign a positive `flex-grow` value to just one flex item.** The flex item grows until there is no more empty space in the flex container. For example, here's a rule that sets `flex-grow` to `1` for the element with class `item1`, and Figure 4-10 shows that item 1 has grown until there is no more empty space in the flex container:

```
.item1 {
    flex-grow: 1;
}
```

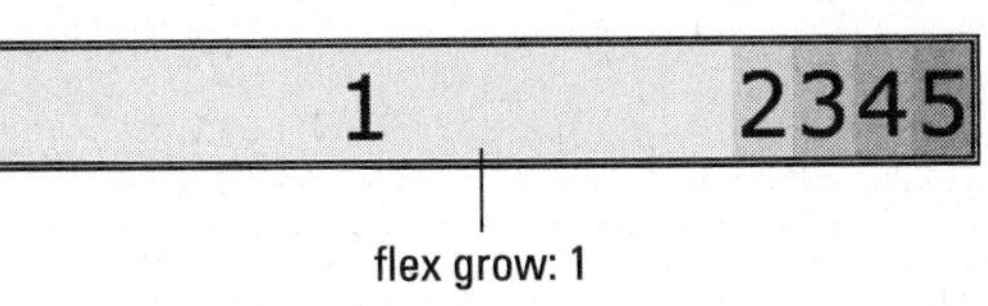

FIGURE 4-10: With `flex-grow: 1`, an item grows until the container has no more empty space.

» **You assign the same positive `flex-grow` value to two or more flex items.** The flex items grow equally until there is no more empty space in the flex container. For example, here's a rule that sets `flex-grow` to `1` for the elements with the classes `item1`, `item2`, and `item3`, and Figure 4-11 shows that items 1, 2, and 3 have grown until there is no more empty space in the flex container:

```
.item1,
.item2,
.item3 {
    flex-grow: 1;
}
```

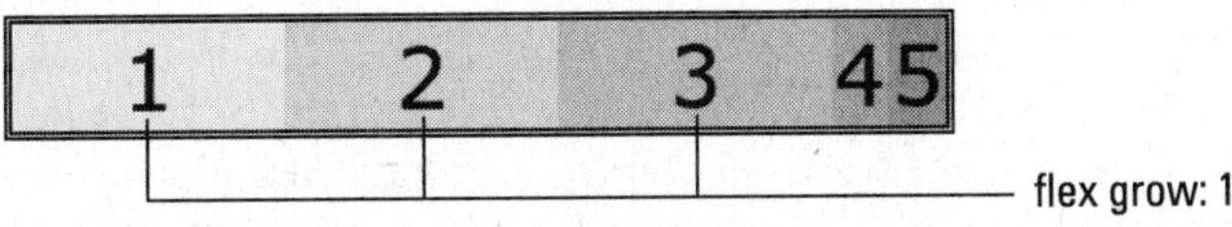

FIGURE 4-11: When items 1, 2, and 3 are styled with `flex-grow: 1`, the items grow equally.

Creating the Page Layout

» **You assign a different positive `flex-grow` value to two or more flex items.** The flex items grow proportionally based on the `flex-grow` values until there is no more empty space in the flex container. For example, if you give one item a `flex-grow` value of `1`, a second item a `flex-grow` value of `2`, and a third item a `flex-grow` value of `1`, then the proportion of the empty space given to each will be, respectively, 25 percent, 50 percent, and 25 percent. Here's some CSS that supplies these proportions to the elements with the classes `item1`, `item2`, and `item3`, and Figure 4-12 shows the results:

```
.item1 {
    flex-grow: 1;
}
.item2 {
    flex-grow: 2;
}
.item3 {
    flex-grow: 1;
}
```

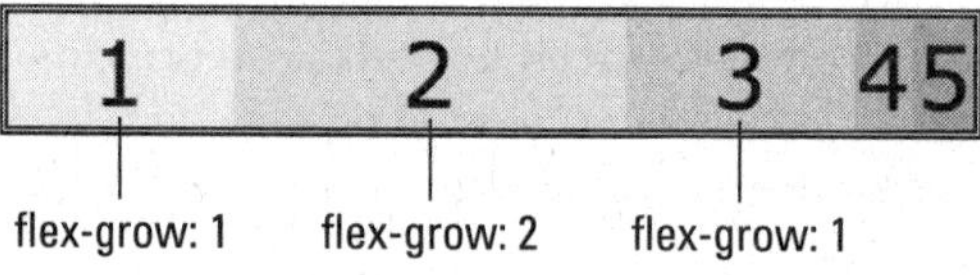

FIGURE 4-12: Items 1 and 3 get 25 percent of the container's empty space, whereas item 2 gets 50 percent.

TECHNICAL STUFF

To calculate what proportion of the flex container's empty space is assigned to each flex item, add up the `flex-grow` values, then divide the individual `flex-grow` values by that total. For example, values of 1, 2, and 1 add up to 4, so the percentages are 25 percent (1/4), 50 percent (2/4), and 25 percent (1/4), respectively.

Allowing flex items to shrink

The flexibility of flexbox means not only that flex items can grow to fill a flex container's empty space, but also that they can shrink if the flex container doesn't have enough space to fit the items. Shrinking flex items to fit inside their container is the default flexbox behavior, but you gain a measure of control over which items shrink and by how much by using the `flex-shrink` property on a flex item:

```
item {
    flex-shrink: value;
}
```

Here, *value* is a number greater than or equal to `0`. The default value is `1`, which tells the browser to shrink all the flex items equally to get them to fit inside the flex container.

For example, consider the following code:

CSS:

```
.container {
    display: flex;
    width: 500px;
    border: 5px double black;
}
.item {
    width: 200px;
}
```

HTML:

```
<div class="container">
    <div class="item item1">1</div>
    <div class="item item2">2</div>
    <div class="item item3">3</div>
    <div class="item item4">4</div>
    <div class="item item5">5</div>
</div>
```

The flex container (the `container` class) is `500px` wide, but each flex item (the item class) is `200px` wide. To get everything the fit, the browser shrinks each item equally, and the result is shown in Figure 4-13.

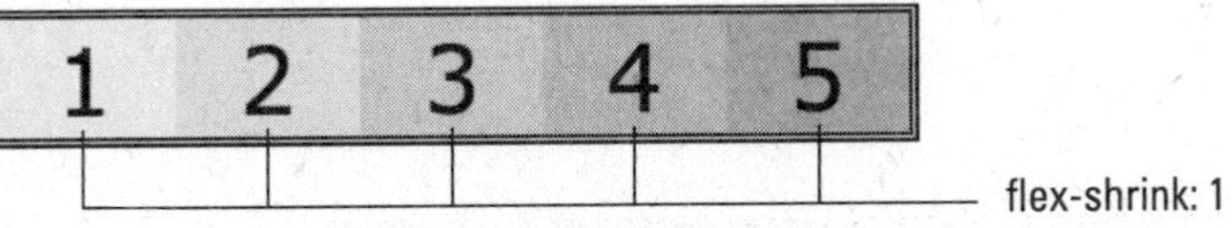

FIGURE 4-13: By default, the browser shrinks the items equally along the primary axis until they fit.

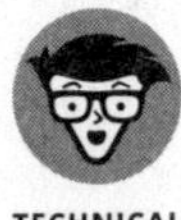

TECHNICAL STUFF

The browser only shrinks each flex item truly equally (that is, by the same amount) when each item has the same size along the primary axis (for example, the same width when the primary axis is horizontal). If the flex items have different sizes, the browser shrinks each item roughly in proportion to its size: Larger items shrink more, whereas smaller items shrink less. I use the word "roughly" here because in fact the calculations the browser uses to determine the shrinkage factor are brain-numbingly complex. If you want to learn more (don't say I didn't warn you!), see `https://madebymike.com.au/writing/understanding-flexbox`.

For positive values of `flex-shrink`, you have three ways to control the shrinkage of a flex item:

» **Assign the item a `flex-shrink` value between 0 and 1.** The browser shrinks the item less than the other flex items. For example, here's a rule that sets `flex-shrink` to `.5` for the element with class `item1`, and Figure 4-14 shows that item 1 has shrunk less than the other items in the container:

```
.item1 {
    flex-shrink: .5;
}
```

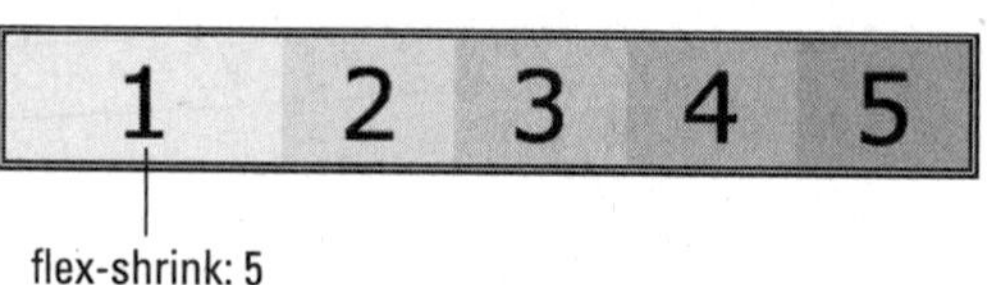

FIGURE 4-14: Styling item 1 with `flex-shrink: .5` shrinks it less than the other items.

» **Assign the item a `flex-shrink` value greater than 1.** The browser shrinks the item more than the other flex items. For example, the following rule sets `flex-shrink` to 2 for the element with class `item1`, and Figure 4-15 shows that item 1 has shrunk more than the other items in the container:

```
.item1 {
    flex-shrink: 2;
}
```

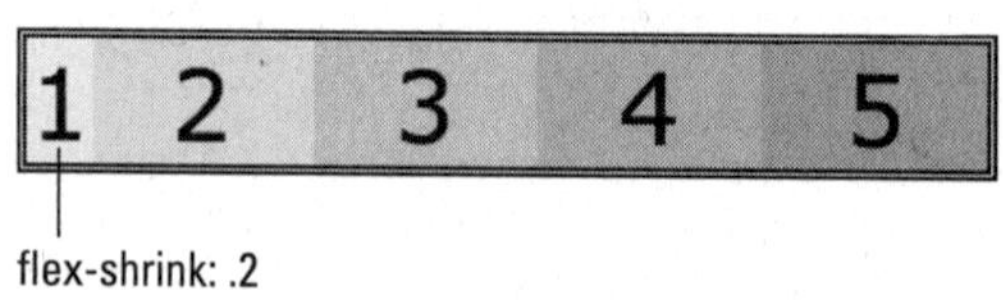

FIGURE 4-15: Styling item 1 with `flex-shrink: 2` shrinks the item more than the others.

» **Assign the item a `flex-shrink` value of 0.** The browser doesn't shrink the item. The following rule sets `flex-shrink` to `0` for the element with class `item1`, and Figure 4-16 shows that the browser doesn't shrink item 1:

```
.item1 {
    flex-shrink: 0;
}
```

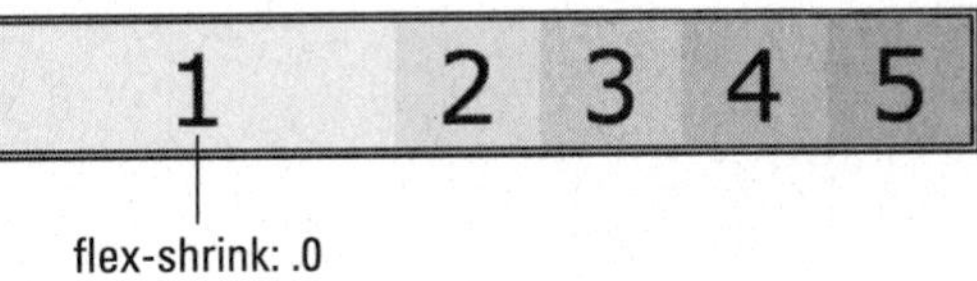

FIGURE 4-16: Styling item 1 with `flex-shrink: 0` doesn't shrink the item.

WARNING

If a flex item is larger along the primary axis than its flex container, and you set `flex-shrink: 0` on that item, ugliness ensues. That is, the flex item breaks out of the container and, depending on where it sits within the container, might take one or more other items with it. If you don't want a flex item to shrink, make sure the flex container is large enough to hold it.

Laying out content columns with flexbox

Flexbox works best when you use it to lay out components along one dimension, but that doesn't mean you can't use it to lay out an entire page. As long as the page structure is relatively simple, then flexbox works great for laying out elements both horizontally and vertically.

A good example is the classic page layout that I discuss earlier: a header and navigation bar across the top of the page, a main section with an article and a sidebar beside it, and a footer across the bottom of the page. Here's some flexbox code that creates this layout, which is shown in Figure 4-17:

CSS:

```
body {
    display: flex;
    flex-direction: column;
    width: 30rem;
    min-height: 100vh;
}
```

```
header {
    height: 2.5rem;
    border: 1px solid black;
}
nav {
    height: 2.5rem;
    margin-top: 1rem;
    border: 1px solid black;
}
main {
    flex-grow: 1;
    display: flex;
    margin-top: 1rem;
}
article {
    flex-grow: 1;
    margin-right: 1rem;
    border: 1px solid black;
    overflow-y: auto;
}
aside {
    flex-grow: 0;
    flex-shrink: 0;
    flex-basis: 10rem;
    border: 1px solid black;
}
footer {
    height: 2.5rem;
    margin-top: 1rem;
    border: 1px solid black;
}
```

HTML:

```
<body>
    <header>
        Header
    </header>
    <nav>
        Navigation
    </nav>
    <main>
        <article>
            Article
        </article>
```

```
        <aside>
            Aside
        </aside>
    </main>
    <footer>
        Footer
    </footer>
</body>
```

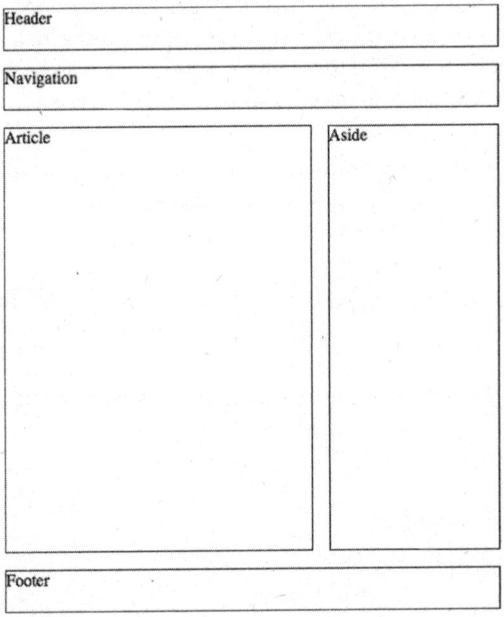

Header

Navigation

Article

Aside

Footer

FIGURE 4-17: The classic page layout, flexbox-style.

Let's take a closer look at what's happening here:

- The `<body>` tag is set up as a flex container, and that container is styled with `flex-direction: column` to create a vertical primary axis for the page as a whole.
- The body element has its `min-height` property set to `100vh`, which makes the flex container always take up at least the entire height of the browser's content area.
- All `header`, `nav`, and `footer` elements are given explicit height values.
- The `main` element is styled with `flex-grow: 1`, which tells the browser to grow the `main` element vertically until it uses up the empty space in the flex

container. This also ensures that the `footer` element appears at the bottom of the content area even if there isn't enough content to fill the `main` element.

- The `main` element is also a flex container styled with `flex-direction: row` to create a horizontal primary axis.
- Inside the `main` flex container, the `article` element is given `flex-grow: 1`, so it grows as needed to take up the remaining width of the `main` element (that is, after the width of the `aside` element is taken into account).
- To get a fixed-width sidebar, the `aside` element's rule has both `flex-grow` and `flex-shrink` set to `0`, and it also includes the declaration `flex-basis: 10rem`. The `flex-basis` property provides the browser with a suggested starting point for the size of the element. In this case, with both `flex-grow` and `flex-shrink` set to `0`, the `flex-basis` value acts like a fixed width.

TIP

There's a shorthand property called `flex` that you can use to combine `flex-grow`, `flex-shrink`, and `flex-basis` into a single declaration:

```
item {
  flex: grow-value shrink-value basis-value;
}
```

For example, I could rewrite the `aside` element's rule in the above example as follows:

```
aside {
    flex: 0 0 10rem;
    border: 1px solid black;
}
```

Flexbox browser support

The good news is that all major web browsers, both desktop and mobile, support flexbox. The bad news is that they haven't always supported flexbox, or, to be accurate, they've supported it, but only with what are known as *vendor prefixes*. A vendor prefix is a label specific to each browser — such as `-webkit-` for browsers that use the WebKit page rendering engine (including Chrome and Safari), `-moz-` for Firefox, and `-ms-` for Microsoft Edge and Internet Explorer — that enabled the browser to implement a CSS feature before knowing the final specification.

So while a declaration such as `display: flex` will work just fine in about 90 percent of today's browsers, to handle the rest you need to include prefixed versions of the same declaration:

```
container {
    display: -webkit-box;
    display: -ms-flexbox;
    display: flex;
}
```

Yuck. Vendor prefixes are one of the great annoyances of modern web development. However, rather than have you memorize the prefixed versions of every flexbox property, I'm going to suggest, instead, that you wait until your CSS code is complete (or nearly so), then run it through the online Autoprefixer tool, which will add all the required prefixes for you lickety-split:

`https://autoprefixer.github.io`

Shaping the Overall Page Layout with CSS Grid

One of the most exciting and anticipated developments in recent CSS history is the advent of a technology called CSS Grid. The Grid specification gives you a straightforward way to divide up a container into one or more rows and one or more columns — that is, as a *grid* — and then optionally assign the container's elements to specific sections of the grid. With CSS Grid, you can give the web browser instructions such as the following:

- Set up the <body> tag as a grid with four rows and three columns.
- Place the `header` element in the first row and make it span all three columns.
- Place the `nav` element in the second row and make it span all three columns.
- Place the `article` element in the third row, columns one and two.
- Place the `aside` element in the third row, column three.
- Place the `footer` element in the fourth row and make it span all three columns.

Before you learn how to do all of this and more, you need to know that a Grid uses two categories of elements:

- **Grid container:** This is a block-level element that acts as a parent to the elements inside it and that you configure with a set number of rows and columns.

» **Grid items:** These are the elements that reside within the grid container and that you assign (or the browser assigns automatically) to specific parts of the grid.

Setting up the grid container

To designate an element as a grid container, you set its `display` property to `grid`:

```
container {
    display: grid;
}
```

With that first step complete, the element's children automatically become grid items.

Specifying the grid rows and columns

Your grid container doesn't do much on its own. To make it useful, you need to create a *grid template,* which specifies the number of rows and columns you want in your grid. You set up your template by adding the `grid-template-columns` and `grid-template-rows` properties to your grid container:

```
container {
    display: grid;
    grid-template-columns: column-values;
    grid-template-rows: row-values
}
```

The *`column-values`* and *`row-values`* are space-separated lists of the sizes you want to use for each column and row in your grid. The sizes can be numbers expressed in any of the standard CSS measurement units (`px`, `em`, `rem`, `vw`, or `vh`), a percentage, or the keyword `auto`, which tells the browser to automatically set the size based on the other values you specify.

Here's an example, and Figure 4-18 shows the result:

CSS:

```
.container {
    display: grid;
    grid-template-columns: 100px 300px 200px;
    grid-template-rows: 100px 200px;
}
```

HTML:

```
<div class="container">
    <div class="item item1">1</div>
    <div class="item item2">2</div>
    <div class="item item3">3</div>
    <div class="item item4">4</div>
    <div class="item item5">5</div>
    <div class="item item6">6</div>
</div>
```

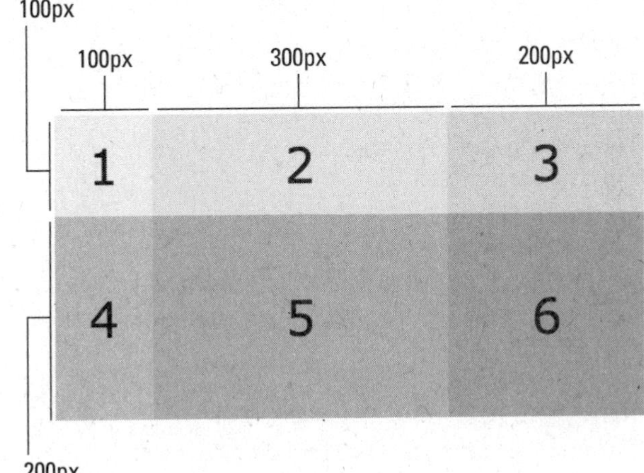

FIGURE 4-18: A basic grid created by setting just three properties: `display`, `grid-template-columns`, and `grid-template-rows`.

TECHNICAL STUFF

You can also specify a column or row size using a new unit called `fr`, which is specific to Grid and represents a fraction of the free space available in the grid container, either horizontally (for columns) or vertically (for rows). For example, if you assign one column `1fr` of space and another column `2fr`, the browser gives one third of the horizontal free space to the first column and two thirds of the horizontal free space to the second column.

TIP

If you leave out the `grid-template-rows` property, the browser automatically configures the row heights based on the height of the tallest element in each row.

Creating grid gaps

By default, the browser doesn't include any horizontal space between each column, or any vertical space between each row. If you'd prefer some daylight between your grid items, you can add the grid-column-gap and grid-row-gap properties to your grid container:

```
container {
    display: grid;
    grid-column-gap: column-gap-value;
    grid-row-gap: row-gap-value
}
```

In both properties, the value is a number expressed in any of the standard CSS measurement units (px, em, rem, vw, or vh). Here's an example:

```
.container {
    display: grid;
    grid-template-columns: 100px 300px 200px;
    grid-template-rows: 100px 200px;
    grid-column-gap: 10px;
    grid-row-gap: 15px;
}
```

TIP

There's a shorthand property called grid-gap that you can use to combine grid-column-gap and grid-row-gap into a single declaration:

```
container {
    display: grid;
    grid-gap: column-gap-value row-gap-value;
}
```

WARNING

While I was writing this book, the CSS Grid overlords declared that the names of the gap-related properties are going to change in the future:

Current Name	Future Name
grid-column-gap	column-gap
grid-row-gap	row-gap
grid-gap	gap

As I write these words, no browser supports the new names, so for now you should include both the current name and the new name when you're styling your grid gaps.

Assigning grid items to rows and columns

Rather than letting the web browser populate the grid automatically, you can take control of the process and assign your grid items to specific rows and columns. For each grid item, you specify four values:

```
item {
    grid-column-start: column-start-value;
    grid-column-end: column-end-value;
    grid-row-start: row-start-value;
    grid-row-end: row-end-value;
}
```

- `grid-column-start`: A number that specifies the column where the item begins.
- `grid-column-end`: A number that specifies the column before which the item ends. For example, if `grid-column-end` is set to 4, the grid item ends in column 3. Some notes:
  - If you omit this property, the item uses only the starting column.
  - If you use the keyword `end`, then the item runs from its starting column through to the last column in the grid.
  - You can use the keyword `span` followed by a space and then a number that specifies the number of columns you want the item to span across the grid. For example, the following two sets of declarations are equivalent:

```
grid-column-start: 1;
grid-column-end: 4;
grid-column-start: 1;
grid-column-end: span 3;
```

- `grid-row-start`: A number that specifies the row where the item begins.
- `grid-row-end`: A number that specifies the row before which the item ends. For example, if `grid-row-end` is set to 3, the grid item ends in row 2. Some notes:
  - If you omit this property, the item uses only the starting row.
  - If you use the keyword `end`, then the item runs from its starting row through to the last row in the grid.

* You can use the keyword span followed by a space and then a number that specifies the number of rows you want the item to span down the grid. For example, the following two sets of declarations are equivalent:

```
grid-row-start: 2;
grid-row-end: 4;
grid-row-start: 2;
grid-row-end: span 2;
```

Here's an example, and the results are shown in Figure 4-19:

CSS:

```
.container {
    display: grid;
    grid-template-columns: repeat(5, 100px);
    grid-template-rows: repeat(3, 150px);
}
.item1 {
    grid-column-start: 1;
    grid-column-end: 3;
    grid-row-start: 1;
    grid-row-end: 1;
}
.item2 {
    grid-column-start: 3;
    grid-column-end: span 3;
    grid-row-start: 1;
    grid-row-end: 1;
}
.item3 {
    grid-column-start: 1;
    grid-column-end: 1;
    grid-row-start: 2;
    grid-row-end: end;
}
.item4 {
    grid-column-start: 2;
    grid-column-end: 4;
    grid-row-start: 2;
    grid-row-end: end;
}
```

```
.item5 {
    grid-column-start: 4;
    grid-column-end: span 2;
    grid-row-start: 2;
    grid-row-end: 2;
}
.item6 {
    grid-column-start: 4;
    grid-column-end: span 2;
    grid-row-start: 3;
    grid-row-end: 3;
}
```

HTML:

```
<div class="container">
    <div class="item item1">1</div>
    <div class="item item2">2</div>
    <div class="item item3">3</div>
    <div class="item item4">4</div>
    <div class="item item5">5</div>
    <div class="item item6">6</div>
</div>
```

Creating the Page Layout

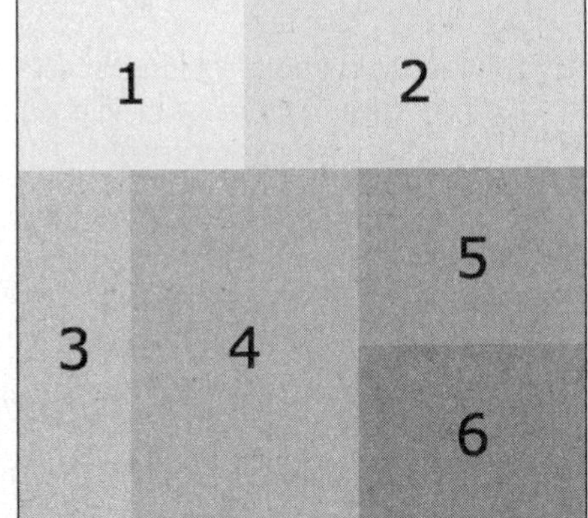

FIGURE 4-19: Some grid items assigned to different columns and rows in the grid.

TIP

In the example, notice that I used a function named `repeat` to specify multiple columns and rows that are the same size. Here's the syntax to use:

```
repeat(number, size)
```

Replace *number* with the number of columns or rows you want to create, and replace *size* with the size you want to use for each of those columns or rows. For example, the following two declarations are equivalent:

```
grid-template-rows: 150px 150px 150px;
grid-template-rows: repeat(3, 150px);
```

TIP

CSS also offers two shorthand properties that you can use to make the process of assigning items to columns and rows a bit more streamlined:

```
item {
    grid-column: column-start-value / column-end-value;
    grid-row: row-start-value / row-end-value;
}
```

Aligning grid items

CSS Grid offers several properties that you can use to align your grid items. For the grid container, you have the `justify-items` and `align-items` properties:

```
container {
    justify-items: start|end|center|stretch;
    align-items: start|end|center|stretch;
}
```

- `justify-items`: Aligns the content inside each grid item horizontally. You can align items to the left (`start`), the right (`end`), in the middle (`center`), or across the width of the item (`stretch`; this is the default value).
- `align-items`: Aligns the content inside each grid item vertically. You can align items to the top (`start`), the bottom (`end`), in the middle (`center`), or across the height of the item (`stretch`; this is the default value).

For a grid item, you have the `justify-self` and `align-self` properties:

```
item {
    justify-self: start|end|center|stretch;
    align-self: start|end|center|stretch;
}
```

- `justify-self`: Aligns the content inside the grid item horizontally. You can align the item to the left (`start`), the right (`end`), in the middle (`center`), or across the width of the item (`stretch`; this is the default value).

» `align-self`: Aligns the content inside the grid item vertically. You can align the item to the top (`start`), the bottom (end), in the middle (`center`), or across the height of the item (`stretch`; this is the default value).

Laying out content columns with Grid

As a two-dimensional layout system, Grid is perfect for laying out an entire page. This includes the classic page layout that I talk about earlier: a header and navigation bar across the top of the page, an article with a sidebar beside it, and a footer across the bottom of the page. Here's some Grid code that creates this layout, which is shown in Figure 4-20:

CSS:

```
body {
    display: grid;
    grid-template-columns: 1fr 10rem;
    grid-template-rows: 2.5rem 2.5rem 1fr 2.5rem;
    grid-gap: 1rem 1rem;
    min-height: 100vh;
}

header {
    grid-column: 1 / end;
    grid-row: 1;
    border: 1px solid black;
}

nav {
    grid-column: 1 / end;
    grid-row: 2;
    border: 1px solid black;
}

article {
    grid-column: 1;
    grid-row: 3;
    border: 1px solid black;
}
```

```
aside {
    grid-column: 2 / end;
    grid-row: 3;
    border: 1px solid black;
}

footer {
    grid-column: 1 / end;
    grid-row: 4;
    border: 1px solid black;
}
```

HTML:

```
<body>
    <header>
        Header
    </header>
    <nav>
        Navigation
    </nav>
    <article>
        Article
    </article>
    <aside>
        Aside
    </aside>
    <footer>
        Footer
    </footer>
</body>
```

Take a closer look at what the code does:

- The `<body>` tag is set up as a grid container, and that container is styled with two columns and four rows.
- The body element has its `min-height` property set to `100vh`, which makes the grid container always take up at least the entire height of the browser's content area.
- All `header`, `nav`, and `footer` elements span from the first column to the end of the grid, and they're assigned rows 1, 2, and 4, respectively.

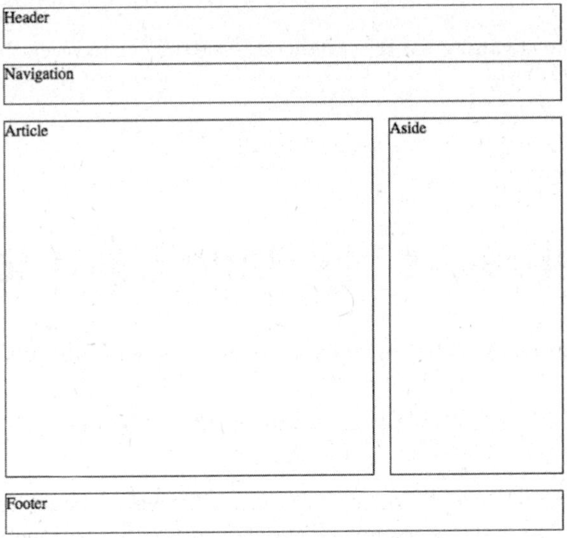

Header

Navigation

Article

Aside

Footer

FIGURE 4-20: The classic page layout, Grid-style.

- This version of the classic layout doesn't include a `main` element, because CSS Grid doesn't offer a mechanism for nesting grids.
- The `article` element uses only column 1 and row 3, both of which were defined with the size `1fr`, which allows the `article` element to take up the free space in the grid.
- The `aside` element uses column 2, which was assigned a width of `10rem`, so its width is fixed.

Grid browser support

CSS Grid offers two pieces of very good news when it comes to browser support:

- All major web browsers, both on the desktop and in mobile devices, support CSS Grid.
- No oddball vendor prefixes are needed in your CSS code.

The fly in the Grid ointment is that, yes, all major browsers are now Grid-friendly, but that support is relatively new, having been implemented in each browser at various points throughout 2017. This means that although Grid has strong browser market share — nearly 80 percent, as I write this — it's not enough for you to write Grid-only layouts. I talk about how you work around this problem in the next section.

TIP

You can take advantage of the handy CanIUse service to track the browser market share for CSS Grid:

```
https://caniuse.com/#search=grid
```

Providing Fallbacks for Page Layouts

Here's a summary of the current state of page layout in today's world:

- Nearly 80 percent of browsers support Grid. This is too small a number to build a Grid-only layout.
- About 85 percent of browsers fully support flexbox, although vendor prefixes are required. This is great support, but if you do a flexbox-only layout, about one in seven visitors will see your page in an ugly light.
- All browsers support both the `float` property and `display: inline-block`.

Does this mean you should just use floats or inline blocks and ignore flexbox and Grid until they have 100-percent browser support? No way! Through a technique called *progressive enhancement*, you can build a layout that uses a newer technology, but also includes an older page layout system that gets used with browsers that don't support the newer CSS. An older technology that a browser uses when it doesn't understand a newer technology is called a *fallback*.

The easiest way to implement fallbacks is to add *feature queries*, which use the `@supports` rule to check whether the web browser supports a CSS feature:

```
@supports (property: value) {
    Code to run if the browser supports the property-value
}
```

Replace *`property`* and *`value`* with the name of the CSS property and its value you want to check. For example, the following feature query-checks for Grid support:

```
@supports (display: grid) {
    Grid CSS goes here
}
```

To put this all together, here's some pseudo-code that shows how you'd implement your progressive enhancement:

```
Float or inline-block CSS comes first

@supports (display: flexbox) {
    Flexbox CSS goes here
}

@supports (display: grid) {
    Grid CSS goes here
}
```

The browser first implements the float or inline-block layout. If the browser supports flexbox, then it will implement the flexbox CSS, which automatically overrides the floats and inline-blocks (although you might have to apply `width: auto` to some elements to override explicit width settings from earlier in your code). If the browser supports Grid, it implements the Grid CSS, which overrides the flexbox code.

3 Coding the Front End, Part 2: JavaScript

Contents at a Glance

» Getting a taste of what you can (and can't) do with JavaScript

» Learning the tools you need to get coding

» Adding JavaScript code to a web page

» Storing your code in a separate JavaScript file

Chapter 1
An Overview of JavaScript

What's in your hands, I think and hope, is intelligence: the ability to see the machine as more than when you were first led up to it, that you can make it more.

— ALAN PERLIS

When we talk about web coding, what we're really talking about is JavaScript. Yep, you need HTML and CSS to create a web page, and you need tools such as PHP and MySQL to convince a web server to give your page some data, but the glue — and sometimes the duct tape — that binds all these technologies together is JavaScript. The result is that JavaScript is now (and has been for a while) the default programming language for web development. If you want to control a page using code (and I know you do), then you must use JavaScript to do it.

It also means that JavaScript is (and has been for a while) universal on the web. Sure, there are plenty of barebones home pages out there that are nothing but HTML and a sprinkling of CSS, but everything else — from humble personal blogs to fancy-pants designer portfolios to bigtime corporate ecommerce operations — relies on JavaScript to make things look good and work the way they're supposed to (most of the time, anyway).

So, when it comes to the care and feeding of your web development education, JavaScript is one of the most important — arguably *the* most important — of all the topics you need to learn. Are you excited to start exploring JavaScript? I *knew* it!

JavaScript: Controlling the Machine

When a web browser is confronted with an HTML file, it goes through a simple but tedious process: It reads the file one line at a time, starting from (usually) the `<html>` tag at the top and finishing with the `</html>` tag at the bottom. Along the way, it might have to break out of this line-by-line monotony to perform some action based on what it has read. For example, if it stumbles over the `<img>` tag, the browser will immediately ask the web server to ship out a copy of the graphics file specified in the `src` attribute.

The point here is that, at its core, a web browser is really just a page-reading machine that doesn't know how to do much of anything else besides follow the instructions (the markup) in an HTML file. (For my own convenience, I'm ignoring the browser's other capabilities, such as saving bookmarks.)

One of the reasons that many folks get hooked on creating web pages is that they realize from the very beginning that they have control over this page-reading machine. Slap some text between a `<b>` tag and its corresponding `</b>` end tag and the browser dutifully displays the text as bold. Create a CSS grid structure and the browser displays your formerly haphazard text in nice, neat rows and columns, no questions asked. In other words, instead of just viewing pages from the outside, you now have a key to get *inside* the machine and start working its controls. *That* is the hook that grabs people and gets them seriously interested in web page design.

Imagine if you could take this idea of controlling the page-reading machine to the next level. Imagine if, instead of ordering the machine to process mere tags and text, you could issue much more sophisticated commands that could actually control the inner workings of the page-reading machine. Who wouldn't want that?

Well, that's the premise behind JavaScript. It's essentially just a collection of commands that you can wield to control the browser. Like HTML tags, JavaScript commands are inserted directly into the web page file. When the browser does its line-by-line reading of the file and it comes across a JavaScript command, it executes that command, just like that.

However, the key here is that the amount of control JavaScript gives you over the page-reading machine is much greater than what you get with HTML tags. The reason is that JavaScript is a full-fledged *programming language*. The "L" in HTML might stand for "language," but there isn't even the tiniest hint of a programming language associated with HTML. JavaScript, though, is the real programming deal.

What Is a Programming Language?

So what does it mean to call something a "programming language"? To understand this term, you need look no further than the language you use to speak and write. At its most fundamental level, human language is composed of two things — words and rules:

- The words are collections of letters that have a common meaning among all the people who speak the same language. For example, the word "book" denotes a type of object, the word "heavy" denotes a quality, and the word "read" denotes an action.
- The rules are the ways in which words can be combined to create coherent and understandable concepts. If you want to be understood by other speakers of the language, then you have only a limited number of ways to throw two or more words together. "I read a heavy book" is an instantly comprehensible sentence, but "book a I read heavy" is gibberish.

The key goal of human language is being understood by someone else who is listening to you or reading something you wrote. If you use the proper words to refer to things and actions, and if you combine words according to the rules, then the other person will understand you.

A programming language works in more or less the same way. That is, it, too, has words and rules:

- The words are a set of terms that refer to the specific things that your program works with (such as the browser window) or the specific ways in which those things can be manipulated (such as sending the browser to a specified address). They're known as *reserved words* or *keywords*.
- The rules are the ways that the words can be combined so as to produce the desired effect. In the programming world, these rules are known as the language's *syntax*.

In JavaScript, many of the words you work with are very straightforward. There are some that refer to aspects of the browser, others that refer to parts of the web page, and some that are used internally by JavaScript. For example, in JavaScript the word `document` refers to a specific object (the web page as a whole), and the word `write()` refers to a specific action (writing data to the page).

The crucial concept here is that just as the fundamental purpose of human language is to be understood by another person, the fundamental purpose of a programming language is to be understood by whatever machine is processing the language. With JavaScript, that machine is the page-reading machine: the web browser.

You can make yourself understood by the page-reading machine by using the proper JavaScript words and by combining them using the proper JavaScript syntax. For example, JavaScript's syntax rules tell you that you can combine the words `document` and `write()` like so: `document.write()`. If you use `write().document` or `document write()` or any other combination, the page-reading machine won't understand you.

The key, however, is that being "understood" by the page-reading machine really means being able to *control* the machine. That is, your JavaScript "sentences" are actually commands that you want the machine to carry out. For example, if you want to add the text "Hello World!" to a web page using JavaScript, you include the following statement in your code:

```
document.write("Hello World!");
```

When the page-reading machine trudges through the HTML file and it comes upon this statement, it will go right ahead and insert it into the page.

Is JavaScript Hard to Learn?

I think there's a second reason why many folks get jazzed about creating web pages: It's not that hard. HTML sounds like it's a hard thing, and certainly if you look at the source code of a typical web page without knowing anything about HTML, the code appears about as intimidating as anything you can imagine.

However, I've found that anyone can learn HTML as long as a person starts with the basic tags, sees lots of examples of how they work, and slowly works one's way up to more complex pages. It's just a matter of creating a solid foundation and then building on it.

I'm convinced that JavaScript can be approached in much the same way. I'm certainly not going to tell you that JavaScript is as easy to learn as HTML. That would be a bald-faced lie. However, I will tell you that there is nothing inherently difficult about JavaScript. Using our language analogy, it just has a few more words to know and a few more rules to learn. But I believe that if you begin with the basic words and rules, see lots of examples of how they work, and then slowly build up to more complex scripts, you can learn JavaScript programming. By the time you finish this book, I predict here and now that you'll even be a little bit amazed at yourself and at what you can do.

What Can You Do with JavaScript?

The people I've taught to create web pages are a friendly bunch who enjoy writing to me to tell me how their pages are coming along. In many cases, they tell me they've hit the web page equivalent of a roadblock. That is, there's a certain thing they want to do, but they don't know how to do it in HTML. So I end up getting lots of questions like these:

- How do I display one of those pop-up boxes?
- How do I add content to the page on-the-fly?
- How can I make something happen when a user clicks a button?
- How can I make an image change when the mouse hovers over it?
- How can I calculate the total for my order form?

For each question, the start of the answer is always this: "Sorry, but you can't do that using HTML; you have to use JavaScript instead." I then supply them with a bit of code that they can "cut and paste" into their web pages and then get on with their lives.

If you're just getting started with JavaScript, then my goal in this book is to help you to move from "cut-and-paste" to "code-and-load." That is, you'll end up being able to create your own scripts to solve your own unique HTML and web page problems. I hope to show you that learning JavaScript is worthwhile because there are many other things you can do with it:

- You can ask a web server for data and then display that data on your page.
- You can add, modify, or remove page text, HTML tags, and even CSS properties.

- You can display messages to the user and ask the user for info.
- You can "listen" for and then perform actions based on events such as visitors clicking their mouse or pressing a key.
- You can send the user's browser to another page.
- You can validate the values in a form before submitting it to the server. For example, you can make sure that certain fields are filled in.
- You can collect, save, and retrieve data for each of your users, such as site customizations.

In this book, you learn how to do all these things and many more.

What Can't You Do with JavaScript?

JavaScript is good, but it's not that good. JavaScript can do many things, but there's a long list of things that it simply can't do. Here's a sampling:

- It can't write data permanently to an existing file. For example, you can't take the data from a guest book and add it to a page that displays the messages.
- It can't access files on the server.
- It can't glean any information about the user, including email or IP addresses.
- It can't submit credit card–based purchases for authorization and payment.
- It can't create multiplayer games.
- It can't get data directly from a server database.
- It can't handle file uploads.

The reason JavaScript can't do most of these things is that it's what's known in the trade as a *client-side* programming language, which means that it runs on the user's browser (which programming types like to call a *client*).

There are so-called *server-side* JavaScript tools that can do some of these things, but they're super-sophisticated and therefore beyond the scope here. The good news is that many of the items in the above list are doable using PHP and MySQL, which I discuss later on. For now, though, just know that there are so many things that client-side JavaScript can do that you'll have no trouble being as busy as you want to be.

What Do You Need to Get Started?

One of the nicest things about HTML and CSS is that the hurdles you have to leap to get started are not only short, but few in number. In fact, you really need only two things, both of which are free: a text editor to enter the text, tags, and properties, and a browser to view the results. (You'll also need a web server to host the finished pages, but the server isn't necessary when you're creating the pages.) Yes, there are high-end HTML editors and fancy graphics programs, but these fall into the "Bells and Whistles" category and you can create perfectly respectable web pages without them.

The basic requirements for JavaScript programming are exactly the same as for HTML: a text editor and a browser. Again, there are programs available to help you write and test your scripts, but you don't need them.

To learn more, check out Book 1, Chapter 2.

Basic Script Construction

Okay, that's more than enough theory. It's time to roll up your sleeves, crack your knuckles, and start coding. This section describes the standard procedure for constructing and testing a script. You'll see a working example that you can try out, and later you'll move on to other examples that illustrate some JavaScript techniques that you'll use throughout this book.

The <script> tag

The basic container for a script is, naturally enough, the HTML `<script>` tag and its associated `</script>` end tag:

```
<script>
    JavaScript statements go here
</script>
```

TECHNICAL STUFF

In HTML5 you can use `<script>` without any attributes, but before HTML5 the tag would look like this:

```
<script type="text/javascript">
```

The `type` attribute told the browser the programming language being used in the script, but JavaScript is the default now, so you no longer need it. You still see the

<script> tag with the type attribute used on a ton of pages, so I thought I better let you know what it means.

Handling browsers with JavaScript turned off

You don't have to worry about web browsers not being able to handle JavaScript, because all modern browsers have supported JavaScript for a very long time. However, you might want to worry about people who don't support JavaScript. Although rare, some folks have turned off their browser's JavaScript functionality. Why would someone do such a thing? Many people disable JavaScript because they're concerned about security, they don't want cookies written to their hard drives, and so on.

To handle these iconoclasts, place the <noscript> tag within the body of the page:

```
<noscript>
    <p>
        Hey, your browser has JavaScript turned off!
    </p>
    <p>
        Okay, cool, perhaps you'll prefer this <a href="no-js.
  html">non-JavaScript version</a> of the page.
    </p>
</noscript>
```

If the browser has JavaScript enabled, the user sees none of the text within the <noscript> tag. However, if JavaScript is disabled, the text and tags within the <noscript> tag are displayed to the user.

Where do you put the <script> tag?

With certain exceptions, it doesn't matter a great deal where you put your <script> tag. Some people place the tag between the page's </head> and <body> tags. The HTML standard recommends placing the <script> tag within the page header (that is, between <head> and </head>), so that's the style I use in this book:

```
<!DOCTYPE html>
<html lang="en">
    <head>
        <meta charset="utf-8">
        <title>Where do you put the script tag?</title>
```

```
        <script>
            JavaScript statements go here
        </script>
    </head>
    <body>
    </body>
</html>
```

Here are the exceptions to the put-your-script-anywhere technique:

- If your script is designed to write data to the page, the `<script>` tag must be positioned within the page body (that is, between the `<body>` and `</body>` tags) in the exact position where you want the text to appear.
- If your script refers to an item on the page (such as a form object), then the script must be placed *after* that item.
- With many HTML tags, you can add one or more JavaScript statements as attributes directly within the tag.

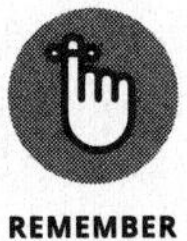

REMEMBER

It's perfectly acceptable to insert multiple `<script>` tags within a single page, as long as each one has a corresponding `</script>` end tag, and as long as you don't put one `<script>` block within another one.

Example #1: Displaying a message to the user

You're now ready to construct and try out your first script. This example shows you the simplest of all JavaScript actions: displaying a simple message to the user. The following code shows the script within an HTML file.

```
<!DOCTYPE html>
<html lang="en">
    <head>
        <meta charset="utf-8">
        <title>Displaying a Message to the User</title>
        <script>
            alert("Hello Web Coding World!");
        </script>
    </head>
    <body>
    </body>
</html>
```

As shown in here, place the script within the header of a page, save the file, and then open the HTML file within your browser.

This script consists of just a single line:

```
alert("Hello Web Coding World");
```

This is called a *statement*, and each statement is designed to perform a single JavaScript task. You might be wondering about the semicolon (`;`) that appears at the end of the statement. Good eye. You use the semicolon to mark the end of each of your JavaScript statements.

Your scripts will range from simple programs with just a few statements, to huge projects consisting of hundreds of statements. In the example, the statement runs the JavaScript `alert()` method, which displays to the user whatever message is enclosed within the parentheses (which could be a welcome message, an announcement of new features on your site, an advertisement for a promotion, and so on). Figure 1-1 shows the message that appears when you open the file.

TECHNICAL STUFF

A *method* is a special kind of JavaScript feature. I discuss methods in detail in Book 3, Chapter 8. For now, however, think of a method as a kind of action you want your code to perform.

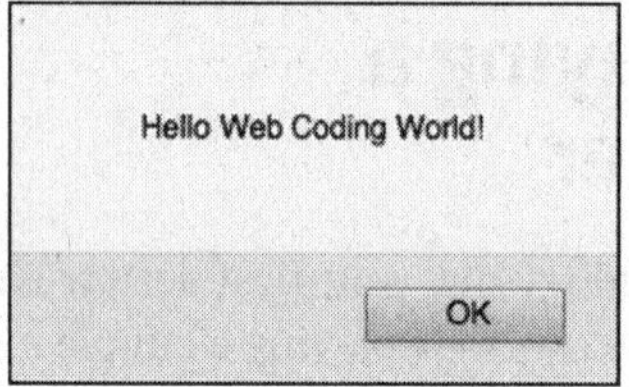

FIGURE 1-1: This "alert" message appears when you open the HTML file containing the example script.

How did the browser know to run the JavaScript statement? When a browser processes (*parses*, in the vernacular) a page, it basically starts at the beginning of the HTML file and works its way down, one line at a time, as I mention earlier. If it trips over a `<script>` tag, then it knows one or more JavaScript statements are coming, and it automatically executes those statements, in order, as soon as it reads them. The exception is when JavaScript statements are enclosed within a *function*, which I explain in Book 3, Chapter 5.

WARNING

One of the cardinal rules of JavaScript programming is "one statement, one line." That is, each statement must appear on only a single line, and there should be no more than one statement on each line. I said "should" in the second part of the previous sentence because it is possible to put multiple statements on a single line, as long as you separate each statement with a semicolon (;). There are rare times when it's necessary to have two or more statements on one line, but you should avoid it for the bulk of your programming because multiple-statement lines are difficult to read and to troubleshoot.

Example #2: Writing text to the page

One of JavaScript's most powerful features is the capability to write text and even HTML tags and CSS properties to the web page on-the-fly. That is, the text (or whatever) gets inserted into the page when a web browser loads the page. What good is that? For one thing, it's ideal for time-sensitive data. For example, you might want to display the date and time that a web page was last modified so that visitors know how old (or new) the page is. Here's some code that shows just such a script:

```
<!DOCTYPE html>
<html lang="en">
    <head>
        <meta charset="utf-8">
        <title>Writing Data to the Page</title>
    </head>
    <body>
        This is a regular line of text.<br>
        <script>
            document.write("This page was last modified on " +
  document.lastModified)
        </script>
        <br>This is another line of regular text.
    </body>
</html>
```

Notice how the script appears within the body of the HTML document, which is necessary whenever you want to write data to the page. Figure 1-2 shows the result.

This is a regular line of text.
This page was last modified on 02/18/2018 15:35:47
This is another line of regular text.

FIGURE 1-2: When you open the file, the text displays the date and time the file was last modified.

This script makes use of the *Document object*, which is a built-in JavaScript construct that refers to whatever HTML file (document) the script resides in (see Book 3, Chapter 8 for more about this). The `document.write()` statement tells the browser to insert whatever is within the parentheses to the web page. The `document.lastModified` portion returns the date and time the file was last changed and saved.

Adding Comments to Your Code

A script that consists of just a few lines is usually easy to read and understand. However, your scripts won't stay that simple for long, and these longer and more complex creations will be correspondingly more difficult to read. (This difficulty will be particularly acute if you're looking at the code a few weeks or months after you first programmed it.) To help you decipher your code, it's good programming practice to make liberal use of comments throughout the script. A *comment* is text that describes or explains a statement or group of statements. Comments are ignored by the browser, so you can add as many as you deem necessary.

For short, single-line comments, use the double-slash (//). Put the // at the beginning of the line, and then type in your comment after it. Here's an example:

```
// Display the date and time the page was last modified
document.write("This page was last modified on " + document.
   lastModified)
```

You can also use // comments for two or three lines of text. If you have more than that, however, then you're better off using multiple-line comments that begin with the /* symbol and end with the */ symbol. Here's an example:

```
/*
This script demonstrates JavaScript's ability
to write text to the web page by using the
document.write() method to display the date and time
the web page file was last modified.

This script is Copyright 2018 Paul McFedries.
*/
```

WARNING

Although it's fine to add quite a few comments when you're just starting out, you don't have to add a comment to everything. If a statement is trivial or if what a statement does is glaringly obvious, forget the comment and move on.

Creating External JavaScript Files

Putting a script inside the page header isn't a problem if the script is relatively short. However, if your script (or scripts) take up dozens or hundreds of lines, it can make your HTML code look cluttered. Another problem you might run into is needing to use the same code on multiple pages. Sure, you can just copy the code into each page that requires it, but if you make changes down the road, you need to update every page that uses the code.

The solution to both problems is to move the code out of the HTML file and into an external JavaScript file. Moving the code reduces the JavaScript presence in the HTML file to a single line (as you'll see shortly), and means that you can update the code by editing only the external file.

Here are some things to note about using an external JavaScript file:

- The file must use a plain text format.
- Use the `.js` extension when you name the file.
- Don't use the `<script>` tag within the file. Just enter your statements exactly as you would within an HTML file.
- The rules for when the browser executes statements within an external file are identical to those used for statements within an HTML file. That is, statements outside of functions are executed automatically when the browser sees your file reference, and statements within a function aren't executed until the function is called.

To let the browser know that an external JavaScript file exists, add the `src` attribute to the `<script>` tag. For example, if the external file is named `myscripts.js`, then your `<script>` tag is set up as follows:

```
<script src="myscripts.js">
```

This example assumes the `myscripts.js` file is in the same directory as the HTML file. If the file resides in a different directory, adjust the `src` value accordingly. For example, if the `myscripts.js` file is in a subdirectory named `scripts`, you'd use this:

```
<script src="scripts/myscripts.js">
```

You can even specify a file from another site (presumably your own!) by specifying a full URL as the `src` value:

```
<script src="http://www.host.com/myscripts.js">
```

As an example, the following code shows a one-line external JavaScript file named `footer.js`:

```
document.write("Copyright " + new Date().getFullYear());
```

This statement writes the text "Copyright" followed by the current year. (I know: This code looks like some real gobbledygook right now. Don't sweat it, because you learn exactly what's going on here when I discuss the JavaScript Date object in Book 3, Chapter 8.)

The following code shows an HTML file that includes a reference for the external JavaScript file:

```
<!DOCTYPE html>
<html lang="en">
    <head>
        <meta charset="utf-8">
        <title>Using an External JS File</title>
    </head>
    <body>
        <hr>
        <footer>
            <script src="footer.js">
            </script>
        </footer>
    </body>
</html>
```

When you load the page, the browser runs through the HTML line by line. When it gets to the `<footer>` tag, it sees the external JavaScript file that's referenced by the `<script>` tag. The browser loads that file and then runs the code within the file, which writes the Copyright message to the page, as you can see in Figure 1-3.

Copyright 2018

FIGURE 1-3: This page uses an external JavaScript file to display a footer message.

» Assigning names to variables

» Introducing JavaScript data types

» Figuring out numbers

» Stringing strings together

Chapter 2 Understanding Variables

You should imagine variables as tentacles, rather than boxes. They do not contain values; they grasp them.

— MARIJN HAVERBEKE

You might have heard about — or perhaps even know — people who, through mishap or misfortune, have lost the ability to retain short-term memories. If you introduce yourself to one of these poor souls, he'll be asking you your name again five minutes later. These unfortunates live in a perpetual present, seeing the world anew every minute of every day.

What, I'm sure you're asking yourself by now, can any of the above possibly have to do with coding? Just that, by default, your JavaScript programs also live a life without short-term memory. The web browser executes your code one statement at a time, until there are no more statements left to process. It all happens in the perpetual present. Ah, but notice that, above, I said this lack of short-term memory was the "default" state of your scripts. It's not the only state, so that means things can be different. You have the power to give your scripts the gift of short-term memory, and you do that by using handy little chunks of code called variables. In this chapter, you delve into variables, which is a fundamental and crucial programming topic. You investigate what variables are, what you can do with them, and how to wield them in your JavaScript code.

What Is a Variable?

Why would a script need short-term memory? Because one of the most common concepts that crops up when coding is the need to store a temporary value for use later on. In most cases, you want to use that value a bit later in the same script. However, you might also need to use it in some other script, to populate an HTML form, or to get data from a server.

For example, your page might have a button that toggles the page text between a larger font size and the regular font size, so you need some way to "remember" that choice. Similarly, if your script performs calculations, you might need to set aside one or more calculated values to use later. For example, if you're constructing a shopping cart script, you might need to calculate taxes on the order. To do that, you must first calculate the total value of the order, store that value, and then later take a percentage of it to work out the tax.

In programming, the way you save a value for later use is by storing it in a *variable*. A variable is a small chunk of computer memory that's set aside for holding program data. The good news is that the specifics of how the data is stored and retrieved from memory happen well behind the scenes, so it isn't something you ever have to worry about. As a coder, working with variables involves just three things:

1. Creating (or *declaring*) variables
2. Assigning values to those variables
3. Including the variables in other statements in your code

The next three sections fill in the details.

Declaring a variable

The process of creating a variable is called *declaring* in programming terms. All declaring really means is that you're supplying the variable with a name and telling the browser to set aside a bit of room in memory to hold whatever value you end up storing in the variable. To declare a variable in JavaScript, you use the `var` keyword, followed by a space, the name of the variable, and the usual line-ending semicolon. For example, to declare a variable named `interestRate`, you'd use the following statement:

```
var interestRate;
```

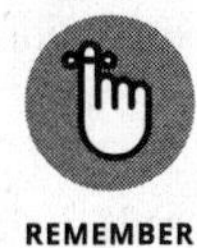

REMEMBER

Although you're free to use a variable as many times as you need to within a script, only declare the variable once, and make sure that declaration occurs before any other uses of the variable. Declaring a variable more than once won't cause an error, but doing so is bad programming practice.

Storing a value in a variable

After your variable is declared, your next task is to give it a value. You use the assignment operator — the equal (=) sign — to store a value in a variable, as in this general statement:

```
variableName = value;
```

Here's an example that assigns the value `0.03` to a variable named `interestRate`:

```
interestRate = 0.03;
```

Note, too, that if you know the initial value of the variable in advance, you can combine the declaration and initial assignment into a single statement, like this:

```
var interestRate = 0.03;
```

It's important to remember that you're free to change a variable's value any time you want. (That's why it's called a *variable,* because its value can vary.) For example, if the value you assign to the `interestRate` variable is an annual rate, later on your code might need to work with a monthly rate, which is the annual rate divided by 12. Rather than calculate that by hand, just put it in your code using the division operator (/):

```
interestRate = 0.03 / 12;
```

As a final note about using variable assignment, take a look at a variation that often causes some confusion among new programmers. Specifically, you can set up a statement that assigns a new value to a variable by changing its existing value. Here's an example:

```
interestRate = interestRate / 12;
```

If you've never seen this kind of statement before, it probably looks a bit illogical. How can something equal itself divided by 12? The secret to understanding such a statement is to remember that the browser always evaluates the right side of the statement — that is, the expression to the right of the equal sign (=) — first. In other words, it takes the current value of `interestRate`, which is `0.03`, and divides it by 12. The resulting value is what's stored in `interestRate` when all is said and done. For a more in-depth discussion of operators and expressions, see Book 3, Chapter 3.

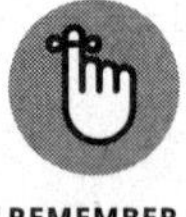

REMEMBER

Because of this evaluate-the-expression-and-*then*-store-the-result behavior, JavaScript assignment statements shouldn't be read as "variable *equals* expression." Instead, it makes more sense to think of them as "variable *is set to* expression" or "variable *assumes the value given by* expression." Reading assignment statements this way helps to reinforce the important concept that the expression result is being stored in the variable.

Using variables in statements

With your variable declared and assigned a value, you can then use that variable in other statements. When the browser sees the variable, it goes to the computer's memory, retrieves the current value of the variable, and then substitutes that value into the statement. The following code presents an example:

```
var interestRate;
interestRate = 0.03;
alert(interestRate);
```

This code declares a variable named `interestRate` and assigns the value `0.03` to that variable. The `alert()` statement then displays the current value of the variable, as shown in Figure 2-1.

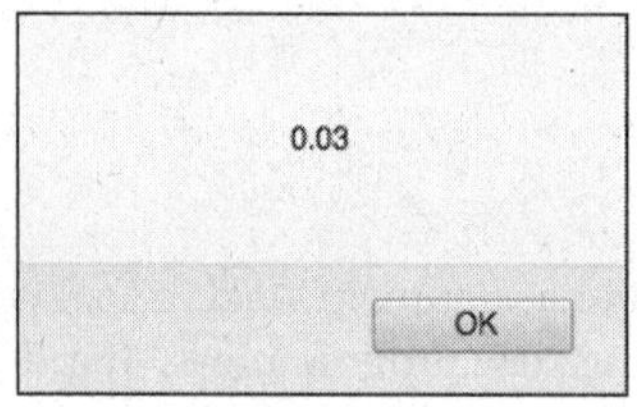

FIGURE 2-1: When you use a variable in a statement, such as the `alert()` statement in the example code, the browser substitutes the current value of that variable.

The following code shows a slightly different example:

```
var firstName;
firstName = prompt("Please tell me your first name:");
alert("Welcome to my website, " + firstName);
```

This script uses the `prompt()` method to ask the user to enter her first name, as shown in Figure 2-2. (To learn more about the `prompt()` method, see Book 3,

Chapter 7.) When the user clicks OK, her name is stored in the `firstName` variable. The script then uses an `alert()` statement to display a personalized welcome message using the value of the `firstName` variable, as shown in Figure 2-3.

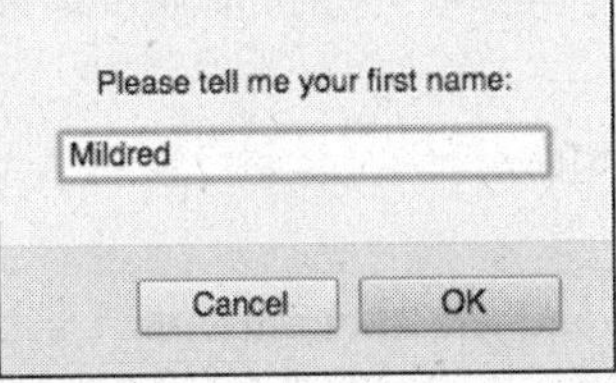

FIGURE 2-2: The script first prompts the user for her first name.

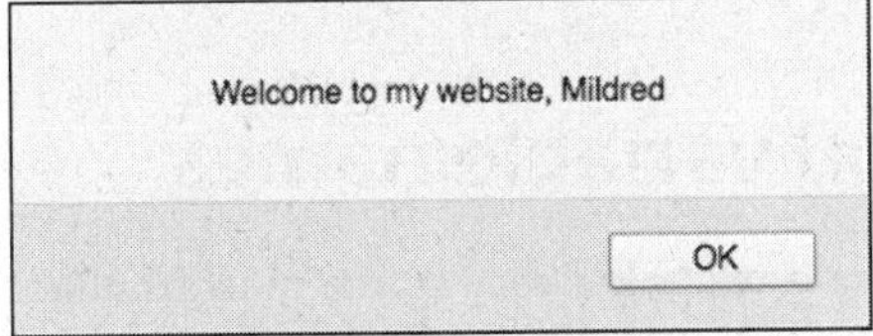

FIGURE 2-3: The script then uses the name to display a personalized welcome message.

WARNING

In these early chapters, I use the `alert()` method quite often because it gives you an easy way to see the results of my example scripts. In practice, however, you'll use `alert()` only rarely because few users want to be pestered by dialog boxes throughout a site.

Naming Variables: Rules and Best Practices

If you want to write clear, easy-to-follow, and easy-to-debug scripts (and who doesn't?), you can go a long way toward that goal by giving careful thought to the names you use for your variables. This section helps by running through the rules you need to follow and by giving you some tips and guidelines for creating good variable names.

Rules for naming variables

JavaScript has only a few rules for variable names:

- The first character must be a letter or an underscore (_). You can't use a number as the first character.

- The rest of the variable name can include any letter, any number, or the underscore. You can't use any other characters, including spaces, symbols, and punctuation marks.
- As with the rest of JavaScript, variable names are case sensitive. That is, a variable named `InterestRate` is treated as an entirely different variable than one named `interestRate`.
- There's no limit to the length of the variable name.
- You can't use one of JavaScript's *reserved words* as a variable name (such as `var`, `alert`, or `prompt`). All programming languages have a supply of words that are used internally by the language and that can't be used for variable names, because doing so would cause confusion (or worse).

Ideas for good variable names

The process of declaring a variable doesn't take much thought, but that doesn't mean you should just type in any old variable name that comes to mind. Take a few extra seconds to come up with a good name by following these guidelines:

- Make your names descriptive. Sure, using names that are just a few characters long makes them easier to type, but I guarantee you that you won't remember what the variables represent when you look at the script down the road. For example, if you want a variable to represent an account number, use `accountNumber` or `accountNum` instead of, say, `acnm` or `accnum`.

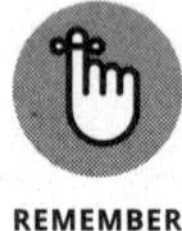
REMEMBER

- Although it's best to avoid single-letter variable names, such short names are accepted in some places, such as when constructing loops as described in Book 3, Chapter 4.
- The best way to create a descriptive variable name is to use multiple words. However, because JavaScript doesn't take kindly to spaces in names, you need some way of separating the words to keep the name readable. The two standard conventions for using multi-word variable names are *camelCase,* where you cram the words together and capitalize all but the first word (for example, `lastName`), or to separate each word with a dash (for example, `last-name`). I prefer the former style, so I use it throughout this book.
- Use one naming convention for JavaScript variables and a different one for HTML identifiers and CSS classes. For example, if you use camelCase for JavaScript variables, use dashes for `id` values and class names.
- Try to make your variable names look as different from JavaScript's keywords and other built-in terms (such as `alert`) as possible. Differentiating variable

names helps avoid the confusion that can arise when you look at a term and you can't remember if it's a variable or a JavaScript word.

- Although short, cryptic variable names are to be shunned in favor of longer, descriptive names, that doesn't mean you should be using entire sentences. Extremely long names are inefficient because they take so long to type, and they're dangerous because the longer the name, the more likely you are to make a typo. Names of 2 to 4 words and 8 to 20 characters should be all you need.

Understanding Literal Data Types

In programming, a variable's *data type* specifies what kind of data is stored within the variable. The data type is a crucial idea because it determines not only how two or more variables are combined (for example, mathematically), but also whether they can be combined at all. *Literals* are a special class of data type, and they cover those values that are fixed (even if only temporarily). For example, consider the following variable assignment statement:

```
todaysQuestion = "What color is your parachute?";
```

Here, the text `"What color is your parachute?"` is a literal string value. JavaScript supports three kinds of literal data types: numeric, string, and Boolean. The next three sections discuss each type.

Working with numeric literals

Unlike many other programming languages, JavaScript treats all numbers the same, so you don't have to do anything special when working with the two basic numeric literals, which are integers and floating-point numbers:

- **Integers:** These are numbers that don't have a fractional or decimal part. So you represent an integer using a sequence of one or more digits, as in these examples:

```
0
42
2001
-20
```

» **Floating-point numbers:** These are numbers that do have a fractional or decimal part. Therefore, you represent a floating-point number by first writing the integer part, followed by a decimal point, followed by the fractional or decimal part, as in these examples:

```
0.07
3.14159
-16.6666667
7.6543e+21
1.234567E-89
```

Exponential notation

The last two floating-point examples require a bit more explanation. These two use *exponential notation*, which is an efficient way to represent really large or really small floating-point numbers. Exponential notation uses an `e` (or `E`) followed by a plus sign (+) or a minus sign (–), followed by a number, which is called the *exponent*.

If the notation contains a plus sign, then you multiply the first part of the number (that is, the part before the `e` or `E`) by 10 to the power of the exponent. Here's an example:

```
9.87654e+5;
```

The exponent is 5, and 10 to the power of 5 is 100,000. So multiplying 9.87654 by 100,000 results in the value 987,654.

If the notation contains a minus sign, instead, then you divide the rest of the number by 10 to the power of the exponent. Here's an example:

```
3.4567e-4;
```

The exponent is 4, and 10 to the power of 4 is 10,000. So dividing 3.4567 by 10,000 results in the value .00034567.

JavaScript has a ton of built-in features for performing mathematical calculations. To get the scoop on these, head for Book 3, Chapter 8.

When I mentioned earlier that JavaScript treats all numeric literals the same, what I really meant was that JavaScript treats the numeric literals as floating-point values. This is fine (after all, there's no practical difference between 2 and 2.0), but it does put a limit on the maximum and minimum integer values that you can work with safely. The maximum is 9007199254740992 and the minimum is -9007199254740992. If you use numbers outside of this range (unlikely, but you never know), JavaScript won't be able to maintain accuracy.

Hexadecimal integer values

You'll likely deal with the usual decimal (base-10) number system throughout most of your JavaScript career. However, just in case you have cause to work with hexadecimal (base-16) numbers, this section shows you how JavaScript deals with them.

The hexadecimal number system uses the digits 0 through 9 and the letters A through F (or a through f), where these letters represent the decimal numbers 10 through 15. So, what in the decimal system would be 16 is actually 10 in hexadecimal. To specify a hexadecimal number in JavaScript, begin the number with a `0x` (or `0X`), as shown in the following examples:

```
0x23;
0xff;
0X10ce;
```

Working with string literals

A *string literal* is a sequence of one or more letters, numbers, or punctuation marks, enclosed either in double quotation marks (`"`) or single quotation marks (`'`). Here are some examples:

```
"Web Coding and Development";
'August 23, 1959';
"";
"What's the good word?";
```

REMEMBER

The string `""` (or `''` — two consecutive single quotation marks) is called the *null string*. It represents a string that doesn't contain any characters.

Using quotation marks within strings

The last example in the previous section shows that it's okay to insert one or more instances of one of the quotation marks (such as `'`) inside a string that's enclosed by the other quotation mark (such as `"`). Being able to nest quotation marks comes in handy when you need to embed one string inside another, which is very common (particularly when using bits of JavaScript within HTML tags). Here's an example:

```
onsubmit="processForm('testing')";
```

However, it's illegal to insert in a string one or more instances of the same quotation mark that encloses the string, as in this example:

```
"This is "illegal" in JavaScript.";
```

Understanding escape sequences

However, what if you must include, say, a double quotation mark within a string that's enclosed by double quotation marks? Having to nest the same type of quotation mark is rare, but it is possible if you precede the double quotation mark with a backslash (\), like this:

```
"The double quotation mark (\") encloses this string.";
```

The \" combination is called an *escape sequence*. You can combine the backslash with a number of other characters to form other escape sequences, and each one enables the browser to represent a character that, by itself, would be illegal or not representable otherwise. Table 2-1 lists the most commonly used escape sequences.

TABLE 2-1 **Common JavaScript Escape Sequences**

Escape Sequence	Character It Represents
\'	Single quotation mark
\"	Double quotation mark
\b	Backspace
\f	Form feed
\n	New line
\r	Carriage return
\t	Tab
\\	Backslash

The following code shows an example script that uses the \n escape sequence to display text on multiple lines with an alert box.

```
alert("This is line 1.\nSo what. This is line 2.");
```

Figure 2-4 shows the result.

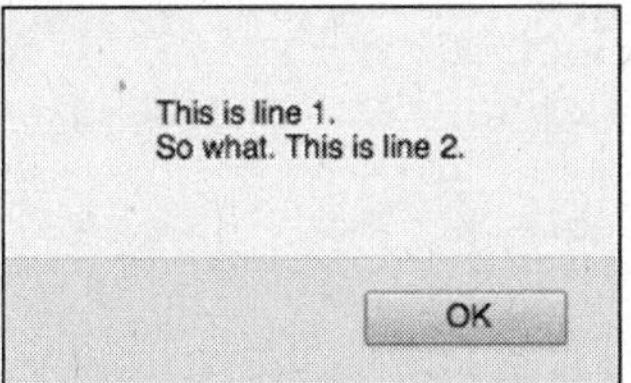

FIGURE 2-4: Using the \n escape sequence enables you to format text so that it displays on different lines.

To learn how to combine two or more string literals, check out Book 3, Chapter 3. Also, JavaScript has a nice collection of string manipulation features, which I discuss in Book 3, Chapter 8.

Working with Boolean literals

Booleans are the simplest of all the literal data types because they can assume only one of two values: `true` or `false`. That simplicity might make it seem as though Booleans aren't particularly useful, but the capability to test whether a particular variable or condition is true or false is invaluable in JavaScript programming.

You can assign Boolean literals directly to a variable, like this:

```
taskCompleted = true;
```

Alternatively, you can work with Boolean values implicitly using expressions:

```
currentMonth === "August"
```

The comparison expression `currentMonth === "August"` asks the following: Does the value of the `currentMonth` variable equal the string `"August"`? If it does, the expression evaluates to the Boolean value `true`; if it doesn't, the expression evaluates to `false`. I discuss much more about comparison expressions in Book 3, Chapter 3.

JavaScript Reserved Words

As I mention earlier, JavaScript has a bunch of reserved words that you need to avoid when naming your variables. Table 2-2 presents a list of the JavaScript keywords. It's illegal to use any of these words as variable or function names.

TABLE 2-2 JavaScript's Reserved Words

abstract	boolean	break	byte
case	catch	char	class
const	continue	debugger	default
delete	do	double	else
enum	export	extends	false
final	finally	float	for
function	goto	if	import
in	instanceof	int	long
native	new	null	return
short	super	switch	synchronized
this	throw	throws	transient
true	try	typeof	var
void	volatile	while	with
yield			

JavaScript Keywords

Table 2-3 presents the complete list of keywords used in JavaScript and HTML that you should avoid using for variable and function names.

TABLE 2-3 JavaScript and HTML Keywords

alert	all	anchor	anchors
area	Array	assign	blur
button	checkbox	clearInterval	clearTimeout
clientInformation	close	closed	confirm
constructor	crypto	Date	decodeURI
decodeURIComponent	defaultStatus	document	element
elements	embed	embeds	encodeURI

encodeURIComponent	escape	eval	event
fileUpload	focus	form	forms
frame	frameRate	frames	function
hasOwnProperty	hidden	history	image
images	Infinity	innerHeight	innerWidth
isFinite	isNaN	isPrototypeOf	layer
layers	length	link	location
Math	mimeTypes	name	NaN
navigate	navigator	Number	Object
offscreenBuffering	onblur	onclick	onerror
onfocus	onkeydown	onkeypress	onkeyup
onload	onmousedown	onmouseover	onmouseup
onsubmit	open	opener	option
outerHeight	outerWidth	packages	pageXOffset
pageYOffset	parent	parseFloat	parseInt
password	pkcs11	plugin	prompt
propertyIsEnum	prototype	radio	reset
screenX	screenY	scroll	secure
select	self	setInterval	setTimeout
status	String	submit	taint
text	textarea	top	toString
undefined	unescape	untaint	valueOf

» **Figuring out numeric expressions**

» **Tying up string expressions**

» **Getting the hang of comparison expressions**

» **Learning about logical expressions**

Chapter 3 Building Expressions

It's not at all important to get it right the first time. It's vitally important to get it right the last time.

— DAVID THOMAS

The JavaScript variables described in the previous chapter can't do all that much by themselves. They don't become useful members of your web code community until you give them something productive to do. For example, you can assign values to them, use them to assign values to other variables, use them in calculations, and so on.

This productive side of variables in particular, and JavaScript-based web code in general, is brought to you by a JavaScript feature known as the expression. This chapter takes you through everything you need to know about expressions. You discover some expression basics and then you explore a number of techniques for building powerful expressions using numbers, strings, and Boolean values.

Understanding Expression Structure

To be as vague as I can be, an *expression* is a collection of symbols, words, and numbers that performs a calculation and produces a result. That's a nebulous definition, I know, so I'll make it more concrete.

When your check arrives after a restaurant meal, one of the first things you probably do is take out your smartphone and use the calculator to figure out the tip amount. The service and food were good, so you're thinking 20 percent is appropriate. With phone in hand, you tap in the bill total, tap the multiplication button, tap 20%, and then tap Equals. Voila! The tip amount appears on the screen and you're good to go.

A JavaScript expression is something like this kind of procedure because it takes one or more inputs, such as a bill total and a tip percentage, and combines them in some way — for example, by using multiplication. In expression lingo, the inputs are called *operands*, and they're combined by using special symbols called *operators*.

- **Operand:** An input value for an expression. It is, in other words, the raw data that the expression manipulates to produce its result. It could be a number, a string, a variable, a function result (see Book 3, Chapter 5), or an object property (see Book 3, Chapter 8).
- **Operator:** A symbol that represents a particular action performed on one or more operands. For example, the * operator represents multiplication, and the + operator represents addition. I discuss the various JavaScript operators throughout this chapter.

For example, here's an expression that calculates a tip amount and assigns the result to a variable:

```
tipAmount = billTotal * tipPercentage;
```

The expression is everything to the right of the equals sign (=). Here, `billTotal` and `tipPercentage` are the operands, and the multiplication sign (*) is the operator.

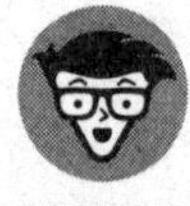

Expression results always have a particular data type — numeric, string, or Boolean. So when you're working with expressions, always keep in mind what type of result you need and then choose the appropriate operands and operators accordingly.

Another analogy I like to use for operands and operators is a grammatical one — that is, if you consider an expression to be a sentence, then the operands are the nouns (the things) of the sentence, and the operators are the verbs (the actions) of the sentence.

Building Numeric Expressions

Calculating a tip amount on a restaurant bill is a mathematical calculation, so you may be thinking that JavaScript expressions are going to be mostly mathematical. If I was standing in front of you and I happened to have a box of gold stars on me, then I'd certainly give you one because, yes, math-based expressions are probably the most common type you'll come across.

This type of calculation is called a *numeric expression*, and it combines numeric operands and arithmetic operators to produce a numeric result. This section discusses all the JavaScript arithmetic operators and shows you how best to use them to build useful and handy numeric expressions.

A quick look at the arithmetic operators

JavaScript's basic arithmetic operators are more or less the same as those found in your smartphone's calculator app or on the numeric keypad of your computer's keyboard, plus a couple of extra operators for more advanced work. Table 3-1 lists the basic arithmetic operators you can use in your JavaScript expressions. (In subsequent sections, I discuss each one in more detail.)

TABLE 3-1 The JavaScript Arithmetic Operators

Operator	Name	Example	Result
+	Addition	10 + 4	14
++	Increment	10++	11
–	Subtraction	10 - 4	6
–	Negation	-10	-10
--	Decrement	10--	9
*	Multiplication	10 * 4	40
/	Division	10 / 4	2.5
%	Modulus	10 % 4	2

JavaScript also comes with a few extra operators that combine some of the arithmetic operators and the assignment operator, which is the humble equal sign (=) that assigns a value to a variable. Table 3-2 lists these so-called *arithmetic assignment* operators.

TABLE 3-2 The JavaScript Arithmetic Assignment Operators

Operator	Example	Equivalent
+=	x += y	x = x + y
-=	x -= y	x = x - y
*=	x *= y	x = x * y
/=	x /= y	x = x / y
^=	x ^= y	x = x ^ y
%=	x %= y	x = x % y

Using the addition (+) operator

You use the addition operator (+) to calculate the sum of two operands. The operands are usually of the numeric data type, which means they can be numeric literals, variables that store numeric values, or methods or functions that return numeric values. Here's an example:

```
widthMax = widthContent + widthSidebar + 100;
```

You could use such an expression in a web app when you need to know the maximum width to assign the app's container. In this case, you take the width of the app's content (represented by the `widthContent` variable), add the width of the app's sidebar (the `widthSidebar` variable), and then add the literal value `100` (which may be a value in pixels).

Using the increment (++) operator

One of the most common programming operations involves adding 1 to an existing value, such as a variable. This operation is called *incrementing* the value, and the standard way to write such a statement is as follows:

```
someVariable = someVariable + 1;
```

However, JavaScript offers a much more compact alternative that uses the increment operator (++):

```
++someVariable;
```

TECHNICAL STUFF

THE PRE- AND POST-INCREMENT OPERATORS

If you need to increment the variable and then assign this new value to another variable, use the following form:

```
someVariable = ++anotherVariable;
```

This is exactly the same as the following two statements:

```
anotherVariable = anotherVariable + 1;
someVariable = anotherVariable;
```

Because the ++ appears before the variable, it is often called the *pre-increment operator*. So far, so good. However, just to confuse you, JavaScript also supports a variation on this theme called the *post-increment operator*:

```
someVariable = anotherVariable++;
```

In this case, the ++ operator appears after the variable. Big whoop, right? Actually, there is a subtle but crucial difference. Take a look at the following two statements that do exactly the same thing as the post-increment operator:

```
someVariable = anotherVariable;
anotherVariable = anotherVariable + 1;
```

As you can see, the first variable is set equal to the second variable and then the second variable is incremented.

Using the subtraction and negation (-) operators

The subtraction operator (–) subtracts the numeric value to the right of the operator from the numeric value to the left of the operator. For example, consider the following statements:

```
var targetYear = 2020;
var birthYear = 1985;
var yearsDifference = targetYear - birthyear;
```

The third statement subtracts 1985 from 2020 and the result — 35 — is stored in the `yearsDifference` variable.

The negation operator (-) is the same symbol, but it works in a totally different way. You use it as a kind of prefix by appending it to the front of an operand. The result is a new value that has the opposite sign of the original value. In other words, applying the negation operator to an operand is exactly the same as multiplying the operand by -1. This means the following two statements are identical:

```
negatedValue = -originalValue;
negatedValue = originalValue * -1;
```

Using the decrement (--) operator

Another common programming operation is subtracting 1 from an existing variable or other operand. This operation is called *decrementing* the value, and the usual way to go about this is with a statement like this one:

```
thisVariable = thisVariable - 1;
```

However (you just knew there was going to be a however), JavaScript offers a much more svelte alternative that takes advantage of the decrement operator (--):

```
--thisVariable;
```

Using the multiplication (*) operator

The multiplication operator (*) multiplies two operands together. Here's an example:

```
var totalColumns = 8;
var columnWidth = 100;
var totalWidth = totalColumns * columnWidth;
```

You might use this code when you want to calculate the width taken up by a web page layout that uses multiple columns. This code assigns literal numeric values to the variables `totalColumns` and `columnWidth`. It then uses a numeric expression to multiply these two values together and assign the result to the `totalWidth` variable.

Using the division (/) operator

The division operator (/) divides one numeric value by another. You can show off at parties by remembering that the number to the left of the slash (/) is called the *dividend*, and the number to the right of the / is called the *divisor*:

```
dividend / divisor
```

TECHNICAL STUFF

THE PRE- AND POST-DECREMENT OPERATORS

If you need to decrement the variable and then assign this new value to another variable, use the *pre-decrement* form:

```
thisVariable = --thatVariable;
```

This is the same as the following two statements:

```
thatVariable = thatVariable - 1;
thisVariable = thatVariable;
```

To assign the value of a variable to another variable and then decrement the first variable, use the *post-decrement* form:

```
thisVariable = thatVariable--;
```

Again, the following two statements do exactly the same thing:

```
thisVariable = thatVariable;
thatVariable = thatVariable - 1;
```

As you can see, the first variable is set equal to the second variable and then the second variable is decremented.

Here's an example:

```
var contentWidth = 600;
var windowWidth = 1200;
var contentRatio = contentWidth / windowWidth;
```

You can use this code to calculate the portion of the browser's window width that the page content is currently using. In this code, the variables `contentWidth` and `windowWidth` are assigned literal numeric values, and then a numeric expression divides the first of the values by the second, the result of which is stored in the `contentRatio` variable.

WARNING

Whenever you use the division operator, you must guard against cases where the divisor is 0. If that happens, your script will produce an `Infinity` result, which is almost certain to wreak havoc on your calculations. Before performing any division, your script should use an `if()` statement (see Book 3, Chapter 4) to check whether the divisor is 0 and, if it is, to cancel the division or perform some kind of work-around.

Using the modulus (%) operator

The modulus operator (`%`) divides one number by another and then returns the remainder as the result:

```
dividend % divisor
```

For example, the following code stores the value `1` in the variable named `myModulus` because 5 (the `myDivisor` value) divides into 16 (the `myDividend` value) three times and leaves a remainder of 1:

```
var myDividend = 16;
var myDivisor = 5;
var myModulus = myDividend % myDivisor;
```

On a more practical level, suppose that you're trying to come up with a web page color scheme, and you want to use two colors that are complements of each other. Complementary means that the two hues are on the opposite side of the color wheel, so one way to calculate the second color is by adding 180 to the first color's hue value. That approach works when the hue of the first color is between 0 and 179, which give second color hue values between 180 and 359. However, an initial hue of 180, 181, and so on produces a second hue of 360, 361, and so on, which are illegal values. You can work around that issue by using a modulus expression like this:

```
complementaryColor = (originalColor + 180) % 360;
```

This statement adds 180 to the original color, but then uses `% 360` to return the remainder when divided by 360 to avoid illegal values.

Using the arithmetic assignment operators

Your web coding scripts will often update the value of a variable by adding to it the value of some other operand. Here's an example:

```
totalInterestPaid = totalInterestPaid + monthlyInterestPaid
```

Coders are an efficiency-loving bunch, so the fact that the `totalInterestPaid` variable appears twice in that statement is like chewing tin foil to your average programmer. The JavaScript brain trust hate that kind of thing, too, so they came up with the addition assignment operator (+=):

```
totalInterestPaid += monthlyInterestPaid
```

Yep, this statement does exactly the same thing as the first one, but it does it with 19 fewer characters. Sweet!

If you need to subtract one operand from another, again you can do it the old-fashioned way:

```
housePrincipleOwing = housePrincipleOwing - monthlyPrincipalPaid
```

To avoid other coders laughing behind your back at your inefficiency, use the subtraction assignment operator (–=):

```
housePrincipleOwing -= monthlyPrincipalPaid
```

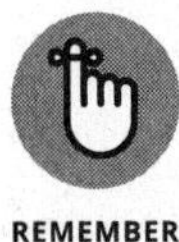

REMEMBER

Like the increment and decrement operators, the arithmetic assignment operators are designed to save wear-and-tear on your typing fingers and to reduce the size of your scripts, particularly if you use long variable names.

Building String Expressions

A string expression is one where at least one of the operands is a string, and the result of the expression is another string. String expressions are straightforward in the sense that there is only one operator to deal with: *concatenation* (+). You use this operator to combine (or *concatenate*) strings within an expression. For example, the expression `"Java" + "Script"` returns the string `"JavaScript"`. Note, however, that you can also use strings with the comparison operators discussed in the next section.

It's unfortunate that the concatenation operator is identical to the addition operator because this similarity can lead to some confusion. For example, the expression `2 + 2` returns the numeric value `4` because the operands are numeric. However, the expression `"2" + "2"` returns the string value `22` because the two operands are strings.

TIP

BREAKING UP LONG STATEMENTS

All your JavaScript statements should appear on a single line (see Book 3, Chapter 1). An exception to that rule is any statement that contains a long expression, which you can break into multiple lines as long as the break occurs immediately before or after an operator. For example, you can display a string expression in multiple lines as long as the break occurs immediately before or after the + operator, as in the following examples:

```
var message1 = "How did the fool and his money " +
               "get together in the first place?";
var message2 = "Never put off until tomorrow that which you "
             + "can put off until the day after tomorrow.";
```

To further complicate matters, JavaScript will often convert numbers into strings depending on the context:

- If the first operand in an expression is a string, JavaScript converts any number in the expression to a string. For example, the following expression returns the string 222:

  ```
  "2" + 2 + 2
  ```

- If the first two or more operands in an expression are numbers and the rest of the expression contains a string, JavaScript handles the numeric part of the expression first and then converts the result into a string. For example, the following expression returns the string 42 because the result of `2 + 2` is 4, which is then concatenated as a string to `"2"`:

  ```
  2 + 2 + "2"
  ```

As an example of how this conversion can be a problem, consider the script in the following code.

```
var preTipTotal = 10.00;
var tipAmount = preTipTotal * 0.15;
var message1 = "Your tip is ";
var message2 = "\nYour total bill is ";
alert(message1 + tipAmount + message2 + preTipTotal +
  tipAmount);
```

The `preTipTotal` variable stores a total for a restaurant bill, and the `tipAmount` variable stores 15 percent of the total. The variables `message1` and `message2` are initialized with strings, and then an alert box is displayed with the results. In particular, the expression `preTipTotal + tipAmount` is included in the `alert()` method to display the total bill. However, as you can see in Figure 3-1, the "total" displayed is actually `101.5` instead of `11.5` (10 plus 1.5 for the tip).

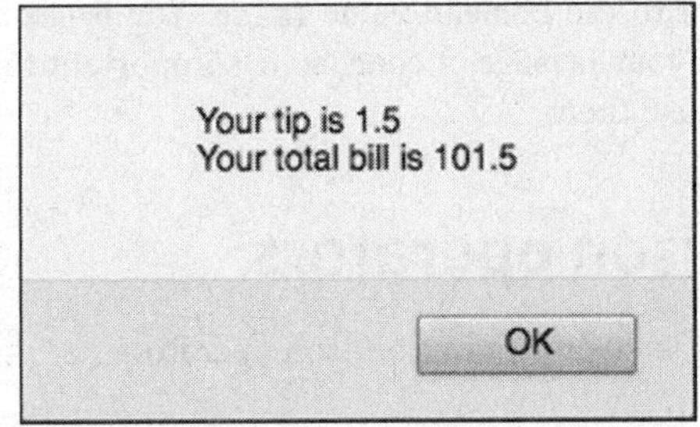

FIGURE 3-1: When the result is displayed, the `preTipTotal` and `tipAmount` values are concatenated instead of added.

What happened here is that because the first part of the expression in the `alert()` method was a string, JavaScript converted the `preTipTotal` and `tipAmount` values to strings and concatenated them instead of adding them.

To fix this, you could perform the addition in a separate statement and then use only this sum in the `alert()` expression. The following code demonstrates this approach:

```
var preTipTotal = 10.00;
var tipAmount = preTipTotal * 0.15;
var totalBill = preTipTotal + tipAmount;
var message1 = "Your tip is ";
var message2 = "\nYour total bill is ";
alert(message1 + tipAmount + message2 + totalBill);
```

A new variable named `totalBill` is declared and is used to store the `preTipTotal + tipAmount` sum. `totalBill` is then used to display the sum in the `alert()` expression, which, as you can see in Figure 3-2, now displays the correct answer.

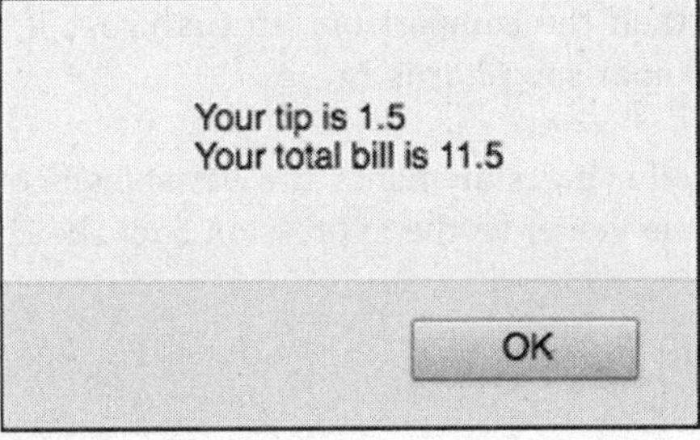

FIGURE 3-2: Calculating `preTipTotal` and `tipAmount` separately fixes the problem.

Building Comparison Expressions

You use comparison expressions to compare the values of two or more numbers, strings, variables, properties, or function results. If the expression is true, the expression result is set to the Boolean value `true`; if the expression is false, the expression result is set to the Boolean value `false`. You'll use comparisons with alarming frequency in your JavaScript code, so it's important to understand what they are and how you use them.

The comparison operators

Table 3-3 summarizes JavaScript's comparison operators.

TABLE 3-3 The JavaScript Comparison Operators

Operator	Name	Example	Result
==	Equal	`10 == 4`	`false`
!=	Not equal	`10 != 4`	`true`
>	Greater than	`10 > 4`	`true`
<	Less than	`10 < 4`	`false`
>=	Greater than or equal	`10 >= 4`	`true`
<=	Less than or equal	`10 <= 4`	`false`
===	Identity	`"10" === 10`	`false`
!==	Non-identity	`"10" !== 10`	`true`

Using the equal (==) operator

You use the equal operator (==) to compare the values of two operands. If both have the same value, then the comparison returns `true`; if the operands have different values, the comparison returns `false`.

For example, in the following statements the variables `booksRead` and `weeksPassed` contain the same value, so the expression `booksRead == weeksPassed` returns `true`:

```
var booksRead = 48;
var weeksPassed = 48;
var bookAWeek = booksRead == weeksPassed;
```

One of the most common mistakes made by beginning and experienced JavaScript programmers alike is to use = instead of == in a comparison expression. If your script isn't working properly or is generating errors, one of the first things you should check is that your equal operator has two equal signs.

Using the not equal (!=) operator

You also use the not equal operator (`!=`) to compare the values of two operands, but in the opposite way. That is, if the operands have different values, the comparison returns `true`; if both operands have the same value, the comparison returns `false`.

In the following statements, for example, the variables `currentFontSize` and `defaultFontSize` contain different values, so the expression `currentFontSize!= defaultFontSize` returns `true`:

```
var currentFontSize = 19;
var defaultFontSize = 16;
var weirdoFontSize = currentFontSize != defaultFontSize;
```

Using the greater than (>) operator

You use the greater than operator (`>`) to compare two operands to see if the operand to the left of `>` has a greater value than the operand to the right of `>`. If it does, then the expression returns `true`; otherwise, it returns `false`.

In the statements below, the value of the `contentWidth` variable is more than that of the `windowWidth` variable, so the expression `contentWidth > windowWidth` returns `true`:

```
var contentWidth = 1000;
var windowWidth = 800;
var tooBig = contentWidth > windowWidth;
```

Using the less than (<) operator

You use the less than operator (`<`) to compare two operands to see if the operand to the left of `>` has a lesser value than the operand to the right of `>`. If it does, then the expression returns `true`; otherwise, it returns `false`.

For example, in the statements that follow, the values of the kumquatsInStock and kumquatsSold variables are the same, so the expression kumquatsInStock < kumquatsSold returns false:

```
var kumquatsInStock = 3;
var kumquatsSold = 3;
var backordered = kumquatsInStock < kumquatsSold;
```

Using the greater than or equal (>=) operator

You use the greater than or equal operator (>=) to compare two operands to see if the operand to the left of >= has a greater value than or an equal value to the operand to the right of >=. If either or both of those comparisons get a thumbs up, then the expression returns true; otherwise, it returns false.

In the following statements, for example, the value of the score variable is more than that of the prize1Minimum variable and is equal to that of the prize2Minimum variable. Therefore, both the expressions score >= prize1Minimum and score >= prize2Minimum return true:

```
var score = 90;
var prize1Minimum = 80;
var prize2Minimum = 90;
var getsPrize1 = score >= prize1Minimum;
var getsPrize2 = score >= prize2Minimum;
```

Using the less than or equal (<=) operator

You use the less than or equal operator (<=) to compare two operands to see if the operand to the left of <= has a lesser value than or an equal value to the operand to the right of <=. If either or both of those comparisons get a nod of approval, then the expression returns true; otherwise, it returns false.

For example, in the following statements, the value of the defects variable is less than that of the defectsMaximumA variable and is equal to that of the defectsMaximumB variable. Therefore, both the expressions defects <= defectsMaximumA and defects <= defectsMaximumB return true:

```
var defects = 5
var defectsMaximumA = 10
var defectsMaximumB = 5
```

```
var getsBonus = defects <= defectsMaximumA
var getsRaise = defects <= defectsMaximumB
```

The comparison operators and data conversion

In the previous examples, I used only numbers to demonstrate the various comparison operators. However, you can also use strings and Boolean values. These comparisons are straightforward if your expressions include only operands of the same data type; that is, if you compare two strings or two Booleans. (Although see my discussion of using strings in comparison expressions a bit later in this chapter.)

TECHNICAL STUFF

Things become less straightforward if you mix data types within a single comparison expression. In this case, you need to remember that JavaScript always attempts to convert each operand into a number before running the comparison. Here's how it works:

- If one operand is a string and the other is a number, JavaScript attempts to convert the string into a number. For example, in the following statements the string "5" gets converted to the number 5, so the comparison `value1 == value2` returns `true`:

  ```
  var value1 = "5"
  var value2 = 5
  var result = value1 == value2
  ```

  If the string can't be converted to a number, then the comparison always returns `false`.

- If one operand is a Boolean and the other is a number, JavaScript converts the Boolean to a number as follows:

  - `true` — This value is converted to `1`.
  - `false` — This value is converted to `0`.

  For example, in the following statements, the Boolean `true` gets converted to the number 1, so the comparison `value1 == value2` returns `true`:

  ```
  var value1 = true
  var value2 = 1
  var result = value1 == value2
  ```

Building Expressions

» If one operand is a Boolean and the other is a string, JavaScript converts the Boolean to a number as in the previous item, and it attempts to convert the string into a number. For example, in the following statements, the Boolean `false` is converted to the number 0 and the string `"0"` is converted to the number 0, so the comparison `value1 == value2` returns `true`:

```
var value1 = false
var value2 = "0"
var result = value1 == value2
```

If the string can't be converted to a number, then the comparison always returns `false`.

Using the identity (===) operator

The identity operator (===) checks whether two operands are identical, which means it checks not only that the operands' values are equal, but also that the operands are of the same data type. (Which is why the identity operator is also sometimes called the *strict equality operator*.)

For example, in the following statements, variable `albumName` contains a string and variable `albumReleaseDate` contains a number. These values are of different data types, so the expression `albumName === albumReleaseDate` returns `false`:

```
var albumName = "1984";
var albumReleaseDate = 1984;
var result = albumName === albumReleaseDate;
```

By comparison, if instead you used the equal operator (==), which doesn't check the operand data types, the expression `albumName == albumReleaseDate` would return `true`.

REMEMBER

So when should you use equal (==) and when should you use identity (===)? Many pro JavaScript coders ignore this question entirely and just use the identity operator all the time. You should, too.

Using the non-identity (!==) operator

The non-identity operator (!==) performs the opposite function, sort of. That is, it checks to see not only if the values of two operands are different, but it also checks to see whether the operand are of different data types. (Which is why the non-identity operator is also sometimes called the *strict inequality operator*.)

In the statements below, variable hasBugs contains the Boolean value true and variable totalBugs contains a number. These values are of different data types, so the expression hasBugs !== totalBugs returns true:

```
var hasBugs = true;
var totalBugs = 1;
var result = hasBugs !== totalBugs;
```

Using strings in comparison expressions

Comparison expressions involving only numbers hold few surprises, but comparisons involving only strings can sometimes raise an eyebrow or two. The comparison is based on alphabetical order, as you might expect, so "A" comes before "B" and "a" comes before "b." Ah, but this isn't your father's alphabetical order. In JavaScript's world, all the uppercase letters come before all the lowercase letters, which means that, for example, "B" comes before "a," so the following expression would return false:

```
"a" < "B"
```

Another thing to keep in mind is that most string comparisons involve multiple-letter operands. In these situations, JavaScript compares each string letter-by-letter. For example, consider the following expression:

```
"Smith" < "Smyth"
```

The first two letters in each string are the same, but the third letters are different. The internal value of the i in Smith is less than the internal value of the y in Smyth, so the comparison above would return true. (Notice, too, that after a point of difference is found, JavaScript ignores the rest of the letters in each string.)

Also, a space is a legitimate character for comparison purposes, and its internal value comes before all other letters and symbols. In particular, if you compare two strings of different lengths, JavaScript will pad the shorter string with spaces so that it's the same length as the longer string. Therefore, the following two expressions are equivalent:

```
"Marg" > "Margaret"
"Marg    " > "Margaret"
```

The second statement returns false because the fifth "letter" of the left operand is a space, whereas the fifth letter of "Margaret" is a.

Using the ternary (?:) operator

TECHNICAL STUFF

Knowing the comparison operators also enables you to use one of my favorite expression tools, a complex but oh-so-handy item called the *ternary operator* (?:). Here's the basic syntax for using the ternary operator in an expression:

```
expression ? result_if_true : result_if_false
```

The *expression* is a comparison expression that results in a true or false value. In fact, you can use any variable, function result, or property that has a true or false Boolean value. The *result_if_true* is the value that the expression returns if the *expression* evaluates to true; the *result_if_false* is the value that the expression returns if the *expression* evaluates to false.

TIP

In JavaScript, by definition, the following values are the equivalent of false:

- 0 (the number zero)
- "" (the empty string)
- null
- undefined (which is, say, the "value" of an uninitialized variable)

Everything else is the equivalent of true.

Here's a simple example:

```
var screenWidth = 768;
var maxPortableWidth = 1024;
var screenType = screenWidth > maxPortableWidth ? "Desktop" :
  "Portable";
```

The variable screenWidth is initialized to 768, the variable maxPortableWidth is initialized to 1024, and the variable screenType stores the value returned by the conditional expression. For the latter, screenWidth > maxPortableWidth is the comparison expression, "Desktop!" is the string that is returned given a true result, and "Portable!" is the string that is returned given a false result. Since screenWidth is less than maxPortableWidth, the comparison will be false, so "Portable!" will be the result.

Building Logical Expressions

You use logical expressions to combine or manipulate Boolean values, particularly comparison expressions. For example, if your code needs to test whether two different comparison expressions are both `true` before proceeding, you can do that with a logical expression.

The logical operators

Table 3-4 lists JavaScript's logical operators.

TABLE 3-4 **The JavaScript Logical Operators**

Operator	Name	General Syntax	Returned Value
&&	AND	*expr1* && *expr2*	`true` if both *expr1* and *expr2* are `true`; `false` otherwise.
||	OR	*expr1* || *expr2*	`true` if one or both of *expr1* and *expr2* are `true`; `false` otherwise.
!	NOT	!*expr*	`true` if *expr* is `false`; `false` if *expr* is `true`.

Using the AND (&&) operator

You use the AND operator (&&) when you want to test two Boolean operands to see if they're both `true`. For example, consider the following statements:

```
var finishedDinner = true;
var clearedTable = true;
var getsDessert = finishedDinner && clearedTable;
```

Since both `finishedDinner` and `clearedTable` are `true`, the logical expression `finishedDinner && clearedTable` evaluates to `true`.

On the other hand, consider these statements:

```
var haveWallet = true;
var haveKeys = false;
var canGoOut = haveWallet && haveKeys;
```

In this example, since haveKeys is false, the logical expression haveWallet && haveKeys evaluates to false. The logical expression would also return false if just haveWallet was false or if both haveWallet and haveKeys were false.

Table 3-5 lists the various operands you can enter and the results they generate (this is called a *truth table*).

TABLE 3-5 Truth Table for the AND (&&) Operator

left_operand	right_operand	left_operand && right_operand
true	true	true
true	false	false
false	true	false
false	false	false

Using the OR (||) operator

You use the OR (||) operator when you want to test two Boolean operands to see if at least one of them is true. For example, consider the following statements:

```
var hasFever = true;
var hasCough = false;
var missSchool = hasFever || hasCough;
```

Since hasFever is true, the logical expression hasFever || hasCough evaluates to true since only one of the operands needs to be true. You get the same result if only hasCough is true or if both operands are true.

On the other hand, consider these statements:

```
var salesOverBudget = false;
var expensesUnderBudget = false;
var getsBonus = salesOverBudget || expensesUnderBudget;
```

In this example, since both salesOverBudget and expensesUnderBudget are false, the logical expression salesOverBudget || expensesUnderBudget evaluates to false.

Table 3-6 displays the truth table for the various operands you can enter.

TABLE 3-6 Truth Table for the OR (||) Operator

left_operand	right_operand	left_operand || right_operand
true	true	true
true	false	true
false	true	true
false	false	false

Using the NOT (!) Operator

The NOT (!) operator is the logical equivalent of the negation operator (-) I cover earlier in this chapter. In this case, NOT returns the opposite Boolean value of an operand. For example, consider the following statements:

```
var dataLoaded = false;
var waitingForData = !dataLoaded;
```

`dataLoaded` is `false`, so `!dataLoaded` evaluates to `true`.

Table 3-7 displays the truth table for the various operands you can enter.

TABLE 3-7 Truth Table for the NOT (!) Operator

Operand	!Operand
true	false
false	true

Advanced notes on the && and || operators

TECHNICAL STUFF

I mention earlier that JavaScript defines various values that are the equivalent of `false` — including `0` and `""` — and that all other values are the equivalent of `true`. These equivalences means that you can use both the AND operator and the OR operator with non-Boolean values. However, if you plan on using non-Booleans, then you need to be aware of exactly how JavaScript evaluates these expressions.

Let's begin with an AND expression:

1. Evaluate the operand to the left of the AND operator.
2. If the left operand's value is `false` or is equivalent to `false`, return that value and stop; otherwise, continue with Step 3.
3. If the left operand's value is `true` or is equivalent to `true`, evaluate the operand to the right of the AND operator.
4. Return the value of the right operand.

This is quirky behavior, indeed, and there are two crucial concepts you need to bear in mind:

- If the left operand evaluates to `false` or its equivalent, the right operand is *never* evaluated.
- The logical expression returns the result of either the left or right operand, which means the expression might *not* return `true` or `false`; instead, it might return a value that's equivalent to `true` or `false`.

To try these concepts out, use the following code:

```
var v1 = true;
var v2 = 10;
var v3 = "testing";
var v4 = false;
var v5 = 0;
var v6 = "";
var leftOperand =
    eval(prompt("Enter the left operand (a value or
  expression):", true));
var rightOperand =
    eval(prompt("Enter the right operand (a value or
  expression):", true));
var result = leftOperand && rightOperand;
alert(result);
```

The script begins by declaring and initializing six variables. The first three (`v1`, `v2`, and `v3`) are given values equivalent to `true` and the last three (`v4`, `v5`, and `v6`) are given values equivalent to `false`. The script then prompts for a left operand and a right operand, which are then entered into an AND expression. The key here is that you can enter any value for each operand, or you can use the `v1` through `v6` variables to enter a comparison expression, such as `v2 > v5`. The use of `eval()` on the `prompt()` result ensures that JavaScript uses the expressions as they're entered.

Table 3-8 lists some sample inputs and the results they generate.

TABLE 3-8 Some Sample Results for the Previous Code

left_operand	right_operand	left_operand && right_operand
true	true	true
true	false	false
5	10	10
false	"Yo"	false
v2	v5	0
true	v3	testing
v5	v4	0
v2 > v5	v5 == v4	true

Like the AND operator, the logic of how JavaScript evaluates an OR expression is strange and needs to be understood, particularly if you'll be using operands that are `true` or `false` equivalents:

1. Evaluate the operand to the left of the OR operator.
2. If the left operand's value is `true` or is equivalent to `true`, return that value and stop; otherwise, continue with Step 3.
3. If the left operand's value is `false` or is equivalent to `false`, evaluate the operand to the right of the AND operator.
4. Return the value of the right operand.

Understanding Operator Precedence

Your JavaScript code will often use expressions that are blissfully simple: just one or two operands and a single operator. But, alas, "often" here doesn't mean "mostly," because many expressions you use will have a number of values and operators. In these more complex expressions, the order in which the calculations are performed becomes crucial. For example, consider the expression `3+5*2`. If you calculate from left to right, the answer you get is `16` (`3+5` equals `8`, and `8*2` equals `16`). However, if you perform the multiplication first and then the addition, the result is 13 (5*2 equals 10, and 3+10 equals 13). In other words, a single expression can produce multiple answers depending on the order in which you perform the calculations.

To control this ordering problem, JavaScript evaluates an expression according to a predefined *order of precedence*. This order of precedence lets JavaScript calculate an expression unambiguously by determining which part of the expression it calculates first, which part second, and so on.

The order of precedence

The order of precedence that JavaScript uses is determined by the various expression operators covered so far in this chapter. Table 3-9 summarizes the complete order of precedence used by JavaScript.

TABLE 3-9 The JavaScript Order of Precedence for Operators

Operator	Operation	Order of Precedence	Order of Evaluation
++	Increment	First	R -> L
--	Decrement	First	R -> L
–	Negation	First	R -> L
!	NOT	First	R -> L
*, /, %	Multiplication, division, modulus	Second	L -> R
+, –	Addition, subtraction	Third	L -> R
+	Concatenation	Third	L -> R
<, <=	Less than, less than, or equal	Fourth	L -> R
>, >=	Greater than, greater than, or equal	Fourth	L -> R
==	Equal	Fifth	L -> R
!=	Not equal	Fifth	L -> R
===	Identity	Fifth	L -> R
!==	Non-identity	Fifth	L -> R
&&	AND	Sixth	L -> R
||	OR	Sixth	L -> R

Operator	Operation	Order of Precedence	Order of Evaluation
?:	Ternary	Seventh	R -> L
=	Assignment	Eighth	R -> L
+=, -=, and so on.	Arithmetic assignment	Eighth	R -> L

For example, Table 3-9 tells you that JavaScript performs multiplication before addition. Therefore, the correct answer for the expression =3+5*2 (just discussed) is 13.

Notice, as well, that some operators in Table 3-9 have the same order of precedence (for example, multiplication and division). Having the same precedence means that the order in which JavaScript evaluates these operators doesn't matter. For example, consider the expression 5*10/2. If you perform the multiplication first, the answer you get is 25 (5*10 equals 50, and 50/2 equals 25). If you perform the division first, you also get an answer of 25 (10/2 equals 5, and 5*5 equals 25).

However, JavaScript does have a predefined order for these kinds of expressions, which is what the Order of Evaluation column tells you. A value of L -> R means that operations with the same order of precedence are evaluated from left-to-right; R -> L means the operations are evaluated from right-to-left.

Controlling the order of precedence

Sometimes you want to take control of the situation and override the order of precedence. That might seem like a decidedly odd thing to do, so perhaps an example is in order. As you probably know, you calculate the total cost of a retail item by multiplying the retail price by the tax rate, and then adding that result to the retail price:

```
Total Price = Retail Price + Retail Price * Tax Rate
```

However, what if you want to reverse this calculation? That is, suppose you know the final price of an item and, given the tax rate, you want to know the original (that is, pre-tax) price. Applying a bit of algebra to the preceding equation, it turns out that you can calculate the original price by dividing the total price by 1 plus the tax rate. So if the total price is $11.00 and the tax rate is 10%, then you divide 11 by 1.1 and get an answer of $10.00.

Okay, now I'll convert this calculation to JavaScript code. A first pass at the new equation might look something like this:

```
retailPrice = totalPrice / 1 + taxRate;
```

The following code implements this formula and Figure 3-3 shows the result:

```
var totalPrice = 11.00;
var taxRate = .1;
var retailPrice = totalPrice / 1 + taxRate;
alert("The pre-tax price is " + retailPrice);
```

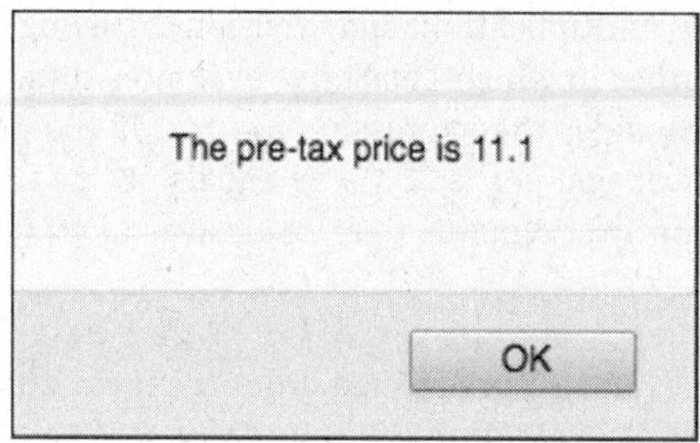

FIGURE 3-3: The result of our first stab at calculating the pre-tax cost of an item.

As you can see, the result is incorrect. What happened? Well, according to the rules of precedence, JavaScript performs division before addition, so the `totalPrice` value first is divided by 1 and then is added to the `taxRate` value, which isn't the correct order.

To get the correct answer, you have to override the order of precedence so that the addition `1 + taxRate` is performed first. You override precedence by surrounding that part of the expression with parentheses, as shown in the following code. Using this revised script, you get the correct answer, as shown in Figure 3-4.

```
var totalPrice = 11.00;
var taxRate = .1;
var retailPrice = totalPrice / (1 + taxRate);
alert("The pre-tax price is " + retailPrice);
```

WARNING

One of the most common mistakes when using parentheses in expressions is to forget to close a parenthetic term with a right parenthesis. To make sure you've closed each parenthetic term, count all the left parentheses and count all the right parentheses. If these totals don't match, you know you've left out a parenthesis.

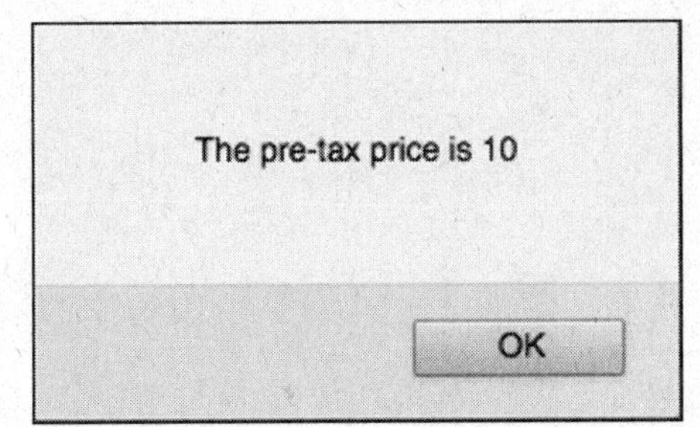

FIGURE 3-4: The revised script calculates the pre-tax cost correctly.

In general, you can use parentheses to control the order that JavaScript uses to calculate expressions. Terms inside parentheses are always calculated first; terms outside parentheses are calculated sequentially (according to the order of precedence). To gain even more control over your expressions, you can place parentheses inside one another; this is called *nesting* parentheses, and JavaScript always evaluates the innermost set of parentheses first.

Using parentheses to determine the order of calculations allows you to gain full control over JavaScript expressions. This way, you can make sure that the answer given by an expression is the one you want.

» Setting up your code to make decisions

» Understanding code looping

» Setting up code loops

» Avoiding the dreaded infinite loop

Chapter 4
Controlling the Flow of JavaScript

In a minute there is time

For decisions and revisions which a minute will reverse.

— T. S. ELIOT

When the web browser comes across a <script> tag, it puts on its JavaScript hat and starts processing the statements. Not surprisingly, the browser doesn't just leap randomly around the script, parsing the statements willy-nilly. That would be silly. No, the browser puts its head down and starts processing the statements one at a time: the first statement, the second statement, and so on until there's no more JavaScript left to parse.

That linear statement-by-statement progression through the code makes sense, but it doesn't fit every situation. Sometimes you want your code to test some condition and then run different chunks of code depending on the result of that test. Sometimes you want your code to repeat a collection of statements over and over again, with some subtle or significant change occurring with each repetition. Code that runs tests and code that repeats itself all fall under the rubric of controlling the flow of JavaScript. In this chapter, you dive into this fascinating and powerful subject.

Understanding JavaScript's Control Structures

There are lots of sites on the web that offer widgets and doodads that you can link to (or sometimes download) to add functionality to your web pages. Easy? For sure. Fast? Absolutely. Recommended? Nope. That's because those doohickeys are black boxes where the code is hidden and unchangeable (at least by the likes of you and me). That, in turn, means you lose out on one of the main advantages of writing your own JavaScript code: that you end up with complete and exquisite control over what your code does and how it performs its tasks.

There are many ways to exert such control over your code, but there are two that you'll find to be the most useful and powerful. The first of these are JavaScript statements that make decisions based on certain conditions, and then depending on the results of those decisions, send your code branching one way or another. The second are JavaScript statements that perform loops, which means that they run one or more statements over and over again, and you control the number of times this happens. The JavaScript statements that handle this kind of processing are known as *control structures* to those in the trade.

Making True/False Decisions with if() Statements

A smart script performs tests on its environment and then decides what to do next based on the results of each test. For example, suppose you've written a function that uses one of its arguments as a divisor in an expression. You should test the argument before using it in the expression to make sure that it isn't 0.

The most basic test is the simple true/false decision (which could also be seen as a yes/no or an on/off decision). In this case, your program looks at a certain condition, determines whether it's currently true or false, and acts accordingly. Comparison and logical expressions (covered in Book 3, Chapter 3) play a big part here because they always return a `true` or `false` result.

In JavaScript, simple true/false decisions are handled by the `if()` statement. You can use either the *single-line* syntax:

```
if (expression) { statement };
```

or the *block* syntax:

```
if (expression) {
    statement1;
    statement2;
    ...
}
```

In both cases, `expression` is a comparison or logical expression that returns `true` or `false`, and `statement(s)` represent the JavaScript statement or statements to run if `expression` returns `true`. If `expression` returns `false`, JavaScript skips over the statements.

TIP

This is a good place to note that JavaScript defines the following values as the equivalent of `false`: `0`, `""` (that is, the empty string), `null`, and `undefined`. Everything else is the equivalent of `true`.

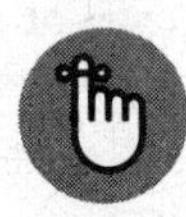

REMEMBER

This is the first time you've seen JavaScript's braces (`{` and `}`), so let's take a second to understand what they do because they come up a lot. The braces surround one or more statements that you want JavaScript to treat as a single entity. This entity is a kind of statement itself, so the whole caboodle — the braces and the code they enclose — is called a *block statement.* Also, any JavaScript construction that consists of a statement (such as `if()`) followed by a block statement is called a *compound statement.* And, just to keep you on your toes, note that the lines that include the braces don't end with semicolons.

Whether you use the single-line or block syntax depends on the statements you want to run if the `expression` returns a `true` result. If you have only one statement, you can use either syntax. If you have multiple statements, use the block syntax.

Consider the following example:

```
if (totalSales != 0) {
    var grossMargin = (totalSales - totalExpenses) / totalSales;
}
```

This code assumes that earlier the script has calculated the total sales and total expenses, which are stored in the `totalSales` and `totalExpenses` variables, respectively. The code now calculates the gross margin, which is defined as gross profit (that is, sales minus expenses) divided by sales. The code uses `if()` to test whether the value of the `totalSales` variable is not equal to zero. If the `totalSales != 0` expression returns `true`, then the `grossMargin` calculation is executed; otherwise, nothing happens. The `if()` test in this example is righteous because it ensures that the divisor in the calculation — `totalSales` — is never zero.

Branching with if(). . .else Statements

Using the `if()` statement to make decisions adds a powerful new weapon to your JavaScript arsenal. However, the simple version of `if()` suffers from an important drawback: A `false` result only bypasses one or more statements; it doesn't execute any of its own. This is fine in many cases, but there will be times when you need to run one group of statements if the condition returns `true` and a different group if the result is `false`. To handle this, you need to use an `if()...else` statement:

```
if (expression) {
    statements-if-true
} else {
    statements-if-false
}
```

The *`expression`* is a comparison or logical expression that returns `true` or `false`. *`statements-if-true`* represents the block of statements you want JavaScript to run if *`expression`* returns `true`, and *`statements-if-false`* represents the block of statements you want executed if *`expression`* returns `false`.

As an example, consider the following code:

```
var discountRate;
if (currMonth === "December") {
    discountRate = 0.2;
} else {
    discountRate = 0.1;
}
var discountedPrice = regularPrice * (1 - discountRate);
```

This code calculates a discounted price of an item, where the discount depends on whether the current month is December. The code assumes that earlier the script set the value of the current month (`currMonth`) and the item's regular price (`regularPrice`). After declaring the `discountRate` variable, an `if()...else` statement checks to see if `currMonth` equals December. If it does, `discountRate` is set to 0.2; otherwise, `discountRate` is set to 0.1. Finally, the code uses the `discountRate` value to calculate `discountedPrice`.

TIP

`if()...else` statements are much easier to read when you indent the statements within each block, as I've done in my examples. This lets you easily identify which block will run if there is a `true` result and which block will run if the result is `false`. I find that an indent of four spaces does the job, but many programmers prefer either two spaces or a tab.

The `if()...else` statements are very similar to the ternary operator (`?:`) that I discuss in Book 3, Chapter 3. In fact, for a very specific subset of `if()...else` statements, the two are identical.

The `?:` operator evaluates a comparison expression and then returns one value if the expression is `true`, or another value if it's `false`. For example, if you have a variable named `currentHour` that contains the hour part of the current time of day, then consider the following statement:

```
var greeting = currentHour < 12 ? "Good morning!" : "Good day!";
```

If `currentHour` is less than 12, then the string `"Good morning!"` is stored in the `greeting` variable; otherwise, the string `"Good day!"` is returned. This statement does exactly the same thing as the following `if()...else` statements:

```
if (currentHour < 12) {
    greeting = "Good morning!";
} else {
    greeting = "Good day!";
}
```

The ternary operator version is clearly more efficient, both in terms of total characters typed and total lines used. So any time you find yourself testing a condition only to store something in a variable depending on the result, use a ternary operator statement instead of `if()...else`.

Making Multiple Decisions

The `if()...else` control structure makes only a single decision. The `if()` part calculates a single logical result and performs one of two actions. However, plenty of situations require multiple decisions before you can decide which action to take.

For example, to calculate the pre-tax price of an item given its total price and its tax rate, you divide the total price by the tax rate plus 1. In real-world web coding, one of your jobs as a developer is to make sure you're dealing with numbers that make sense. What makes sense for a tax rate? Probably that it's greater than or equal to 0 and less than 1 (that is, 100%). That's two things to test about any tax rate value in your code, and JavaScript offers multiple ways to handle this kind of thing.

Using the AND (??) and OR (||) operators

One solution to a multiple-decision problem is to combine multiple comparison expressions in a single `if()` statement. As I discuss in Book 3, Chapter 3, you can combine comparison expressions by using JavaScript's AND (`??`) and OR (`||`) operators.

The following code shows an example `if()` statement that combines two comparison expressions using the `&&` operator:

```
var retailPrice;
if (taxRate >= 0 && taxRate < 1) {
    retailPrice = totalPrice / (1 + taxRate);
    alert(retailPrice);
} else {
    alert("Please enter a tax rate between 0 and 1.");
}
```

The key here is the `if()` statement:

```
if (taxRate >= 0 && taxRate < 1);
```

This tells the browser that only if the `taxRate` value is greater than or equal to `0` and less than `1` should the statements in the true block be executed. If either one is `false` (or if both are `false`), the user sees the message in the false block instead.

Nesting multiple if() statements

There is a third syntax for the `if()...else` statement that lets you string together as many logical tests as you need:

```
if (expression1) {
   statements-if-expression1-true
} else if (expression2) {
   statements-if-expression2-true
}
etc.
else {
   statements-if-false
}
```

JavaScript first tests *`expression1`*. If *`expression1`* returns `true`, JavaScript runs the block represented by *`statements-if-expression1-true`* and skips over everything else. If *`expression1`* returns `false`, JavaScript then tests *`expression2`*. If *expression2* returns `true`, JavaScript runs the block represented by *statements-if-expression2-true* and skips over everything else. Otherwise, JavaScript runs the block represented by *statements-if-false*. The second `if()` statement is said to be *nested* within the first `if()` statement.

The following code shows a script that uses a nested `if()` statement:

```
var greeting;
if (currentHour < 12) {
    greeting = "Good morning!";
} else if (currentHour < 18) {
    greeting = "Good afternoon!";
} else {
    greeting = "Good evening!";
}
alert(greeting);
```

The code assumes that earlier in the script the current hour value was stored in the `currentHour` variable. The first `if()` checks to see if `currentHour` is less than 12. If so, then the string `"Good morning!"` is stored in the `greeting` variable; if not, the next `if()` checks to see if `currentHour` less than 18 (that is, less than 6:00 PM). If so, then `greeting` is assigned the string `"Good afternoon!"`; if not, `greeting` is assigned `"Good evening"` instead.

Using the switch() statement

Performing multiple tests with `if()...else if` is a handy technique — it's a JavaScript tool you'll reach for quite often. However, it quickly becomes unwieldy as the number of tests you need to make gets larger. It's okay for two or three tests, but any more than that makes the logic harder to follow.

For situations where you need to make a whole bunch of tests (say, four or more), JavaScript's `switch()` statement is a better choice. The idea is that you provide an expression at the beginning and then list a series of possible values for that expression. For each possible result — called a *case* — you provide one or more JavaScript statements to execute should the case prove to be true. Here's the syntax:

```
switch(expression) {
    case Case1:
        Case1 statements
        break;
    case Case2:
        Case2 statements
        break;
```

```
    etc.
    default:
        Default statements
}
```

The *expression* is evaluated at the beginning of the structure. It must return a value (numeric, string, or Boolean). *Case1*, *Case2*, and so on are possible values for *expression*. JavaScript examines each case value to see whether one matches the result of *expression*. If *expression* returns the *Case1* value, the code represented by *Case1 statements* is executed, and the `break` statement tells JavaScript to stop processing the rest of the `switch()` statement. Similarly, if *expression* returns the *Case2* value, the code represented by *Case2 statements* is executed, JavaScript stops processing the rest of the `switch()` statement. Finally, the optional `default` statement is used to handle situations where none of the cases matches *expression*, so JavaScript executes the code represented by *Default statements*.

If you do much work with dates in JavaScript, it's likely that your code will eventually need to figure out how many days are in any month. There's no built-in JavaScript property or method that tells you this, so you need to construct your own code, as shown here:

```
var daysInMonth;
switch(monthName) {
    case "January":
        daysInMonth = 31;
        break;
    case "February":
        if (yearValue % 4 === 0) {
            daysInMonth = 29;
        }
        else {
            daysInMonth = 28;
        }
        break;
    case "March":
        daysInMonth = 31;
        break;
    case "April":
        daysInMonth = 30;
        break;
    case "May":
        daysInMonth = 31;
        break;
```

```
        case "June":
            daysInMonth = 30;
            break;
        case "July":
            daysInMonth = 31;
            break;
        case "August":
            daysInMonth = 31;
            break;
        case "September":
            daysInMonth = 30;
            break;
        case "October":
            daysInMonth = 31;
            break;
        case "November":
            daysInMonth = 30;
            break;
        case "December":
            daysInMonth = 31;
    }
```


This code assumes that the variable `monthName` is the name of the month you want to work with, and `yearValue` is the year. (You need the latter to know when you're dealing with a leap year.) The `switch()` is based on the name of the month:

```
switch(monthName)
```

Then `case` statements are set up for each month. For example:

```
case "January":
    daysInMonth = 31;
    break;
```

If `monthName` is `"January"`, this case is `true` and the `daysInMonth` variable is set to 31. All the other months are set up the same, with the exception of February:

```
case "February":
    if (yearValue % 4 === 0) {
        daysInMonth = 29;
    }
    else {
        daysInMonth = 28;
    }
    break;
```

Here you need to know whether you're dealing with a leap year, so the modulus (`%`) operator checks to see if `yearValue` is divisible by four. If so, it's a leap year, so `daysInMonth` is set to 29; otherwise, it's set to 28.

TECHNICAL STUFF

Time geeks will no doubt have their feathers ruffled by my assertion that a year is a leap year if it's divisible by four. In fact, that only works for the years 1901 to 2099, which should take care of most people's needs. The formula doesn't work for 1900 and 2100 because, despite being divisible by 4, these years aren't leap years. The general rule is that a year is a leap year if it's divisible by 4 and it's not divisible by 100, unless it's also divisible by 400.

Understanding Code Looping

There are some who would say that the only real goal of the programmer should be to get the job done. As long as the code produces the correct result or performs the correct tasks in the correct order, everything else is superfluous. Perhaps, but *real* programmers know that the true goal of programming is not only to get the job done, but to get it done *as efficiently as possible*. Efficient scripts run faster, take less time to code, and are usually (not always, but usually) easier to read and troubleshoot.

One of the best ways to introduce efficiency into your coding is to avoid reinventing too many wheels. For example, consider the following code fragment:

```
var sum = 0;
var num = prompt("Type a number:", 1);
sum += Number(num);
num = prompt("Type a number:", 1);
sum += Number(num);
num = prompt("Type a number:", 1);
sum += Number(num);
alert("The total of your numbers is " + sum);
```

This code first declares a variable named `sum`. The code prompts the user for a number (see Book 3, Chapter 7 for a discussion of `prompt()` method) that gets stored in the `num` variable, adds that value to `sum`, and then repeats this prompt-and-sum routine two more times. (Note my use of the `Number()` function, which ensures that the value returned by `prompt()` is treated as a number rather than a string.) Finally, the sum of the three numbers is displayed to the user.

Besides being a tad useless, this code just reeks of inefficiency because most of the code consists of the following two lines appearing three times:

```
num = prompt("Type a number:", 1);
sum += Number(num);
```

Wouldn't it be more efficient if you put these two statements just once in the code and then somehow get JavaScript to repeat these statements as many times as necessary?

Why, yes, it would, and the good news is that not only is it possible to do this, but JavaScript also gives you a number of different methods to perform this so-called *looping*. I spend the rest of this chapter investigating each of these methods.

Using while() Loops

The most straightforward of the JavaScript loop constructions is the `while()` loop, which uses the following syntax:

```
while (expression) {
    statements
}
```

Here, *`expression`* is a comparison or logical expression (that is, an expression that returns `true` or `false`) that determines how many times the loop gets executed, and *`statements`* represents a block of statements to execute each time through the loop.

Essentially, JavaScript interprets a `while()` loop as follows: "Okay, as long as *`expression`* remains `true`, I'll keep running through the loop statements, but as soon as *`expression`* becomes `false`, I'm out of there."

Take a closer look at this. Here's how a `while()` loop works:

1. Evaluate the *`expression`* in the `while()` statement.
2. If *`expression`* is `true`, continue with Step 3; if *`expression`* is `false`, skip to Step 5.
3. Execute each of the statements in the block.
4. Return to Step 1.
5. Exit the loop (that is, execute the next statement that occurs after the `while()` block).

The following code demonstrates how to use `while()` to rewrite the inefficient code I show in the previous section:

```
var sum = 0;
var counter = 1;
var num;
while (counter <= 3) {
    num = prompt("Type a number:", 1);
    sum += Number(num);
    counter++;
}
alert("The total of your numbers is " + sum);
```

To control the loop, the code declares a variable named `counter` and initializes it to `1`, which means the expression `counter <= 3` is `true`, so the code enters the block, does the prompt-and-sum thing, and then increments `counter`. This is repeated until the third time through the loop when `counter` is incremented to `4`, at which point the expression `counter <- 3` becomes `false` and the loop is done.

TIP

To make your loop code as readable as possible, always use a two- or four-space indent for each statement in the `while()` block. This also applies to the `for()` and `do...while()` loops that I talk about later in this chapter.

The `while()` statement isn't the greatest loop choice when you know exactly how many times you want to run through the loop. (For that, use the `for()` statement, described in the next section.) The best use of the `while()` statement is when your script has some naturally occurring condition that you can turn into a comparison expression. A good example is when you're prompting the user for input values. You'll often want to keep prompting the user until she clicks the Cancel button. The easiest way to set that up is to include the prompt inside a `while()` loop, as shown here:

```
var sum = 0;
var num = prompt("Type a number or click Cancel:", 1);
while (num != null) {
    sum += Number(num);
    num = prompt("Type a number or click Cancel:", 1);
}
alert("The total of your numbers is " + sum);
```

The first `prompt()` method displays a dialog box like the one shown in Figure 4-1 to get the initial value, and stores it in the `num` variable.

FIGURE 4-1: When prompting the user for multiple values, set up your `while()` expression so that the prompting stops when the user clicks the Cancel button.

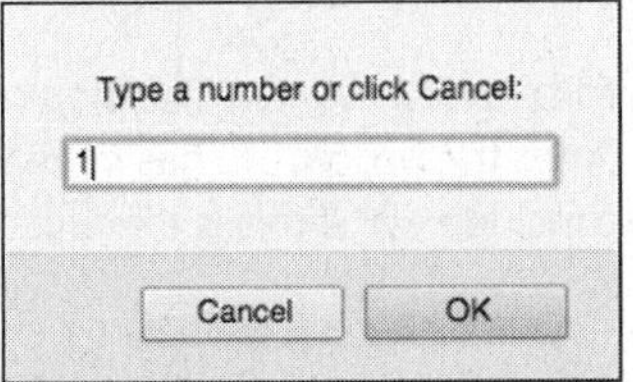

Then the `while()` statement checks the following expression:

```
while (num != null);
```

Two things can happen here:

- If the user enters a number, this expression returns `true` and the loop continues. In this case, the value of `num` is added to the `sum` variable, and the user is prompted for the next number.
- If the user clicks Cancel, the value returned by `prompt()` is `null`, so the expression becomes `false` and the looping stops.

Using for() Loops

Although `while()` is the most straightforward of the JavaScript loops, the most common type by far is the `for()` loop. This is slightly surprising when you consider (as you will shortly) that the `for()` loop's syntax is a bit more complex than that of the `while()` loop. However, the `for()` loop excels at one thing: looping when you know exactly how many times you want to repeat a group of statements. This is extremely common in all types of programming, so it's no wonder `for()` is so often seen in scripts.

The structure of a `for()` loop looks like this:

```
for (var counter = start; counterExpression; counter++) {
    statements
}
```

There's a lot going on here, so I take it one bit at a time:

- *counter*: A numeric variable used as a *loop counter*. The loop counter is a number that counts how many times the procedure has gone through the loop. (Note that you only need to include `var` if this is the first time you've used the variable in the script.)
- *start*: The initial value of *counter*. This is usually 1, but you can use whatever value makes sense for your script.
- *counterExpression*: A comparison or logical expression that determines the number of times through the loop. This expression usually compares the current value of *counter* to some maximum value.
- *counter*++: The increment operator applied to the *counter* variable. This can be any expression that changes the value of *counter*, and this expression is run after each turn through the loop.
- *statements*: The statements you want JavaScript to execute each time through the loop.

When JavaScript sees the `for()` statement, it changes into its for-loop outfit and follows this seven-step process:

1. Set *counter* equal to *start*.
2. Evaluate the *counterExpression* in the `for()` statement.
3. If *counterExpression* is `true`, continue with Step 4; if *counterExpression* is `false`, skip to Step 7.
4. Execute each of the statements in the block.
5. Increment (or whatever) *counter*.
6. Return to Step 2.
7. Exit the loop (that is, execute the next statement that occurs after the `for()` block).

As an example, the following code shows how to use `for()` to rewrite the inefficient code shown earlier in this chapter:

```
var sum = 0;
var num;
for (var counter = 1; counter <= 3; counter++) {
    num = prompt("Type a number:", 1);
    sum += Number(num);
}
alert("The total of your numbers is " + sum);
```

This is the most efficient version yet because the declaring, initializing, and incrementing of the counter variable all take place within the for() statement.

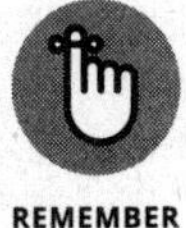
REMEMBER

To keep the number of variables declared in a script to a minimum, always try to use the same name in all your for() loop counters. The letters i through n traditionally are used for counters in programming. For greater clarity, you might prefer full words such as count or counter.

Here's a slightly more complex example:

```
var sum = 0;
var num, ordinal;
for (var counter = 1; counter < 4; counter++) {
    switch (counter) {
        case 1:
            ordinal = "first";
            break;
        case 2:
            ordinal = "second";
            break;
        case 3:
            ordinal = "third";
    }
    num = prompt("Enter the " + ordinal + " number:", 1);
    sum += Number(num);
}
alert("The average is " + sum / 3);
```

The purpose of this script is to ask the user for three numbers and then to display the average of those values. The for() statement is set up to loop three times. (Note that counter < 4 is the same as counter <= 3.) The first thing the loop block does is use switch to determine the value of the ordinal variable: If counter is 1, ordinal is set to "first", if counter is 2, ordinal becomes "second", and so on. These values enable the script to customize the prompt() message with each pass through the loop (see Figure 4-2). With each loop, the user enters a number and that value is added to the sum variable. When the loop exits, the average is displayed.

It's also possible to use for() to count down. You do this by using the decrement operator instead of the increment operator:

```
for (var counter = start; counterExpression; counter--) {
    statements
}
```

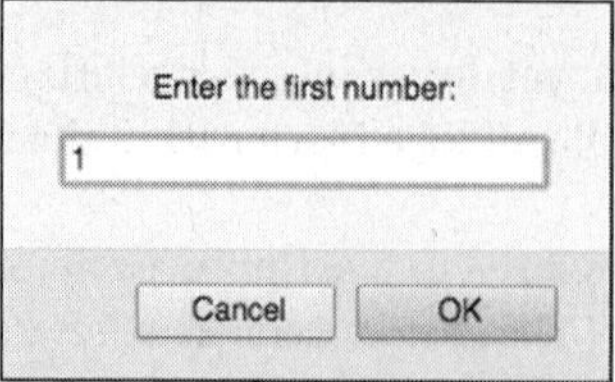

FIGURE 4-2: This script uses the current value of the `counter` variable to customize the prompt message.

In this case, you must initialize the *`counter`* variable to the maximum value you want to use for the loop counter, and use the *`counterExpression`* to compare the value of *`counter`* to the minimum value you want to use to end the loop.

In the following example, I use a decrementing counter to ask the user to rank, in reverse order, his top three CSS colors:

```
var ordinal, color;
for (var rank = 3; rank >= 1; rank--) {
    switch (rank) {
        case 1:
            ordinal = "first";
            break;
        case 2:
            ordinal = "second";
            break;
        case 3:
            ordinal = "third";
    }
    color = prompt("What is your " + ordinal + "-favorite
  CSS color?", "");
    document.write(rank + ". " + color + "<br>");
}
```

The `for()` loop runs by decrementing the `rank` variable from `3` down to `1`. Each iteration of the loop prompts the user to type a favorite CSS color, and that color is written to the page, with the current value of `rank` being used to create a reverse-ordered list, as shown in Figure 4-3.

FIGURE 4-3: The decrementing value of the rank variable is used to create a reverse-ordered list.

3. rebeccapurple
2. lemonchiffon
1. peachpuff

TIP

There's no reason why the `for()` loop counter has to be only incremented or decremented. You're actually free to use any expression to adjust the value of the loop counter. For example, suppose you want the loop counter to run through only the odd numbers 1, 3, 5, 7, and 9. Here's a `for()` statement that will do that:

```
for (var counter = 1; counter <= 9; counter += 2)
```

The expression `counter += 2` tells JavaScript to increment the `counter` variable by 2 each time.

Using do. . .while() Loops

JavaScript also has a third and final type of loop that I've left until the last because it isn't one that you'll use all that often. To understand when you might use it, consider this code snippet:

```
var num = prompt("Type a number or click Cancel:", 1);
while (num != null) {
    sum += Number(num);
    num = prompt("Type a number or click Cancel:", 1);
}
```

The code needs the first `prompt()` statement so that the `while()` loop's expression can be evaluated. The user may not feel like entering *any* numbers, and they can avoid it by clicking Cancel in the first prompt box so that the loop will be bypassed.

That seems reasonable enough, but what if your code requires that the user enter at least one value? The following presents one way to change the code to ensure that the loop is executed at least once:

```
var sum = 0;
var num = 0;
while (num !== null || sum === 0) {
    num = prompt("Type a number; when you're done, click
  Cancel:", 1);
    sum += Number(num);
}
alert("The total of your numbers is " + sum);
```

The changes here are that the code initializes both `sum` and `num` as `0`. This ensures that the `while()` expression — `num !== null || sum === 0` — returns `true` the first time through the loop, so the loop will definitely execute at least once. If the user clicks Cancel right away, `sum` will still be `0`, so the `while()` expression — `num !== null || sum === 0` — still returns `true` and the loop repeats once again.

This works fine, but you can also turn to JavaScript's third loop type, which specializes in just this kind of situation. It's called a `do...while()` loop, and its general syntax looks like this:

```
do {
    statements
}
while (expression);
```

Here, *`statements`* represents a block of statements to execute each time through the loop, and *`expression`* is a comparison or logical expression that determines how many times JavaScript runs through the loop.

This structure ensures that JavaScript executes the loop's statement block at least once. How? Take a closer look at how JavaScript processes a `do...while()` loop:

1. Execute each of the statements in the block.
2. Evaluate the *`expression`* in the `while()` statement.
3. If *`expression`* is `true`, return to Step 1; if *`expression`* is `false`, continue with Step 4.
4. Exit the loop.

For example, the following shows you how to use `do...while()` to restructure the prompt-and-sum code I show you earlier:

```
var sum = 0;
var num;
do {
    num = prompt("Type a number; when you're done, click
  Cancel:", 1);
    sum += Number(num);
}
while (num !== null || sum === 0);
alert("The total of your numbers is " + sum);
```

This code is very similar to the `while()` code I show earlier in this section. All that's really changed is that the `while()` statement and its expression have been moved after the statement block so that the loop must be executed once before the expression is evaluated.

Controlling Loop Execution

Most loops run their natural course and then the procedure moves on. There might be times, however, when you want to exit a loop prematurely or skip over some statements and continue with the next pass through the loop. You can handle each situation with, respectively, the `break` and `continue` statements.

Exiting a loop using the break statement

You use `break` when your loop comes across some value or condition that would either prevent the rest of the statements from executing properly, or that satisfies what the loop was trying to accomplish. The following code demonstrates `break` with a simple example:

```
var sum = 0;
var num;
for (var counter = 1; counter <= 3; counter++) {
    num = prompt("Type a positive number:", 1);
    if (num < 0) {
        sum = 0;
        break;
    }
    sum += Number(num);
}
if (sum > 0) {
    alert("The average of your numbers is " + sum / 3);
}
```

This script sets up a `for()` loop to prompt the user for positive numbers. For the purposes of this section, the key code is the `if()` test:

```
if (num < 0) {
    sum = 0;
    break;
}
```

If the user enters a negative number, the `sum` variable is reset to `0` (to prevent the alert box from appearing later in the script). Also, a `break` statement tells JavaScript to bail out of the loop altogether.

Here's a more complex example:

```
var numberToGuess = Math.ceil(Math.random() * 10);
var promptMessage = "Guess a number between 1 and 10:";
```

```
var totalGuesses = 1;
var guess;

do {
    guess = Number(prompt(promptMessage, ""));
    if (guess === null) {
        break;
    } else if (guess === numberToGuess) {
        alert("You guessed it in " + totalGuesses +
              (totalGuesses === 1 ? " try." : " tries."));
        break;
    } else if (guess < numberToGuess) {
        promptMessage = "Sorry, your guess was too low. Try
  again:";
    } else {
        promptMessage = "Sorry, your guess was too high. Try
  again:";
    }
    totalGuesses++;
}
while (true);
```

This script is a game in which a number between 1 and 10 is generated and the user has to try and guess what it is. The first four lines set up some variables. The head-scratcher here is the expression for the `numberToGuess` variable. This uses a couple of methods of the `Math` object, which I discuss in Book 3, Chapter 8. For now, suffice it to say that this expression generates a random integer between (and including) 1 and 10.

Then a `do...while()` loop is set up with the following structure:

```
do {
    statements
}
while (true);
```

This tells JavaScript just to run the loop without bothering with a comparison expression. As you'll see, the loop itself will take care of exiting the loop by using the `break` statement.

Next the user is prompted to enter a guess, which is stored in the `guess` variable. The script then checks to see if `guess` equals `null`, which would mean the user clicked Cancel. If so, then `break` is used to stop the game by exiting the loop:

```
guess = Number(prompt(promptMessage,""));
if (guess === null) {
    break;
}
```

Otherwise, a series of if() statements tests the guessed number against the actual number. The first one checks to see if they're the same. If so, a message is displayed and then another break statement exits the loop because the game is finished:

```
else if (guess === numberToGuess) {
    alert("You guessed it in " + totalGuesses +
          (totalGuesses === 1 ? " try." : " tries."));
    break;
}
```

TIP

Notice that the alert() statement contains a ternary operator expression:

```
totalGuesses === 1 ? " try." : " tries."
```

This illustrates an extremely common programming situation: You have to display a word to the user, but that word may be either singular or plural depending on the value of some variable or expression. In this case, if totalGuesses equals 1, you want to display the word try (as in 1 try); if totalGuesses is more than 1, you want to display the word tries (as in 2 tries). This is what the conditional expression does.

The other two tests check to see if the guess was lower or higher than the actual number, and a message to that effect is displayed, as shown in Figure 4-4.

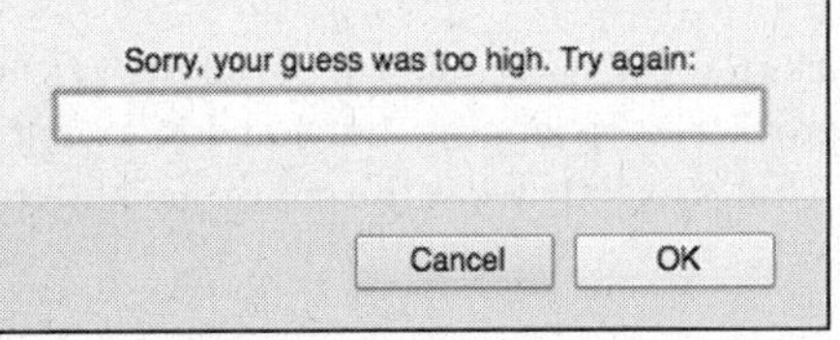

FIGURE 4-4: When the user clicks Cancel or guesses the correct number, the break statement exits the loop.

Bypassing loop statements using the continue statement

The continue statement is similar to break, but instead of exiting a loop entirely, continue tells JavaScript to bypass the rest of the statements in the loop block and begin a new iteration of the loop.

A good use for `continue` is when you want the user to enter one or more values no matter what. If they click Cancel in the prompt box, you want the script to keep on looping until the user enters the correct number of values. The following code shows one way to do this:

```
var counter = 0;
var sum = 0;
var num;
while (counter < 3) {
    num = prompt("Type a number:", 1);
    if (num === null) {
        continue;
    }
    sum += Number(num);
    counter++;
}
alert("The average of your numbers is " + sum / 3);
```

Because you don't know in advance how many times the code will have to run through the loop, a `while()` loop is a better choice than a `for()` loop. You need to count the number of values entered, however, so a variable named `counter` is initialized for that purpose. The script requires three numbers, so the `while()` statement is set up to continue looping as long as `counter` is less than 3. The `prompt()` result is stored in the `num` variable, which is then tested:

```
if (num === null) {
    continue;
}
```

If the user enters a number, the `if()` expression returns `false` and the rest of the loop executes: `sum` is updated and `counter` is incremented.

However, if the user clicks Cancel, `num` equals `null`, so the `if()` expression returns `true`. What you want here is to keep looping, but you don't want the rest of the loop statements to execute. That's exactly what the `continue` statement accomplishes.

Avoiding Infinite Loops

Whenever you use a `while()`, `for()`, or `do...while()` loop, there's always the danger that the loop will never terminate. This is called an *infinite loop*, and it has been the bugbear of programmers for as long as people have been programming. Here are some notes to bear in mind to help you avoid infinite loops:

- The statements in the `for()` block should never change the value of the loop counter variable. If they do, then your loop may either terminate prematurely or it may end up in an infinite loop.
- In `while()` and `do...while()` loops, make sure you have at least one statement within the loop that changes the value of the comparison variable. (That is, the variable you use in the loop's comparison statement.) Otherwise, the statement might always return `true` and the loop will never end.
- In `while()` and `do...while()` loops, never rely on the user to enter a specific value to end the loop. She might cancel the prompt box or do something else that prevents the loop from terminating.
- If you have an infinite loop and you're not sure why, insert one or more `debugger` and/or `console.log()` statements within the loop statement block to display the current value of the counter or comparison variable. (Wondering what the heck "debugger" and "console.log" might be? I cover them in Book 3, Chapter 9.) This enables you to see what happens to the variable with each pass through the loop.

» Creating and using custom functions

» Passing and returning function values

» Understanding recursive functions

» Introducing JavaScript's built-in functions

Chapter 5
Harnessing the Power of Functions

To iterate is human, to recurse divine.

— L. PETER DEUTSCH

As I demonstrate throughout this book, JavaScript comes with a huge number of built-in features that perform specific tasks. For example, something called the `Math` object has a built-in method for calculating the square root of a number. Similarly, a feature called the `String` object has a ready-made method for converting a string value to all lowercase letters.

There are, in fact, hundreds of these ready-to-roll features that perform tasks that range from the indispensable to the obscure. But JavaScript can't possibly do everything that you'd like or need it to do. What happens if your web development project requires a particular task or calculation that isn't part of the JavaScript language? Are you stuck? Not even close! The solution is to roll up your sleeves and then roll your own code that accomplishes the task or runs the calculation.

This chapter shows you how to create such do-it-yourself code. In the pages that follow, you explore the powerful and infinitely useful realm of custom functions, where you craft reusable code that performs tasks that out-of-the-box JavaScript can't do.

What Is a Function?

A *function* is a group of related JavaScript statements that are separate from the rest of the script and that perform a designated task. (Technically, a function can perform any number of chores, but as a general rule it's best to have each function focus on a specific task.) When your script needs to perform that task, you tell it to run the function.

Functions are also useful for those times when you need to control exactly when a particular task occurs (if ever). If you just enter some statements between your web page's `<script>` and `</script>` tags, the browser executes those statements automatically when the page loads. However, the statements within a function aren't executed by the browser automatically. Instead, the function doesn't execute until either your code asks the function to run, or some event occurs — such as the user clicking a button — and you've set up your page to run the function in response to that event.

The Structure of a Function

The basic structure of a function looks like this:

```
function functionName([arguments]) {
    JavaScript statements
}
```

Here's a summary of the various parts of a function:

- `function`: Identifies the block of code that follows it as a function.
- *`functionName`*: A unique name for the function. The naming rules and guidelines that I outline for variables in Book 3, Chapter 2 also apply to function names.
- *`arguments`*: One or more optional values that are passed to the function and that act as variables within the function. Arguments (or *parameters,* as they're sometimes called) are typically one or more values that the function uses as the raw materials for its tasks or calculations. You always enter arguments between parentheses after the function name, and you separate multiple arguments with commas. If you don't use arguments, you must still include the parentheses after the function name.
- *`JavaScript statements`*: This is the code that performs the function's tasks or calculations.

TIP

Notice how the *JavaScript statements* line in the example is indented slightly from the left margin. This is a standard and highly recommended programming practice because it makes your code easier to read. This example is indented four spaces, which is enough to do the job, but isn't excessive.

Note, too, the use of braces ({ and }). These are used to enclose the function's statements within a block, which tells you (and the browser) where the function's code begins and ends. There are only two rules for where these braces appear:

- The opening brace must appear after the function's parentheses and before the first function statement.
- The closing brace must appear after the last function statement.

There is no set-in-stone rule that specifies exactly where the braces appear. The positions used in the previous function syntax are the traditional ones, but you're free to try other positions, if you want. For example:

```
function functionName([arguments])
{
    JavaScript statements
}
```

Where Do You Put a Function?

For most applications, it doesn't matter where you put your functions, as long as they reside within a `<script>` block. However, one of the most common uses of functions is to handle events when they're triggered. It's possible that a particular event might fire when the page is loading, and if that happens before the browser has parsed the corresponding function, you could get strange results or an error. To prevent that, it's good practice to place the script containing all your functions within the page's header section (or within an external JavaScript file).

Note, as well, that you can add as many functions as you want within a single `<script>` block, but there are two things to watch out for:

- Each function must have a unique name. In fact, all the functions that exist in or are referenced by a page must have unique names.
- You can't embed one function inside another function.

Calling a Function

After your function is defined, you'll eventually need to tell the browser to execute it, or *call* it. There are three main ways to do this:

- When the browser parses the `<script>` tag.
- After the page is loaded.
- In response to an event, such as the user clicking a button.

The next three sections cover each of these scenarios.

Calling a function when the <script> tag is parsed

The simplest way to call a function is to include in your script a statement consisting of only the function name, followed by parentheses (assuming for the moment that your function uses no arguments.) The following code provides an example. (I've listed the entire page so you can see where the function and the statement that calls it appear in the page code.)

```
<!DOCTYPE html>
<html lang="en">
<head>
    <meta charset="utf-8">
    <title>Calling a function when the &lt;script&gt; tag is
  parsed</title>
    <script>
        function displayGreeting() {
            var currentHour = new Date().getHours();
            if (currentHour < 12) {
                console.log("Good morning!");
            } else {
                console.log("Good day!");
            }
        }
        displayGreeting();
    </script>
</head>
<body>
</body>
</html>
```

The <script> tag includes a function named displayGreeting, which determines the current hour of the day, and then writes a greeting to the console based on whether it's currently morning. The function is called by the displayGreeting() statement that appears just after the function.

Calling a function after the page is loaded

If your function references a page element, then calling the function from within the page's head section won't work because when the browser parses the script, the rest of the page hasn't loaded yet, so your element reference will fail.

To work around this problem, place another <script> tag at the end of the body section, just before the closing </body> tag, as shown here:

```
<!DOCTYPE html>
<html lang="en">
<head>
    <meta charset="utf-8">
    <title>Calling a function after the page is loaded</title>
    <script>
        function makeBackgroundRed() {
            document.body.style.backgroundColor = "red";
            console.log("The background is now red.");
        }
    </script>
</head>
<body>
    <!-- Other body elements go here -->

    <script>
        makeBackgroundRed();
    </script>
</body>
</html>
```

The makeBackgroundRed() function does two things: It uses document.body.style.backgroundColor to change the background color of the body element to red, and it uses console.log() to write a message to that effect on the console.

In the function, document.body is a reference to the body element, which doesn't "exist" until the page is fully loaded. That means if you try to call the function with the initial script, you'll get an error. To execute the function properly, a second <script> tag appears at the bottom of the body element and that script calls the function with the following statement:

```
makeBackgroundRed();
```

Since by the time the browser executes that statement the body element exists, the function runs without an error.

Calling a function in response to an event

One of the most common ways that JavaScript functions are called is in response to some event. This is such an important topic that I devote an entire chapter to it later in the book (see Book 4, Chapter 2). For now, take a look at a relatively straightforward application: executing the function when the user clicks a button. The following code shows one way to do it.

```
<!DOCTYPE html>
<html lang="en">
<head>
    <meta charset="utf-8">
    <title>Calling a function in response to an event</title>;
    <script>
        function makeBackgroundRed() {
            document.body.style.backgroundColor= "red";
        }

        function makeBackgroundWhite() {
            document.body.style.backgroundColor= "white";
        }
    </script>
</head>
<body>
    <button onclick="makeBackgroundRed()">
        Make Background Red
    </button>
    <button onclick="makeBackgroundWhite()">
        Make Background White
    </button>
</body>
</html>
```

What I've done here is place two functions in the script: `makeBackgroundRed()` changes the page background to red, as before, and `makeBackgroundWhite()` changes the background color back to white.

The buttons are standard HTML `button` elements, each of which includes the `onclick` attribute. This attribute defines a *handler* — that is the function to execute — for the event that occurs when the user clicks the button. For example, consider the first button:

```
<button onclick="makeBackgroundRed()">
```

The `onclick` attribute here says, in effect, "When somebody clicks this button, call the function named `makeBackgroundRed()`."

Passing Values to Functions

One of the main reasons to use functions is to gain control over when some chunk of JavaScript code gets executed. The previous section, for example, discusses how easy it is to use functions to set things up so that code doesn't run until the user clicks a button.

However, there's another major reason to use functions: to avoid repeating code unnecessarily. To see what I mean, consider the two functions from the previous section:

```
function makeBackgroundRed() {
    document.body.style.backgroundColor= "red";
}
function makeBackgroundWhite() {
    document.body.style.backgroundColor= "white";
}
```

These functions perform the same task — changing the background color — and the only difference between them is one changes the color to red and the other changes it to white. Whenever you end up with two or more functions that do essentially the same thing, then you know that your code is inefficient.

So how do you make the code more efficient? That's where the arguments that I mention earlier come into play. An *argument* is a value that is "sent" — or *passed*, in programming terms — to the function. The argument acts just like a variable, and it automatically stores whatever value is sent.

Passing a single value to a function

As an example, you can take the previous two functions, reduce them to a single function, and set up the color value as an argument. Here's a new function that does just that:

```
function changeBackgroundColor(newColor) {
    document.body.style.backgroundColor = newColor;
}
```

The argument is named newColor and it's added between the parentheses that occur after the function name. JavaScript declares newColor as a variable automatically, so there's no need for a separate var statement. The function then uses the newColor value to change the background color. So how do you pass a value to the function? The following code presents a sample file that does this.

```
<!DOCTYPE html>
<html lang="en">
<head>
    <meta charset="utf-8">
    <title>Passing a single value to a function</title>;
    <script>
        function changeBackgroundColor(newColor) {
            document.body.style.backgroundColor = newColor;
        }
    </script>
</head>
<body>
    <button onclick="changeBackgroundColor('red')">
        Make Background Red
    </button>
    <button onclick="changeBackgroundColor('white')">
        Make Background White
    </button>
</body>
</html>
```

The key here is the onclick attribute that appears in both <button> tags. For example:

```
onclick="changeBackgroundColor('red')"
```

The string 'red' is inserted into the parentheses after the function name, so that value is passed to the function itself. The other button passes the value 'white', and the function result changes accordingly.

WARNING

In the two onclick attributes in the example code, notice that the values passed to the function are enclosed in single quotation marks ('). This is necessary because the onclick value as a whole is enclosed in double quotation marks (").

Passing multiple values to a function

For more complex functions, you might need to use multiple arguments so that you can pass different kinds of values. If you use multiple arguments, separate each one with a comma, like this:

```
function changeColors(newBackColor, newForeColor) {
    document.body.style.backgroundColor = newBackColor;
    document.body.style.color = newForeColor;
}
```

In this function, the document.body.style.color statement changes the foreground color (that is, the color of the page text). The following code shows a revised page where the buttons pass two values to the function.

```
<!DOCTYPE html>
<html lang="en">
<head>
    <meta charset="utf-8">
    <title>Passing multiple values to a function</title>;
    <script>
        function changeColors(newBackColor, newForeColor) {
            document.body.style.backgroundColor = newBackColor;
            document.body.style.color = newForeColor;
        }
    </script>
</head>
<body>
    <h1>Passing Multiple Values to a Function</h1>
    <button onclick="changeColors('red', 'white')">
        Red Background, White Text
    </button>
    <button onclick="changeColors('white', 'red')">
        White Background, Red Text
    </button>
</body>
</html>
```

WARNING

If you define a function to have multiple arguments, then you must always pass values for each of those arguments to the function. If you don't, then the "value" `undefined` is passed, instead, which can cause problems.

TECHNICAL STUFF

If you use a variable to pass data to a function, only the current value of that variable is sent, not the variable itself. Therefore, if you change the value of the argument within the function, the value of the original variable isn't changed. Here's an example:

```
var passThis = 10;
function sendMe(acceptThis) {
    acceptThis = 5;
}
sendMe(passThis);
console.log(passThis);
```

The variable `passThis` starts off with a value of `10`. The function `sendMe()` is then defined to accept an attribute named `acceptThis`, and to then change the value of that attribute to `5`. `sendMe()` is then called and the value of the `passThis` variable is passed to it. Then a `console.log()` statement displays the value of `passThis`. If you run this code, the displayed value will be `10`, the original value of `passThis`. In other words, changing the value of `acceptThis` within the function had no effect on the value of the `passThis` variable.

Returning a Value from a Function

So far I've outlined two major advantages of using functions:

- You can use them to control when code is executed.
- You can use them to consolidate repetitive code into a single routine.

The third major benefit that functions bring to the JavaScript table is that you can use them to perform calculations and then return the result. As an example, I construct a function that calculates the tip on a restaurant bill:

```
var preTipTotal = 100.00;
var tipPercentage = 0.15;
function calculateTip(preTip, tipPercent) {
```

```
    var tipResult = preTip * tipPercent;
    return (tipResult);
}

var tipCost = calculateTip(preTipTotal, tipPercentage);
var totalBill = preTipTotal + tipCost;
console.log("Your total bill is $" + totalBill);
```

The function named `calculateTip()` takes two arguments: `preTip` is the total of the bill before the tip, and `tipPercent` is the percentage used to calculate the tip. The function then declares a variable named `tipResult` and uses it to store the calculation — `preTip` multiplied by `tipPercent`. The key for this example is the second line of the function:

```
return (tipResult);
```

The `return` statement is JavaScript's way of sending a value *back* to the statement that called the function. That statement comes after the function:

```
tipCost = calculateTip(preTipTotal, tipPercentage);
```

This statement first passes the value of `preTipTotal` (initialized as `100.00` earlier in the script) and `tipPercentage` (initialized as `0.15` earlier) to the `calculateTip()` function. When that function returns its result, the entire expression `calculateTip(preTipTotal, tipPercentage)` is replaced by that result, meaning that it gets stored in the `tipCost` variable. Then `preTipTotal` and `tipCost` are added together, the result is stored in `totalBill`, and a `console.log` statement displays the final calculation.

Understanding Local versus Global Variables

In the example I give in the previous section, notice that there are four variables declared outside the function (`preTipTotal`, `tipPercentage`, `tipCost`, and `totalBill`) and one variable declared inside the function (`tipPercent`). That might not seem like an important distinction, but there's a big difference between variables declared outside of functions and those declared inside of functions. This section explains this crucial difference.

In programming, the *scope* of a variable defines where in the script a variable can be used and where it can't be used. To put it another way, a variable's scope determines which statements and functions can access and work with the variable. There are two main reasons you need to be concerned with scope:

- **You might want to use the same variable name in multiple functions.** If these variables are otherwise unrelated, you'll want to make sure that there is no confusion about which variable you're working with. In other words, you'll want to restrict the scope of each variable to the function in which it is declared.
- **You might need to use the same variable in multiple functions.** For example, your function might use a variable to store the results of a calculation, and other functions might also need to use that result. In this case, you'll want to set up the scope of the variable so that it's accessible to multiple functions.

JavaScript lets you establish two types of scope for your variables:

- Local (or function-level) scope
- Global (or page-level) scope

The next two sections describe each type in detail.

Working with local scope

When a variable has *local* scope, it means the variable was declared inside a function and the only statements that can access the variable are the ones in that same function. (That's why local scope also is referred to as *function-level* scope.) Statements outside the function and statements in other functions can't access the local variable.

To demonstrate this, consider the following code:

```
function A() {
    var myMessage;
    myMessage = "I'm in the scope!";
    console.log("Function A: " + myMessage);
}

function B() {
    console.log("Function B: " + myMessage);
}
```

```
A();
B();
```

There are two functions here, named `A()` and `B()`. Function `A()` declares a variable named `myMessage`, sets its value to a text string, and uses JavaScript's `console.log()` method to display the string in the console.

Function `B()` also uses `console.log()` to attempt to display the `myMessage` variable. However, as you can see in Figure 5-1, JavaScript generates an error that says `myMessage is not defined`. Why? Because the scope of the `myMessage` variable extends only to function `A()`; function `B()` can't "see" the `myMessage` variable,

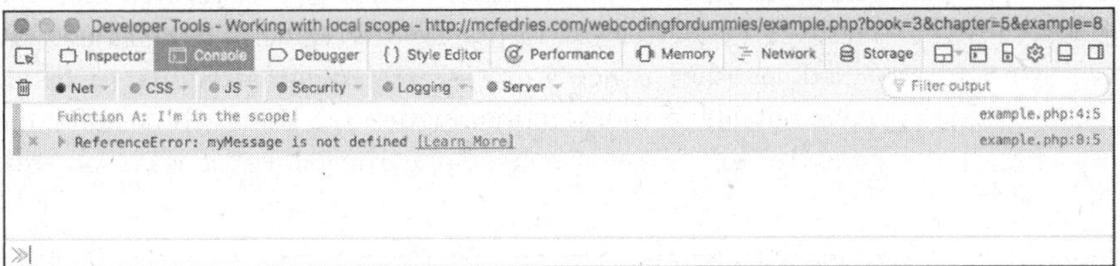

FIGURE 5-1: Attempting to display the myMessage variable in function `B()` results in an error.

so it has nothing to display. In fact, after function `A()` finishes executing, JavaScript removes the `myMessage` variable from memory entirely, so that's why the `myMessage` variable referred to in function `B()` is undefined.

The same result occurs if you attempt to use the `myMessage` variable outside of any function, as in the following code:

```
function A() {
    var myMessage;
    myMessage = "I'm in the scope!";
    console.log("Function A: " + myMessage);
}
A();
// The following statement generates an error:
console.log(myMessage);
```

Working with global scope

What if you want to use the same variable in multiple functions or even in multiple script blocks within the same page? In that case, you need to use *global* scope, which makes a variable accessible to any statement or function on a page. (That's why global scope is also called *page-level* scope.) To set up a variable with global scope, declare it outside any function. The following code gives this a whirl:

```
var myMessage = "I've got global scope!";

function C() {
    console.log("Function C: " + myMessage);
}
C();
console.log("Outside the function: " + myMessage);
```

The script begins by declaring the `myMessage` variable and setting it equal to a string literal. Then a function named `C()` is created and it displays a console message that attempts to display the value of `myMessage`. After the function is called, another `console.log()` statement attempts to display the `myMessage` value outside of the function. Figure 5-2 shows the results. As you can see, both `console.log()` statements display the value of `myMessage` without a problem.

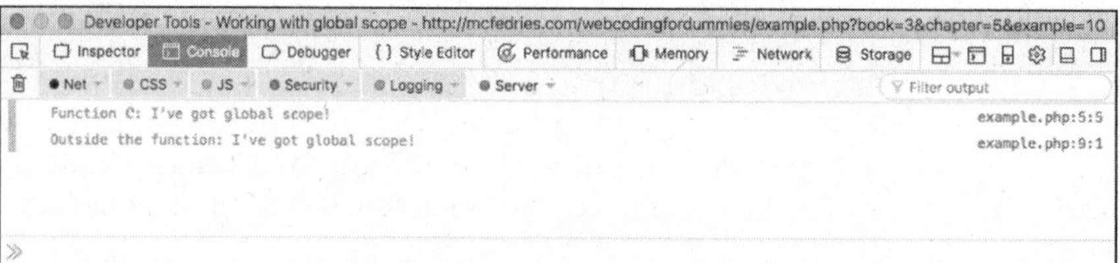

FIGURE 5-2: When you declare a global variable, you can access its value both inside and outside of a function.

Using Recursive Functions

One of the stranger things you can do with a function is have it execute itself. That is, you place a statement within the function that calls the function. This is called *recursion*, and such a function is called a *recursive function*.

Before trying out a practical example, I begin with a simple script that demonstrates the basic procedure:

```
var counter = 0;
addOne();

function addOne() {
    counter++;
    if (confirm("counter is now " + counter + ". Add another
  one?")) {
```

```
        addOne();
    }
}

console.log("Counter ended up at " + counter);
```

The script begins by declaring a variable named `counter` and initializing it to `0`. Then a function named `addOne()` is called. This function increments the value of `counter`. It then displays the current value of `counter` and asks if you want to add another. If you click OK, the `addOne()` function is called again, but this time it's called from within `addOne()` itself! This just means that the whole thing repeats itself until you eventually click Cancel in the dialog box. After the function is exited for good, a `console.log()` statement shows the final `counter` total.

What possible use is recursion in the real world? That's a good question. Consider a common business problem: calculating a profit-sharing plan contribution as a percentage of a company's net profits. This isn't a simple multiplication problem, because the net profit is determined, in part, by the profit-sharing figure. For example, suppose that a company has sales of $1,000,000 and expenses of $900,000, which leaves a gross profit of $100,000. The company also sets aside 10 percent of net profits for profit sharing. The net profit is calculated with the following formula:

```
Net Profit = Gross Profit - Profit Sharing Contribution;
```

That looks straightforward enough, but it's really not because the `Profit Sharing Contribution` value is derived with the following formula:

```
Profit Sharing Contribution = Net Profit * 10%;
```

In other words, the `Net Profit` value appears on both sides of the equation, which complicates things considerably.

One way to solve the Net Profit formula is to guess at an answer and see how close you come. For example, because profit sharing should be 10 percent of net profits, a good first guess might be 10 percent of *gross* profits, or $10,000. If you plug this number into the Net Profit formula, you get a value of $90,000. This isn't right, however, because you'd end up with a profit sharing value — 10 percent of $90,000 — of $9,000. Therefore, the original profit-sharing guess is off by $1,000.

So you can try again. This time, use $9,000 as the profit-sharing number. Plugging this new value into the Net Profit formula returns a value of $91,000. This number translates into a profit-sharing contribution of $9,100. This time you're off by only $100, so you're getting closer.

If you continue this process, your profit-sharing guesses will get closer to the calculated value (this process is called *convergence*). When the guesses are close enough (for example, within a dollar), you can stop and pat yourself on the back for finding the solution.

This process of calculating a formula and then continually recalculating it using different values is what recursion is all about, so let's see how you'd go about writing a script to do this for you. Take a look at the following code.

```
var grossProfit = 100000;
var netProfit;
var profitSharingPercent = 0.1;

// Here's the initial guess
var profitSharing = grossProfit * profitSharingPercent;

calculateProfitSharing (profitSharing);

function calculateProfitSharing(guess) {

    // First, calculate the new net profit
    netProfit = grossProfit - guess;

    // Now use that to guess the profit sharing value again
    profitSharing = Math.ceil(netProfit * profitSharingPercent);

    // Do we have a solution?
    if ((netProfit + profitSharing) != grossProfit) {
        // If not, plug it in again
        calculateProfitSharing (profitSharing);
    }
}

console.log("Gross Profit:\t" + grossProfit + "\nNet Profit:
   \t" + netProfit + "\nProfit Sharing:\t" + profitSharing);
```

The `grossProfit` variable is initialized at `100000`, the `netProfit` variable is declared, the `profitSharingPercent` variable is set to `0.1` (10 percent), and the `profitSharing` variable is set to the initial guess of 10 percent of gross profits. Then the `calculateProfitSharing()` function is called, and the `profitSharing` guess is passed as the initial value of the `guess` argument.

TECHNICAL STUFF

AVOIDING INFINITE RECURSION

If you're trying to call a function recursively, you might see error messages such as `Stack overflow` or `Too much recursion`. These error messages indicate that you have no "brakes" on your recursive function so, if not for the errors, it would call itself forever. This is called *infinite recursion,* and the actual maximum number of recursive calls depends on the browser and operating system, but the range is between about 75 and about 1,000.

In any case, it's important to build in some kind of test that ensures the function will stop calling itself after a certain number of calls:

- The addOne( ) function in the previous section avoided infinite recursion by asking the user if she wanted to continue or stop.
- The `calculateProfitSharing()` function in the previous section avoided infinite recursion by testing the sum of `netProfit` and `profitSharing` to see if this sum was equal to `grossProfit`.

If you don't have a convenient or obvious method for stopping the recursion, then you can set up a counter that tracks the number of function calls. When that number hits a predetermined maximum, the script should bail out of the recursion process. The following code presents such a script:

```
var currentCall = 1;
var maximumCalls = 3;

recursionTest();

function recursionTest() {
    if (currentCall <= maximumCalls) {
        console.log(currentCall);
        currentCall++;
        recursionTest();
    }
}
```

The `currentCall` variable is the counter, and the `maximumCalls` variable specifies the maximum number of times the recursive function can be called. In the function, the following statement compares the value of `currentCall` and `maximumCalls`:

```
if (currentCall <= maximumCalls);
```

(continued)

Harnessing the Power of Functions

(continued)

> If `currentCall` is less than or equal to `maximumCalls`, then all is well and the script can continue. In this case, a console message displays the value of `currentCall`, that value is incremented, and the `recursionTest()` function is called again. When `currentCall` becomes greater than `maximumCalls`, the function exits and the recursion is done.

The function first calculates the `netProfit` and then uses that value to calculate the new `profitSharing` number. Remember your goal here is to end up with the sum of `netProfit` and `profitSharing` being equal to `grossProfit`. The `if` statement tests that, and if the sum is not equal to `grossProfit`, the `calculateProfitSharing()` function is called again (here's the recursion), and this time the new `profitSharing` value is passed. When the correct values are finally found, the function exits and a console message displays the results, as shown in Figure 5-3.

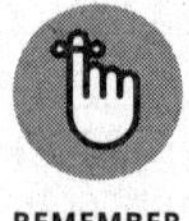

REMEMBER

Note that all the variables in previous example are declared as globals. That's because if you declared them within the `calculateProfitSharing()` function, they would get wiped out and reset with each call, which is not what you want when doing recursion.

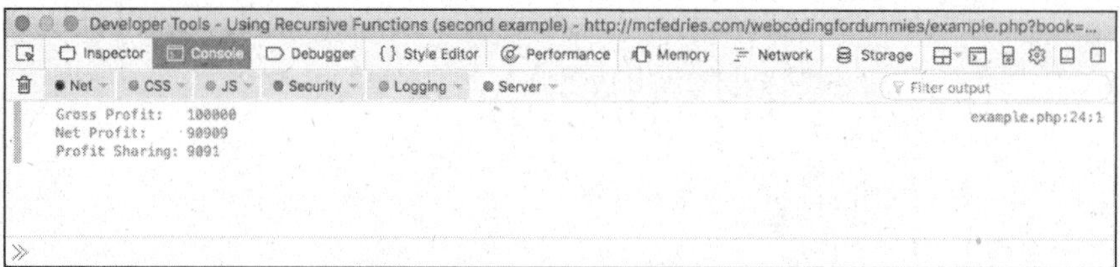

FIGURE 5-3: Using recursion to calculate a profit sharing value.

» Messing with object properties

» Running object methods

» Giving the Windows object a whirl

» Interacting with your site visitors

Chapter 6
Working with Objects

The problem with object-oriented languages is they've got all this implicit environment that they carry around with them. You wanted a banana but what you got was a gorilla holding the banana and the entire jungle.

— JOE ARMSTRONG

JavaScript derives most of its power, flexibility, and utility from its extensive collection of methods for reading, changing, adding, and deleting web page doodads and bric-a-brac. It could be HTML elements, CSS properties, form controls, or internal programming resources such as strings and numbers. Whatever it is, JavaScript has an amazing and seemingly endless collection of powerful tools — called objects — that enable you to monitor and control almost every aspect of the web page. This chapter represents a major step forward in your JavaScript education as you explore the wide and fascinating world of objects. You discover what objects are and how to use them in your code. You also get your object feet wet by taking an up close and personal look at one of the most important webpage objects.

What Is an Object?

Only the simplest JavaScript programs will do nothing but assign values to variables and calculate expressions. To go beyond these basic script beginnings — that is, to write truly useful scripts — you have to do what JavaScript was designed to do from the start: Manipulate the web page that it's displaying. That's what JavaScript is all about, and that manipulation can come in many different forms:

- » Add text and HTML tags to an **element.**
- » Modify a CSS **property** of a class or other selector.
- » Store some data in the browser's internal **storage.**
- » Read **JSON** data returned by the server.
- » Validate a **form's** data before submitting it.

The bold items in this list are examples of the "things" that you can work with, and they're special for no other reason than they're programmable. In JavaScript parlance, these "programmable things" are called *objects.*

You can manipulate objects in JavaScript in any of the following three ways:

- » You can make changes to the object's *properties.*
- » You can make the object perform a task by activating a *method* associated with the object.
- » You can define a procedure that runs whenever a particular *event* happens to the object.

To help you understand objects and their properties, methods, and events, I put things in real-world terms. Specifically, consider your computer as though it were an object:

- » If you wanted to describe your computer as a whole, you'd mention things like the name of the manufacturer, the price, and the amount of RAM. Each of these items is a *property* of the computer.
- » You also can use your computer to perform tasks such as writing letters, crunching numbers, and coding web pages. These are the *methods* associated with your computer.
- » There are also a number of things that happen to the computer that cause it to respond in predefined ways. For example, when the On button is pressed, the computer runs through its Power On Self-Test, initializes its components, and so on. The actions to which the computer responds automatically are its *events.*

The sum total of all these properties, methods, and events gives you an overall description of your computer.

But your computer is also a collection of objects, each with its own properties, methods, and events. The hard drive, for example, has various properties, including its speed and data transfer rate. The hard drive's methods would be actions such as storing and retrieving data. A hard drive event might be a scheduled maintenance task, such as defragmenting the drive's data or checking the drive for errors.

In the end, you have a complete description of the computer: what it looks like (its properties), how you interact with it (its methods), and to what actions it responds (its events).

The JavaScript Object Hierarchy

Sticking with the computer metaphor for just a moment longer, when you think about how the computer's hardware is put together, you see there is a kind of hierarchy to the organization. The computer itself is at the top, and then below that are major components such as the system unit and the monitor. Drilling down, you see that these also have their own subcomponents. For example, the system unit has the motherboard, the hard drive, and the power supply, to name just a few. Taking things down just one more level, the motherboard (for example) also holds smaller components such as the microprocessor and the memory chips.

JavaScript's objects are also organized in a hierarchical way. The top-level represents the main JavaScript objects, including the Array object (which I cover in Book 3, Chapter 7), and the Date, Math, Number, and String objects (which I talk about in Book 3, Chapter 8). These are shown in Figure 6-1, which represents only a partial view of the JavaScript object hierarchy.

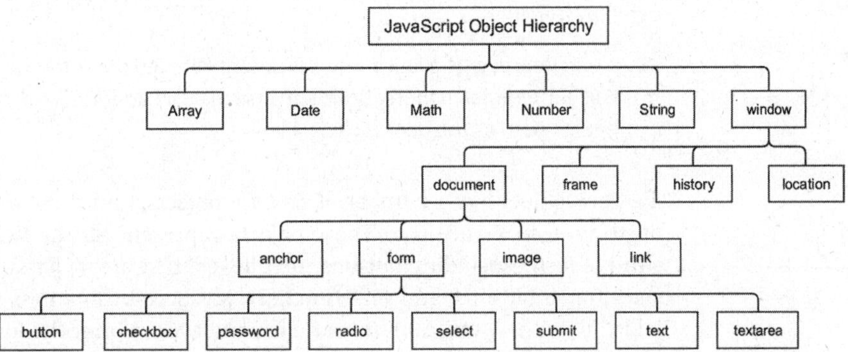

FIGURE 6-1: A partial look at the JavaScript object hierarchy.

Also in the first level of Figure 6-1 is the `window` object, which represents the browser window. Notice that the `window` object has four "subobjects":

- » `document`: Refers to whatever document is currently loaded in the browser window. Because you use this object to control such fundamental page items as links, images, and forms, this is probably the object you'll use most often in your JavaScript career.
- » `frame`: Represents a frame (if any) that's used to display multiple pages in the browser window. For example, you can use this object to display a different page inside a particular frame.
- » `history`: Represents an item in the list of pages that the user has visited in the current browser session. One common use for this object is to send the user back to the page she was on before coming to the current page.
- » `location`: Represents the address of the page that's displayed in the browser. You can use this object to determine the current address, send the user to a different address, refresh the browser display, and more.

The `document` object has its own objects, which are displayed in the third level in Figure 6-1. There are four in all:

- » `anchor`: Represents an anchor in the document, created using the `<a id>` tag. For example, you can use this object to check if a document contains an anchor that uses a particular name.
- » `form`: Represents a form in the document, created with the `<form>` tag. You can use this object to work with all the various form controls, as well as to submit a form.
- » `image`: Represents an image in the document, created using the `<img>` tag. You can use this object to change the image that's displayed within a particular `<img>` tag.
- » `link`: Represents a link in the document, created using the `<a href>` tag. You can gather information about a link (such as its address) and you can handle events such as the user clicking a link.

The `form` object has a number of its own objects, and these are displayed as the fourth level in Figure 6-1. These objects represent all the fields you can insert within a form, including buttons, text boxes, text areas, password boxes, check-boxes, radio buttons, and selection lists. JavaScript can access the values in form fields, insert new values in form fields, and even submit the form for the user.

Manipulating Object Properties

All these JavaScript objects have at least one property, and some of them have a couple of dozen or more. What you do with these properties depends on the object, but you generally use them for the following tasks:

- **Gathering information about an object's current settings:** With the `text` object, for example, you can use the `value` property to get whatever string is currently in the text box.
- **Changing an object's current settings:** For example, you can use the `window` object's `location` property to send the web browser to a different URL.
- **Changing an object's appearance:** With the `document` object, for example, you can use the `backgroundColor` property to change the background color of the page.

Referencing a property

Whatever the task, you refer to a property by using the syntax in the following generic expression:

```
object.property
```

- *`object`:* The object that has the property.
- *`property`:* The name of the property you want to work with.

The dot (`.`) in between is called the *property access operator.*

For example, consider the following expression:

```
window.location
```

This refers to the `window` object's `location` property, which holds the address of the document currently displayed in the browser window. (In conversation, you'd pronounce this expression as "window dot location.") The following code shows a simple one-line script that displays this property in the console, as shown in Figure 6-2.

```
console.log(window.location);
```

Because the property always contains a value, you're free to use property expressions in just about any type of JavaScript statement and as an operand in a

JavaScript expression. For example, the following statement assigns the current value of the `window.location` property to a variable named `currentUrl`:

```
var currentUrl = window.location;
```

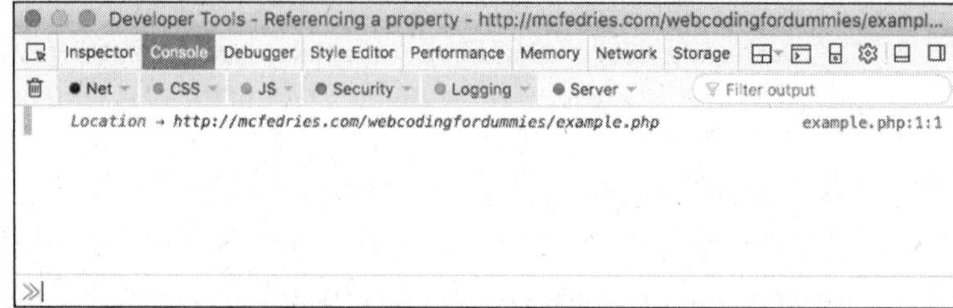

FIGURE 6-2: This script displays the `window.location` property in a console message.

Similarly, the following statement includes `window.location` as part of a string expression:

```
var message = "The current address is " + window.location + ".";
```

Some objects are properties

You might be wondering if the `window` object's `location` property is related to the `location` object that I discuss earlier. Yep, it is. Good eye! In fact, they're the same thing! This is one of the most confusing aspects of the relationship between objects and properties, but it's also one of the most important, so I'll dive into this a bit deeper to make sure you understand what's going on.

The basic idea is that in the JavaScript object hierarchy shown in Figure 6-1, any object that is subordinate to another object is automatically a property of that other object. So, for example, the `location` object is subordinate to the `window` object; therefore, it's a property of the `window` object. This means you can reference the `location` object by using the *`object.property`* syntax.

Because `location` is an object, it also has its own properties. For example, it has a `hostname` property that references just the host name part of the address (for example, `mcfedries.com`). To work with this property, you extend the expression syntax accordingly:

```
window.location.hostname
```

TIP

When you're dealing with the four second-level objects — `document`, `frame`, `history`, and `location` — it's understood that these are properties of the `window` object. Therefore, you don't have to include `window` at the front of the property expression. For example, the following two statements are equivalent:

```
window.location.hostname
location.hostname
```

Changing the value of a property

Some properties are "read-only," which means your code can only read the current value and can't change it. However, many properties are "read/write," which means you can also change their values. To change the value of a property, use the following generic syntax:

```
object.property = value
```

- *object*: The object that has the property
- *property*: The name of the property you want to change
- *value*: A literal value (such as a string or number) or an expression that returns the value to which you want to set the property

Here's an example:

```
var newAddress = prompt("Enter the address you want to surf
  to:");
window.location = newAddress;
```

This script prompts the user for a web page address and stores the result in the `newAddress` variable. This value is then used to change the `window.location` property, which in this case tells the browser to open the specified address.

Working with Object Methods

Each one of the JavaScript objects I mention earlier has at least one or two methods that you can wield to make the object do something. These actions generally fall into the following categories:

- **Simulate a user's action.** For example, the `form` object's `submit()` method submits a form to the server just as though the user clicked the form's submit button.
- **Perform a calculation.** For example, the `Math` object's `sqrt()` method calculates the square root of a number.

- **Manipulate an object.** For example, the `String` object's `toLowercase()` method changes all of a string's letters to lowercase.

To run a method, begin with the simplest case, which is a method that takes no arguments:

```
object.method()
```

- *`object`:* The object that has the method you want to work with
- *`method`:* The name of the method you want to execute

For example, consider the following statement:

```
history.back();
```

This runs the `history` object's `back()` method, which tells the browser to go back to the previously visited page. The following code shows this method at work:

```
var goBack = confirm("Do you want to go back?");
if (goBack === true) {
    history.back();
}
```

The user is first asked if she wants to go back. If she clicks OK, the Boolean value `true` is stored in the `goBack` variable, the comparison expression `goBack === true` becomes `true`, so the `history.back()` method runs.

I mention in Book 3, Chapter 5 that it's possible to define a function so that it accepts one or more arguments, and that these arguments are then used as input values for whatever calculations or manipulations the function performs. Methods are similar in that they can take one or more arguments and use those values as raw data.

If a method requires arguments, you use the following generic syntax:

```
object.method (argument1, argument2, ...)
```

For example, consider the `confirm()` method, used in the following statement, which takes a single argument — a string that specifies the text to display to the user:

```
confirm("Do you want to go back?")
```

Finally, as with properties, if the method returns a value, you can assign that value to a variable (as I did with the `confirm()` method in the earlier example) or you can incorporate the method into an expression.

Playing Around with the window Object

It's time you get practical with all this object stuff by tackling some actual objects. This section gets you started by examining one of the top-level objects in the hierarchy of the JavaScript object model: the `window` object. This object refers to the browser window *viewport*, which is the content area where the web page appears (not the full window of the browser application). This makes the `window` object the topmost object in the web page object hierarchy, so you'll be using the `window` object a great deal as you progress in web development.

Referencing the window object

When you need to reference the `window` object, the fact that it's the topmost item in the web page hierarchy gives you far greater flexibility than with the other objects on the lower levels.

For starters, you can combine the `window` keyword with the standard notation for properties and methods:

```
window.propertyName
window.methodName()
```

However, the `window` object is the default object in JavaScript. This means that if JavaScript comes across a property or method that doesn't have a specified object, it automatically assumes the property or method is part of the `window` object. Therefore, you can almost always get away with not using the `window` keyword. In other words, the previous two statements are equivalent to the following two:

```
propertyName
methodName()
```

Some window object properties you should know

The `window` object comes with a few dozen properties, most of which are too obscure or arcane to worry about. However, several `window` object properties are essential to all web developers, and those are listed in Table 6-1.

TABLE 6-1 **Useful Properties of the window Object**

Property	What It Does
`console`	Returns a reference to the `console` object, which you use to log text to the console with `console.log()`.
`document`	Returns a reference to the `document` object (that is, the web page) contained in the window.
`frames`	Returns a reference to the frames (if any) that are used to display multiple pages in the browser window.
`history`	Returns a reference to the list of pages that the user has visited in the current browser session. Your code can navigate these pages — for example, by calling the `back()` method to go back one page — but your code can't access the URLs of these pages.
`innerHeight`	Returns the height, in pixels, of the browser window viewport.
`innerWidth`	Returns the width, in pixels, of the browser window viewport.
`localStorage`	Returns a reference to the local `Storage` object, which you can use to store and retrieve data in the browser indefinitely.
`location`	Returns a reference to the `location` object, which contains info about the current web page URL.
`navigator`	Returns a reference to the `navigator` object, which provides data on the browser application the visitor is using.
`scrollX`	Returns the distance, in pixels, that the window's document has been scrolled horizontally.
`scrollY`	Returns the distance, in pixels, that the window's document has been scrolled vertically.
`sessionStorage`	Returns a reference to the session `Storage` object, which you can use to store and retrieve data in the browser temporarily (that is, the data gets deleted automatically when the user shuts down the current browser session).

Rather than providing you with a similar table for the `window` object's methods, I use the rest of the chapter to discuss a few useful methods in detail.

Working with JavaScript timeouts and intervals

In the scripts I've presented so far in this book, the code has executed in one of three ways:

- Automatically when the page loads
- When your script calls a function

» In response to some event, such as the user clicking a button

JavaScript also offers a fourth execution method that's based on time. There are two possibilities:

» Have some code run once after a specified number of milliseconds. This is called a *timeout*.

» Have some code run after a specified number of milliseconds, and then repeat each time that number of milliseconds expires. This is called an *interval*.

The next couple of sections show you how to set up both procedures.

Using a timeout to perform a future action once

To set up a JavaScript timeout, use the `window` object's `setTimeout()` method:

```
setTimeout(function, delay, arg1, arg2, ...)
```

» *`function`*: The name of a function that you want JavaScript to run when the timeout expires. Instead of a function, you can also use a JavaScript statement, surrounded by quotation marks.

» *`delay`*: The number of milliseconds that JavaScript waits before executing *`function`*.

» *`arg1, arg2, ...`*: Optional arguments to pass to *`function`*.

Note that `setTimeout()` returns a value that uniquely identifies the timeout. You can store this value just in case you want to cancel the timeout (as described later in this section).

Here's some code that shows how `setTimeout()` works:

```
// Create a message
var str = "Hello World!";

// Set the timeout
var timeoutId = setTimeout(logIt, 2000, str);

// Run this function when the timeout occurs
function logIt(msg) {
```

```
    // Display the message
    console.log(msg);
}
```

The script begins by creating a message string and storing it in the `str` variable. Then the `setTimeout()` method runs:

```
setTimeout(logIt, 2000, str);
```

This tells JavaScript to run the function named `logIt()` after two seconds (2,000 milliseconds) have elapsed, and to pass the `str` variable to that function. The `logIt()` function takes the `msg` argument and displays it in the console.

If you've set up a timeout and then decide that you don't want the code to execute after all for some reason, you can cancel the timeout by running the `clearTimeout()` method:

```
clearTimeout(id);
```

» *`id`:* The name of the variable that was used to store the `setTimeout()` method's return value

For example, suppose you set a timeout with the following statement:

```
var timeoutId = setTimeout(logIt, 2000, str);
```

Then you'd cancel the timeout using the following statement:

```
clearTimeout(timeoutId);
```

Using an interval to perform a future action repeatedly

Running code once after a specified number of seconds is only an occasionally useful procedure. A much more practical skill is being able to repeat code at a specified interval. This enables you to set up countdowns, timers, animations, image slide shows, and more. To set up an interval, use the window object's `setInterval()` method:

```
setInterval(function, delay, arg1, arg2, ...)
```

» *`function`:* The name of a function that you want JavaScript to run at the end of each interval. Instead of a function, you can also use a JavaScript statement, surrounded by quotation marks.

- *delay:* The number of milliseconds in each interval, after which JavaScript executes *function*
- *arg1, arg2, ...:* Optional arguments to pass to *function*

As with setTimeout(), the setInterval() method returns a value that uniquely identifies the interval. You use that value to cancel the interval with the clearInterval() method:

```
clearInterval(id);
```

- *id:* The name of the variable that was used to store the setInterval() method's return value

For example, suppose you set an interval with the following statement:

```
var intervalId = setInterval(countdown, 5000);
```

Then you'd cancel the interval using the following statement:

```
clearInterval(intervalId);
```

Note that although the clearTimeout() method is optional with setTimeout(), you should always use clearInterval() with setInterval(). Otherwise, the interval will just keep executing.

The following code demonstrates both setInterval() and clearInterval().

```
var counter = 10;

// Set the interval
var intervalId = setInterval(countdown, 1000);

// Run this function at the end of each interval
function countdown() {

    // Display the countdown and then decrement the counter
    console.log(counter--);

    // Cancel the interval when we hit 0
    if (counter < 0) {
        clearInterval(intervalId);
        console.log("All done!");
    }
}
```

The purpose of this script is to display a countdown from 10 to 0 in the console. The script begins by declaring a variable named `counter` and initializing it to `10`. Then the `setInterval()` method sets up a function named `countdown()` to run at intervals of one second (1,000 milliseconds). The `countdown()` function displays the current value of `counter` in the console and then decrements `counter`. Then an `if()` test checks the value of `counter`. If it's negative, it means that `counter` was just `0`, so it's done. The `clearInterval()` method cancels the interval, and then a final console message is logged.

Interacting with the user

Many of your scripts will do all of their work "behind the scenes," and your page visitors will probably never even know what programming wonders are happening beneath their noses. That's a good thing because a well-crafted script should neither be seen nor heard.

However, that's not to say that all your scripts must remain mute servants who blend into the background. There are plenty of good reasons to interact with the user:

- **To display a message to the user:** This message might include navigation instructions, help information, or warnings about improperly entered data.
- **To ask the user a simple yes/no question:** Such a question could be used to confirm a pending action, ask permission to perform a task, or cancel a form submission.
- **To get data from the user:** This data could be used to populate form fields, personalize the page, or gather information about the user.

For all these purposes and many more, JavaScript has three tools you can use: the `alert()`, `confirm()`, and `prompt()` methods. I discuss each one in the sections that follow.

Displaying messages using the alert() method

When you need to display a simple text message to the user, the `alert()` method is your best choice:

```
alert(string);
```

- *`string`*: A string literal or string expression containing the message you want to display

The *string* argument must be plain text; you can't format the text using HTML tags. The only formatting control you have is to use the \n escape character to start a new line, and the \t escape character to insert a tab character. The following code demonstrates the use of both characters, and Figure 6-3 shows the result.

```
// Build the message
var msg = "Some location properties:\n";
msg += "Protocol:\t" + location.protocol + "\n";
msg += "Host:\t" + location.hostname + "\n";
msg += "Path:\t" + location.pathname + "\n";
msg += "Search:\t" + location.search + "\n";

// Display the message
alert(msg);
```

Some location properties:
Protocol: http:
Host: mcfedries.com
Path: /webcodingfordummies/example.php
Search: ?book=3&chapter=7&example=6
OK

FIGURE 6-3: An alert box formatted with the \n and \t escape characters.

Asking questions using the confirm() method

When you need to ask the user a yes/no question or have the user accept or reject an action, use the `confirm()` method:

```
confirm(string);
```

- *string:* A string literal or string expression containing the question or action you need the user to confirm

The *string* argument must be plain text, so don't use HTML tags. However, as with `alert()`, you can use the \n and \t escape characters to format the string.

The `confirm()` method displays a dialog box with OK and Cancel buttons:

- If the user clicks OK, `confirm()` returns the value `true`.
- If the user clicks Cancel, `confirm()` returns `false`.

If you need the `confirm()` result later in your script, include it as part of a variable assignment statement to save the result:

```
var goOrWhoa = confirm("Do you want to proceed?");
```

Alternatively, if you only need to use the `confirm()` result immediately after it's displayed, include it in a comparison or logical expression. The following code provides a simple example, and Figure 6-4 shows the dialog box that appears.

```
if (confirm("Are you sure about this?") === true) {
    console.log("You clicked OK.");
} else {
    console.log("You clicked Cancel.");
}
```

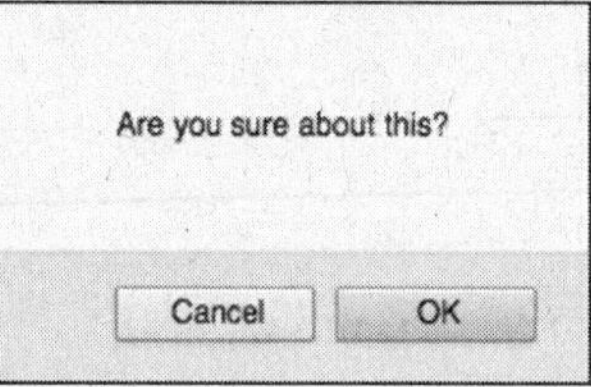

FIGURE 6-4: Use the `confirm` method to ask the user for yes/no input.

Actually, since `confirm()` returns `true` or `false`, you don't have to set up a full comparison expression to test if the result equals one of those values. Instead, just use `confirm()` by itself. For example, this `if()` test returns `true` if `confirm()` returns `true`:

```
if (confirm("Are you sure about this?"))
```

Similarly, the following `if()` test returns `true` if `confirm()` returns `false`:

```
if (!confirm("Are you sure about this?"))
```

Getting input using the prompt() method

When you need to get data from the user, run the `prompt()` method:

```
prompt(string, default);
```

- *`string`*: A string literal or string expression that instructs the user what to enter into the prompt box

- *default*: An optional string literal or string expression that represents the initial value that appears in the prompt box

Both the *string* and *default* arguments must be plain text, so don't use HTML tags. For the *string* argument, you can include the \n and \t escape characters.

If you don't include the *default* argument, the browser leaves the text box blank. If your code requires a non-blank return value, then you should include a default value.

The prompt() method always returns a value:

- If the user clicks OK, prompt() returns the value entered into the prompt text box.
- If the user clicks Cancel, prompt() returns null.

As with confirm(), you can either store the prompt() method's return value in a variable or use it in an expression. In most cases, you'll want to set up your script to check the return value and make sure that it isn't null, as shown in the following code:

```
var bgColor = prompt("Type a color to use for the background:
  \nSome examples: azure, linen, gainsboro");

if (bgColor !== null) {;
    document.body.style.backgroundColor = bgColor;
} else {
    document.body.style.backgroundColor = "white";
}
```

TIP

Prompt boxes are fine if you just need a single bit of data from the user. If you need multiple items from the user, don't bother using multiple prompt boxes. Instead, set up a form and use JavaScript to read and manipulate the form data. My coverage of forms appears in Book 6, Chapter 2.

Don't overdo it

There are few things in this world as annoying as an unnecessary dialog box, and a page that includes a number of such annoyances will likely cause much disgruntlement. So when designing your scripts, bear in mind the following points concerning the alert(), confirm(), and prompt() methods:

- Don't set up an alert box or other dialog box to display automatically when your page loads. If people realize that the dialog box is going to show up every time they load your page, there's a good chance they won't load the page again.

- Similarly, don't set up a message to display when the user leaves your site. When they're leaving, most people just want to leave and be done with it.
- If you must display a message automatically when a page loads or unloads, use the browser's local storage to record that the user has seen it once. Then check for that stored value as part of your script: If the value tells you that the user has already seen the message, don't display it again. I talk about local storage in Book 8, Chapter 1.
- Don't use alert boxes to display welcome messages, `"This site works best with..."` recommendations, or other unnecessary notes to the user. If you have something to say, put it on your page.
- Make your dialog box text as short and as clear as possible. Assume every user is a busy person with a quick mouse trigger finger. If what you make users read is too long or too convoluted, they'll head for the next site.

Programming the document Object

One of JavaScript's most fundamental features is the capability it offers you as a web developer to read and change the elements of a web page, even after the page is loaded. I show you how this works in detail in Book 4, Chapter 1, but that material uses jQuery to manipulate the web page elements. jQuery is a fantastic tool, but you should also know how to program page stuff using vanilla JavaScript. To that end, this section presents you with a quick tour of some extremely useful and powerful JavaScript techniques for dealing with the `document` object.

Specifying an element

Elements represent the tags in a document, so you'll be using them constantly in your code. This section shows you several methods for referencing an element.

Specifying an element by id

If it's a specific element you want to work with in your script, you can reference the element directly by assigning it an "id" using the `id` attribute:

```
<div id="my-div">
```

With that done, you can then refer to the element in your code by using the `document` object's `getElementById()` method:

```
document.getElementById(id)
```

» *id:* A string representing the `id` attribute of the element you want to work with

For example, the following statement returns a reference to the previous `<div>` tag (the one that has `id="my-div"`):

```
document.getElementById("my-div")
```

WARNING

When you're coding the `document` object, don't put your `<script>` tag in the web page's head section (that is, between the `<head>` and `</head>` tags). If you place your code there, the web browser will run the code before it has had a chance to create the `document` object, which means your code with fail, big-time. Instead, place your `<script>` tag at the bottom of the web page, just before the `</body>` tag.

Specifying elements by tag name

Besides working with individual elements, it's also possible to work with collections of elements. One such collection is the set of all elements in a page that use the same tag name. For example, you could reference all the `<a>` tags or all the `<div>` tags. This is a handy way to make large-scale changes to these tags (such as changing all the `target` attributes in your links).

The mechanism for returning a collection of elements that have the same tag is the `getElementsByTagName()` method:

```
document.getElementsByTagName(tag)
```

» *tag:* A string representing the HTML name used by the tags you want to work with

This method returns an arraylike collection that contains all the elements in the document that use the specified tag. (See Book 3, Chapter 7 to learn how arrays work.) The collection order is the same as the order in which the elements appear in the document. For example, consider the following HTML pseudo-code:

```
<div id="div1">
Other elements go here
```

```
</div>
<div id="div2">
Other elements go here
</div>
<div id="div3">
Other elements go here
</div>
```

Now consider the following statement:

```
divs = document.getElementsByTagName("div");
```

In the resulting collection, the first item (`divs[0]`) will be the `<div>` element with `id` equal to `div1`, the second item (`divs[1]`) will be the `<div>` element with `id` equal to `div2`, and the third item (`divs[2]`) will be the `<div>` element with `id` equal to `div3`.

Specifying elements by class name

Another collection you can work with is the set of all elements in a page that use the same class. The JavaScript tool for returning all the elements that share a specific class name is the `getElementsByClassName()` method:

```
document.getElementsByClassName(class)
```

» *`class`*: A string representing the class name used by the elements you want to work with

This method returns an arraylike collection that contains all the elements in the document that use the specified class name. The collection order is the same as the order in which the elements appear in the document. Here's an example:

```
var keywords = document.getElementsByClassName("keyword");
```

Specifying elements by selector

In Book 2, Chapter 2, I discuss CSS selectors, including the id, tag, class, descendant, and child selectors. You can use those same selectors in your JavaScript code to reference page elements by using the `document` object's `querySelector()` and `querySelectorAll()` methods:

```
document.querySelector(selector)
document.querySelectorAll(selector)
```

» *selector*: A string representing the selector for the element or elements you want to work with

The difference between these methods is that `querySelectorAll()` returns a collection of all the elements that match your selector, whereas `querySelector()` returns only the first element that matches your selector.

For example, the following statement returns the collection of all `section` elements that are direct children of an `article` element:

```
var articles = document.querySelectorAll("article > section");
```

REMEMBER

Rather than using three distinct `document` object methods to reference page elements by id, tag, and class — that is, `getElementById()`, `getElementsByTagName()`, and `getElementsByClassName()` — many web developers prefer the more generic approach offered by `querySelector()` and `querySelectorAll()`.

Working with elements

Once you've got a reference to one or more elements, you can then use code to manipulate those elements in various ways, as shown in the next few sections.

Adding an element to the page

To add an element to the page, you follow three steps:

1. Create an object for the type of element you want to add.
2. Add the new object from Step 1 as a child element of an existing element.
3. Insert some text and tags into the new object from Step 1.

Step 1: Creating the element

For Step 1, you use the `document` object's `createElement()` method:

```
document.createElement(elementName)
```

» *elementName*: A string containing the HTML tag name for the type of the element you want to create

This method creates the element and then returns it, which means you can store the new element in a variable. Here's an example:

```
newArticle = createElement("article");
```

Step 2: Appending the new element as a child

With your element created, Step 2 is to append it to an existing parent element using the appendChild() method:

```
parent.appendChild(child)
```

- *parent*: A reference to the parent element to which the new element will be appended
- *child*: A reference to the child element you're adding

Here's an example that creates a new article element and then appends it to the main element:

```
newArticle = document.createElement("article");
document.querySelector("main").appendChild(newArticle);
```

Note that the child element is added to the *end* of the parent element's collection of child elements, so be sure to add the child elements in the appropriate order.

Step 3: Adding text and tags to the new element

With your element created and appended to a parent, the final step is to add some text and tags using the innerHTML property:

```
element.innerHTML = text
```

- *element*: A reference to the new element within which you want to add the text and tags
- *text*: A string containing the text and HTML tags you want to insert

In this example, the code creates a new article element, appends it to the main element, and then adds some text and tags:

```
newArticle = document.createElement("article");
document.querySelector("main").appendChild(newArticle);
newArticle.innerHTML = "Hello <code>document</code> Object
  World!";
```

Changing an element's styles

Most HTML tags can have a style attribute that you use to set inline styles. Since standard attributes all have corresponding element object properties, you won't be surprised to learn that most elements also have a `style` property that enables you to get and modify a tag's styles. The way it works is that the `style` property actually returns a `style` object that has properties for every CSS property. When referencing these style properties, you need to keep two things in mind:

- For single-word CSS properties (such as `color` and `visibility`), use all-lowercase letters.
- For multiple-word CSS properties, drop the hyphen and use uppercase for the first letter of the second word and for each subsequent word if the property has more than two. For example, the `font-size` and `border-left-width` CSS properties become the `fontSize` and `borderLeftWidth` `style` object properties.

Here's an example:

```
var pageTitle = document.querySelector("h1");
pageTitle.style.fontSize = "64px";
pageTitle.style.color = "maroon";
pageTitle.style.textAlign = "center";
pageTitle.style.border = "1px solid black";
```

This code gets a reference to the page's first `<h1>` element. With that reference in hand, the code then uses the `style` object to style four properties of the heading: `fontSize`, `color`, `text-align`, and `border`.

Adding a class to an element

Besides changing an element's styles, you can also assign a class to an element. First, you can get a list of an element's assigned classes by using the `classList` property:

```
element.classList
```

- *`element`:* The element you're working with

The returned list of classes is an arraylike object that includes an `add` method that you can use to add a new class to the element's existing classes:

```
element.classList.add(class)
```

- *`element`:* The element you're working with.
- *`class`:* A string representing the name of the class you want to add to *`element`*. You can add multiple classes by separating each class name with a comma.

Here's an example:

```
var articleSections = document.querySelectorAll("article >
  section");
for (var i = 0; i < articleSections.length; i++) {
    articleSections[i].classList.add("sectionText");
}
```

This code uses `querySelectorAll` to return all the `section` elements that are direct children of an `article` element, and those `section` elements are stored in the `articleSections` variable. `articleSections` is an arraylike object, so we can iterate through it using a `for` loop. Inside the loop, the code uses `classList.add` to add the class named `sectionText` to each `section` element.

» Declaring an array variable

» Populating an array with data

» Trying out multidimensional arrays

» Working with JavaScript's Array object

Chapter 7 Working with Arrays

I choose a lazy person to do a hard job. Because a lazy person will find an easy way to do it.

— BILL GATES

In this chapter, you discover one of JavaScript's most important concepts: the array. Arrays are important not only because they're extremely powerful, but because once you know how to use them, you'll think of a thousand and one uses for them. To make sure you're ready for your new array-filled life, this chapter explains what they are and why they're so darn useful, and then explores all the fantastic ways that arrays can make your coding life easier.

What Is an Array?

I talk quite a bit about efficient programming in this book because I believe (okay, I know) that efficient scripts run faster and take less time to program and debug. As I've said, efficiency in programming really means eliminating unnecessary repetition, whether it's consolidating statements into a loop that can be repeated as often as required, or moving code into a function that can be called as often as you need.

Another source of unnecessary repetition involves variables. For example, consider the following declarations:

```
var dog1 = "dog-1";
var dog2 = "dog-2";
var dog3 = "dog-3";
var dog4 = "dog-4";
var dog5 = "dog-5";
```

These are string variables and they store the names of some dog photos. Now suppose you want to write a script that asks the user for a dog number and then displays the corresponding photo as the page background. The following code shows such a script:

```
var dog1 = "dog-1";
var dog2 = "dog-2";
var dog3 = "dog-3";
var dog4 = "dog-4";
var dog5 = "dog-5";
var promptNum = prompt("Enter the dog you want to see
  (1-5):", "");

if (promptNum !== "" && promptNum !== null) {
    var promptDog = "dog-" + promptNum;
    if (promptDog === dog1) {
        document.body.style.backgroundImage = "url('/images/" +
  dog1 + ".png')";
    } else if (promptDog === dog2) {
        document.body.style.backgroundImage = "url('/images/" +
  dog2 + ".png')";
    } else if (promptDog === dog3) {
        document.body.style.backgroundImage = "url('/images/" +
  dog3 + ".png')";
    } else if (promptDog === dog4) {
        document.body.style.backgroundImage = "url('/images/" +
  dog4 + ".png')";
    } else if (promptDog === dog5) {
        document.body.style.backgroundImage = "url('/images/" +
  dog5 + ".png')";
    }
}
```

After declaring and initializing the variables, the script uses `prompt()` to get a number between 1 and 5, which is stored in the `promptNum` variable. An `if()` test ensures that promptNum isn't the empty string (no value entered) or null (Cancel was clicked). The code then adds the number to the string dog-, which is then stored in the promptDog variable.

Now the code runs through five separate if() tests, each of which checks to see if promptDog is equal to one of the variables. If a match is found, the document.body.style.backgroundImage property is set to the URL of the image.

This might not seem outrageously inefficient, but what if instead of five images you actually had to take 10 or 20 or even 100 images into account? I'm sure the idea of typing 100 if() tests isn't your idea of a good time.

To understand the solution to this problem, first understand that the variables dog1 through dog5 all contain related values. That is, each variable holds part of the filename of a dog photo, which in turn is part of the full URL for that image. In JavaScript (or, indeed, in just about any programming language), whenever you have a collection of variables with related data, it's possible to group them together into a single variable called an *array*. You can enter as many values as you want into the array, and JavaScript tracks each value by the use of an *index number*. For example, the first value you add is given the index 0. (For obscure reasons, programmers since time immemorial have started numerical lists with 0 instead of 1.) The second value you put into the array is given the index 1, the third value gets 2, and so on. You can then access any value in the array by specifying the index number you want.

The next couple of sections flesh out this theory with the specifics of creating and populating an array, and then you'll see how to rewrite a much more efficient version of the above code using arrays.

Declaring an Array

Because an array is a type of variable, you need to declare it before using it. In fact, unlike regular numeric, string, or Boolean variables that don't really need to be declared (but always should be), JavaScript insists that you declare an array in advance. You use the var statement again, but this time with a slightly different syntax. Actually, there are four syntaxes you can use. Let's start with the simplest:

```
var arrayName =  new Array();
```

Here, *arrayName* is the name you want to use for the array variable.

In JavaScript, an array is actually an object, so what the new keyword is doing here is creating a new Array object. The Array() part of the statement is called a *constructor* because its job is to construct the object in memory. For example, to create a new array named dogPhotos, you'd use the following statement:

```
var dogPhotos = new Array();
```

The second syntax is useful if you know in advance the number of values (or *elements*) you'll be putting into the array:

```
var arrayName = new Array(num);
```

- *arrayName:* The name you want to use for the array variable
- *num:* The number of values you'll be placing into the array

For example, here's a statement that declares a new dogPhotos array with 5 elements:

```
var dogPhotos = new Array(5);
```

If you're not sure how many elements you need, don't worry about it because JavaScript is happy to let you add elements to and delete elements from the array as needed, and it will grow or shrink the array to compensate. I talk about the other two array declaration syntaxes in the next section.

Populating an Array with Data

Once your array is declared, you can start populating it with the data values you want to store. Here's the general syntax for doing this:

```
arrayName[index] = value;
```

- *arrayName:* The name of the array variable
- *index:* The array index number where you want the value stored
- *value:* The value you're storing in the array

JavaScript is willing to put just about any type of data inside an array, including numbers, strings, Boolean values, and even other arrays! You can even mix multiple data types within a single array.

As an example, here are a few statements that declare a new array named dogPhotos and then enter five string values into the array:

```
var dogPhotos = new Array(5);
dogPhotos[0] = "dog-1";
dogPhotos[1] = "dog-2";
dogPhotos[2] = "dog-3";
dogPhotos[3] = "dog-4";
dogPhotos[4] = "dog-5";
```

To reference an array value (say, to use it within an expression), you specify the appropriate index:

```
strURL + dogPhotos[3]
```

The following code offers a complete example:

HTML:

```
<div id="output">
</div>
```

JavaScript:

```
// Declare the array
var dogPhotos = new Array(5);

// Initialize the array values
dogPhotos[0] = "dog-1";
dogPhotos[1] = "dog-2";
dogPhotos[2] = "dog-3";
dogPhotos[3] = "dog-4";
dogPhotos[4] = "dog-5";

// Display an example
document.getElementById('output').innerHTML = '/images/' +
  dogPhotos[0] + '.png';
```

Declaring and populating an array at the same time

Earlier I mention that JavaScript has two other syntaxes for declaring an array. Both enable you to declare an array *and* populate it with values by using just a single statement.

The first method uses the `Array()` constructor in the following general format:

```
var arrayName =  new Array(value1, value2, ...);
```

» *arrayName*: The name you want to use for the array variable

» *value1, value2, ...*: The initial values with which you want to populate the array

Here's an example:

```
var dogPhotos = new Array("dog-1", "dog-2", "dog-3", "dog-4",
    "dog-5");
```

JavaScript also supports the creation of *array literals*, which are similar to string, numeric, and Boolean literals. In the same way that you create, say, a string literal by enclosing a value in quotation marks, you create an array literal by enclosing one or more values in square brackets. Here's the general format:

```
var arrayName = [value1, value2, ...];
```

» *arrayName*: The name you want to use for the array variable

» *value1, value2, ...*: The initial values with which you want to populate the array

An example:

```
var dogPhotos= ["dog-1", "dog-2", "dog-3", "dog-4", "dog-5"];
```

Using a loop to populate an array

So far, you probably don't think arrays are all that much more efficient than using separate variables. That's because you haven't yet learned about the single most powerful aspect of working with arrays: using a loop and some kind of counter variable to access an array's index number programmatically.

For example, here's a `for()` loop that replaces the six statements I used earlier to declare and initialize the `dogPhotos` array:

```
var dogPhotos = new Array(5);
for (var counter = 0; counter < 5; counter++) {
    dogPhotos[counter] = "dog-" + (counter + 1);
}
```

The statement inside the for() loop uses the variable counter as the array's index. For example, when counter is 0, the statement looks like this:

```
dogPhotos[0] = "dog-" + (0 + 1);
```

In this case, the expression to the right of the equals sign evaluates to "dog-1", which is the correct value. The following code shows this loop technique at work:

HTML:

```
<div id="output">
</div>
```

JavaScript:

```
// Declare the array
var dogPhotos = new Array(5);

// Initialize the array values using a loop
for (var counter = 0; counter < 5; counter++) {
    dogPhotos[counter] = "dog-" + (counter + 1);
}

// Display an example
document.getElementById('output').innerHTML = '/images/' +
   dogPhotos[0] + '.png';
```

Using a loop to insert data into an array works best in two situations:

- When the array values can be generated using an expression that changes with each pass through the loop
- When you need to assign the same value to each element of the array

REMEMBER

If you declare your array with a specific number of elements, JavaScript doesn't mind at all if you end up populating the array with more than that number.

Using a loop to work with array data

The real problem with using a large number of similar variables isn't so much declaring them, but working with them in your code. In this chapter's original code example, the script had to use five separate if() tests to check the input value against all five variables.

Arrays can really help make your code more efficient by enabling you to reduce these kinds of long-winded checking procedures to a much shorter routine that fits inside a loop. As with populating the array, you use the loop counter or some other expression to generate new array values to work with.

For example, here's a `for()` loop that replaces all those `if()` tests from the earlier script:

```
for (var counter = 0; counter < 5; counter++) {
    if (promptDog === dogPhotos[counter]) {
        document.body.style.backgroundImage = "url('/images/" +
  dogPhotos[counter] + ".png')";
        break;
    }
}
```

Each time through the loop, a new array value is generated by `dogPhotos[counter]`, and this value is compared with `promptDog`. If a match is found, `dogPhotos[counter]` is used in an expression to generate the new `backgroundImage` property, and then `break` takes the code out of the loop.

Putting it all together, the following code presents the full and very efficient replacement for the earlier script:

```
// Declare the array
var dogPhotos = new Array(5);

// Initialize the array values using a loop
for (var counter = 0; counter < 5; counter++) {
    dogPhotos[counter] = "dog-" + (counter + 1);
}

// Get the photo number
var promptNum = prompt("Enter the dog you want to see
  (1-5):", "");

if (promptNum !== "" && promptNum !== null) {

    // Construct the primary part of the filename
    var promptDog = "dog-" + promptNum;

    // Work with the array values using a loop
    for (counter = 0; counter < 5; counter++) {
```

```
        if (promptDog === dogPhotos[counter] {
            document.body.style.backgroundImage =
    "url('/images/" + dogPhotos[counter] + ".png')";
            break;
        }
    }
}
```

Creating Multidimensional Arrays

A *multidimensional array* is one where two or more values are stored within each array element. For example, if you wanted to create an array to store user data, you might need each element to store a first name, a last name, a user name, a password, and more. The bad news is that JavaScript doesn't support multidimensional arrays. The good news is that it's possible to use a trick to simulate a multidimensional array.

The trick is to populate your array in such a way that each element is itself an array. To see how such an odd idea might work, first recall the general syntax for an array literal:

```
[value1, value2, ...]
```

Now recall the general syntax for assigning a value to an array element:

```
arrayName[index] = value;
```

In a one-dimensional array, the `value` is usually a string, number, or Boolean. Now imagine, instead, that `value` is an array literal. For a two-dimensional array, the general syntax for assigning an array literal to an array element looks like this:

```
arrayName[index] = [value1, value2];
```

As an example, say you want to store an array of background and foreground colors. Here's how you might declare and populate such an array:

```
var colorArray = new Array(3);
colorArray[0] = ['white', 'black'];
colorArray[1] = ['aliceblue', 'midnightblue'];
colorArray[2] = ['honeydew', 'darkgreen'];
```

Alternatively, you can declare and populate the array using only the array literal notation:

```
var colorArray = [['white', 'black'], ['aliceblue',
   'midnightblue'], ['honeydew', 'darkgreen']];
```

Either way, you can then refer to individual elements using double square brackets, as in these examples:

```
colorArray[0][0]; // Returns 'white'
colorArray[0][1]; // Returns 'black'
colorArray[1][0]; // Returns 'aliceblue'
colorArray[1][1]; // Returns 'midnightblue'
colorArray[2][0]; // Returns 'honeydew'
colorArray[2][1]; // Returns 'darkgreen'
```

The number in the left set of square brackets is the index of the overall array, and the number in the right set of square brackets is the index of the element array.

Using the Array Object

In JavaScript, an array is actually an object. That's what the `Array()` constructor does: It creates a new object based on the arguments (if any) that you supply within the parentheses. So, like any good object, `Array` comes with a collection of properties and methods that you can work with and manipulate. The rest of this chapter takes a look at these properties and methods.

The length property

The Array object has just a couple of properties, but the only one of these that you'll use frequently is the `length` property:

```
array.length
```

The `length` property returns the number of elements that are currently in the specified array. This is very useful when looping through an array because it means you don't have to specify a literal as the maximum value of the loop counter. For example, consider the following `for()` statement:

```
for (var counter = 0; counter < 5; counter++) {
    dogPhotos[counter] = "dog-" + (counter + 1);
}
```

This statement assumes the dogPhotos array has five elements, which might not be the case. To enable the loop to work with any number of elements, replace 5 with dogPhotos.length:

```
for (var counter = 0; counter < dogPhotos.length; counter++)
    dogPhotos[counter] = "dog-" + (counter + 1);
}
```

Note, too, that the loop runs while the counter variable is *less than* dogPhotos.length. That's because array indexes run from 0 to the array's length value minus 1. In other words, the previous for() loop example is equivalent to the following:

```
for (var counter = 0; counter <= dogPhotos.length - 1;
  counter++)
```

Concatenating to create a new array: concat()

The concat() method takes the elements of an existing array and concatenates one or more specified values onto the end to create a new array:

```
array.concat(value1, value2, ...)
```

- *array:* The name of the array you want to work with.
- *value1, value2, ...:* The values you want to concatenate to *array*. This can also be another array.

Note that the original array remains unchanged. The following code demonstrates using concat() to concatenate two arrays into a third array, each element of which is printed to the page, as shown in Figure 7-1.

HTML:

```
<div id="output">
</div>
```

JavaScript:

```
var array1 = new Array("One", "Two", "Three");
var array2 = new Array("A", "B", "C");
var array3 = array1.concat(array2);
var str = "";
```

```
for (var counter = 0; counter < array3.length; counter++) {
    str += array3[counter] + "<br>";
}
document.getElementById("output").innerHTML = str;
```

```
One
Two
Three
A
B
C
```

FIGURE 7-1: Concatenating array1 and array2 produces array3 with the values shown here.

Creating a string from an array's elements: join()

The `join()` method enables you to take the existing values in an array and concatenate them together to form a string. Check out the syntax:

```
array.join(separator)
```

- *array*: The name of the array you want to work with.
- *separator*: An optional character or string to insert between each array element when forming the string. If you omit this argument, a comma is inserted between each element.

In the following code, three arrays are created and then `join()` is applied to each one using a space as a separator, then the null string (`""`), and then no separator. Figure 7-2 shows the resulting page output.

HTML:

```
<div id="output">
</div>
```

JavaScript:

```
var array1 = new Array("Make", "this", "a", "sentence.");
var array2 = new Array("antid", "isest", "ablis", "hment",
   "arian", "ism");
var array3 = new Array("John", "Paul", "George", "Ringo");
var string1 = array1.join(" ");
```

```
var string2 = array2.join("");
var string3 = array3.join();

document.getElementById('output').innerHTML = string1 + '<br>' +
  string2 + '<br>' + string3;
```

FIGURE 7-2: Joining the arrays with a space, null string (""), and default comma.

```
Make this a sentence.
antidisestablishmentarianism
John,Paul,George,Ringo
```

REMEMBER

The Array object's toString() method performs a similar function to the join() method. Using *array*.toString() takes the values in *array*, converts them all to strings, and then concatenates them into a single, comma-separated string. In other words, *array*.toString() is identical to *array*.join(","), or just *array*.join().

Removing an array's last element: pop()

The pop() method removes the last element from an array and returns the value of that element. Here's the syntax:

```
array.pop()
```

For example, consider the following statements:

```
var myArray = new Array("First", "Second", "Third");
var myString = myArray.pop();
```

The last element of myArray is "Third", so myArray.pop() removes that value from the array and stores it in the myString variable.

REMEMBER

After you run the pop() method, JavaScript reduces the value of the array's length property by one.

Adding elements to the end of an array: push()

The push() method is the opposite of pop(): It adds one or more elements to the end of an array. Here's the syntax to use:

```
array.push(value1, value2, ...)
```

» *array*: The name of the array you want to work with.

» *value1, value2, ...*: The values you want to add to the end of *array*. This can also be another array.

push() differs from the concat() method in that it doesn't return a new array. Instead, it changes the existing array by adding the new values to the end of the array. For example, consider the following statements:

```
var myArray = new Array("First", "Second", "Third");
var pushArray = new Array("Fourth", "Fifth", "Sixth");
for (var i = 0; i < pushArray.length; i++) {
    myArray.push(pushArray[i]);
}
```

After these statements, myArray contains six values: "First", "Second", "Third", "Fourth", "Fifth", and "Sixth". Why didn't I just add the entire pushArray in one fell swoop? That is, like so:

```
myArray.push(pushArray);
```

That's perfectly legal, but it would mean myArray would contain the following four elements: "First", "Second", "Third", and pushArray, which means you've created a kind of hybrid multidimensional array; which is probably not what you want in this situation.

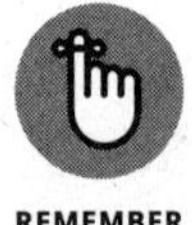

REMEMBER

After you run the push() method, JavaScript increases the value of the array's length property by the number of new elements added.

Reversing the order of an array's elements: reverse()

The reverse() method takes the existing elements in an array and reverses their order: The first moves to the last, the last moves to the first, and so on. The syntax takes just a second to show:

```
array.reverse()
```

The following code puts the reverse() method to work, and Figure 7-3 shows what happens.

```
var myArray = new Array("Show", "Place", "Win");
myArray.reverse();
```

```
var str = "";
for (var counter = 0; counter < myArray.length; counter++) {
    str += myArray[counter] + "<br>";
}
document.getElementById("output").innerHTML = str;
```

```
Win
Place
Show
```

FIGURE 7-3: Use the `reverse()` method to reverse the order of elements in an array.

Removing an array's first element: shift()

The `shift()` method removes the first element from an array and returns the value of that element:

```
array.shift()
```

For example, consider the following statements:

```
var myArray = new Array("First", "Second", "Third");
var myString = myArray.shift();
```

The first element of `myArray` is `"First"`, so `myArray.shift()` removes that value from the array and stores it in the `myString` variable.

REMEMBER

After you run the `shift()` method, JavaScript reduces the value of the array's `length` property by one.

Returning a subset of an array: slice()

The `slice()` method returns a new array that contains a subset of the elements in an existing array. Take a look at the syntax:

```
array.slice(start, end);
```

- *array:* The name of the array you want to work with.
- *start:* A number that specifies the index of the first element in *array* that you want to include in the subset. If this number is negative, the subset

starting point is counted from the end of *array* (for example, -1 is the last element of the array).

» *end:* An optional number that specifies the index of the element in *array* *before which* you want the subset to end. If you leave out this value, the subset includes all the elements in *array* from *start* to the last element. This value can be negative.

WARNING

If you use a negative number for the `start` value, the *end* value must also be negative, but it must be larger than `start`. For example, if you use `-4` for `start`, then *end* can only be -1, -2, or -3.

The following code defines an array and then tries out various values for the `slice()` arguments. The results are shown in Figure 7-4.

```
var myArray = new Array("A", "B", "C", "D", "E", "F");
var array1 = myArray.slice(0, 4);
var array2 = myArray.slice(3);
var array3 = myArray.slice(-3, -1);
var str = "array1: " + array1 + "<br>";
str += "array2: " + array2 + "<br>";
str += "array3: " + array3;
document.getElementById('output').innerHTML = str;
```

FIGURE 7-4: The `slice()` method creates a new array from a subset of another array.

```
array1: A,B,C,D
array2: D,E,F
array3: D,E
```

Ordering array elements: sort()

The `sort()` method is an easy way to handle a common programming problem: rearranging an array's elements to put them in alphabetical, numerical, or some other order. Here's the syntax:

```
array.sort(function)
```

» *array:* The name of the array you want to work with.

» *function:* An optional name of a function that specifies the sort order. If you leave out this argument, the elements of *array* are sorted alphabetically.

Using `sort()` without an argument gives you a straightforward alphabetical sort:

```
myArray.sort();
```

If you want to sort the array based on some other criterion, then you need to create a function to define the sort order. Your function must be set up as follows:

- » The function must accept two arguments. For the purposes of this list, I'll call these arguments `a` and `b`.
- » Using these arguments, the function must define an expression that returns a numeric value.
- » For those cases where you want `a` sorted before `b`, the function must return a negative value.
- » For those cases where you want `a` sorted after `b`, the function must return a positive value.
- » For those cases where you want `a` and `b` to be treated equally, the function must return zero.

The following code shows a function named `numericSort` that you can use if you want a numeric sort from lowest to highest. Figure 7-5 displays the original array and then the sorted array.

```
// This function sorts numbers from lowest to highest
function numericSort(a, b) {
    return (a - b);
}

var myArray = [3, 5, 1, 6, 2, 4];

// Write the array before sorting it
var str = "myArray (before sorting): " + myArray + "<br>";

// Sort the array
myArray.sort(numericSort);

// Write the array after sorting it
str+= "myArray (after sorting): " + myArray;

document.getElementById('output').innerHTML = str;
```

TIP

To get a numeric sort from highest to lowest, use the following `return` expression, instead:

```
return (b - a);
```

FIGURE 7-5: Using `sort()` and a function to sort items numerically from lowest to highest.

```
myArray (before sorting): 3,5,1,6,2,4
myArray (after sorting): 1,2,3,4,5,6
```

TIP

What if you want a reverse alphabetical sort? Here's a function that will do it:

```
function reverseAlphaSort(a, b) {
    if (a > b) {
        return -1
    }
    else if (a < b) {
        return 1
    }
    else {
        return 0
    }
}
```

Removing, replacing, and inserting elements: splice()

The `splice()` method is a complex function that comes in handy in all kinds of situations. First, here's the syntax:

```
array.splice(start, elementsToDelete, value1, value2, ...)
```

- *`array`*: The name of the array you want to work with.
- *`start`*: A number that specifies the index of the element where the splice takes place.
- *`elementsToDelete`*: An optional number that specifies how many elements to delete from *`array`* beginning at the *`start`* position. If you don't include this argument, elements are deleted from *`start`* to the end of the array.

- *value1, value2, ...*: Optional values to insert into *array* beginning at the *start* position.

With splice() at your side, you can perform one or more of the following tasks:

- **Deletion:** If *elementsToDelete* is greater than zero or unspecified and no insertion values are included, splice() deletes elements beginning at the index *start*. The deleted elements are returned in a separate array.
- **Replacement:** If *elementsToDelete* is greater than zero or unspecified and one or more insertion values are included, splice() first deletes elements beginning at the index *start*. It then inserts the specified values before the element with index *start*.
- **Insertion:** If *elementsToDelete* is 0, splice() inserts the specified values before the element with index *start*.

The following code demonstrates all three tasks, and the results are shown in Figure 7-6.

```
var array1 = new Array("A", "B", "C", "D", "E", "F");
var array2 = new Array("A", "B", "C", "D", "E", "F");
var array3 = new Array("A", "B", "C", "D", "E", "F");

// DELETION
// In array1, start at index 2 and delete to the end
// Return the deleted elements to the delete1 array
var delete1 = array1.splice(2);

// Write array1
var str = "array1: " + array1 + "<br>";

// Write delete1
str += "delete1: " + delete1 + "<br>";

// REPLACEMENT
// In array2, start at index 3 and delete 2 elements
// Insert 2 elements to replace them
// Return the deleted elements to the delete2 array
var delete2 = array2.splice(3, 2, "d", "e");

// Write array2
str += "array2: " + array2 + "<br>";
```

```
// Write delete2
str += "delete2: " + delete2 + "<br>";

// INSERTION
// In array3, start at index 1 and insert 3 elements
array3.splice(1, 0, "1", "2", "3")

// Write array3
str += "array3: " + array3;

document.getElementById('output').innerHTML = str;
```

FIGURE 7-6: The `splice()` method can delete, replace, and insert array elements.

```
array1: A,B
delete1: C,D,E,F
array2: A,B,C,d,e,F
delete2: D,E
array3: A,1,2,3,B,C,D,E,F
```

Inserting elements at the beginning of an array: unshift()

The `unshift()` method is the opposite of the `shift()` method: It inserts one or more values at the beginning of an array. When it's done, `unshift()` returns the new `length` of the array. Here's the syntax:

```
array.unshift(value1, value2, ...)
```

- *array*: The name of the array you want to work with
- *value1*, *value2*, ...: The values you want to add to the beginning of *array*

For example, consider the following statements:

```
var myArray = new Array("First", "Second", "Third");
var newLength = myArray.unshift("Fourth", "Fifth", "Sixth");
```

After these statements, `myArray` contains six values — `"Fourth"`, `"Fifth"`, and `"Sixth"`, `"First"`, `"Second"`, and `"Third"` — and the value of `newLength` is 6.

» **Working with dates and times**

» **Performing math calculations**

Chapter 8

Manipulating Strings, Dates, and Numbers

First learn computer science and all the theory. Next develop a programming style. Then forget all that and just hack.

— GEORGE CARRETTE

Although your JavaScript code will spend much of its time dealing with web page knickknacks such as HTML tags and CSS properties, it will also perform lots of behind-the-scenes chores that require manipulating strings, dealing with dates and times, and performing mathematical calculations. To help you through these tasks, in this chapter you explore three of JavaScript's built-in objects: the String object, the Date object, and the Math object. You investigate the most important properties of each object, master the most used methods, and see lots of useful examples along the way.

Manipulating Text with the String Object

I've used dozens of examples of strings so far in this book. These have included not only string literals (such as `"Web Coding and Development for Dummies"`), but also methods that return strings (such as the `prompt()` method). So it should be clear by now that strings play a major role in all JavaScript programming, and it will be a rare script that doesn't have to deal with strings in some fashion.

For this reason, it pays to become proficient at manipulating strings, which includes locating text within a string and extracting text from a string. You learn all of that and more in this section.

Any string you work with — whether it's a string literal or the result of a method or function that returns a string — is a `String` object. So, for example, the following two statements are equivalent:

```
var bookName = new String("Web Coding and Development for
   Dummies");
var bookName = "Web Coding and Development for Dummies";
```

This means that you have quite a bit of flexibility when applying the properties and methods of `String` objects. For example, the `String` object has a `length` property that I describe in the next section. The following are all legal JavaScript expressions that use this property:

```
bookName.length;
"Web Coding and Development for Dummies".length;
prompt("Enter the book name:").length;
myFunction().length;
```

The last example assumes that `myFunction()` returns a string value.

Determining the length of a string

The most basic property of a `String` object is its `length`, which tells you how many characters are in the string:

```
string.length
```

All characters within the string — including spaces and punctuation marks — are counted toward the length. The only exceptions are escape sequences (such as `\n`), which always count as one character. The following code grabs the length property value for various String object types.

```
function myFunction() {
    return "filename.htm";
}
```

```
var bookName = "Web Coding and Development for Dummies";

length1 = myFunction().length; // Returns 12
length2 = bookName.length; // Returns 38
length3 = "123\n5678".length; // Returns 8
```

What the `String` object lacks in properties it more than makes up for in methods. There are over two dozen, and they enable your code to perform many useful tasks, from converting between uppercase and lowercase letters, to finding text within a string, to extracting parts of a string.

Finding substrings

A *substring* is a portion of an existing string. For example, substrings of the string `"JavaScript"` would be `"Java"`, `"Script"`, `"vaSc"`, and `"v"`. When working with strings in your scripts, you'll often have to determine whether a given string contains a given substring. For example, if you're validating a user's email address, you should check that it contains an @ symbol.

Table 8-1 lists the two `String` object methods that find substrings within a larger string.

TABLE 8-1 **String Object Methods for Finding Substrings**

Method	What It Does
string.indexOf(*substring*, *start*)	Searches *string* for the first instance of *substring*
string.lastIndexOf(*substring*, *start*)	Searches *string* for the last instance of *substring*

You'll use both of these methods quite often in your scripts, so I take a closer look at each one.

When you want to find the first instance of a substring, or if all you want to know is whether a string contains a particular substring, use the `indexOf()` method; if you need to find the last instance of a substring, use the `lastIndexOf()` method:

```
string.indexOf(substring, start)
string.lastIndexOf(substring, start)
```

- *string*: The string in which you want to search.
- *substring*: The substring that you want to search for in *string*.

- *start:* An optional character position from which the search begins. If you omit this argument, JavaScript starts the search from the beginning of the string.

Here are some notes you should keep in mind when using `indexOf()` or `lastIndexOf()`:

- Each character in a string is given an index number, which is the same as the character's position within the string.
- Strings, like arrays, are *zero-based,* which means that the first character has index 0, the second character has index 1, and so on.
- Both methods are case-sensitive. For example, if you search for `B`, neither method will find any instances of `b`.
- If either method finds *substring,* they return the index position of the first character of *substring*.
- If either method doesn't find *substring*, they return -1.

The following code tries out these methods in a few different situations.

HTML:

```
<pre>
Web Coding and Development for Dummies
01234567890123456789012345678901234567
</pre>
<div id="output"></div>
```

JavaScript:

```
var bookName = "Web Coding and Development for Dummies";

var str = "\"C\" is at index " + bookName.indexOf("C") + "<br>";
str += "\"v\" is at index " + bookName.indexOf("v") + "<br>";
str += "The first space is at index " + bookName.indexOf(" ") +
   "<br>";
str += "The first \"D\" is at index " + bookName.indexOf("D") +
   "<br>";
str += "The last \"D\" is at index " + bookName.lastIndexOf("D")
   + "<br>";
str += "The first \"e\" after index 2 is at index " + bookName.
   indexOf("e", 2) + "<br>";
```

```
str += "The substring \"Develop\" begins at index " + bookName.
   indexOf("Develop");

document.getElementById("output").innerHTML = str;
```

As you can see in Figure 8-1, the numbers show you the index positions of each character in the script.

```
Web Coding and Development for Dummies
01234567890123456789012345678901234567

"C" is at index 4
"v" is at index 17
The first space is at index 3
The first "D" is at index 15
The last "D" is at index 31
The first "e" after index 2 is at index 16
The substring "Develop" begins at index 15
```

FIGURE 8-1: The `indexOf()` and `lastIndexOf()` methods search for substrings within a string.

On a more practical note, the following code presents a simple validation script that uses `indexOf()`.

```
var emailAddress = "";
do {
    emailAddress = prompt("Enter a valid email address:");
}
while (emailAddress.indexOf("@") === -1);
```

The script prompts the user for a valid email address, which is stored in the `emailAddress` variable. Any valid address will contain the @ symbol, so the `while()` portion of a `do...while()` loop checks to see if the entered string contains @:

```
while (emailAddress.indexOf("@") === -1);
```

If not (that is, if `emailAddress.indexOf("@")` returns -1), the loop continues and the user is prompted again.

Methods that extract substrings

Finding a substring is one thing, but you'll often have to extract a substring, as well. For example, if the user enters an email address, you might need to extract just the username (the part to the left of the @ sign) or the domain name (the part to the right of @). For these kinds of operations, JavaScript offers six methods, listed in Table 8-2.

TABLE 8-2 String Object Methods for Extracting Substrings

Method	What It Does
`string``.charAt(`*`index`*`)`	Returns the character in *`string`* that's at the index position specified by *`index`*
`string``.charCodeAt(`*`index`*`)`	Returns the code of the character in *`string`* that's at the index position specified by *`index`*
`string``.slice(`*`start`*`, `*`end`*`)`	Returns the substring in *`string`* that starts at the index position specified by *`start`* and ends immediately before the index position specified by *end*
`string``.split(`*`separator`*`, `*`limit`*`)`	Returns an array where each item is a substring in *`string`*, where those substrings are separated by the *`separator`* character
`string``.substr(`*`start`*`, `*`length`*`)`	Returns the substring in *`string`* that starts at the index position specified by *`start`* and is *`length`* characters long
`string``.substring(`*`start`*`, `*`end`*`)`	Returns the substring in *`string`* that starts at the index position specified by *`start`* and ends at the index position specified by *end*

The charAt() method

You use the `charAt()` method to return a single character that resides at a specified position within a string:

```
string.charAt(index)
```

- *`string`*: The string that contains the character
- *`index`*: The position within *`string`* of the character you want

Here are some notes about this method:

- To return the first character in *`string`*, use the following:

  ```
  string.charAt(0)
  ```

- To return the last character in *`string`*, use this:

  ```
  string.charAt(string.length - 1)
  ```

- If the *`index`* value is negative or if it's greater than or equal to *`string`*`.length`, JavaScript returns the empty string ("").

The following code presents an example.

HTML:

```
<div id="output"></div>
```

JavaScript:

```
// Set up an array of test strings
var stringArray = new Array(4);
stringArray[0] = "Not this one.";
stringArray[1] = "Not this one, either.";
stringArray[2] = "1. Step one.";
stringArray[3] = "Shouldn't get this far.";

var firstChar;

// Loop through the array
for (var i = 0; i < 4; i++) {

    // Get the first character of the string;
    firstChar = stringArray[i].charAt(0);

    // If it's a number, break because that's the one we want
    if (!isNaN(firstChar)) { break }
}
document.getElementById("output").innerHTML = "Here's the one:
  \"" + stringArray[i] + "\"";
```

The idea here is to examine a collection of strings and find the one that starts with a number. The collection is stored in the array named `stringArray`, and a `for()` loop is set up to run through each item in the array. The `charAt()` method is applied to each array item to return the first character, which is stored in the `firstChar` variable. In the `if()` test, the logical expression `!isNaN(firstChar)` returns `true` if the first character is a number, at which point the loop breaks and the correct string is displayed in the web page.

```
Web Coding and Development for Dummies
01234567890123456789012345678901234567

slice(0, 3) = Web
slice(4, 10) = Coding
slice(15) = Development for Dummies
slice(0, -12) = Web Coding and Development
```

FIGURE 8-2: Some examples of the `slice()` method in action.

The slice() method

Use the `slice()` method to carve out a piece of a string:

```
string.slice(start, end)
```

- *`string`:* The string you want to work with.
- *`start`:* The position within *`string`* of the first character you want to extract.
- *end:* An optional position within *`string`* immediately after the last character you want to extract. If you leave out this argument, JavaScript extracts the substring that runs from *`start`* to the end of the string. Also, this argument can be negative, in which case it specifies an offset from the end of the string.

To be clear, `slice()` extracts a substring that runs from the character at *`start`* up to, but not including, the character at *end*.

The following code runs through a few examples (see Figure 8-2).

HTML:

```
<pre>
Web Coding and Development for Dummies
01234567890123456789012345678901234567
</pre>
<div id="output"></div>
```

JavaScript:

```
var bookName = "Web Coding and Development for Dummies";

var str = "slice(0, 3) = " + bookName.slice(0, 3) + "<br>";
str += "slice(4, 10) = " + bookName.slice(4, 10) + "<br>";
str += "slice(15) = " + bookName.slice(15) + "<br>";
str += "slice(0, -12) = " + bookName.slice(0, -12);
document.getElementById("output").innerHTML = str;
```

The split() method

The `split()` method breaks up a string and stores the pieces inside an array:

```
string.split(separator, limit)
```

- *string:* The string you want to work with.
- *separator:* The character used to mark the positions at which *string* is split. For example, if *separator* is a comma, the splits will occur at each comma in *string*.
- *limit:* An optional value that sets the maximum number of items to store in the array. For example, if *limit* is 5, split() stores the first 5 pieces in the array and then ignores the rest of the string.

TIP

If you want each character in the string stored as an individual array item, use the empty string ("") as the *separator* value.

The split() method is useful for those times when you have a "well-structured" string. This means that the string contains a character that acts as a delimiter between each string piece that you want set up as an array item. For example, it's fairly common to have to deal with *comma-delimited* strings:

```
string1 = "Sunday,Monday,Tuesday,Wednesday,Thursday,Friday,
  Saturday";
```

As you can see, each day in the string is separated by a comma. This makes using the split() method a no-brainer:

```
var string1Array = string1.split(",");
```

When you run this statement, string1Array[0] will contain "Sunday", string1Array[1] will contain "Monday", and so on. Note, too, that JavaScript sets up the array for you automatically. You don't have to declare the array using new Array().

The following code tries out split() with a couple of example strings.

HTML:

```
<div id="output"></div>
```

JavaScript:

```
var string1 = "Sunday,Monday,Tuesday,Wednesday,Thursday,Friday,
  Saturday";
var string2 = "ABCDEF";
var str = "";
```

```
var string1Array = string1.split(",");
for (var i = 0; i < string1Array.length; i++) {
    str += "string1Array[" + i + "] = " + string1Array[i] +
   "<br>";
}

var string2Array = string2.split("", 4);
for (i = 0; i < string2Array.length; i++) {
    str += "string2Array[" + i + "] = " + string2Array[i] +
   "<br>";
}

document.getElementById("output").innerHTML = str;
```

After `string1` is split into `string1Array`, a `for()` loop runs through the array and writes the items to the web page. For `string2`, the empty string is used as the separator and a limit of 4 is placed on the size of the `string2Array`. Again, a `for()` writes the array values to the page. Figure 8-3 shows what happens.

```
string1Array[0] = Sunday
string1Array[1] = Monday
string1Array[2] = Tuesday
string1Array[3] = Wednesday
string1Array[4] = Thursday
string1Array[5] = Friday
string1Array[6] = Saturday
string2Array[0] = A
string2Array[1] = B
string2Array[2] = C
string2Array[3] = D
```

FIGURE 8-3: Some examples of the `split()` method.

The substr() method

If you want to extract a substring and you know how long you want that substring to be, then the `substr()` method is often the best approach:

```
string.substr(index, length)
```

- *`string`:* The string you want to work with.
- *`index`:* The position within *`string`* of the first character you want to extract.
- *`length`:* An optional value that specifies the length of the substring. If you omit this argument, JavaScript extracts all the way to the end of the string.

The following code runs `substr()` through some examples; the results appear in Figure 8-4.

HTML:

```
<pre>
Web Coding and Development for Dummies
01234567890123456789012345678901234567
</pre>
<div id="output"></div>
```

JavaScript:

```
var bookName = "Web Coding and Development for Dummies";

var str = "substr(0, 10) = " + bookName.substr(0, 10)+"<br>";
str += "substr(15, 11) = " + bookName.substr(15, 11) + "<br>";
str += "substr(27) = " + bookName.substr(27);

document.getElementById("output").innerHTML = str;
```

```
Web Coding and Development for Dummies
01234567890123456789012345678901234567

substr(0, 10) = Web Coding
substr(15, 11) = Development
substr(27) = for Dummies
```

FIGURE 8-4: Some examples of the `substr()` method.

Manipulating Strings, Dates, and Numbers

The substring() method

Use the `substring()` method to extract a substring from a string:

```
string.substring(start, end)
```

- *string:* The string you want to work with.
- *start:* The position within *string* of the first character you want to extract.
- *end:* An optional value that specifies the position within *string* immediately after the last character you want to extract. If you leave out this argument, JavaScript extracts the substring that runs from *start* to the end of the string.

The following code gives the `substring()` method a whirl, and the results are shown in Figure 8-5.

HTML:

```
<pre>
Web Coding and Development for Dummies
01234567890123456789012345678901234567
</pre>

<div id="output"></div>
```

JavaScript:

```
var bookName = "Web Coding and Development for Dummies";

var str = "substring(0, 10) = " + bookName.substring(0, 10) +
    "<br>";
str += "substring(11, 14) = " + bookName.substring(11, 14) +
    "<br>";
str += "substring(31) = " + bookName.substring(31);

document.getElementById("output").innerHTML = str;
```

```
Web Coding and Development for Dummies
01234567890123456789012345678901234567

substring(0, 10) = Web Coding
substring(11, 14) = and
substring(31) = Dummies
```

FIGURE 8-5: Some examples of the `substring()` method.

Understanding the differences between splice(), substr(), and substring()

The `splice()`, `substr()`, and `substring()` methods are very similar and are often confused by even experienced JavaScript programmers. Here are some notes to help you understand the differences between these three string extraction methods:

- The `splice()` and `substring()` methods perform the same task. The only difference is that `splice()` enables you to use a negative value for the *end* argument. This is handy if you want to leave out a certain number of characters from the end of the original string. For example, if you want to extract everything but the last three characters, you'd use this:

  ```
  string.splice(0, -3)
  ```

- Use either `splice()` or `substring()` when you're not sure how long the extracted string will be. This usually means that you'll use the `indexOf()` and `lastIndexOf()` methods to find particular characters that mark the starting and ending points of the substring you want. You then use those values as the *`start`* and *end* arguments of `splice()` or `substring()`. For example, suppose you have a string of the form `www.domain.com` and you want to extract just the `domain` part. Here's a short routine that will do it:

```
var hostName = "www.domain.com";
var firstDot = hostName.indexOf(".");
var lastDot = hostName.lastIndexOf(".");
var domainName = hostName.substring(firstDot + 1, lastDot);
```

- On the other hand, if you know in advance exactly how long the extracted string must be, use the `substr()` method.

Dealing with Dates and Times

Dates and times seem like the kind of things that ought to be straightforward programming propositions. After all, there are only 12 months in a year, 28 to 31 days in a month, seven days in a week, 24 hours in a day, 60 minutes in an hour, and 60 seconds in a minute. Surely something so set in stone couldn't get even the least bit weird, could it?

You'd be surprised. Dates and times *can* get strange, but they get much easier to deal with if you always keep three crucial points in mind:

- JavaScript time is measured in milliseconds, or thousandths of a second. More specifically, JavaScript measures time by counting the number of milliseconds that elapsed between January 1, 1970 and the date and time in question. So, for example, *you* might see the date January 1, 2001 and think, "Ah, yes, the start the new millennium." *JavaScript,* however, sees that date and thinks "978307200000."
- In the JavaScript world, time began on January 1, 1970, at midnight Greenwich Mean Time. Dates before that have *negative* values in milliseconds.
- Since your JavaScript programs run inside a user's browser, dates and times are almost always the user's *local* dates and times. That is, the dates and times your scripts will manipulate will *not* be those of the server on which your page resides. This means that you can never know what time the user is viewing your page.

Arguments used with the Date object

Before getting to the nitty-gritty of the `Date` object and its associated methods, I'll take a second to run through the various arguments that JavaScript requires for many date-related features. This will save me from repeating these arguments tediously later on. Table 8-3 has the details.

TABLE 8-3 Arguments Associated with the Date Object

Argument	What It Represents	Possible Values
date	A variable name	A `Date` object
yyyy	The year	Four-digit integers
yy	The year	Two-digit integers
month	The month	The full month name from `"January"` to `"December"`
mth	The month	Integers from 0 (January) to 11 (December)
dd	The day of the month	Integers from 1 to 31
hh	The hour of the day	Integers from 0 (midnight) to 23 (11:00 PM)
mm	The minute of the hour	Integers from 0 to 59
ss	The second of the minute	Integers from 0 to 59
ms	The milliseconds of the second	Integers from 0 to 999

Working with the Date object

Whenever you work with dates and times in JavaScript, you work with an instance of the `Date` object. More to the point, when you deal with a `Date` object in JavaScript, you deal with a specific moment in time, down to the millisecond. A `Date` object can never be a block of time, and it's not a kind of clock that ticks along while your script runs. Instead, the `Date` object is a temporal snapshot that you use to extract the specifics of the time it was taken: the year, month, date, hour, and so on.

Specifying the current date and time

The most common use of the `Date` object is to store the current date and time. You do that by invoking the `Date()` function, which is the constructor function for creating a new `Date` object. Here's the general format:

```
var dateToday = new Date();
```

Specifying any date and time

If you need to work with a specific date or time, you need to use the `Date()` function's arguments. There are five versions of the `Date()` function syntax (see the list of arguments near the beginning of this chapter):

```
var date = new Date("month dd, yyyy hh:mm:ss");
var date = new Date("month dd, yyyy");
var date = new Date(yyyy, mth, dd, hh, mm, ss);
var date = new Date(yyyy, mth, dd);
var date = new Date(ms);
```

The following statements give you an example for each syntax:

```
var myDate = new Date("August 23, 2018 3:02:01");
var myDate = new Date("August 23, 2018");
var myDate = new Date(2018, 8, 23, 3, 2, 1);
var myDate = new Date(2018, 8, 23);
var myDate = new Date(1408777321000);
```

Manipulating Strings, Dates, and Numbers

Extracting information about a date

When your script just coughs up whatever `Date` object value you stored in the variable, the results aren't particularly appealing. If you want to display dates in a more attractive format, or if you want to perform arithmetic operations on a date, then you need to dig a little deeper into the `Date` object to extract specific information such as the month, year, hour, and so on. You do that by using the `Date` object methods listed in Table 8-4.

One of the ways you can take advantage of these methods is to display the time or date to the user using any format you want. Here's an example:

HTML:

```
<div id="output"></div>
```

TABLE 8-4 **Date Object Methods That Extract Date Values**

Method Syntax	What It Returns
date.getFullYear()	The year as a four-digit number (1999, 2000, and so on)
date.getMonth()	The month of the year; from 0 (January) to 11 (December)
date.getDate()	The date in the month; from 1 to 31
date.getDay()	The day of the week; from 0 (Sunday) to 6 (Saturday)
date.getHours()	The hour of the day; from 0 (midnight) to 23 (11:00 PM)
date.getMinutes()	The minute of the hour; from 0 to 59
date.getSeconds()	The second of the minute; from 0 to 59
date.getMilliseconds()	The milliseconds of the second; from 0 to 999
date.getTime()	The milliseconds since January 1, 1970 GMT

JavaScript:

```
var timeNow = new Date();
var hoursNow = timeNow.getHours();
var minutesNow = timeNow.getMinutes();
var message = "It's ";
var hoursText;

if (minutesNow <= 30) {
    message += minutesNow + " minutes past ";
    hoursText = hoursNow;
} else {
    message += (60 - minutesNow) + " minutes before ";
    hoursText = hoursNow + 1;
}

if (hoursNow == 0 && minutesNow <= 30) {
    message += "midnight.";
} else if (hoursNow == 11 && minutesNow > 30) {
    message += "noon.";
} else if (hoursNow < 12) {
    message += hoursText + " in the morning.";
} else if (hoursNow == 12 && minutesNow <= 30) {
    message += "noon.";
} else if (hoursNow < 18) {
    message += parseInt(hoursText - 12) + " in the afternoon.";
```

```
} else if (hoursNow == 23 && minutesNow > 30) {
    message += "midnight.";
} else {
    message += parseInt(hoursText - 12) + " in the evening.";
}
document.getElementById("output").innerHTML = message;
```

This script begins by storing the user's local time in the `timeNow` variable. Then the current hour is extracted using `getHours()` and stored in the `hoursNow` variable, and the current minute is extracted using `getMinutes()` and stored in the `minutesNow` variable. A variable named `message` is initialized and will be used to store the message that's displayed in the web page. The variable `hoursText` will hold the non-military hour (for example, 4 instead of 16).

Then the value of `minutesNow` is checked to see if it's less than or equal to 30, because this determines the first part of the message, as well as the value of `hoursText`. Here are two examples of what the message will look like:

```
It's 20 minutes past 10 // minutesNow is less than or equal to
   30 (10:20)
It's 20 minutes to 11 // minutesNow is greater than 30 (10:40)
```

Then the script checks the value of `hoursNow`:

- » If it equals 0 and `minutesNow` is less than or equal to 30, then the string `midnight` is added to the message.
- » If it equals 11 and `minutesNow` is greater than 30, then the string noon is added to the message.
- » If it's less than 12, the value of `hoursText` and the string `in the morning` are added to the message.
- » If it equals 12 and `minutesNow` is less than or equal to 30, then the string noon is added to the message.
- » If it's less than 18 (6:00 PM), the result of `hoursText - 12` and the string `in the afternoon` are added.
- » If it equals 23 and `minutesNow` is greater than 30, then the string `midnight` is added to the message.
- » Otherwise, `hoursText - 12` and the string `in the evening` are added.

Finally, the result is written to the page, as shown in Figure 8-6.

FIGURE 8-6: The results of the script.

```
It's 5 minutes before 4 in the afternoon.
```

Converting getMonth() into a month name

If you want to use the month in a nicer format than the standard `Date` object display, there's one problem: The `getMonth()` method returns a number instead of the actual name of the month: 0 for January, 1 for February, and so on. If you prefer to use the name, you need some way to convert the number returned by `getMonth()`.

There are two ways you can go about this: an array or a function. The following code shows the array route:

HTML:

```
<div id="output"></div>
```

JavaScript:

```
var monthNames =
   ["January","February","March","April","May","June","July",
   "August","September","October","November","December"];
var dateNow = new Date();
var monthNow = dateNow.getMonth();
document.getElementById("output").innerHTML = "getMonth() is " +
   monthNow + "; the name is " + monthNames[monthNow];
```

The script declares a 12-item array named `monthNames` that stores the names of the months. The key here is that the array index matches the return value of `getMonth()`. For example, `getMonth()` returns 0 for January, so the array index 0 is assigned the string `"January"`. Then the current date is stored in `dateNow`, and the month is stored in `monthNow`. Finally, in the `getElementById()` statement, the month name is displayed by using the `monthNow` value as the array index: `monthNames[monthNow]`.

The following code shows how to do it using a function.

HTML:

```
<div id="output"></div>
```

JavaScript:

```
function monthName(monthValue) {
    switch (monthValue) {
        case 0 : return "January";
        case 1 : return "February";
        case 2 : return "March";
        case 3 : return "April";
        case 4 : return "May";
        case 5 : return "June";
        case 6 : return "July";
        case 7 : return "August";
        case 8 : return "September";
        case 9 : return "October";
        case 10 : return "November";
        case 11 : return "December";
    }
}

var dateNow = new Date();
var monthNow = dateNow.getMonth();
document.getElementById("output").innerHTML = "getMonth() is " +
  monthNow + "; the name is " + monthName(monthNow);
```

With this technique, you pass the `getMonth()` value as an argument to the `monthName()` function, which then uses a `switch()` statement to test the value and return the appropriate string.

So which method should you use? Neither one has any glaringly obvious benefits over the other. The array method is a bit quicker to set up and it probably executes a bit faster than the function, so it's probably the (slightly) better choice.

Converting getDay() into a day name

You face a similar problem with `getDay()` as you do with `getMonth()`: converting the returned number into a "friendly" name such as, in this case, Sunday for 0, Monday for 1, and so on. The solution, as you can imagine, is also similar. The following code shows how to return a day name from a `getDay()` value using an array.

HTML:

```
<div id="output"></div>
```

JavaScript:

```
var dayNames = ["Sunday","Monday","Tuesday",
"Wednesday","Thursday","Friday","Saturday"];

var dateNow = new Date();
var dayNow = dateNow.getDay();
document.getElementById("output").innerHTML = "getDay() is " +
  dayNow + "; the name is "+dayNames[dayNow];
```

This time, the script declares a seven-item array named `dayNames` and initializes each item to a name of a day (again, making sure each array index corresponds with the return value of `getDay()`).

A function to return the day name from a `getDay()` value would be almost identical to the one I listed earlier for month names, so I'll leave that as an exercise.

Setting the date

When you perform date arithmetic, you often have to change the value of an existing `Date` object. For example, an ecommerce script might have to calculate a date that is 90 days from the date that a sale occurs. It's usually easiest to create a `Date` object and then use an expression or literal value to change the year, month, or some other component of the date. You do that by using the `Date` object methods listed in Table 8-5.

TABLE 8-5 **Date Object Methods That Set Date Values**

Method Syntax	What It Sets
date.`setFullYear(`*yyyy*`)`	The year as a four-digit number (1999, 2000, and so on)
date.`setMonth(`*mth*`)`	The month of the year; from 0 (January) to 11 (December)
date.`setDate(`*dd*`)`	The date in the month; from 1 to 31
date.`setHours(`*hh*`)`	The hour of the day; from 0 (midnight) to 23 (11:00 PM)
date.`setMinutes(`*mm*`)`	The minute of the hour; from 0 to 59
date.`setSeconds(`*ss*`)`	The second of the minute; from 0 to 59
date.`setMilliseconds(`*ms*`)`	The milliseconds of the second; from 0 to 999
date.`setTime(`*ms*`)`	The milliseconds since January 1, 1970 GMT

To try out some of these methods, the following code presents a script that specifies a date (year, month, and day in the month) and then displays what day of the week it was, is, or will be.

HTML:

```
<div id="output"></div>
```

JavaScript:

```
var monthNames =
   ["January","February","March","April","May","June","July",
   "August","September","October","November","December"];

var dayNames = ["Sunday","Monday","Tuesday",
"Wednesday","Thursday","Friday","Saturday"];

// Set the year, month, and day
var userYear = 2018;
var userMonth = 11;
var userDay = 31;

// Make a date object then use the data to change the date
var userDate = new Date();
userDate.setFullYear(userYear);
userDate.setMonth(userMonth);
userDate.setDate(userDay);

// Convert the numbers into names
var dayName = dayNames[userDate.getDay()];
var monthName = monthNames[userDate.getMonth()];

// Display the message
document.getElementById("output").innerHTML = "The date you
  entered was: "
monthName + " " + userDay + ", " + userYear + "<br>The day of
  the week is: " + dayName;
```

The script opens by declaring and initializing the arrays for converting the values returned by `getMonth()` and `getDate()`. Then three variables are declared to store the year, month (as a number), and day.

The next four statements are the keys to this example. A new `Date` object is stored in the `userDate` variable. It begins with the current date, but, as you'll see,

Manipulating Strings, Dates, and Numbers

this doesn't matter. Then the script runs the `setFullYear()`, `setMonth()`, and `setDate()` methods.

At this point, the `userDate` variable contains a new date that corresponds to the supplied date. This means you can apply any of the "get" methods to that date. In particular, you can figure out which day of the week corresponds to the new date by running the `getDay()` method — `userDate.getDay()`. So the next two statements in the script use `getDay()` and `getMonth` to return the day and month values, and the arrays are used to convert them into names. Once that's done, the script displays the date and the day of the week that it corresponds to (see Figure 8-7).

```
The date you entered was: December 31, 2018
The day of the week is: Monday
```

FIGURE 8-7: The script displays the day of the week for a given year, month, and day.

REMEMBER

All the "set" methods also return values. Specifically, they return the number of milliseconds from January 1, 1970 GMT to whatever new date is the result of the method. Therefore, you can use the return value of a "set" method to create a new `Date` object:

```
newDate = new Date(userDate.SetFullYear(userYear));
```

Performing date calculations

Many of your date-related scripts will need to make arithmetic calculations. For example, you might need to figure out the number of days between two dates, or you might need to calculate the date that is six weeks from today. The methods you've seen so far and the way JavaScript represents dates internally serve to make most date calculations straightforward.

The simplest calculations are those that involve whole numbers of the basic JavaScript date and time units: years, months, days, hours, minutes, and seconds. For example, suppose you need to calculate a date that's five years from the current date. Here's a code snippet that will do it:

```
var myDate = new Date();
var myYear = myDate.getFullYear() + 5;
myDate.setFullYear(myYear);
```

You use getFullYear() to get the year, add 5 to it, and then use setFullYear() to change the date.

Determining a person's age

As a practical example, the following code presents a script that calculates a person's age.

HTML:

```
<div id="output"></div>
```

JavaScript:

```
var userAge;

// Set the birth date: year, month, and day
var userYear = 1990;
var userMonth = 7;
var userDay = 23;

// Make a Date object and change it
// to the user's birthday this year
var birthdayDate = new Date();
birthdayDate.setMonth(userMonth);
birthdayDate.setDate(userDay);

// Store the current date
var currentDate = new Date();
var currentYear = currentDate.getFullYear();

// Check to see if the birthday has yet to occur this year
if (currentDate < birthdayDate) {
    userAge = currentYear - userYear - 1;
} else {
    userAge = currentYear - userYear;
}

document.getElementById("output").innerHTML = "You are " +
  userAge + " years old.";
```

The script prompts the user for the year, month, and day of her birth date. Then it creates a new Date object and stores it in `birthdayDate`. The date is changed using `setMonth()` and `setDate()`, but *not* `setFullYear()`. This gives you the user's birthday for this year. Then the current date is stored in `currentDate` and the year is stored in `currentYear`.

Now the script compares `currentDate` and `birthdayDate`: If `currentDate` is less, it means the user's birthday hasn't happened, so her age is the difference between `currentYear` and `userYear` (the year she was born), minus one. Otherwise, her age is the difference between `currentYear` and `userYear`.

Performing complex date calculations

Other date calculations are more complex. For example, you might need to calculate the number of days between two dates. For this kind of calculation, you need to take advantage of the fact that JavaScript stores dates internally as millisecond values. They're stored, in other words, as numbers, and once you're dealing with numeric values, you can use numeric expressions to perform calculations on those values.

The key here is converting the basic date units — seconds, minutes, hours, days, and weeks — into milliseconds. Here's some code that will do it:

```
var ONESECOND = 1000;
var ONEMINUTE = ONESECOND * 60;
var ONEHOUR = ONEMINUTE * 60;
var ONEDAY = ONEHOUR * 24;
var ONEWEEK = ONEDAY * 7;
```

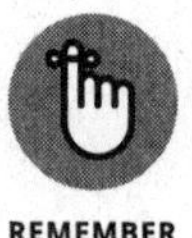
REMEMBER

In programming, whenever you have variables that are *constants* — that is, they have values that will never change throughout the script — it's traditional to write them entirely in uppercase letters to help differentiate them from regular variables.

Because one second equals 1,000 milliseconds, the `ONESECOND` variable is given the value 1000; because one minute equals 60 seconds, the `ONEMINUTE` variable is given the value `ONESECOND * 60`, or 60,000 milliseconds. The other values are derived similarly.

Calculating the days between two dates

A common date calculation involves figuring out the number of days between any two dates. The following code presents a function that performs this calculation.

```
function daysBetween(date1, date2) {

    // The number of milliseconds in one day
    var ONEDAY = 1000 * 60 * 60 * 24;

    // Convert both dates to milliseconds
    var date1Ms = date1.getTime();
    var date2Ms = date2.getTime();

    // Calculate the difference in milliseconds
    var differenceMs = Math.abs(date1Ms - date2Ms);

    // Convert to days and return
    return Math.round(differenceMs/ONEDAY);
}
```

This function accepts two `Date` object arguments — `date1` and `date2`. Note that it doesn't matter which date is earlier or later because this function calculates the absolute value of the difference between them. The constant `ONEDAY` stores the number of milliseconds in a day, and then the two dates are converted into milliseconds using the `getTime()` method. The results are stored in the variables `date1Ms` and `date2Ms`.

Next, the following statement calculates the absolute value, in milliseconds, of the difference between the two dates:

```
var differenceMs = Math.abs(date1Ms - date2Ms);
```

This difference is then converted into days by dividing it by the `ONEDAY` constant. `Math.round()` (which I discuss in the next section) ensures an integer result.

Working with Numbers: The Math Object

It's a rare JavaScript programmer who never has to deal with numbers. Most of us have to cobble together scripts that process order totals, generate sales taxes and shipping charges, calculate mortgage payments, and perform other number-crunching duties. To that end, it must be said that JavaScript's numeric tools aren't the greatest in the programming world, but there are plenty of features to keep most scripters happy. This section tells you about those features, with special emphasis on the `Math` object.

The first thing you need to know is that JavaScript likes to keep things simple, particularly when it comes to numbers. For example, JavaScript is limited to dealing with just two numeric data types: *integers* — numbers without a fractional or decimal part, such as 1, 759, and -50 — and *floating-point numbers* — values that have a fractional or decimal part, such as 2.14, 0.01, and -25.3333.

Converting between strings and numbers

When you're working with numeric expressions in JavaScript, it's important to make sure that all your operands are numeric values. For example, if you prompt the user for a value, you need to check the result to make sure it's not a letter or `undefined` (the default `prompt()` value). If you try to use the latter, for example, JavaScript will report that its value is `NaN` (not a number).

Similarly, if you have a value that you know is a string representation of a number, then you need some way of converting that string into its numerical equivalent.

For these situations, JavaScript offers several techniques that ensure your operands are numeric.

The parseInt() function

I begin with the `parseInt()` function, which you use to convert a string into an integer:

```
parseInt(string, base);
```

- *`string`*: The string value you want to convert.
- *base*: An optional base used by the number in *`string`*. If you omit this value, JavaScript uses base 10.

Note that if the *`string`* argument contains a string representation of a floating-point value, `parseInt()` returns only the integer portion. Also, if the string begins with a number followed by some text, `parseInt()` returns the number (or, at least, its integer portion). The following table shows you the `parseInt()` results for various *`string`* values.

string	parseInt(string)
"5"	5
"5.1"	5

string	parseInt(string)
"5.9"	5
"5 feet"	5
"take 5"	NaN
"five"	NaN

The parseFloat() function

The `parseFloat()` function is similar to `parseInt()`, but you use it to convert a string into a floating-point value:

```
parseFloat(string);
```

Note that if the *string* argument contains a string representation of a integer value, `parseInt()` displays just an integer. Also, like `parseInt()`, if the string begins with a number followed by some text, `parseInt()` returns the number. The following table shows you the `parseFloat()` results for some *string* values.

string	parseFloat(string)
"5"	5
"5.1"	5.1
"5.9"	5.9
"5.2 feet"	5.2
"take 5.0"	NaN
"five-point-one"	NaN

The + operator

For quick conversions from a string to a number, I most often use the + operator, which tells JavaScript to treat a string that contains a number as a true numeric value. For example, consider the following code:

```
var numOfShoes = '2';
var numOfSocks = 4;
var totalItems = +numOfShoes + numOfSocks;
```

By adding + in front of the numOfShoes variable, I force JavaScript to set that variable's value to the number 2, and the result of the addition will be 6.

The Math object's properties and methods

The Math object is a bit different than most of the other objects you come across in this book. That's because you never create an instance of the Math object that gets stored in a variable. Instead, the Math object is a built-in JavaScript object that you use as-is. The rest of this chapter explores some properties and methods associated with the Math object.

Properties of the Math object

The Math object's properties are all constants that are commonly used in mathematical operations. Table 8-6 lists all the available Math object properties.

TABLE 8-6 Some Properties of the Math Object

Property Syntax	What It Represents	Approximate Value
Math.E	Euler's constant	2.718281828459045
Math.LN2	The natural logarithm of 2	0.6931471805599453
Math.LN10	The natural logarithm of 10	2.302585092994046
Math.LOG2E	Base 2 logarithm of E	1.4426950408889633
Math.LOG10E	Base 10 logarithm of E	0.4342944819032518
Math.PI	The constant pi	3.141592653589793
Math.SQRT12	The square root of 1/2	0.7071067811865476
Math.SQRT2	The square root of 2	1.4142135623730951

Methods of the Math object

The Math object's methods enable you to perform mathematical operations such as square roots, powers, rounding, trigonometry, and more. Many of the Math object's methods are summarized in Table 8-7.

TABLE 8-7 Some Methods of the Math Object

Method Syntax	What It Returns
`Math.abs(`*number*`)`	The absolute value of *number* (that is, the number without any sign)
`Math.ceil(`*number*`)`	The smallest integer greater than or equal to *number*
`Math.cos(`*number*`)`	The cosine of *number*; returned values range from -1 to 1 radians
`Math.exp(`*number*`)`	E raised to the power of *number*
`Math.floor(`*number*`)`	The largest integer that is less than or equal to *number*
`Math.log(`*number*`)`	The natural logarithm (base E) of *number*
`Math.max(`*number1*, *number2*`)`	The larger of *number1* and *number2*
`Math.min(`*number1*, *number2*`)`	The smaller of *number1* and *number2*
`Math.pow(`*number1*, *number2*`)`	*number1* raised to the power of *number2*
`Math.random()`	A random number between 0 and 1
`Math.round(`*number*`)`	The integer closest to *number*
`Math.sin(`*number*`)`	The sine of *number*; returned values range from -1 to 1 radians
`Math.sqrt(`*number*`)`	The square root of *number* (which must be greater than or equal to 0)
`Math.tan(`*number*`)`	The tangent of *number*, in radians

IN THIS CHAPTER

» Learning JavaScript's error types

» Debugging errors using the Console

» Setting breakpoints

» Watching variable and expression values

» Learning JavaScript's most common errors and error messages

Chapter 9
Debugging Your Code

Sometimes it pays to stay in bed on Monday, rather than spending the rest of the week debugging Monday's code.

— CHRISTOPHER THOMPSON

It usually doesn't take too long to get short scripts and functions up and running. However, as your code grows larger and more complex, errors inevitably creep in. In fact, it has been proven mathematically that any code beyond a minimum level of complexity will contain at least one error, and probably quite a bit more than that.

Many of the bugs that creep into your code will be simple syntax problems you can fix easily, but others will be more subtle and harder to find. For the latter — whether the errors are incorrect values being returned by functions or problems with the overall logic of a script — you'll need to be able to look "inside" your code to scope out what's wrong. The good news is that JavaScript and modern web browsers offer a ton of top-notch debugging tools that can remove some of the burden of program problem-solving. In this chapter, you delve into these tools to explore how they can help you find and fix most programming errors. You also investigate a number of tips and techniques that can go a long way to helping you avoid coding errors in the first place.

Understanding JavaScript's Error Types

When a problem occurs, the first thing you need to determine is what kind of error you're dealing with. There are three basic types: syntax errors, runtime errors, and logic errors.

Syntax errors

Syntax errors arise from misspelled or missing keywords or incorrect punctuation. JavaScript almost always catches these errors when you load the page (which is why syntax errors are also known as *load-time errors*). That is, as JavaScript reads the script's statements, it checks each one for syntax errors. If it finds an error, it stops processing the script and displays an error message. Here's an example statement with a typical syntax error (can you spot it?) and Figure 9-1 shows how the error gets flagged in the Firefox Console window.

```
pageFooter = document.querySelector("footer');
```

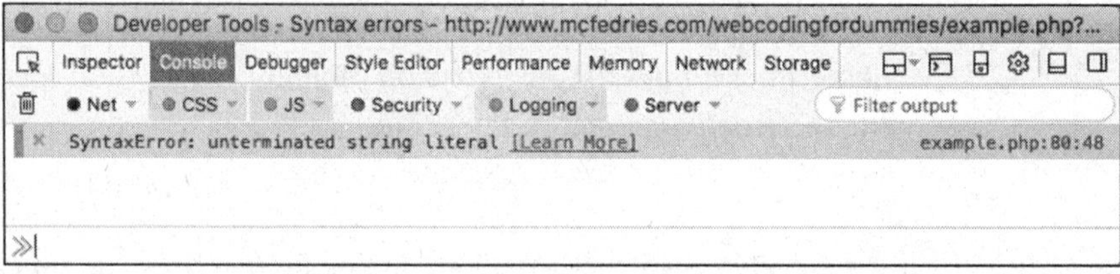

FIGURE 9-1: The Firefox Console window displaying data about a typical syntax error.

Runtime errors

Runtime errors occur during the execution of a script. They generally mean that JavaScript has stumbled upon a statement that it can't figure out. It might be caused by trying to use an uninitialized variable in an expression or by using a property or method with the wrong object.

If your script has statements that execute as the page loads, and there have been no syntax errors, JavaScript will attempt to run those statements. If it comes across a statement with a problem, it halts execution of the script and displays the error. If your script has one or more functions, JavaScript doesn't look for runtime errors in those functions until you call them.

Here's some code where I misspelled a variable name in the third line (`pagefooter` instead of `pageFooter`), and Figure 9-2 shows the Firefox Console window displaying the runtime error that results.

```
pageFooter = document.querySelector("footer");
currDate = new Date();
pagefooter.innerHTML = "Copyright " + currDate.getFullYear() +
   " Logophilia Limited.";
```

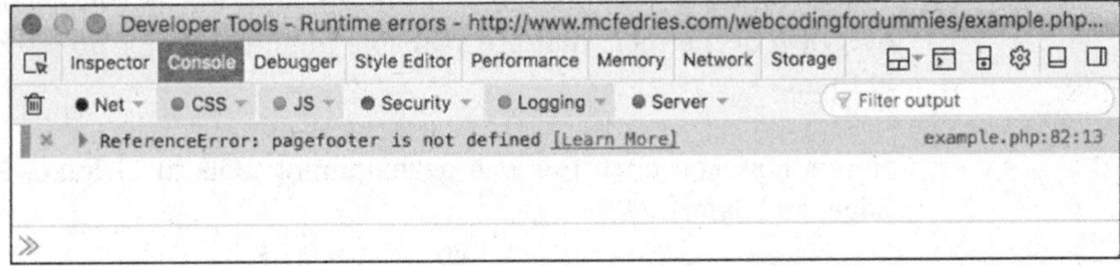

FIGURE 9-2: The Firefox Console displaying data about a typical runtime error.

Logic errors

If your code zigs instead of zags, the cause is usually a flaw in the logic of your script. It might be a loop that never ends or a `switch` test that doesn't switch to anything.

Logic errors are the toughest to pin down because you don't get any error messages to give you clues about what went wrong and where. What you usually need to do is set up *debugging code* that helps you monitor values and trace the execution of your program. I go through the most useful debugging techniques later in this chapter.

WHY ARE PROGRAM ERRORS CALLED BUGS?

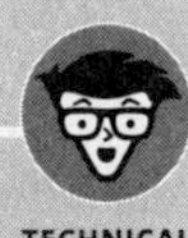

TECHNICAL STUFF

The computer scientist Edsger Dijkstra once quipped, "If debugging is the process of removing bugs, then programming must be the process of putting them in." But why on Earth do we call programming errors "bugs"? There's a popular and appealing tale that claims to explain how the word "bug" came about. Apparently, the early computer pioneer Grace Hopper was working on a machine called the Mark II in 1947. While investigating a glitch, she found a moth among the vacuum tubes, so from then on glitches were called *bugs*. Appealing, yes, but true? Not quite. In fact, engineers had already been referring to mechanical defects as "bugs" for at least 60 years before Ms. Hopper's discovery. As proof, the *Oxford English Dictionary* offers the following quotation from an 1889 edition of the Pall Mall Gazette:

> Mr. Edison, I was informed, had been up the two previous nights discovering 'a bug' in his phonograph — an expression for solving a difficulty, and implying that some imaginary insect has secreted itself inside and is causing all the trouble.

Getting to Know Your Debugging Tools

All the major web browsers come with a sophisticated set of debugging tools that can make your life as a web developer much easier and much saner. Most web developers debug their scripts using either Google Chrome or Mozilla Firefox, so I focus on those two browsers in this chapter. But in this section, I give you an overview of the tools that are available in all the major browsers and how to get at them.

Here's how you open the web development tools in Chrome, Firefox, Microsoft Edge, and Safari:

- **Chrome for Windows:** Click Customize and Control Google Chrome (the three vertical dots to the right of the address bar), then choose More Tools⇨Developer Tools. Shortcut: Ctrl+Shift+I.
- **Chrome for Mac:** Choose View⇨Developer⇨Developer Tools. Shortcut: Option+⌘+I.
- **Firefox for Windows:** Choose Menu⇨Developer⇨Toggle Tools. Shortcut: Ctrl+Shift+I.
- **Firefox for Mac:** Choose Tools⇨Web Developer⇨Toggle Tools. Shortcut: Option+⌘+I.
- **Microsoft Edge:** Choose Settings and More⇨Developer Tools. Shortcut: F12.
- **Safari:** Choose Develop⇨Show Web Inspector. Shortcut: Option+⌘+I. If you don't see the Develop menu, choose Safari⇨Preferences, click the Advanced tab, and then select the Show Develop Menu in Menu Bar checkbox.

These development tools vary in the features they offer, but each one offers the same set of basic tools, which are the tools you'll use most often. These basic web development tools include the following:

- **HTML viewer:** This tab (it's called Inspector in Firefox and Elements in the other browsers) shows the HTML tags used in the web page. When you hover the mouse pointer over a tag, the browser highlights the element in the displayed page and shows its width and height, as shown in Figure 9-3. When you click a tag, the browser shows the CSS styles applied with the tag, as well as the tag's box dimensions (again, see Figure 9-3).
- **Console:** This tab enables you to view error messages, log messages, test expressions, and execute statements. I cover the Console in more detail in the next section.

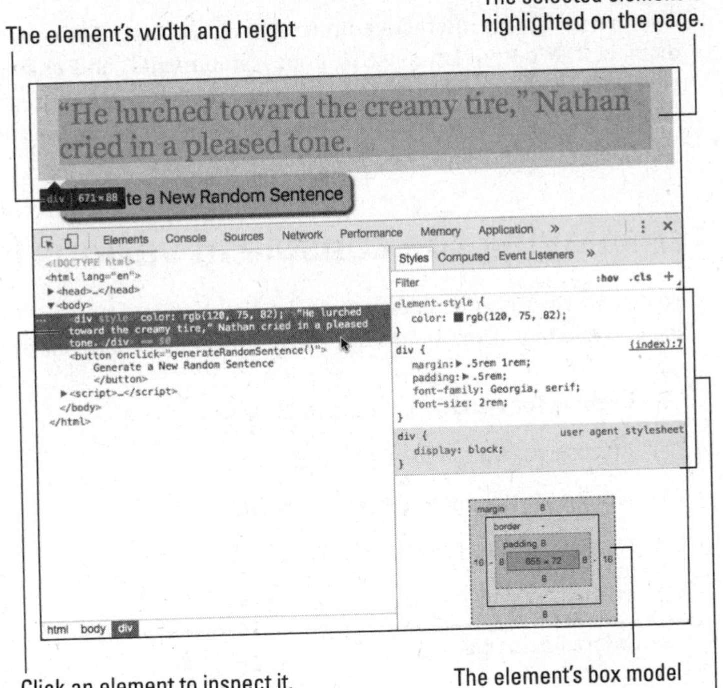

FIGURE 9-3: The HTML viewer, such as Chrome's Elements tab, enables you to inspect each element's styles and box dimensions.

- **Debugging tool:** This tab (it's called Debugger in Firefox and Safari, and Sources in Chrome and Edge) enables you to pause code execution, step through your code, watch the values of variables and properties, and much more. This is the most important JavaScript debugging tool, so I cover it in detail later in this chapter.
- **Network:** This tab tells you how long it takes to load each file referenced by your web page. If you find that your page is slow to load, this tab can help you find the bottleneck.

Debugging with the Console

If your web page is behaving strangely — for example, the page is blank or missing elements — you should first check your HTML code to make sure it's correct. (Common HTML errors are not finishing a tag with a greater than sign (>), not including a closing tag, and missing a closing quotation mark for an attribute value.) If your HTML checks out, then there's a good chance that your JavaScript code is wonky. How do you know? A trip to the Console window is your first step.

The Console is an interactive browser window that shows warnings and errors, displays the output of `console.log()` statements, and enables you to execute expressions and statements without having to run your entire script. The Console is one of the handiest web browser debugging tools, so you need to know your way around it.

Displaying the console in various browsers

To display the Console, open your web browser's development tools and then click the Console tab. You can also use the following keyboard shortcuts:

- **Chrome for Windows:** Press Ctrl+Shift+J.
- **Chrome for Mac:** Press Option+⌘+J.
- **Firefox for Windows:** Press Ctrl+Shift+K.
- **Firefox for Mac:** Press Option+⌘+K.
- **Microsoft Edge:** Press F12 and then Ctrl+2.
- **Safari:** Press Option+⌘+C.

Logging data to the Console

You can use the `console.log()` method of the special `Console` object to print text and expression values in the Console:

```
console.log(output)
```

- *output:* The expression you want to print in the Console, formatted as a string

The *output* expression can be a text string, a variable, an object property, a function result, or any combination of these, as long as the expression result is a string.

TIP

You can also use the handy `console.table()` method to output the values of arrays or objects in an easy-to-read tabular format:

```
console.table(output)
```

- *output:* The array or object (as a variable or as a literal) you want to view in the Console

For debugging purposes, you most often use the Console to keep an eye on the values of variables, object properties, and expressions. That is, when your code sets or changes the value of something, you insert a `console.log()` (or `console.table()`) statement that outputs the new value. When the script execution is complete, you can open the Console and then check out the logged value or values.

Executing code in the Console

One of the great features of the Console is that it's interactive, which means not only can you see messages generated by the browser or by your `console.log()` statements, but you can also type code directly into the Console. That is, you can use the Console to execute expressions and statements. There are many uses for this feature:

- You can try some experimental expressions or statements to see their effect on the script.
- When the script is paused, you can output the current value of a variable or property.
- When the script is paused, you can change the value of a variable or property. For example, if you see that a variable with a value of zero is about to be used as a divisor, you could change that variable to a nonzero value to avoid crashing the script.
- When the script is paused, you can run a function or method to see if it operates as expected under the current conditions.

Each browser's Console tab includes a text box (usually marked by a greater-than > prompt) that you can use to enter your expressions or statements.

TIP

You can execute multiple statements in the Console by separating each statement with a semicolon. For example, you can test a `for...` loop by entering a statement similar to the following:

```
for (var i=1; i < 10; i++){console.log(i**2); console.log(i**3);}
```

TIP

If you want to repeat an earlier code execution in the Console, or if you want to run some code that's very similar to code you ran earlier, you can recall statements and expressions that you used in the current browser session. Press the Up Arrow key to scroll back through your previously executed code; press the Down Arrow key to scroll forward through your code.

Debugging Your Code

Pausing Your Code

Pausing your code midstream lets you see certain elements such as the current values of variables and properties. It also lets you execute program code one statement at a time so you can monitor the flow of the script.

When you pause your code, JavaScript enters *break mode*, which means the browser displays its debugging tool and highlights the current statement (the one that JavaScript will execute next). Figure 9-4 shows a script in break mode in Chrome's debugger (the Sources tab).

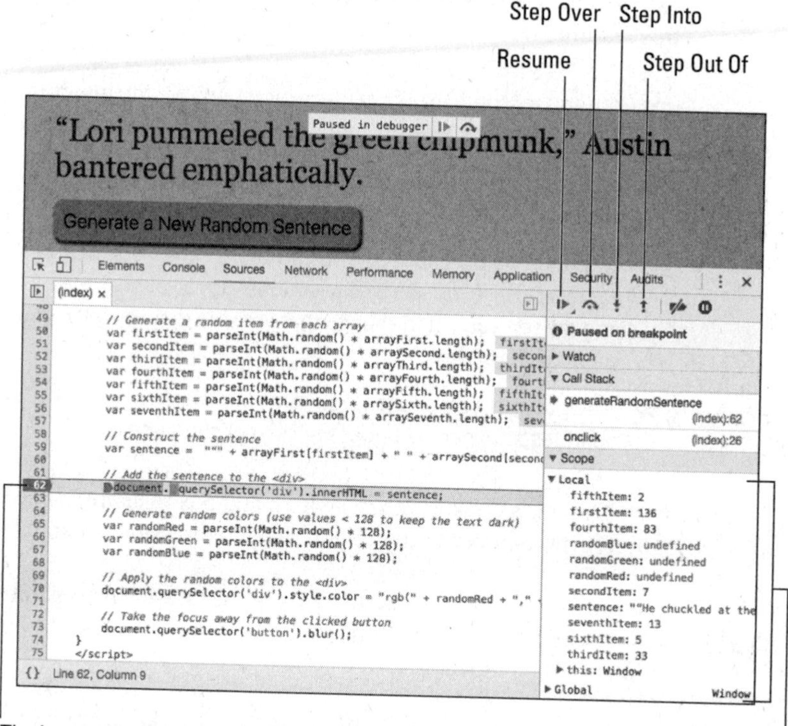

FIGURE 9-4: When you invoke break mode, the web browser displays its debugging tool and highlights the statement that it will execute next.

Entering break mode

JavaScript gives you two ways to enter break mode:

- By setting breakpoints
- By using a `debugger` statement

Setting a breakpoint

If you know approximately where an error or logic flaw is occurring, you can enter break mode at a specific statement in the script by setting up a *breakpoint*. Here are the steps to follow:

1. **Display your web browser's developer tools and switch to the debugging tool.**
2. **Open the file that contains the JavaScript code you want to debug.**

   How you do this depends on the browser: In Chrome and Firefox, press Ctrl+P (Windows) or ⌘+P (Mac).
3. **Locate the statement where you want to enter break mode.**

   JavaScript will run every line of code up to, but not including, this statement.
4. **Click the line number to the left of the statement to set the breakpoint (see Figure 9-5).**

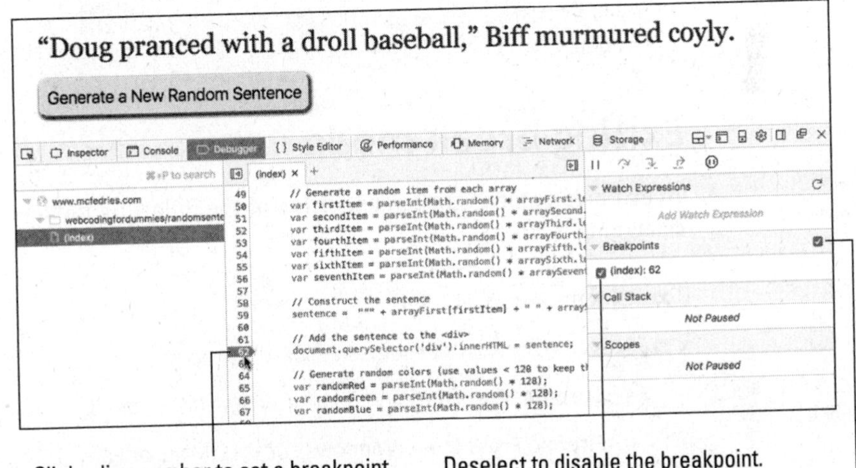

FIGURE 9-5: In the browser's debugging tool, click a line number to set a breakpoint on that statement.

To remove a breakpoint, most browsers give you three choices:

- To disable a breakpoint temporarily, deselect the breakpoint's checkbox in the Breakpoints list.
- To disable all your breakpoints temporarily, deselect the Breakpoints checkbox.
- To remove a breakpoint completely, click the statement's line number.

Debugging Your Code

Entering break mode using a debugger statement

When developing your web pages, you'll often test the robustness of a script by sending it various test values or by trying it out under different conditions. In many cases, you'll want to enter break mode to make sure things look okay. You could set breakpoints at specific statements, but you lose them if you close the file. For something a little more permanent, you can include a `debugger` statement in a script. JavaScript automatically enters break mode whenever it encounters a `debugger` statement.

Here's a bit of code that includes a `debugger` statement:

```
// Add the sentence to the <div>
document.querySelector('div').innerHTML = sentence;

// Generate random colors (use values < 128 to keep the text
   dark)
var randomRed = parseInt(Math.random() * 128);
var randomGreen = parseInt(Math.random() * 128);
var randomBlue = parseInt(Math.random() * 128);
debugger;
```

Exiting break mode

To exit break mode, you can use either of the following methods in the browser's debugging tool:

- Click the Resume button.
- Press the browser's Resume keyboard shortcut:
  - **Chrome:** Press Ctrl+\ (Windows), or ⌘+\ (Mac), or F8.
  - **Firefox:** Press Ctrl+\ (Windows), or ⌘+\ (Mac), or F8.

Stepping through Your Code

One of the most common (and most useful) debugging techniques is to step through the code one statement at a time. This lets you get a feel for the program flow to make sure that things such as loops and function calls are executing properly. You can use three techniques:

- Stepping into some code
- Stepping over some code
- Stepping out of some code

Stepping into some code

In break mode, stepping into some code means two things:

- You execute the code one line at a time.
- If the next statement to run is a function call, stepping into it takes you into the function and pauses at the function's first statement. You can then continue to step through the function until you execute the last statement, at which point the browser returns you to the statement after the function call.

To step into your code, set a breakpoint and then after your code is in break mode, do one of the following to step through a single statement:

- Click the Step Into button.
- Press the browser's Step Into keyboard shortcut:
  - **Chrome:** Press Ctrl+; or F11 (Windows) or ⌘+; or F11 (Mac).
  - **Firefox:** Press F11 (Windows) or ⌘+; or F11 (Mac).

Keep stepping through until the script ends or until you're ready to resume normal execution.

Stepping over some code

Some statements call other functions. If you're not interested in stepping through a called function, you can step over it. This means that JavaScript executes the function normally and then resumes break mode at the next statement *after* the function call.

To step over a function, first either step through your code until you come to the function call you want to step over, or set a breakpoint on the function call and refresh the web page. Once you're in break mode, you can step over the function using any of the following techniques:

- Click the Step Over button.

» Press the browser's Step Over keyboard shortcut:
  - **Chrome:** Press Ctrl+' or F10 (Windows) or ⌘+' or F10 (Mac).
  - **Firefox:** Press F10 (Windows) or ⌘+' or F10 (Mac).

Stepping out of some code

I'm always accidentally stepping into functions I'd rather step over. If the function is short, I just step through it until I'm back in the original code. If the function is long, however, I don't want to waste time stepping through every statement. Instead, I invoke the Step Out feature using any of these methods:

» Click the Step Out button.

» Press the browser's Step Out keyboard shortcut:
  - **Chrome:** Press Ctrl+Shift+; or Shift+F11 (Windows) or ⌘+Shift+; or Shift+F11 (Mac).
  - **Firefox:** Press Shift+F11 (Windows) or ⌘+Shift+; or Shift+F11 (Mac).

JavaScript executes the rest of the function and then reenters break mode at the first line after the function call.

Monitoring Script Values

Many runtime and logic errors are the result of (or, in some cases, can result in) variables or properties assuming unexpected values. If your script uses or changes these elements in several places, you'll need to enter break mode and monitor the values of these elements to see where things go awry. The browser developer tools offer three main ways to keep an eye on your script values:

» View the current value of a single variable.

» View the current values of all the variables in both the local and global scopes.

» View the value of a custom expression or object property.

Viewing a single variable value

If you just want to eyeball the current value of a variable, the developer tools in both Chrome and Firefox make this straightforward:

1. **Enter break mode in the code that contains the variable you want to check.**
2. **If the script hasn't yet set the value of the variable, step through the code until you're past the statement that supplies the variable with a value.**

   If you're interested in how the variable's value changes during the script, step through the script until you're past any statement that changes the value.
3. **Hover the mouse over the variable name.**

   The browser pops up a tooltip that displays the variable's current value. Figure 9-6 shows an example.

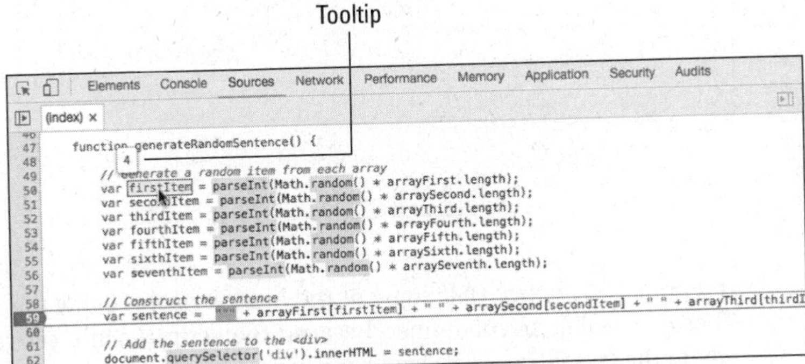

FIGURE 9-6: In break mode, hover the mouse pointer over a variable name to see the variable's current value.

Viewing all variable values

Most of the values you'll want to monitor will be variables, which come in two flavors (or *scopes*):

- **Local scope:** These are variables declared in the current function and are available only to that function.
- **Global scope:** These are variables declared outside of any function, which makes them available to any script or function on the page.

For a more detailed look at variable scope, see Book 3, Chapter 5.

When you're in break mode, the debugging tool in both Chrome and Firefox displays a pane on the right that includes a section that shows the current values of all your declared variables:

- **Chrome:** The section is named Scope and it includes two lists: Local (for local variables) and Global (for global variables). I pointed out Chrome's Scope section back in Figure 9-4.

» **Firefox:** The section is named Scopes and it includes two lists: one named after the current function that includes the function's local variables, and one named Window: Global that includes the script's global variables. Figure 9-7 shows an example.

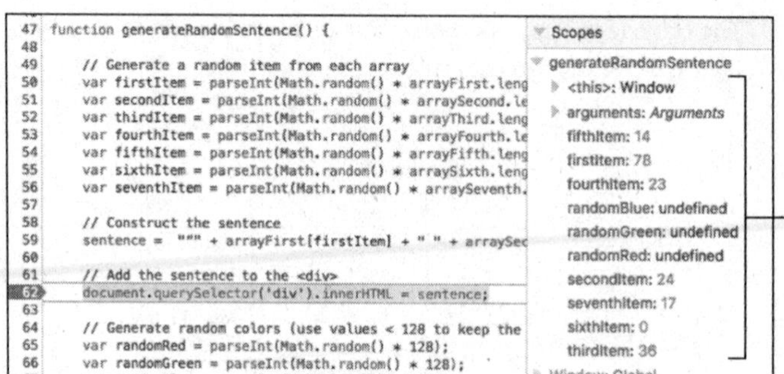

FIGURE 9-7: In break mode, Firefox's Scopes section shows the current values of the local and global variables.

In Figure 9-7, notice that some of the local variables show the value `undefined`. Those variables are undefined because the script hasn't yet reached the point where the variables are assigned a value.

Adding a watch expression

Besides monitoring variable values, JavaScript also lets you monitor the results of any expression or the current value of an object property. To do this, you need to set up a *watch expression* that defines what you want to monitor. These watch expressions appear in a special section of the browser's debugging tools. Here's how to add a watch expression in Chrome and Firefox:

» **Chrome:** In break mode, open the Watch section in the right pane, then click Add Expression (+). Type your expression in the text box that appears, and then press Enter or Return.

» **Firefox:** In break mode, open the Watch Expressions section in the right pane, then click Add Watch Expression (+). Type your expression in the text box that appears, and then press Enter or Return.

The browser adds the expression and then displays the current value of the expression to the right. Figure 9-8 shows an example in Firefox.

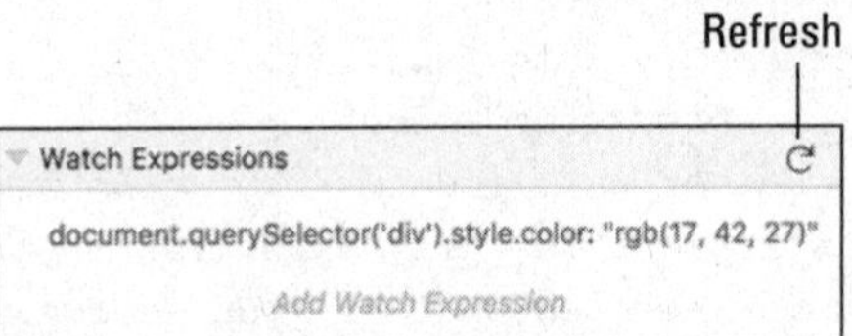

FIGURE 9-8: In Firefox, click Add Watch Expression to define a watch expression for your code.

You can use the following techniques to work with your watch expressions:

- **Edit a watch expression.** Double-click the expression, edit it, and then press Enter or Return.
- **Update the values of your watch expressions.** Click the Refresh button (located in the upper- right corner of Figure 9-8).
- **Delete a watch expression.** Hover the mouse over the watch expression you want to remove, then click the Delete icon that appears to the right of the expression.

More Debugging Strategies

Debugging your scripts can be a frustrating job, even during the best of times. Here are a few tips to keep in mind when tracking down programming problems:

- **Indent your code for readability.** JavaScript code is immeasurably more readable when you indent the code within each statement block. Readable code is that much easier to trace and decipher, so your debugging efforts have one less hurdle to negotiate. How far you indent is a matter of personal style, but two or four spaces is typical:

```
function myFunction() {
    Each statement in this function
    block is indented four spaces.
}
```

If you nest one block inside another, indent the nested block by another four spaces:

```
function myFunction() {
    Each statement in this function
    block is indented four spaces.
    for (var counter = 1; counter < 5; counter++) {
        Each statement in this nested for()
        block is indented another four spaces.
    }
}
```

- **Break down complex tasks.** Don't try to solve all your problems at once. If you have a large script or function that isn't working right, test it in small chunks to try to narrow down the problem.
- **Break up long statements.** One of the most complicated aspects of script debugging is making sense out of long statements (especially expressions). The Console window can help (you can use it to print parts of the statement), but it's usually best to keep your statements as short as possible. Once you get things working properly, you can often recombine statements for more efficient code.
- **Comment out problem statements.** If a particular statement is giving you problems, you can temporarily deactivate it by placing two slashes (\\) at the beginning of the line. This tells JavaScript to treat the line as a comment. If you have a number of statements you want to skip, place * at the beginning of the first statement and *\ at the end of the last statement.
- **Use comments to document your scripts.** Speaking of comments, it's a programming truism that you can never add enough explanatory comments to your code. The more comments you add, the easier your scripts will be to debug.

Top Ten Most Common JavaScript Errors

When you encounter a script problem, the first thing you should do is examine your code for the most common errors. To help you do that, here's a list of the ten most common errors made by both beginning and experienced programmers:

- **JavaScript keywords as variable names:** JavaScript has many reserved words and keywords that are built into the language, so it's common to accidentally use one of these words as a variable or function name.

Double-check your names to make sure you're not using any reserved words, or the names of any objects, properties, or methods.

- **Misspelled variables and other names:** Check your variable and function names to make sure you spell them consistently throughout the script. Also, check the spelling of the objects, properties, and methods you use.
- **Misused uppercase and lowercase letters:** JavaScript is a *case-sensitive* language, which means that it treats each letter differently depending on whether it's uppercase or lowercase. For example, consider the following two statements:

```
var firstName = "Millicent";
var message = "Welcome " + firstname;
```

  The first statement declares a variable named `firstName`, but the second statement uses `firstname`. This code would generate the error `firstname is not defined` (or something similar, depending on the browser) because JavaScript thinks that `firstname` is a different (and uninitialized) variable.

- **Mismatched quotation marks:** In any statement where you began a string literal with a quotation mark (" or '), always check to make sure that you included the corresponding closing quotation mark at the end of the string. Also, check to see if you used one or more instances of the same quotation mark within the string. If so, edit the string to use the proper escape sequence (\" or \'), instead:

```
// This is illegal
var myString1 = "There are no "bad" programs.";

// This is legal
var myString2 = "There are no \"bad\" programs.";
```

- **Mismatched parentheses:** Look for statements that contain a left parenthesis — (— and make sure there's a corresponding right parenthesis —). This also applies to square brackets — [and].

TIP

For complex expressions that include three or more sets of parentheses, a quick match-up check is to count the number of left parenthesis in the expression, and then count the number of right parentheses. If these numbers don't match, then you know you have a mismatch somewhere in the expression.

Debugging Your Code

- **Missed parentheses after function names:** Speaking of parentheses, if your script calls a function or method that doesn't take any arguments, check that you included the parentheses — `()` — after the name of the function or method:

```
function tryThis() {
    alert("Parentheses travel in pairs!");
}

// This won't work
tryThis;

// This will
tryThis();
```

- **Improper use of braces:** JavaScript uses braces to mark the start (`{`) and end (`}`) of statement blocks associated with functions, tests involving `if()` and `switch()`, and loops, including `for()`, `while()`, and `do...while()`. It's very easy to miss one or both braces in a block, and it's even easier to get the braces mixed up when nesting one test or loop inside another. Double-check your braces to make sure each block has both an opening and a closing brace.

TIP

One way to ensure that you don't miss any braces is to position them consistently throughout your script. For example, many people prefer to use the traditional style for brace positions:

```
keyword {
    statements
}
```

(Here, *`keyword`* means the statement — such as `function` or `if()` — that defines the block.) If you prefer this style, use it all through your script so that you know exactly where to look for each brace.

An easy way to ensure that you never forget a closing brace is to enter it immediately after entering the opening brace. That is, you type `{`, press Enter twice, and then type `}`.

Also, use indentation consistently for the statements within the block. This makes it much easier to see the braces, particularly when you have one block nested within another.

- **Using = or == instead of ===:** The identity operator (===) is one of the least intuitive JavaScript features, because the assignment operator (=) feels so much more natural. The equality operator (==) can cause problems because it often converts the data types before making the comparison. Therefore,

check all your comparison expressions to make sure you always use ===
instead of = or ==.

- **Conflicts between local and global variables:** A global variable is available throughout the entire page, even within functions. So, within a function, make sure that you don't declare and use a variable that has the same name as a global variable.
- **The use of an page element before it's loaded:** JavaScript runs through a page's HTML one line at a time and checks the syntax of each JavaScript statement as it comes to it. If your code refers to an element (such as a form field) that JavaScript hasn't come to yet, it will generate an error. Therefore, if your code deals with an element, always place the script after the element in the HTML file.

Top Ten Most Common JavaScript Error Messages

To help you decipher the error messages that JavaScript throws your way, here's a list of the ten most common errors and what they mean:

- `Syntax error`: This load-time error means that JavaScript has detected improper syntax in a statement. The error message almost always tells you the exact line and character where the error occurs (see Figure 9-1).
- `Expected (` or `Missing (`: These messages mean that you forgot to include a left parenthesis:

  ```
  function changeBackgroundColor newColor) {
  ```

  If you forget a right parenthesis, instead, you'll see `Expected )` or `Missing )`:

  ```
  function changeBackgroundColor (newColor{
  ```

- `Expected {` or `Missing { before function body`: These errors tell you that your code is missing the opening brace for a function:

  ```
  function changeBackgroundColor (newColor)
    statements
  }
  ```

Debugging Your Code

If you're missing the closing brace, instead, you'll see the errors `Expected }` or `Missing } after function body`.

- `Unexpected end of input` or `Missing } in compound statement`: These messages indicate that you forgot the closing brace in an `if()` block or other compound statement:

```
if (currentHour < 12) {
    console.log("Good morning!");
} else {
    console.log("Good day!");
```

  If you forget the opening brace, instead, you'll get a `Syntax error` message that points, confusingly, to the block's closing brace.

- `Missing ;` or `Missing ; after for-loop initializer|condition`: These errors mean that a `for()` loop definition is missing a semicolon (`;`), either because you forgot the semicolon or because you used some other character (such as a comma):

```
for (var counter = 1; counter < 5, counter++) {
```

- `Unexpected identifier` or `Missing ; before statement`: These errors tell you that the previous statement didn't end properly for some reason, or that you've begun a new statement with an invalid value. In JavaScript, statements are supposed to end with a semicolon (`;`), but this is optional. So if JavaScript thinks you haven't finished a statement properly, it assumes it's because a semicolon is missing. For example, this can happen if you forget to include the opening `/*` to begin a multiple-line comment:

```
Start the comment (oops!)
Close the comment */
```

- *`X`* `is not defined`: This message most often refers to a variable named *`X`* that has not been declared or initialized, and that you're trying to use in an expression. If that's the case, declare and initialize the variable. Another possible cause is a string literal that isn't enclosed in quotation marks. Finally, also check to see if you misspelled the variable name:

```
var grossProfit = 100000;
var profitSharing = grossPrifit * profitSharingPercent;
```

» *X* `is not an object` or *X* `has no properties`: These messages mean that your code refers to an object that doesn't exist, or to a property that doesn't belong to the specified object. Check to see if you misspelled the object or property or, for the second case, that you're using the wrong object:

```
document.alert("Nope!")
```

» `Unterminated string constant` or `Unterminated string literal`: Both of these messages mean that you began a string literal with a quotation mark, but forgot to include the closing quotation mark:

```
var greeting = "Welcome to my Web site!
```

» `A script on this page is causing [browser name] to run slowly. Do you want to abort the script?` or `Lengthy JavaScript still running. Continue?`: These errors tell you that your code has probably fallen into an infinite loop. You don't get any specific information about what's causing the problem, so you'll need to scour your code carefully for the possible cause.

4

Coding the Front End, Part 3: jQuery

Contents at a Glance

» Selecting page elements with jQuery

» Adding, populating, and removing page elements

» Reading and setting HTML attributes

» Manipulating CSS properties and classes

Chapter 1

Developing Pages Faster with jQuery

jQuery is an amazing tool that's made JavaScript accessible to developers and designers of all levels of experience.

— SCOTT KOSMAN

An old programming adage tells us that you shouldn't reinvent the wheel — unless you really want to learn how to make a wheel. That is, there's nothing wrong with coding something that someone else has already made, because the experience can help give you a deeper understanding of that aspect of programming. That said, most web development projects don't offer the luxury of limitless hacking time. Quite the opposite, in fact: You almost always have a large amount of code to write and what seems like an impossibly short amount of time in which to write it.

So if someone else has already built a programming wheel, it's a wise coder who takes advantage of it. In this chapter, you explore one of the most powerful and popular web development wheels: jQuery. You discover what jQuery is and how it can make your web development life much easier and far more efficient. You then take a satisfyingly deep dive into jQuery's powerful and accessible tools for selecting and manipulating page elements, reading and setting tag attributes, and messing with CSS classes and properties, all with very little code.

Getting Started with jQuery

In programming parlance, a *library* is a set of pre-fab code that you can add to your project and then use as part of your own code — for example, by calling the functions provided by the library. jQuery is a JavaScript library, which means it's a set of JavaScript functions that give you access to sophisticated and powerful techniques that would otherwise require hours of programming on your part. jQuery's slogan is "Write less, do more," and that's exactly what it delivers.

Surely having access to such power must cost a fortune, right? Nope. jQuery is and always will be completely free. It's an open-source project maintained by the jQuery Foundation, and it's by far the most popular JavaScript library out there. How popular is it? Some estimates show jQuery in use on over 70 percent of all websites. That's popular!

Okay, but jQuery must be massive, right? Nope. The current version is only about 260KB, and you can get a compressed version that weighs in at a mere 86KB!

Cool, but this thing sounds complicated. jQuery must be hard to learn, right? Again, nope. The syntax is designed to be straightforward and to not require a steep (or even a moderate) learning curve. And if you know how to wield CSS selectors (which I describe in Book 2, Chapter 2), then you're practically a jQuery master already since it takes advantage of those same selectors.

How to include jQuery in your web page

You might think that given jQuery's power and sophistication that it must require some time-consuming, multi-step procedure to install and configure. Fortunately, that's not the case. jQuery is nothing but a JavaScript (`.js`) file, so you can add it to your page by using a `<script>` tag with a reference to the jQuery external script file.

How do you get this file? You have two ways to go about it:

- **Download the file.** In this case, surf to `jquery.com/download` and click the link for the "compressed, production" version. The file you get will have a name like `jquery-3.`*`x`*`.`*`y`*`.min.js`, where *x* and *y* denote the current version.

Copy the downloaded file to your web app folder and then set up your `<script>` tag to reference the file:

```
<script src="jquery-3.x.y.min.js"></script>
```

» (Remember to replace *x* and *y* with the actual version numbers of your downloaded file.) If you put the file in a subfolder, be sure to include the folder path:

```
<script src="/js/jquery-3.x.y.min.js"></script>
```

» **Link to a remote version of the file.** Several *content delivery networks* (CDNs, for short) store the jQuery file and let you link to it. Since these CDNs have multiple servers based around the world, they can deliver the file really fast. Here's the tag to use for Google's CDN:

```
<script src="https://ajax.googleapis.com/ajax/libs/
   jquery/3.x.y/jquery.min.js"></script>
```

Here's the version to use from the jQuery site:

```
<script src="http://code.jquery.com/ajax/jquery-3.x.y.min.
   js"></script>
```

Again, in both cases, be sure to replace *x* and *y* with the actual version numbers of the latest version of jQuery (see `https://code.jquery.com`).

Which route should you take? The CDN path is better for most people because the remote servers almost always deliver the file faster than your own web server will.

WARNING

jQuery version 3 supports all the major web browsers, so it's safe to use in your code. Or, I should say, it's safe to use in your code if you don't need or want to support Internet Explorer 8 and earlier. Support for versions 6 through 8 of Internet Explorer was dropped way back in jQuery 2 (which was released in 2013). Internet Explorer 8 currently has between 0.25 and 1 percent of browser market share, so most web developers have moved on. If you need to support it, however, use jQuery 1.12.4:

```
<script src="https://ajax.googleapis.com/ajax/libs/
   jquery/1.12.4/jquery.min.js"></script>
```

or:

```
<script src="http://code.jquery.com/ajax/jquery-1.12.4.min.
  js"></script>
```

Understanding the $ function

When you first start learning about jQuery, one of the weirdest things to get your head around is that everything you do in jQuery begins with a dollar sign ($). Here are some examples:

```
$(document).ready();
$('header').html('<h1>Hello World!</h1>');
$('.warning').css('color','red');
$('#mainArticle').append('<section></section>');
```

That $ symbol you see at the beginning of each statement is actually the name of a function! Technically, it's an alias for the main jQuery function, which is named `jQuery`. That is, the previous four statements could also be written like so:

```
jQuery(document).ready();
jQuery('header').html('<h1>Hello World!</h1>');
jQuery('.warning').css('color','red');
jQuery('#mainArticle').append('<section></section>');
```

However, almost no one uses the `jQuery` function name, preferring the shorter and easier-to-type $ moniker.

Where to put jQuery code

The *Document Object Model* (DOM) looks at a page as a kind of tree where the `document` object is the "trunk" and the page elements — `body`, `header`, `main`, `div`, `p`, and so on — are branches or sub-branches. The HTML "family" elements that I discuss in Book 2, Chapter 2 — that is, the parent, child, ancestor, and descendant elements — define the structure of the DOM.

jQuery is, at heart, a DOM-manipulation library, meaning that all your jQuery code will read or change some aspect of the DOM. However, that means you can't use any jQuery code until your page is fully ready — that is, until the web browser has loaded the `document` object.

Therefore, when deciding where to put your jQuery code, you have two considerations:

- **Your jQuery code resides in a function that you don't need to run right away.** For example, you might have a function that will be called only in response to a button click or some other event. In this case, it's best to put your jQuery code in an external JavaScript file and then make sure your `<script>` tag comes after the jQuery `<script>` tag. Here's an example:

```
<script src="https://ajax.googleapis.com/ajax/libs/
   jquery/3.1.2/jquery.min.js"></script>
<script src="/js/my-code.js"></script>
```

- **Your jQuery code needs to be executed immediately after the `document` object is loaded.** For example, you might have some code that adds tags or text to the page. In this case, you have to put your jQuery code in a place where the browser will read it only after the `document` object is loaded. With vanilla JavaScript code, this means adding the `<script>` tag at the end of the body element (that is, just before the `</body>` tag). That works with jQuery code, too, but jQuery gives you a better way:

```
$(document).ready(function() {
     Your jQuery code goes here
});
```

  This code listens for the `document` object to fire the `ready` event, which only happens after the `document` object is fully loaded. (See Book 4, Chapter 2 to get your head around jQuery events.) The code then defines an anonymous (that is, unnamed) function that's called automatically in response to the `ready` event, which means that the function code executes only after the page is loaded. You can put this code anywhere in the page, as long as it's in a `<script>` tag that comes after the `<script>` that loads jQuery. Here's an example:

```
<script src="https://ajax.googleapis.com/ajax/libs/
   jquery/3.1.2/jquery.min.js"></script>
<script>
     $(document).ready(function() {
          Your jQuery code goes here
     });
</script>
```

Selecting Elements with jQuery

jQuery is a DOM-manipulation library, so that means almost all your jQuery-related statements begin with an expression that selects the DOM element or elements you want to mess with. Here's the basic syntax to use for this expression:

```
$(selector)
```

- *selector:* This is a CSS-style selector that specifies the page element or elements. The selector is sent to jQuery's $ function as an argument.

I talk about the basic CSS selectors in Book 2, Chapter 2, and one of the great advantages of jQuery is that it uses the same selectors; so if you know your CSS selectors, you're well on your way with jQuery.

Using the basic selectors

Most of your jQuery work will involve the five basic selectors that I outline in Book 2, Chapter 2:

- **The tag selector: `$('tagName')`:** Selects all the elements in the page that use the specified HTML tag name. This example selects all the <p> tags:

  ```
  $('p')
  ```

- **The class selector: `$('.class-name')`:** Selects all the elements in the page that use the specified `class` attribute. This example selects all the elements that use the `caption` class:

  ```
  $('.caption')
  ```

- **The id selector: `$('#id-name')`:** Selects the page element that uses the specified `id` attribute. This example selects the tag with the `subtitle` id:

  ```
  $('#subtitle')
  ```

- **The descendant selector: `$('ancestor descendant')`.** Selects all the elements in the page that are the descendants of a specified ancestor element. The following example selects all the <a> tags that are contained within an <aside> tag:

  ```
  $('aside a')
  ```

» **The child selector: `$('parent > child')`:** Selects all the elements in the page that are the direct children of a specified parent element. Here's an example that selects all the <a> tags that are direct children of an <aside> tag:

```
$('aside > a')
```

TIP

jQuery also lets you make multiple selections in a single expression by separating the selectors with commas. For example, the following selects all the page elements that use the `caption` class, plus the element that has the id `subtitle`:

```
$('.caption, #subtitle')
```

Working with jQuery sets

When you supply jQuery with a selector, what jQuery sends back is a set of page elements that match the selector. With that set in hand, jQuery offers straightforward techniques for doing a large number of tasks:

- » Adding and removing elements
- » Inserting HTML tags and text into an element
- » Reading and setting CSS properties
- » Adding and removing classes
- » Reading, setting, and removing HTML attributes

I cover all these tasks and more in this chapter, but first you also need to know about three other useful techniques that are available with jQuery sets: looping, chaining, and filtering.

TIP

To get the number of elements in a jQuery set, use the `length` property:

```
$(selector).length
```

Automatic looping through jQuery sets

In Book 3, Chapter 6, I talk about the `document` object's `querySelectorAll()` method, which returns an arraylike set of elements. Once you have that set, you work with its elements by looping through the set. Here's an example:

```
var captions = document.querySelectorAll('.caption');
for (var i = 0; i < captions.length; i++) {
    captions[i].style.fontSize = '.75rem';
}
```

This code selects all the elements with the class `caption`, then loops through the elements, setting the `font-size` property for each element to `.75rem`.

This basic technique — returning a set of elements and then looping through the set to manipulate the elements in some way — is such a common web development task that jQuery decided to automate it for you. That is, when you apply a jQuery method to a set, jQuery automatically applies that method to every element in the set. No need to loop! Here's the jQuery equivalent of the previous code:

```
$('.caption').css('font-size', '.75rem');
```

Chaining jQuery methods

jQuery lets you operate on a set by offering various methods that you can run on the set. For example, the `append` method lets you add an element to each item in the set, and the `css` method lets you apply a CSS property and value to each item in the set.

What if you want to run both methods on the same set? No problem:

```
$('.menuitem a').append('<span>(Click to expand)</span>');
$('.menuitem a').css('color', 'tomato');
```

However, you don't need to use multiple statements here because jQuery supports method *chaining*, where you place each method in a single statement, like so:

```
$('.menuitem a').append('<span>(Click to expand)</span>').
  css('color', 'tomato');
```

Filtering jQuery sets

jQuery offers a number of ways that you can *filter* the selected elements. You won't use filters all that often, but they can be very handy when you need them. Here's quick look at the more useful filters:

- **The even filter: `$('selector:even')`:** Returns every second element in the set, beginning with the first element (that is, it returns elements with the set indexes 0, 2, 4, and so on). Here's an example that selects the even-numbered <p> tags:

```
$('p:even')
```

- **The odd filter: `$('selector:odd')`:** Selects every second element in the set, beginning with the second element (that is, it returns elements with the set indexes 1, 3, 5, and so on). Here's an example that selects odd-numbered elements that use the `caption` class:

```
$('.caption:odd')
```

- **The `first` filter: `$('selector:first')`:** Selects the first element in the set. Here's an example that selects the first <p> tag from the set of <p> tags that are children of a <section> tag:

```
$('section > p:first')
```

- **The `last` filter: `$('selector:last')`:** Selects the last element in the set. Here's an example that selects the last <a> tag from the set of <a> tags that are descendants of elements that use the class `social`:

```
$('.social a:last')
```

- **The `not()` filter: `$('selector1:not(selector2)')`:** Selects all the elements that match *selector1*, except for those that also match *selector2*. Here's an example that selects all the <h2> tags, except for those <h2> tags that have the class `subtitle`:

```
$('h2:not(.subtitle)')
```

Manipulating Page Elements with jQuery

Now it's time to experience the true power and ease of the jQuery way of doing things. jQuery's mission is to make it easier and faster for you to work with page elements, and that includes inserting elements into the DOM, adding HTML tags and text to an element, and removing elements from the DOM. The next few sections provide the not-even-close-to-gritty details.

Adding an element

One of the most common web development chores is to add elements to a web page on-the-fly. For example, if your code asks the server for some data, you almost certainly won't want to just dump the raw data onto the page. Instead, it's better to use code to add HTML tags and then populate those tags with the server data.

When you add an element, you always specify the parent element to which it will be added, then you decide whether you want the new element added to the end or to the beginning of the parent.

To use jQuery to add an element to the end of a parent element's DOM hierarchy, use the `append()` method, and to add an element to the beginning of a parent element's DOM hierarchy, use the `prepend()` method:

```
$('parent').append(content);
$('parent').prepend(content);
```

- *parent:* A selector that specifies the parent element to which the child element will be added.
- *content:* The content you want to add. This can be any of the following:
  - A string containing the HTML tags for the type of the element you want to add. For example:

    ```
    $('article').append('<section></section>');
    ```

  - A string containing text. For example:

    ```
    $('.caption').prepend('Figure: ');
    ```

  - A jQuery selector. (Note that jQuery moves the returned element or elements into the parent container.) For example:

    ```
    $('header').append($('h1'));
    ```

  - An array containing any of the previous. For example:

    ```
    $('#section1').prepend([$('h2'),'<p></p>']);
    ```

  - A comma-separated list of any of the previous. For example:

    ```
    var domArray = ['<header></header>','<main></main>'];
    $('body').append(domArray, '<footer></footer>');
    ```

Here's a longer example that adds `header`, `nav`, `main`, and `footer` elements to the `<body>` tag, and then appends tags and/or text to each of these elements:

```
var domArray = ['<header></header>', '<nav></nav>',
   '<main></main>', '<footer></footer>'];
$('body').append(domArray);
$('header').append('<h1>This is the header.</h1>');
$('nav').append('Nav links will go here.');
$('main').append('<h2>This is the main part of the page.</h2>');
$('footer').append('This is the footer.');
```

Figure 1-1 shows the results.

This is the header.

Nav links will go here.

This is the main part of the page.

This is the footer.

FIGURE 1-1: A complete web page structure, created using nothing but jQuery.

Replacing an element's HTML

You can use jQuery's `append()` and `prepend()` methods to insert HTML tags into one or more elements, as I describe in the previous section. However, it's often the case that you want to completely overwrite an element's HTML tags and text, and you do that using jQuery's `html()` method:

```
$(selector).html(content);
```

- *`selector`:* The element (or elements) you want to work with
- *`content`:* The HTML tags and text that you want to use to replace the element's existing content

Here's an example:

```
$('body').append('<header></header>');
$('header').append('<h2>This is the header.</h2>');

// Replace the header content
$('header').html('<h1>No, <em>this</em> is the header!</h1>');
```

This code adds a `<header>` tag to the body element, then sets the header's tags and text using `append()`. In the final statement, the header's tags and text are replaced using the `html()` method. Figure 1-2 shows that, indeed, the replacement tags and text are what the user sees.

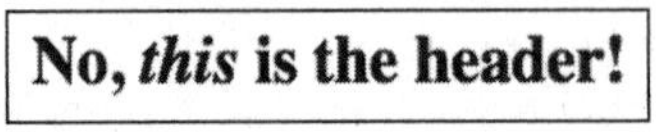

No, *this* is the header!

FIGURE 1-2: The `html()` method completely replaces any existing tags and text with new content.

Replacing an element's text

If you want to replace an element's text content — that is, just plain text without any HTML tags — use jQuery's `text()` method:

```
$(selector).text(content);
```

- *`selector`*: The element (or elements) you want to work with
- *`content`*: The text that you want to replace the element's existing content

If you include tags in *`content`*, jQuery doesn't ignore them. Instead, it encodes them by changing < to `<` and > to `>`. This is very handy if you want to display the angle brackets on your page, as shown in the following example:

HTML:

```
<h1>Placeholder Title</h1>
```

jQuery:

```
$('h1').text('Advanced Uses of the <div> Tag');
```

As you can see in Figure 1-3, jQuery encodes the angle brackets so they are displayed in the page.

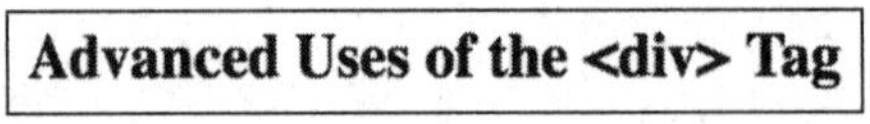

Advanced Uses of the <div> Tag

FIGURE 1-3: The `text()` method completely replaces any existing text with new content.

Removing an element

If you no longer require one or more elements on your page, you can use jQuery's `remove()` method to delete them from the DOM:

```
$(selector1).remove(selector2);
```

- » *selector1:* The element (or elements) you want to remove
- » *selector2:* The optional subset of *selector1* elements that you want to remove

For example, the following statement removes all the `h3` elements from the page:

```
$('h3').remove();
```

By contrast, the following statement only removes those `h3` elements that have the class `temp`:

```
$('h3').remove('.temp');
```

Modifying CSS with jQuery

Although you specify your CSS rules in a static stylesheet (`.css`) file, that doesn't mean the rules themselves have to be static. With jQuery on the job, you can modify an element's CSS in a number of ways. You can:

- » Read the current value of a CSS property.
- » Change the value of a CSS property.
- » Add or remove a class.
- » Toggle a class on or off.

Why would you want to make these changes to your CSS? You already know that a big part of a well-designed web page is a strong CSS component that uses typography, colors, and spacing to create a page that's easily readable, sensibly navigable, and pleasing to the eye. But all of that applies to the initial page the user sees. In the sorts of dynamic web apps that you learn how to build in this book, your page will change in response to data obtained from the server or the user clicking a button or pressing a key. This dynamic behavior needs to be matched with dynamic changes to the page, including changes to the CSS to highlight or reflect what's happening.

Working with CSS properties

jQuery makes it straightforward to read or modify CSS properties by offering a single method to use for most of your CSS chores: the `css()` method. The `.css()` method replaces the vanilla JavaScript `style` property that I discuss in Book 3, Chapter 6 and brings with it a significant advantage: You can use the CSS property names as they are. That's right: no need to convert, say, the `background-color` property to `backgroundColor`. Nice!

Reading a CSS property value

If you want to read the current value of a CSS property for an element, use the following syntax for the `css()` method:

```
$(selector).css(property);
```

- *`selector`:* The element you want to work with. If *`selector`* returns a set of elements, jQuery uses only the first element in the set.
- *`property`:* The name of the CSS property you want to read.

Here's an example:

CSS:

```
h1 {
    font-family: Verdana, serif;
    font-size: 2.5rem;
}
```

HTML:

```
<h1>Welcome to the css() Method!</h1>
<div></div>
```

jQuery:

```
// Get the font-size value for the h1 element
var h1FontSize = $('h1').css('font-size');

// Display the size in the div
$('div').html('The <code>h1</code> element is using a
   <code>font-size</code> value of ' + h1FontSize);
```

In the CSS, you see that the h1 element has a font-size value of 2.5rem, which, assuming the default font size is 16px, corresponds to 40px. The jQuery code uses the css() method to return the font-size value of the h1 element, which it then displays in the empty div element, as shown in Figure 1-4. Notice that the property value returned by the css() method includes the unit of measurement (px, in this case).

FIGURE 1-4: The css() method returns the current value of the specified property.

Welcome to the css() Method!

The h1 element is using a font-size value of 40px

Setting a CSS property value

To set a CSS property value on an element or a set of elements, use the following syntax for the css() method:

```
$(selector).css(property, value);
```

- *selector*: The element or elements you want to work with.
- *property*: The name of the CSS property you want to set.
- *value*: The value you want to assign to *property*. The value can either be a string that includes the unit of measurement, if any (such as '50vw') or a number. If you use a number for *value*, jQuery automatically adds the px measurement unit.

Here's an example:

HTML:

```
<h1>Welcome to the css() Method!</h1>
<div></div>
```

jQuery:

```
// Set the font-size value for the h1 element
$('h1').css('font-size', '3rem');

// Display the new size in the div
$('div').html('The <code>h1</code> element is now using a
   <code>font-size</code> value of ' + $('h1').css('font-size'));
```

The jQuery code uses the `css()` method to set the `font-size` value of the `h1` element to `3rem`, and then displays the new value in the empty `div` element, as shown in Figure 1-5.

Welcome to the css() Method!

The `h1` element is using a `font-size` value of 48px

FIGURE 1-5: The `css()` method can also set the value of a property.

Setting multiple CSS property values

TIP

You can save a bit of wear-and-tear on your typing fingers by setting multiple CSS properties on a single element or set. For example, the long-winded way to change the text color, background color, and font size on an element would be to use three separate statements:

```
$('#my-div').css('color', 'lemonchiffon');
$('#my-div').css('background-color', 'maroon');
$('#my-div').css('font-size', '2rem');
```

Instead, you can convert multiple property-value pairs into a single *object literal* that uses the following syntax:

```
{
    property1: value1,
    property2: value2,
    etc.
    propertyn: valuen
}
```

Here's an example:

```
{
    'color': 'lemonchiffon',
    'background-color': 'maroon',
    'font-size': '2rem'
}
```

You can use this object literal as the `css()` method argument in a single jQuery statement:

```
$('#my-div').css({
    'color': 'lemonchiffon',
    'background-color': 'maroon',
    'font-size': '2rem'
});
```

Working with width and height: A better method

Have a look at the following code and see if you can figure out what it does:

```
var currWidth = $('#my-div').css('width');
var newWidth = currWidth + 100;
$('#my-div').css('width', newWidth);
```

What the code is trying to do is take the current width of an element, add 100 pixels to that value, and then apply that new width value to the element. However, if you run this code, the width of the element doesn't budge one pixel. Why not? The problem is that `css('width')` doesn't return a number. Instead, it returns a string that combines the element width and the `px` measurement unit. So if the element is 250 pixels wide, the `css()` method returns the string `250px` for the element's width value. Adding `100` to this value gives the nonsense string `250px100`, so trying to set the element's `width` property with this value fails.

You could work around this problem by converting the string returned by `css('width')` to a floating-point value by using JavaScript's `parseFloat` function:

```
var currWidth = parseFloat($('#my-div').css('width'));
var newWidth = currWidth + 100;
$('#my-div').css('width', newWidth);
```

That works fine, but it's not only a pain to have remember to add the `parseFloat` function each time you need a number instead of a string, but it also makes your code a teensy bit harder to decipher.

Fortunately, the jQuery programmers, no doubt having bumped up against this same problem a few thousand times in their coding careers, implemented a solution: the `width()` method. `width()` returns just the numeric portion of the `width` property, in pixels. You can also use `width()` to set the element's width to a pixel value. Here's the syntax:

```
$(selector).width(value);
```

» *`selector`*: The element you want to work with

» *value:* An optional numeric value used to set the width of the element in pixels

Here's the example code rewritten with the `width()` method:

```
var currWidth = $('#my-div').width();
var newWidth = currWidth + 100;
$('#my-div').width(newWidth);
```

jQuery also offers a `height()` method that performs a similar function:

```
$(selector).height(value);
```

» *selector:* The element you want to work with

» *value:* An optional numeric value used to set the height of the element in pixels

Manipulating classes

Rather than fiddling with individual CSS properties, you might prefer to work with entire classes. jQuery offers several methods that enable you to do just that.

Adding a class

If you have a class rule defined in your CSS, you can apply that rule to an element by adding the `class` attribute to the element's tag and setting the value of the `class` attribute equal to the name of your class rule.

To add the `class` attribute using code, or, if the `class` attribute already exists, to add another class name to its value, jQuery offers the `addClass()` method:

```
$(selector).addClass(class);
```

» *selector:* The element you want to work with.

» *class:* A string with the name of the class you want to add to the element. To add two or more classes, separate each class name with a space.

Here's an example, and Figure 1-6 shows the result.

CSS:

```
.my-class {
    display: flex;
    justify-content: center;
    align-items: center;
    border: 6px dotted black;
    font-family: Verdana, serif;
    font-size: 2rem;
    background-color: lightgray;
}
```

HTML:

```
<div id="my-div">
Hello World!
</div>
```

jQuery:

```
$('#my-div').addClass('my-class');
```

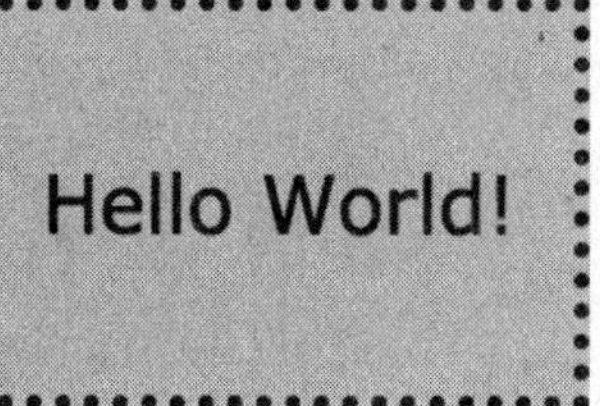

FIGURE 1-6: This code uses the `addClass()` method to add the class named `my-class` to the `<div>` tag.

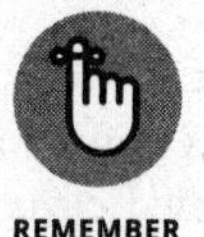

REMEMBER

If the `class` attribute doesn't exist in the element, the `addClass()` method inserts it into the tag. So in the previous example, after the code executes, the `<div>` tag now looks like this:

```
<div id="my-div" class="my-class">
```

Removing a class

To remove a class from an element's `class` attribute, jQuery offers the `removeClass()` method:

```
$(selector).removeClass(class);
```

» *selector:* The element you want to work with.

» *class:* A string specifying the name of the class you want to remove from the element. To remove two or more classes, separate each class name with a space.

Here's an example:

```
$('#my-div').removeClass('my-class');
```

Toggling a class

One very common web development scenario is switching a web page element between two different states. For example, you might want to change an element's styles depending on whether a check box is selected or deselected, or you might want to alternate between showing and hiding an element's text when the user clicks the element's heading.

One way to handle this would be to use `addClass()` to add a particular class when the element is in one state (for example, the user clicks the element's header for the first time) and then use `removeClass()` to remove that class when the element is in the other state (for example, the user clicks the element's header for a second time).

That would work, but it would mean that your code would somehow have to check the element's current state, something like this pseudo-code:

```
if (the element has the class applied) {
    remove the class
} else {
    add the class
}
```

That's a lot of extra work, but fortunately it isn't work you have to worry about because jQuery has got your back on this one. The `toggleClass()` method does the testing for you. That is, it checks the element for the specified class; if the class is there, jQuery removes it; if the class isn't there, jQuery adds it. Sweet! Here's the syntax:

```
$(selector).toggleClass(class);
```

» *selector:* The element you want to work with.

» *class:* A string specifying the name of the class you want to toggle for the element. To toggle two or more classes, separate each class name with a space.

Here's an example:

```
$('#my-div').toggleClass('my-class');
```

Tweaking HTML Attributes with jQuery

In the previous section, I went on and on about jQuery's `addClass()`, `removeClass()`, and `toggleClass()` methods, one of the characteristics of which is that these methods add, modify, or remove the element's `class` attribute. So you won't be even a tad surprised that jQuery offers a similar set of techniques for manipulating any HTML attribute. These techniques mostly center around the `attr()` method, and the next few sections tell all.

Reading an attribute value

If you want to read the current value of an attribute for an element, use the following syntax for the `attr()` method:

```
$(selector).attr(attribute);
```

» *selector:* The element you want to work with. If *selector* returns a set of elements, jQuery uses only the first element in the set.

» *attribute:* The name of the attribute you want to read.

Here's an example that reads the `href` attribute of the first `a` element that's a child of the `footer` element:

```
var firstLink = $('footer > a').attr('href');
```

Setting an attribute value

To set an attribute value on an element, use the following syntax for the `attr()` method:

```
$(selector).attr(attribute, value);
```

» *selector:* The element you want to work with

» *attribute:* The name of the attribute you want to set

» *value:* The string value you want to assign to *attribute*

Here's an example that sets the `title` attribute for the `footer` element's first `a` child element:

```
$('footer > a').attr('title', 'Like us on Facebook!');
```

Removing an attribute

To remove an attribute from an element, jQuery offers the `removeAttr()` method:

```
$(selector).removeAttr(attribute);
```

» *selector:* The element you want to work with.

» *attribute:* A string specifying the name of the attribute you want to remove from the element. To remove two or more attributes, separate each class name with a space.

Here's an example:

```
$('footer > a').removeAttr('title');
```

» Handling mouse clicks, key presses, and more

» Showing, hiding, and fading elements

» Moving elements around the page

» Animating CSS properties

Chapter 2
Livening Up Your Page with Events and Animation

Today's web animation can be built with the same tools we've always used to design and build the web: CSS and JavaScript. That is a huge amount of power and a vast arena in which to be creative.

— VAL HEAD

HTML, CSS, JavaScript, and jQuery are among the web development world's most powerful tools, enabling you to create pages and entire sites that look great and work flawlessly (well, as close to flawlessly as the complexity of the web allows). But there's a problem with most of the web pages built using these tools: The pages just kind of sit there. Once the page loads, its content and its structure are fixed, immutable. You can't click anything, you can't change anything, nothing moves or jiggles, spins or flips, fades in or fades out. Sure, the page doesn't distract, but neither does it delight, and that's a no-no in the modern web. Fortunately, you've come to the right place because this chapter shows you how to liven up even the most moribund page. Here you delve into two techniques for injecting some dynamism into dead pages: events and animation. These powerful tools not only give your page a dose of adrenaline, but they offer you endless possibilities for exploring and expressing your creativity.

Building Reactive Pages with Events

When you buy a car, no matter how much you paid for it or how technologically advanced it is, the car just sits there unless you do something. (If you're reading this in a future where all the cars are autonomous, my apologies.) That might be fine if it's a good-looking car, but it's much more likely you'll want the car to do something, anything. Here's a short list of actions you can take to achieve that goal:

- Start the car.
- Put the transmission into gear.
- Press the accelerator.
- Turn on the radio.

The common denominator for all these actions is that they set up a situation to which the car must respond in some way: turning on, engaging the gears, moving, playing sounds. Looked at it from this angle, the car is a machine that responds to external stimuli, or, in a word, to events.

Somewhat surprisingly, a web page is also a machine that responds to external stimuli. I'll describe what I mean.

What's an event?

In web development, an *event* is an action that occurs when a user interacts with a web page. Here are some examples:

- Loading the page
- Clicking a button
- Pressing a key
- Scrolling the page

How can your web page possibly know when any of these actions occur? The secret is that JavaScript was built with events in mind. As the computer science professors would say, JavaScript is an *event-driven* language.

So why don't web pages respond to events automatically? Why do they just sit there? Because web pages are *static* by default, meaning that they ignore the events that are firing all around them. Your job as a web developer is to change that behavior by making your web pages "listen" for particular events to occur. You do that by setting up special chunks of code called *event handlers* that say, in effect, "Be a dear and watch out for event X to occur, will you? When it does, be so kind as to execute the code that I've placed here for you. Thanks so much." An event handler consists of two parts:

- **Event listener:** An instruction to the web browser to watch out for ("listen" for) a particular event occurring on a particular element
- **Callback function:** The code that the web browser executes when it detects that the event has occurred

I said earlier that events are baked into JavaScript, but in this book I'm not going to talk about vanilla JavaScript event handling. That's because jQuery offers straightforward event-handling methods that are easier to use and more flexible that those offered by pure JavaScript, so it makes sense to learn about events the jQuery way.

Understanding the event types

There are dozens of possible events your web page can respond to, but lucky for you only a small subset of these events is needed in most day-to-day web development. I break these down into the following five categories:

- **Document:** Events that fire in relation to the loading of the `document` object. The only event you need to worry about here is `ready`, which fires when the `document` object has completed loading.
- **Mouse:** Events that fire when the user does something with the mouse (or a similar device, such as a trackpad or touchscreen). The most important events in this category are `click` (the user clicks the mouse), `dblclick` (the user double-clicks the mouse), and `mouseover` (the user moves the mouse pointer over an element).
- **Keyboard:** Events that fire when the user interacts with the keyboard. The main event in this category is `keypress`, which is fired when the user presses a key.
- **Form:** Events associated with web page forms. The important ones are `focus` (an element gains the focus, for example, when the user tabs to a form control), `blur` (an element loses the focus), `change` (the user changes the value of a form control), and `submit` (the user submits the form). See Book 6, Chapters 2 and 3 to learn about forms and form events.

» **Browser window:** Events that fire when the user interacts with the browser window. The two main events here are `scroll`, which fires when the user scrolls the window vertically or horizontally, and `resize`, which fires when the user changes the window width or height.

Setting up an event handler

You configure your code to listen for and react to an event by setting up an *event handler* using jQuery's `on()` method. Here's the syntax:

```
$(selector).on(event, function() {
    This code runs when the event fires
});
```

» *`selector`:* A jQuery selector that specifies the web page element or set to be monitored for the event. The event is said to be *bound* to the element or set.

» *event:* A string specifying the name of the event you want the browser to listen for. For the main events I mention in the previous section, use one of the following, enclosed in quotation marks: `ready`, `click`, `dblclick`, `mouseover`, `keypress`, `focus`, `blur`, `change`, `submit`, `scroll`, or `resize`.

» `function()`: The callback function that jQuery executes when the event occurs.

Here's an example:

HTML:

```
<div id="my-div"></div>
<button id="my-button">Click to add some text, above</button>
```

jQuery:

```
$('#my-button').on('click', function() {
    $('#my-div').html('<h1>Hello Click World!</h1>');
});
```

The HTML sets up an empty `div` element and a `button` element. The jQuery code attaches a `click` event listener to the button, and the callback function adds the HTML string `<h1>Hello Click World!</h1>` to the `div`. Figure 2-1 shows the resulting page after the button has been clicked.

FIGURE 2-1: The `click` event callback function adds some HTML and text to the `div` element.

Hello Click World!

Click to add some text, above

Using jQuery's shortcut event handlers

jQuery also offers some shortcut methods for setting up event handlers. Here's the syntax:

```
$(selector).event(function() {
    This code runs when the event fires
});
```

- `selector`: A jQuery selector that specifies the web page element to be monitored for the event.
- *event:* The name of event you want to handle. This defines a jQuery method as the event listener.
- `function()`: The callback function that jQuery executes when the event occurs.

For example, the `ready` event fires when the `document` object has finished loading, so here's some code that handles that event:

```
$(document).ready(function() {
    $('body').prepend('<h1>Hello Event World!</h1>');
});
```

As another example, here's a rewrite of the earlier code I used to demonstrate the `on()` method:

HTML:

```
<div id="my-div"></div>
<button id="my-button">Click to add some text, above</button>
```

jQuery:

```
$('#my-button').click(function() {
    $('#my-div').html('<h1>Hello Click World!</h1>');
});
```

As a third example, the following code uses the `dblclick()` method to swap a `div` element's text and background colors when the `div` is double-clicked:

CSS:

```
div {
    color: lemonchiffon;
    background-color: darkgreen;
}
```

HTML:

```
<div id="my-div">
   Double-click to switch the text and background colors.
</div>
```

jQuery:

```
$('#my-div').dblclick(function() {
    if($('#my-div').css('color') === 'rgb(255, 250, 205)') {
        $('#my-div').css('color', 'darkgreen');
        $('#my-div').css('background-color', 'lemonchiffon');
    } else {
        $('#my-div').css('color', 'lemonchiffon');
        $('#my-div').css('background-color', 'darkgreen');
    }
});
```

In the `dblclick` callback function, an `if()` statement checks to see if the current `color` value of the `div` element equals `rgb(255, 250, 205)`, which corresponds to the `lemonchiffon` color keyword. If so, the text and background colors are swapped.

TIP

When the user clicks a button or other web page element, the browser sets the focus on that element, which almost always means that, post-click, the element ends up with an unsightly "Look ma, I've got the focus" border around it. To remove this border, trigger the `blur` event by running the `blur()` method on the clicked element:

```
$('#my-button').on('click', function() {
    $('#my-div').html('<h1>Hello Click World!</h1>');
    $('#my-button').blur();
});
```

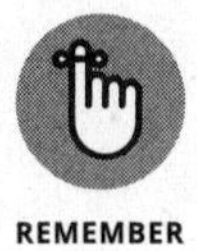

REMEMBER

For many events, you can use your code to trigger that event by running the corresponding jQuery shortcut event method without any arguments.

Getting data about the event

When an event fires, jQuery creates an `Event` object, the properties of which contain info about the event, including the following:

- `target`: The web page element to which the event occurred. For example, if you set up a `click` handler for a `div` element, that `div` is the target of the click.
- `which`: A numeric code that specifies the key that was pressed during a `keypress` event.
- `pageX`: The distance (in pixels) that the mouse pointer was from the left edge of the browser's content area when the event fired.
- `pageY`: The distance (in pixels) that the mouse pointer was from the top edge of the browser's content area when the event fired.
- `metaKey`: A Boolean value that equals `true` if the user had the Windows key (⊞) or the Mac Command key (⌘) held down when the event fired.
- `shiftKey`: A Boolean value that equals `true` if the user had the Shift key held down when the event fired.

To access these properties, you insert a name for the `Event` object as an argument in your event handler's callback function:

```
$(selector).on(event, function(e) {
    This code runs when the event fires
});
```

- `e`: A name for the `Event` object that jQuery generates when the event fires. You can use whatever name you want, but most coders use `e` (although `evt` and `event` are also common).

For example, when handling the `keypress` event, you need access to the `which` property to find out the code for the key the user pressed. Here's an example page that can help you determine which code value to look for:

HTML:

```
<div>
    Type a key:
</div>
```

```
<input id="key-input" type="text">
<div>
    Here's the code of the key you pressed:
</div>
<div id="key-output">
</div>
```

jQuery:

```
$('#key-input').keypress(function(e) {
    $('#key-output').text(e.which);
});
```

The HTML sets up an `<input>` tag to accept a keystroke, and a `<div>` tag with `id="key-output"` to use for the output. The jQuery code adds a `keypress` event listener to the `input` element, and when the event fires, the callback function writes `e.which` to the output `div`. Figure 2-2 shows the page in action.

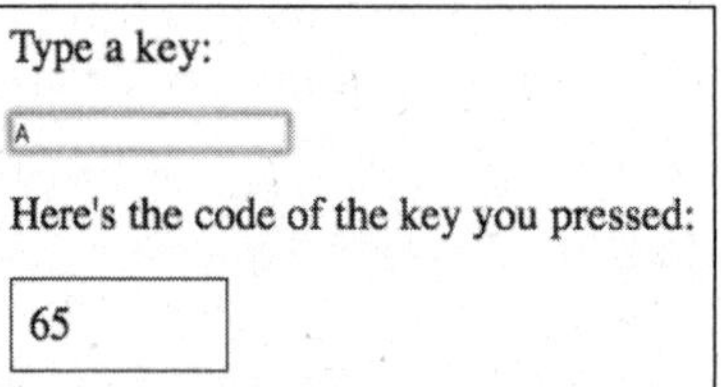

FIGURE 2-2: Type a key in the input box, and the `keypress` event callback function uses `e.which` to write the numeric code of the pressed key to the `div` element.

Preventing the default event action

TIP

Some events come with default actions that they perform when the event fires. For example, a link's `click` event opens the target URL, whereas a form's `submit` event sends the form data to a script on the server. Most of the time these default actions are exactly what you want, but that's not always the case. For example, you might want to intercept a link click to perform some custom action, such as displaying a menu. Similarly, rather than letting the browser submit a form, you might prefer to massage the form data and then send the data via your script.

For these and many similar situations, you can tell the web browser not to perform an event's default action by running the `Event` object's `preventDefault()` method:

```
event.preventDefault();
```

- *event:* A reference to the Event object that jQuery creates when an event fires

For example, take a peek at the following code:

HTML:

```
<a href="http://wiley.com/">Wiley</a>
<a href="http://wordspy.com/">Word Spy</a>
<a href="http://webcodingplayground.io/">Web Coding
  Playground</a>
<div id="output">
    Link URL:
<div>
```

jQuery:

```
$('a').click(function(e) {
    e.preventDefault();
    strURL = e.target.href
    $('#output').text('Link URL: ' + strURL);
});
```

The HTML defines three links (styled as inline blocks, which I haven't shown here) and a div element. The jQuery sets up a click event listener for all the a elements, and the callback function does three things:

- It uses the e.preventDefault() method to tell the browser not to navigate to the link address.
- It uses e.target.href to get the URL of the link.
- It displays that URL in the div element. Figure 2-3 shows an example.

FIGURE 2-3: You can use e.preventDefault() to stop the browser from navigating to the link URL.

Getting your head around event delegation

TECHNICAL STUFF

One of the brow-furrowing problems you run into when using jQuery is trying to get an event handler to work on an element that you create with code. To see what I mean, take a look at an example:

HTML:

```
<button id="add-div-button">
    Click to add the div
</button>
```

jQuery:

```
// Build the div element as a string and then prepend it
$('#add-div-button').click(function() {
    var strDiv = '<div id="my-div">';
    strDiv += 'Double-click to switch the text and background
  colors.';
    strDiv += '</div>'
    $('body').prepend(strDiv);
});

// Set up the div with a double-click event handler
$('#my-div').on('dblclick', function() {
    if($('#my-div').css('color') === 'rgb(255, 250, 205)') {
        $('#my-div').css('color', 'darkgreen');
        $('#my-div').css('background-color', 'lemonchiffon');
    } else {
        $('#my-div').css('color', 'lemonchiffon');
        $('#my-div').css('background-color', 'darkgreen');
    }
});
```

When you click the button, the first jQuery event handler builds a `div` element as a string and then uses `prepend` to add it to the `body` element. That `div` element uses the `id` value `my-div`. However, the second jQuery event handler is for a `dblclick` event on that same `my-div` element. Theoretically, the `dblclick` handler switches the element's text and background colors, but if you try this example, you can double-click the `div` until your finger falls off and nothing will happen.

Why doesn't the event handler handle anything? Because when the browser was loading the page and came upon the code for the `dblclick` event handler, the target — that is, the `div` with the `id` value `my-div` — didn't yet exist, so the browser ignored that event handler.

To fix this problem, you use a jQuery technique called *event delegation*, which means you do two things:

- You bind the event handler not to the element itself, but to an ancestor element higher up in the web page hierarchy. This needs to be an element that exists when the web browser parses the event handler.
- Add an extra parameter to the `on()` method that specifies which element your click handler actually applies to.

Here's the new syntax for the `on()` method:

```
$(ancestor).on(event, descendant, function() {
    This code runs when the event fires
});
```

- *ancestor*: A selector that specifies the ancestor element that is delegated to be monitored for the event
- *event*: A string specifying the name of event you want the browser to listen for
- *descendant*: A selector that specifies the descendant element of *ancestor* that's the actual target of the event
- `function()`: The callback function that jQuery executes when the event occurs

This version of the `on()` method *delegates* the event handler to the *ancestor* element. When the event fires, the *ancestor* element looks through its descendants until it finds the element or set given by *descendant*, and it then runs the handler with that element or set as the event target.

To fix the previous example, you could use the `document` object as the *ancestor* argument, and add `#my-div` as the *descendant* argument:

```
$(document).on('dblclick', '#my-div', function() {
```

WARNING

When choosing which ancestor to use as the delegate, the best practice is to use the closest ancestor that exists when the browser processes the event handler. For example, if in our example we were appending the `div` to, say, an existing `article` element, it would be better to use that `article` element as the delegate than the `document` object. Why is it better, you ask? Because the further away the ancestor, the more descendants the ancestor has to run through before it finds the event target, which can be a real drag on performance.

Turning off an event handler

Most of the time you'll want to leave an event handler on the job full-time so it's always available for your page visitors. However, sometimes you only want an event handler available part-time. For example, if clicking a button loads some HTML and text that you want to leave on the page, then it's best to remove both the button and its event handler to avoid confusing the user.

To remove an event handler, run jQuery's `off()` method:

```
$(selector).off(event);
```

- *`selector`:* A jQuery selector that specifies the web page element or set from which you want the event removed
- *`event`:* A string specifying the name of the event you want to remove

Here's an example that removes the `click` event from the element with the `id` value `my-button`:

```
$('#my-button').off('click');
```

Building Lively Pages with Animation

When you attend a speech or talk, nothing will put you to sleep faster — or, if you remain awake, make you want to head for the exit quicker — than listening to someone speak in a flat, affectless, monotone. The best orators use intonation, gestures, and the dramatic pause for effect to keep listeners not only in, but on the edge of, their seats.

Web pages, too, can appear flat and lifeless. Even if you've applied lots of color and top-notch typography, that's like dressing up a deadly dull speaker in a flattering dress or sharp suit: The deadly dullness remains. Web page liveliness comes not only from an attractive appearance, but also from the judicious use of animation, the digital equivalent of voice modulation and hand gestures.

That might sound like a lot of extra effort to put in for a bit of eye candy, but interface animations aren't just for show: When used properly they help the reader navigate and use your site, keep the reader engaged, and provide delight. But what about the work involved? Forget about it: jQuery offers a few ready-made tools that enable you to add sophisticated animation effects with just a few lines of code.

Hiding and showing elements

One of the most common web page effects is hiding something and then showing it when the user clicks a heading, a button, or some other page element. These effects are used for drop-down menus, navigation bars, image captions, question-and-answer sections (where clicking the question shows and hides the answer), and many other scenarios.

To hide an element, use jQuery's `hide()` method:

```
$(selector).hide();
```

» *selector*: A jQuery selector that specifies the web page element or set you want to hide

For example, the following statement hides the web page's `header` element:

```
$('header').hide();
```

To show a hidden element, use jQuery's `show()` method:

```
$(selector).show();
```

» *selector*: A jQuery selector that specifies the hidden web page element or set you want to show

For example, the following statement shows the web page's `header` element:

```
$('header').show();
```

Finally, you can toggle an element between shown and hidden by using jQuery's `toggle()` method:

```
$(selector).toggle();
```

» *selector*: A jQuery selector that specifies the hidden web page element or set you want to toggle between shown and hidden

For example, the following statement toggles the web page's `header` element:

```
$('header').toggle();
```

Fading elements out and in

The `hide()`, `show()`, and `toggle()` methods that I cover in the previous section change the display of the element immediately. If the suddenness of these effects seems a bit harsh to you, then you might prefer the jQuery animations that fade an element out or in.

To fade an element out, use jQuery's `fadeOut()` method:

```
$(selector).fadeOut();
```

- *`selector`:* A jQuery selector that specifies the web page element or set you want to fade out

For example, the following statement fades out the web page's `aside` element:

```
$('aside').fadeOut();
```

To fade an element in, use jQuery's `fadeIn()` method:

```
$(selector).fadeIn();
```

- *`selector`:* A jQuery selector that specifies the web page element or set you want to fade in

For example, the following statement fades in the web page's `aside` element:

```
$('aside').fadeIn();
```

And, yes, you can toggle the fading by running jQuery's `fadeToggle()` method:

```
$(selector).fadeToggle();
```

- *`selector`:* A jQuery selector that specifies the web page element or set you want to toggle between fading in and fading out

For example, the following statement toggles fading for the web page's `aside` element:

```
$('aside').fadeToggle();
```

Sliding elements

As an alternative to the fade animations that I cover in the previous section, you can also make an element show or hide itself gradually by sliding into or out of its position on the page.

To hide an element by sliding it up from its bottom edge until it disappears, use jQuery's `slideUp()` method:

```
$(selector).slideUp();
```

» *selector*: A jQuery selector that specifies the web page element or set you want to slide up

For example, the following statement slides up the web page's `nav` element:

```
$('nav').slideUp();
```

To show an element by sliding it down from its top edge, use jQuery's `slideDown()` method:

```
$(selector).slideDown();
```

» *selector*: A jQuery selector that specifies the web page element or set you want to slide down

For example, the following statement slides down the web page's `nav` element:

```
$('nav').slideDown();
```

I know, you're way ahead of me: You can toggle the slide effect by running jQuery's `slideToggle()` method:

```
$(selector).slideToggle();
```

» *selector*: A jQuery selector that specifies the web page element or set you want to toggle between sliding up and sliding down

For example, the following statement toggles sliding for the web page's `nav` element:

```
$('nav').slideToggle();
```

Controlling the animation duration and pace

When you use any of jQuery's animation methods — `hide()`, `show()`, `toggle()`, `fadeOut()`, `fadeIn()`, `fadeToggle()`, `slideUp()`, `slideDown()`, or `slideToggle()` — without parameters, jQuery runs the animation using its default settings:

- **Duration:** The animation take 400 milliseconds to complete.
- **Pace:** The animation starts slow, speeds up in the middle, and then slows down at the end. The pace is also called the animation's *easing* function and the default easing function is named `swing`.

You have quite a bit of control over the duration, and a bit of control over the pace, by using jQuery's animations with the addition of two parameters that set the duration and the easing function:

```
$(selector).animation(duration, easing);
```

- *`selector`:* A jQuery selector that specifies the web page element or set you want to work with.
- *`animation`:* The name of the animation method you want to run.
- *`duration`:* The length of the animation, in milliseconds. You can also use the keywords `slow` (equivalent to 600ms) or `fast` (equivalent to 200ms).
- *`easing`:* A string that specifies the easing function you want to use for the animation. The default is `swing`, but you can also specify `linear` to have the animation run at a constant pace.

For example, the following statement toggles the `nav` element between hidden and shown, where the animation takes one second and uses the `linear` easing function.

```
$('nav').toggle(1000, 'linear');
```

WARNING

Resist the temptation to extend the duration of an animation beyond a second or two. Your web visitors are busy people, and no one wants to sit through a ten-second fade or slide animation. As a general rule, your animations should be quick: around half a second in most cases.

Example: Creating a web page accordion

A common web design pattern is the *accordion*, a menu or list of items, each of which contains extra content that is hidden by default. When you click an item in the accordion, that item's hidden content is displayed. Click the item again, and the content returns to being hidden. An accordion is useful when you have a long series or list of items, and to display everything at once would be overwhelming for the reader. Instead, you can display just the headings, menu commands, or similar top-level items, and you can hide the rest of the content associated with each item, thus making the list or menu easier to read and navigate.

Take a look at an example. First, here's some CSS and HTML code to mull over:

CSS:

```
.sentence {
    display: none;
}
```

HTML:

```
<header>
    <h1>Some Food Words to Chew On</h1>
</header>
<main>
    <p>
        Click a word or its definition to see that term's sample
      sentence.
</p>
<section id="alamode" class="word">
        <b>à la mode</b> (al·uh·MODE, adjective). Describes a
      dish that's served with ice cream.
        <p class="sentence">
            Give her a big spoon and a piece of apple pie <b>à
      la mode</b> the size of her head, and Moira had her own little
      slice of heaven.
        </p>
    </section>
    <section id="appetizer" class="word">
        <b>appetizer</b> (AP·uh·tye·zur, noun). Food or drink
      that's served before the main meal and is meant to stimulate
      the appetite.
        <p class="sentence">
            A slow eater, Karen was only halfway through her
      salad <b>appetizer</b> when the waiter showed up with the main
      course.
```

Livening Up Your Page with Events and Animation

```
        </p>
    </section>
    <section id="comestible" class="word">
        <b>comestible</b> (kuh·MES·tuh·bul, noun). An item that
can be eaten as food.
        <p class="sentence">
            After picking up bread, meat, cheese, and a few
other <b>comestibles</b>, Deirdre was ready for the weekend-
long Three Stooges festival.
        </p>
    </section>
    <section id="cuisine" class="word">
        <b>cuisine</b> (kwi·ZEEN, noun). A style of cooking as
well as the food cooked in that style.
        <p class="sentence">
            His local restaurant was supposed to specialize in
French <b>cuisine</b>, so Sean wondered why they didn't serve
french fries.
        </p>
    </section>
    <section id="epicure" class="word">
        <b>epicure</b> (EP·uh·kyoor, noun). A person with
sophisticated tastes, especially when it comes to food and
wine.
        <p class="sentence">
            Being able to tell beef stroganoff from beef
Wellington and a Bordeaux from a Beaujolais convinced Dominic
that he was quite the <b>epicure</b>.
        </p>
    </section>
    <section id="ingest" class="word">
        <b>ingest</b> (in·JEST, verb). To take food into the
body.
        <p class="sentence">
            Not at all hungry, but also unwilling to displease
his wife, Mr. Tortellini <b>ingested</b> her spaghetti with
grim determination.
        </p>
    </section>
    <section id="nosh" class="word">
        <b>nosh</b> (nawsh, verb). To eat a light meal or a
snack.
```

```
      <p class="sentence">
          Wanda would guiltily <b>nosh</b> on a pepperoni
  stick before going in to her vegetarian cooking class.
      </p>
    </section>
</main>
```

The HTML consists mostly of a series of <section> tags, each of which contains a word, its pronunciation, its definition, and a <p> tag that contains a sample sentence that uses the word. Each of these <p> tags is given the class named sentence, and in the CSS code, you can see that the sentence class is hidden by default by styling it with the declaration `display: none`. Figure 2-4 shows the initial state of the page.

Some Food Words to Chew On

Click a word or its definition to see that term's sample sentence.

à la mode (al·uh·MODE, adjective). Describes a dish that's served with ice cream.

appetizer (AP·uh·tye·zur, noun). Food or drink that's served before the main meal and is meant to stimulate the appetite.

comestible (kuh·MES·tuh·bul, noun). An item that can be eaten as food.

cuisine (kwi·ZEEN, noun). A style of cooking as well as the food cooked in that style.

epicure (EP·uh·kyoor, noun). A person with sophisticated tastes, especially when it comes to food and wine.

ingest (in·JEST, verb). To take food into the body.

nosh (nawsh, verb). To eat a light meal or a snack.

FIGURE 2-4: When you first load the page, you see only each word and its pronunciation and definition. The sample sentences are hidden by default with the `display: none` declaration.

The goal here is to display a word's sample sentence when the reader clicks the word (or its pronunciation or definition). One way to do this would be to set up a `click` event handler on each word and then have that handler's callback function use a method such as `slideToggle()` or `fadeToggle()` to show and hide the sample sentence. That would do the job, but it requires a lot of work. Sure, it's not bad with the seven items in my list, but what if there were 70 items, or 700?

Instead, I'm going to take advantage of three timesaving features of my HTML code:

- Each <section> tag uses the class named word, so I can set up a single click event handler that is bound to that class name.
- Each <section> tag also uses a unique id value that is based on its word. I can use that id value to know which term was clicked.
- Each <p> tag is a direct child of its parent <section> tag, which lets me target the <p> tag using the child selector.

Given all this, the jQuery code required to show and hide the sample sentences is remarkably compact:

```
$('.word').click(function(e) {
    var wordID = e.target.id;
    $('#' + wordID + ' > p').slideToggle('slow');
});
```

Three things are going on here:

- The `click` event method is bound to the class named `word`, so it fires any time the reader clicks a `<section>` tag's content.
- To figure out which `<section>` tag was clicked, the code gets the value of `e.target.id`, which returns the `id` value of the clicked `section` element. That `id` value is stored in the `wordID` variable.
- To build the jQuery selector for the sample sentence, the code appends `#` to `wordID`, and then adds the child selector for the `p` element: `> p`. With the `section` element's sample sentence selected, the code runs the `slideToggle()` animation to slide the sample sentence in and out of view.

Figure 2-5 shows the page with one of the sample sentences displayed.

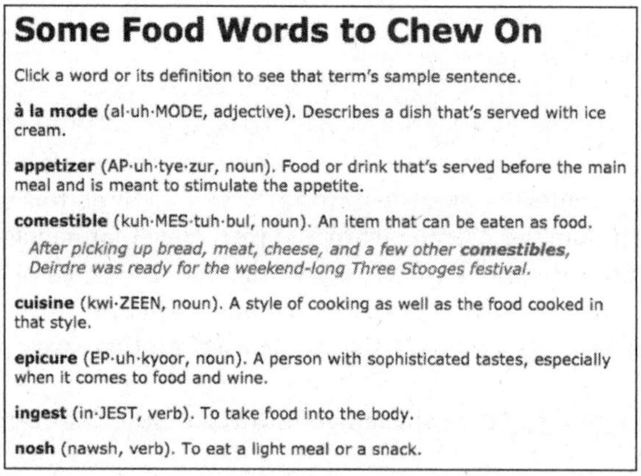

Some Food Words to Chew On

Click a word or its definition to see that term's sample sentence.

à la mode (al·uh·MODE, adjective). Describes a dish that's served with ice cream.

appetizer (AP·uh·tye·zur, noun). Food or drink that's served before the main meal and is meant to stimulate the appetite.

comestible (kuh·MES·tuh·bul, noun). An item that can be eaten as food.

*After picking up bread, meat, cheese, and a few other **comestibles**, Deirdre was ready for the weekend-long Three Stooges festival.*

cuisine (kwi·ZEEN, noun). A style of cooking as well as the food cooked in that style.

epicure (EP·uh·kyoor, noun). A person with sophisticated tastes, especially when it comes to food and wine.

ingest (in·JEST, verb). To take food into the body.

nosh (nawsh, verb). To eat a light meal or a snack.

FIGURE 2-5: Click any word (or its pronunciation or definition) and our four-line jQuery code slides the sample sentence in or out.

Animating CSS properties

One of the most interesting and exciting jQuery methods is `animate()`, which enables you to apply an animation to any CSS property that accepts a numeric value: `font-size`, `padding`, `border-width`, `opacity`, and many more. Here's the syntax to use:

```
$(selector).animate(properties, duration, easing);
```

- *selector:* A jQuery selector that specifies the web page element or set you want to work with.
- *properties:* An object literal that specifies the CSS property-value pairs that you want to animate.
- *duration:* An optional length of the animation, in milliseconds. You can also use the keywords `slow` (equivalent to 600ms) or `fast` (equivalent to 200ms). The default is 400ms.
- *easing:* An optional string that specifies the easing function you want to use for the animation. The default is `swing`, but you can also specify `linear` to have the animation run at a constant pace.

The *properties* parameter requires a bit more elaboration. It requires an object literal, which is a collection of property-value pairs, separated by commas and surrounded by braces. Here's the general form:

```
{
    property1: value1,
    property2: value2,
    etc.
    propertyN: valueN
}
```

Each *property* is a CSS property name, which needs to be enclosed in quotation marks if it contains a hyphen (-). Each *value* is a number, followed by a measurement unit, if needed. (Some CSS properties, such as `opacity` and `line-spacing`, take unitless numeric values.) If the value has a measurement unit, surround the number and unit with quotation marks. For example, here's the object literal to use if you want your animation to change the left position to `425px`, the font size to `1rem`, and the opacity to `1`:

```
{
    left: '425px',
    'font-size': '1rem',
    opacity: 1
}
```

You then insert the object literal into the `animate()` method as the *properties* parameter:

```
$('aside').animate(
    {
```

```
        left: '425px',
        'font-size': '1rem',
        opacity: 1
    },
    1500,
    'linear'
);
```

This example animates the page's `aside` element with a duration of 1.5 seconds and linear easing. Notice that I arranged the `animate()` arguments vertically for easier reading.

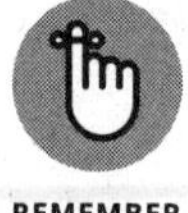
REMEMBER

For an animation to actually animate something, the property values you specify in the `animate()` method's object literal must be different than the values the element already has. For the example just described, the initial CSS rule for the `aside` element might look like this:

```
aside {
    position: absolute;
    left: -20rem;
    font-size: .1rem;
    opacity: 0;
}
```

Given this initial rule, you can see that the animation does three things:

- Moves the element from its initial position offscreen to 425px from the left edge of the content area
- Increases the font size from `.1rem` to `1rem`
- Increases the opacity from `0` (transparent) to `1` (fully visible)

Running code when an animation ends

Most of the time you'll want your jQuery animations to run their course without further ado. However, there might be times when some further ado is exactly what you want. For example, at the completion of an animation, you might want to adjust the text on a button (for example, from "Hide the nav bar" to "Show the nav bar") or you might want to run another animation (a technique known as animation *chaining*).

You can perform these and similar post-animation tasks by adding a callback function to the animation method. First, here's the syntax to use for one of jQuery's built-in animation effects:

```
$(selector).animation(function() {
    Code to run when the animation is done
});
```

- `selector`: A jQuery selector that specifies the web page element or set you want to work with.
- `animation`: The name of the animation method you want to run.
- `function()`: The callback function. jQuery executes the code inside this function after the animation ends.

Here's an example:

HTML:

```
<nav>
    <a href="#">Home</a>
    <a href="#">What's New</a>
    <a href="#">What's Old</a>
    <a href="#">What's What</a>
</nav>
<main>
    <button id="slide-nav">Hide the nav bar</button>
</main>
```

jQuery:

```
$('#slide-nav').click(function() {
    $('nav').slideToggle(function() {

        // Get the current button text
        var btnText = $('#slide-nav').text();

        // Check the first four letters of the button text
        // and then change the button text accordingly
        if (btnText.substr(0, 4) === 'Hide') {
            $('#slide-nav').text('Show the nav bar');
        } else {
            $('#slide-nav').text('Hide the nav bar');
        }
```

```
    });
});
```

The HTML defines a `button` element that, when clicked, hides and shows the `nav` element. The jQuery code sets up a `click` event handler for the button, and that handler's callback function runs the `slideToggle()` animation on the `nav` element. The `slideToggle()` animation also includes a callback function that gets the button text, checks to see if the first four characters are `Hide`, and then changes the button text according to the result.

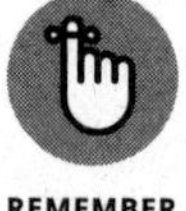

REMEMBER

You can specify a duration and easing value along with the callback function. Here's the complete syntax:

```
$(selector).animation(duration, easing, function() {
    Code to run when the animation is done
});
```

For the `animate()` method, you can also include a callback function by using the following syntax:

```
$(selector).animate(properties, duration, easing, function() {
    Code to run when the animation is done
});
```

Here's an example that runs a second `animate()` method after the first one is complete:

```
$('#animate-aside').click(function() {
    $('aside').animate(
        {
            left: '425px'
        },
        500,
        'linear',
        function() {
            $('aside > p').animate(
                {
                    opacity: 1
                },
                2000
            ); // End of the second animate() method
        } // End of the first animate() method's callback
  function
    ); // End of the first animate() method
}); // End of the click() method
```

» Creating a custom version of jQuery UI

» Including the jQuery UI code in your page

» Trying out a few jQuery UI widgets

» Playing around with jQuery UI interactions and effects

Chapter 3

Getting to Know jQuery UI

Because jQuery UI runs on top of jQuery, the syntax used to initialize, configure, and manipulate the different components is in the same comfortable, easy-to-use, and short-hand style that we've all come to know and love through using jQuery. Therefore, getting used to it is incredibly easy.

— DAN WELLMAN

In Chapters 1 and 2 of this minibook, I go through the basics of jQuery and showed how easy jQuery makes it to select elements, manipulate tags, CSS properties, and HTML attributes, and build interactive and fun pages with events and animations. jQuery's ease and power make it an indispensable tool in the modern web developer's workshop, but as powerful as it is, jQuery can't do everything. In particular, jQuery doesn't offer much — okay, anything — in the way of tools to help ease the chore of building user interface components such as menus, dialog boxes, and tabs. Sure, jQuery gives you the technology to build these things, but the coding is still often time-consuming and laborious.

But it doesn't have to be. That's because the jQuery Foundation — the same group that brings you jQuery — is also behind a sister project called jQuery UI (jQuery User Interface), which offers an impressive set of pre-fab user interface components. In this chapter, you explore what jQuery UI has to offer and investigate a number of the most useful and powerful jQuery UI components.

What's the Deal with jQuery UI?

Have you ever seen one of those homemade Little Free Libraries that people put up on their properties and allow anyone to take (and, ideally, add) books? The jQuery library is a bit like that because it allows third-party developers to create extensions to jQuery called *plug-ins*. These are small bits of code that piggyback on jQuery's syntax, making them intuitive to learn and use. For example, if a plug-in extended jQuery with a method named `doohickey()`, you'd run the plug-in on an element, like so:

```
$(element).doohickey();
```

There are hundreds of available plug-ins (check out `http://plugins.jquery.com` to see the complete list). However, one plug-in in particular is the most popular: jQuery UI, which offers a set of components related to building a web page user interface. jQuery UI itself breaks down its components into ten categories, but for purposes in this chapter, there are three main categories that you explore:

- **Widgets:** Ready-to-use user interface components such as menus, dialog boxes, tabs, and sliders
- **Effects:** Animations that go well beyond built-in jQuery effects, such as `hide()` and `fadeIn()`
- **Interactions:** Mouse-centric tools that enable you to configure web page elements to be resizable, draggable, sortable, and more

jQuery UI has a Download Builder tool that enables you to select just the components you want, a ThemeRoller tool that lets you customize the look of the components you download, and a consistent set of class names that you can access via CSS rules or your jQuery code.

Getting Started with jQuery UI

Getting up and running with jQuery UI involves the following steps:

1. **Surf to the jQuery UI's Download Builder page, at** `https://jqueryui.com/download`**.**

   Figure 3-1 shows the top part of the Download Builder page.

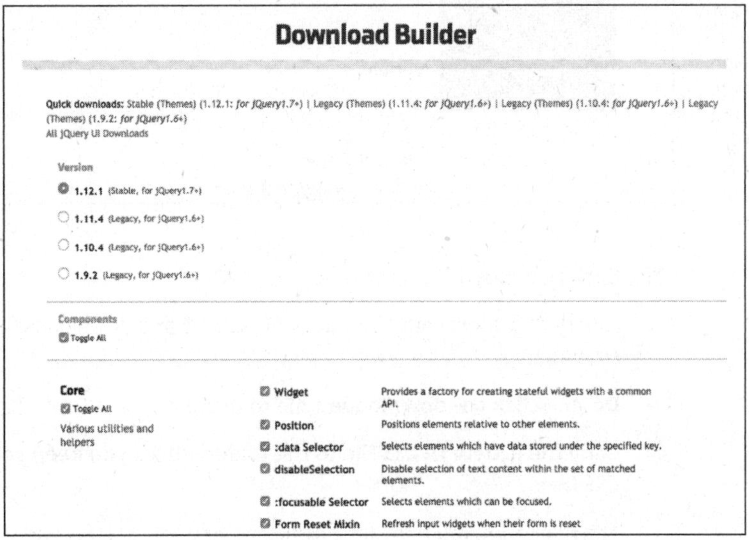

FIGURE 3-1: Use the jQuery UI Download Builder page to create your custom jQuery UI download.

2. **Leave the Version option with the most recent version selected.**
3. **Use the check boxes to choose which jQuery UI components you want to use.**

   If you don't yet know which components you want to use, leave them all selected for now. The resulting file will be quite big (over 250KB), but you can always come back and select just the components you want to use when you're more familiar with what jQuery UI has to offer.

4. **Near the bottom of the page, use the Theme list to select a CSS theme for your components.**

   If you want to roll your own theme, click Design a Custom Theme to open the ThemeRoller, shown in Figure 3-2. Use the ThemeRoller widget on the left to customize your fonts, colors, and more. Then click Download Theme to return to the Download Builder with `Custom Theme` now showing in the Theme list.

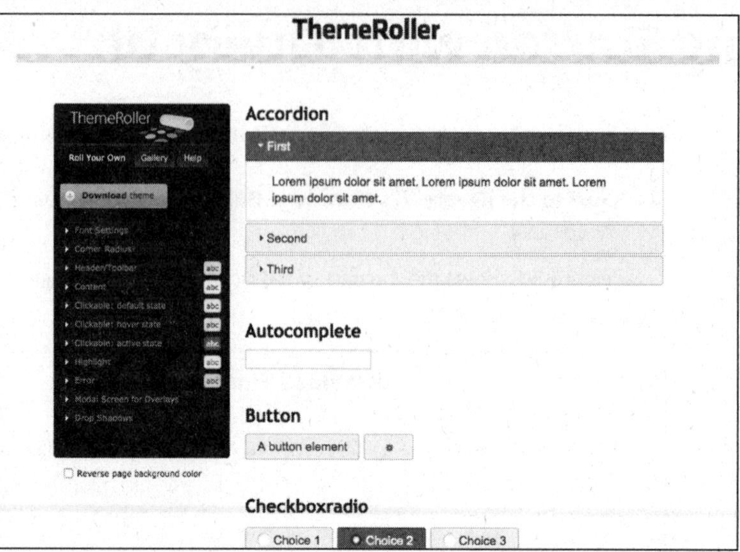

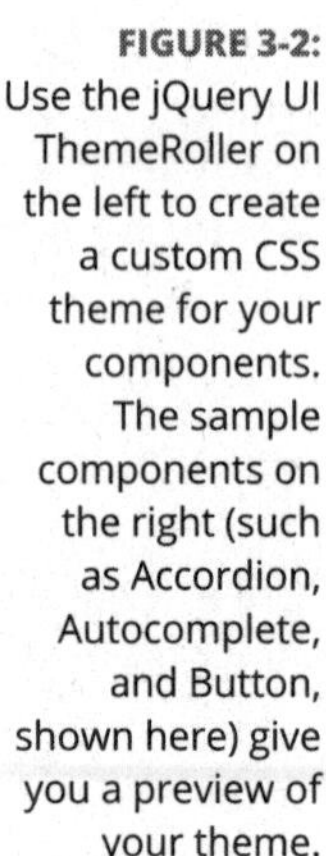

FIGURE 3-2: Use the jQuery UI ThemeRoller on the left to create a custom CSS theme for your components. The sample components on the right (such as Accordion, Autocomplete, and Button, shown here) give you a preview of your theme.

5. **Click Download.**

   jQuery UI gathers your files into a ZIP archive and downloads the file to your computer.

6. **Double-click the downloaded file to unzip it.**

7. **Copy the jQuery UI CSS file to the folder where you keep your web page CSS files.**

   At a minimum, you need to copy the `jquery-ui.css` file and the `images` subfolder. You might also want to copy the minified version of the CSS — `jquery-ui.min.css` — to use with your production code.

8. **Copy the jQuery UI JavaScript file to the folder where you keep your web page JavaScript files.**

   You need to copy the `jquery-ui.js` file. You might also want to copy the minified version — `jquery-ui.min.js` — to use with your production code.

9. **Incorporate the jQuery UI code into your web page.**

   For the CSS file, set up a `<link>` tag (adjusting the path to the file as needed for your own folder structure):

```
<link rel="stylesheet" href="/css/jquery-ui.css">
```

For the JavaScript file, set up a <script> tag and place it after the <script> tag you use for jQuery (again, be sure to adjust the path to the file as needed):

```
<script src="https://ajax.googleapis.com/ajax/libs/
   jquery/3.3.1/jquery.min.js"></script>
<script src="/js/jquery-ui.js">
```

Working with the jQuery UI Widgets

A jQuery UI *widget* is a ready-to-use web page user interface component. jQuery UI offers 15 or so of these widgets, most of which are related to forms, so I won't cover them in this chapter. (See Book 6, Chapter 2 to get the details on forms and form controls.) However, that still leaves you with a fistful of remarkably useful widgets — tabs, menus, dialog boxes, and accordions — that you can put to good use right away to make your web pages stand out from the herd.

Dividing content into tabs

In a web browser, the tabs that run across the window just above the content area each contain a web page, and you switch between the pages by clicking the tabs.

You can offer that same convenience in your web pages by implementing jQuery UI's tabs widget, which displays a series of two or more tabs, each of which is loaded with content. The user switches between the content by clicking the tabs. When you have a lot of content to display, but not a lot of room to display it, tabs are your best choice.

A good example of the tabs widget in action is on jQuery UI's ThemeRoller page (`http://jqueryui.com/themeroller`), where the ThemeRoller tool offers three tabs: Roll Your Own, Gallery, and Help, as pointed out in Figure 3-3.

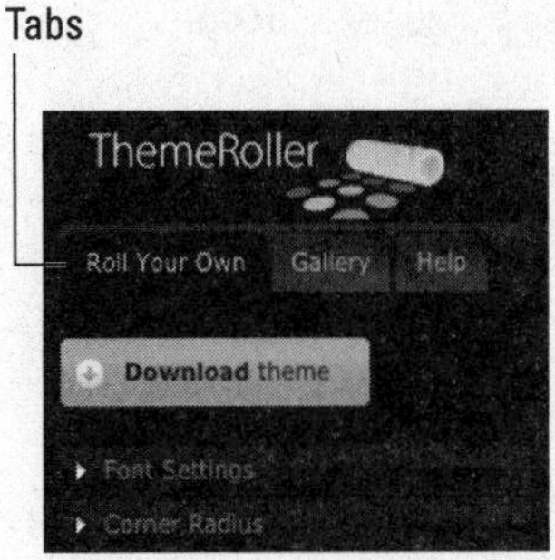

FIGURE 3-3: jQuery UI's ThemeRoller tool makes good use of jQuery UI's tabs widget.

To create tabs on your page, you need to set up your HTML using the following steps:

1. **Add a block-level element to use as the parent for the entire tab structure, and include an `id` value.**

   You can use a semantic element such as `<article>` or `<aside>`, if it fits your content, or a generic `<div>` container:

   ```
   <div id="my-tabs">
   </div>
   ```

2. **The tabs themselves are enclosed in a list (which can be unordered or ordered), where the text for each list item is the text that appears on each tab.**

   ```
   <div id="my-tabs">
       <ul>
           <li>This</li>
           <li>That</li>
           <li>The Other</li>
       </ul>
   </div>
   ```

3. **For each tab, add a block-level element to hold the tab's content, and include a unique `id` value.**

   Again, you can use a semantic element such as `<section>` or `<p>`, if that works for you, or a generic `<div>`:

   ```
   <div id="my-tabs">
       <ul>
           <li>This</li>
           <li>That</li>
           <li>The Other</li>
       </ul>
       <div id="my-tab-1">
           This is the first tab's content.
       </div>
       <div id="my-tab-2">
           This is the second tab's content.
       </div>
       <div id="my-tab-3">
           Yep, this is the third tab's content.
       </div>
   </div>
   ```

4. **Return to your list of items and convert each item's text into a link that points to the `id` value of the tab's content block.**

   Be sure to precede each `id` with a hash symbol (#). Here's the final HTML code:

```
<div id="my-tabs">
    <ul>
        <li><a href="#my-tab-1">This</a></li>
        <li><a href="#my-tab-2">That</a></li>
        <li><a href="#my-tab-3">The Other</a></li>
    </ul>
    <div id="my-tab-1">
        This is the first tab's content.
    </div>
    <div id="my-tab-2">
        This is the second tab's content.
    </div>
    <div id="my-tab-3">
        Yep, this is the third tab's content.
    </div>
</div>
```

With your HTML set up, you turn it into tabs by applying jQuery UI's `tabs()` method to the parent container:

```
$('#my-tabs').tabs();
```

Figure 3-4 shows the result.

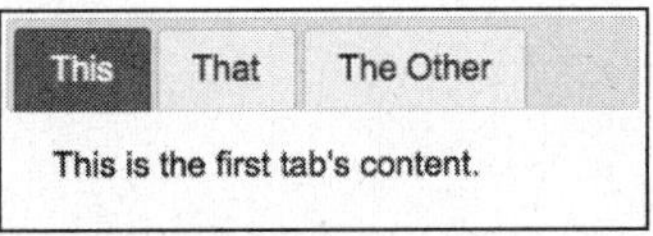

FIGURE 3-4: Some tabs created using jQuery UI's tabs widget.

TIP

You can style the tabs widget by overriding the rules that come with jQuery UI's CSS. There are four main classes you can use to style the tabs widget:

- `ui-tabs`: The parent container. For example, I styled the tabs widget shown in Figure 3-4 to have a width of `300px` as follows:

```
.ui-tabs {
    width: 300px;
}
```

» `ui-tabs-nav`: The list container (the `<ul>` or `<ol>` element).

» `ui-tabs-tab`: Each `<li>` item in the list (that is, each tab).

» `ui-tabs-panel`: The content container for each tab.

Creating a navigation menu

If your page navigation includes quite a few links — especially if those links can be divided into categories — you can tidy things up and make your navigation easier and more comprehensible for page visitors by converting your links into a drop-down menu with submenus.

Creating a menu normally requires quite a bit of coding, but jQuery UI's menu widget simplifies things considerably. Here are the steps to follow to build a menu widget for your page:

1. **Create a parent element to hold the menu widget structure, and include an `id` value.**

   You can use any block-level element, but most developers use an unordered list (`<ul>`):

   ```
   <ul id="my-menu">
   </ul>
   ```

2. **For each menu item, add a list item element (`<li>`), where the item text is your menu item text surrounded by a block-level element, such as `<div>`.**

   To add a menu separator (a horizontal line across the menu), use a dash as the menu item text:

   ```
   <ul id="my-menu">
       <li>
           <div>Menu Item #1</div>
       </li>
       <li>
           <div>Menu Item #2</div>
       </li>
       <li>
           <div>-</div>
       </li>
       <li>
           <div>Menu Item #3</div>
       </li>
   </ul>
   ```

3. To create a submenu within an existing menu item, insert a new unordered list between the menu item's `<li>` and `</li>` tags, after the menu item text element.

Note that the submenu's `<ul>` tag doesn't need an `id` value. Here's the final HTML code:

```
<ul id="my-menu">
    <li>
        <div>Menu Item #1</div>
    </li>
    <li>
        <div>Menu Item #2</div>
        <ul>
            <li>
                <div>Submenu Item #2-A</div>
            </li>
            <li>
                <div>Submenu Item #2-B</div>
            </li>
        </ul>
    </li>
    <li>
        <div>-</div>
    </li>
    <li>
        <div>Menu Item #3</div>
    </li>
</ul>
```

Now you turn your HTML tags into a menu by applying jQuery UI's `menu()` method to the parent container:

```
$('#my-menu).menu();
```

Figure 3-5 shows the finished menu.

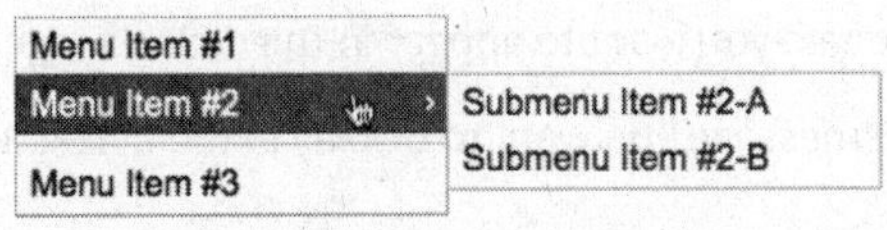

FIGURE 3-5: A drop-down menu with a submenu, created using jQuery UI's menu widget.

Getting to Know jQuery UI

TIP

You can style the menu widget by overriding the rules that come with jQuery UI's CSS. There are three main classes you can use to style the menu widget:

- ui-menu: The parent container (the <ul> element). For example, I styled the menu widget shown in Figure 3-5 to have a width of 200px, as follows:

```
.ui-menu {
    width: 200px;
}
```

- ui-menu-item: Each <li> item in the list (that is, each menu item).
- ui-menu-wrapper: The content container for each menu item (the <div> elements in my example).

Displaying a message in a dialog

In Book 3, Chapter 6, I talk about JavaScript's alert() method, which you can use to display a message to the user. As long as you don't overdo it, displaying messages is a handy trick to have up your web development sleeve. The problem, however, is that JavaScript's alert() boxes are plain to a fault and aren't customizable. If you're going to subject your page visitors to the occasional message, then why not make the message at least look nice?

You can get a better-looking message by foregoing JavaScript's alert() method in favor of jQuery UI's dialog widget. The dialog widget creates a floating window that offers a title bar, a content area for the message, and a button that closes the window.

To set up the dialog widget, create a <div> element that uses the following format:

```
<div id="dialog-id" title="dialog-title">
    Dialog message
</div>
```

- *dialog-id:* A unique id value for the dialog widget
- *dialog-title:* The text you want to appear in the dialog widget's title bar
- *Dialog message:* The message you want to display in the dialog widget's content area

Once that's done, you turn your HTML into a dialog widget by applying jQuery UI's dialog() method to the <div>:

```
$('#dialog-id').dialog({
    autoOpen: false
});
```

Notice that I've included the object literal `{autoOpen: false}`, which tells jQuery UI not to display the dialog automatically when you first run the `dialog()` method. To open the dialog (say, in response to a button click), run the `dialog()` method with the string `open` as the parameter:

```
$('#dialog-id').dialog('open');
```

Here's an example, and Figure 3-6 shows the dialog that appears when the button is clicked:

HTML:

```
<div id="my-dialog" title="Hello Dialog World!">
     Welcome to my dialog widget!
</div>

<button id="my-button">
    Display the dialog
</button>
```

jQuery:

```
// Initialize the dialog widget
$('#my-dialog').dialog({
    autoOpen: false}
);

// Display the dialog when the button is clicked
$('#my-button').click(function() {
    $('#my-dialog').dialog('open');
});
```

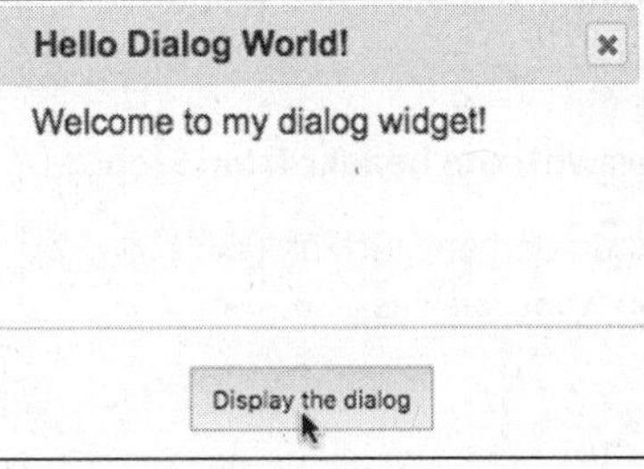

FIGURE 3-6: The jQuery UI dialog widget that appears when you click the button.

Getting to Know jQuery UI

TIP

You can style the dialog widget by overriding the rules that come with jQuery UI's CSS. There are four main classes you can use to style the menu widget:

- `ui-dialog`: The parent container (the `<div>` element)
- `ui-dialog-titlebar`: The dialog widget's title bar
- `ui-dialog-title`: The dialog widget's title text
- `ui-dialog-container`: The dialog widget's content area

Hiding and showing content with an accordion

An *accordion* is a series of headings, each with an associated chunk of content, where only one heading/content combo is shown at a time. Accordions are a great way to display multiple items without overwhelming the reader with all the content at once.

I talk about how to use jQuery to build a simple accordion in Book 4, Chapter 2, but jQuery UI offers a more sophisticated accordion widget. To create an accordion, you first need to set up some HTML tags as follows:

1. **Add a block-level element to use as the parent for the entire accordion structure, and include an `id` value.**

   You can use a semantic element such as `<main>` or `<article>`, if it fits your content, or a generic `<div>` container:

   ```
   <div id="my-accordion">
   </div>
   ```

2. **Add a header.**

   You can use any element you want, but a heading tag makes sense semantically:

   ```
   <div id="my-accordion">
       <h6>Header A</h6>
   </div>
   ```

3. **Add the content that goes with the header from Step 2.**

   Again, you can use a semantic element such as `<section>` or `<p>`, if that works for you, or any element you want, such as a `<div>`:

```
<div id="my-accordion">
    <h6>Header A</h6>
    <div>This is the content panel for Header A</div>
</div>
```

4. **Repeat Steps 2 and 3 for each header/content pair you want to include in your accordion.**

   Here's the final HTML code for my example:

```
<div id="my-accordion">
    <h6>Header A</h6>
    <div>This is the content panel for Header A</div>
    <h6>Header B</h6>
    <div>This is the content panel for Header B</div>
    <h6>Header C</h6>
    <div>This is the content panel for Header C</div>
</div>
```

With your HTML ready to go, you turn that code into an accordion by applying jQuery UI's `accordion()` method to the parent container:

```
$('#my-accordion').accordion();
```

Figure 3-7 shows the result.

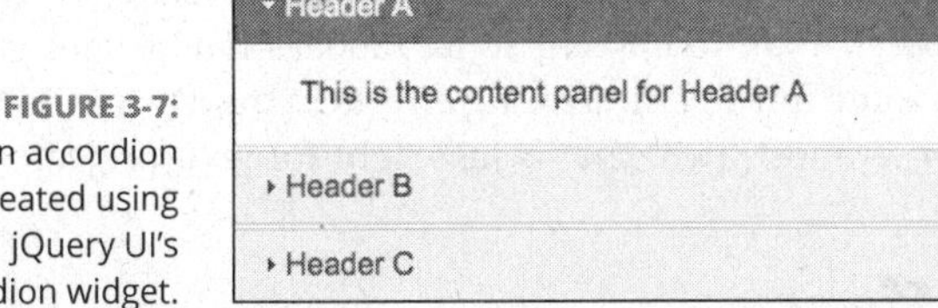

FIGURE 3-7: An accordion created using jQuery UI's accordion widget.

TIP

Note that with jQuery UI's accordion, one content panel is always visible. If you'd prefer that the accordion allow all the content panels to be hidden, initialize the `accordion()` method with an object literal that sets the `collapsible` property to `true`:

```
$('#my-accordion').accordion({
    collapsible: true
});
```

TIP

You can style the accordion widget by overriding the rules that come with jQuery UI's CSS. There are three main classes you can use to style the accordion widget:

- ui-accordion: The parent container. For example, I styled the accordion widget shown in Figure 3-7 to have a width of 400px, as follows:

```
.ui-accordion {
    width: 400px;
}
```

- ui-accordion-header: The accordion headers.
- ui-accordion-content: The accordion content panels.

Introducing jQuery UI Effects

As I go on and on about in Book 4, Chapter 2, jQuery offers half a dozen animation effects: hide(), show(), fadeOut(), fadeIn(), slideUp(), and slideDown(), as well as their toggle versions: toggle(), fadeToggle(), and slideToggle(). That's a decent palette to work with, but apparently it wasn't good enough for the jQuery UI team, who've stuffed no less than 14 extra animations into the Effects category.

WARNING

Do you need all those effects? No, you don't. As with all things related to animation, too little is always better than too much, so let moderation be your watchword. That said, there are some fun and interesting effects in the jQuery UI library, so perhaps there's one (or, at most, two) that is just right for your project.

Applying an effect

Before I describe the available animations, let's see how you apply them to an element. The most straightforward way is to use jQuery UI's effect() method. Here's the syntax:

```
$(selector).effect(effect, options, duration, function() {
    Code to run when the effect is done
});
```

- *selector:* A jQuery selector that specifies the web page element you want to work with.
- *effect:* A string that specifies the name of the jQuery UI effect you want to apply to the element.
- *options:* An object literal that includes one or more property-value pairs that specify the effect options you want to use. These options vary with the effect, but the most common property is `easing`, which sets the easing function. jQuery UI offers more than 30 easings; see `https://api.jqueryui.com/easings` for the complete list and to try out each one.
- *duration:* The length of the effect, in milliseconds. You can also use the keywords `slow` (equivalent to 600ms) or `fast` (equivalent to 200ms). The default duration is 400ms.
- `function()`: A callback function that jQuery UI executes after the effect ends.

For example, the following statement applies jQuery UI's `bounce` effect with a `slow` duration to the element that has an `id` value of `my-div`:

```
$('#my-div').effect('bounce', 'slow');
```

The `effect()` method works best with effects that perform some action on an element, while leaving that element in place (such as bouncing the element). If you want to hide or show an element, then you're better off working with jQuery UI's extensions to jQuery's `hide()`, `show()`, and `toggle()` methods. These use the same syntax as the `effect()` method:

```
$(selector).hide(effect, options, duration, function() {
    Code to run when the effect is done
});
```

```
$(selector).show(effect, options, duration, function() {
    Code to run when the effect is done
});
```

```
$(selector).toggle(effect, options, duration, function() {
    Code to run when the effect is done
});
```

Checking out the effects

Here's a quick look at the available effects offered by jQuery UI:

- `blind`: Hides or shows an element as though the element was a window blind that you pull up or down. As an option, you can set the `direction` property to up, down, `left`, `right`, `vertical`, or `horizontal`.

```
$('#my-div').toggle('blind',{direction: 'left'});
```

- `bounce`: Bounces an element up and down. As options, you can use the `distance` property to set the maximum bounce height (in pixels), and the `times` property to set the number of bounces.

```
$('#my-div').effect('bounce',
    {
        distance: 200,
        times: 10
    },
    1500
);
```

- `clip`: Hides or shows an element by shrinking the element vertically from the top and bottom. Set the `direction` property to `horizontal` to clip the element horizontally.

```
$('#my-div').toggle('clip');
```

- `drop`: Hides or shows an element by fading the element out or in while simultaneously sliding the element left or right. As an option, you can set the `direction` property to up, down, `left`, or `right`.

```
$('#my-div').toggle('drop',{direction: 'up'});
```

- `explode`: Hides an element by exploding it into pieces that fly off in all directions; shows an element by restoring the exploded pieces to their original configuration. You can set the `pieces` property to the number of pieces to explode; the value should be a square, such as `16` or `25` (the default is `9`).

```
$('#my-div').toggle('explode',{pieces: 16});
```

- `fade`: Hides or shows an element by fading the element out or in.

```
$('#my-div').toggle('fade', 'slow');
```

» fold: Hides an element by first shrinking it vertically to a 15-pixel height (the first "fold"), and then shrinking it horizontally until it disappears (the second "fold"); shows an element by reversing the folding procedure. For options, you can use the size property to set the height, in pixels, after the first fold (the default is 15); you can set the horizFirst property to true to make the first fold horizontal rather than vertical.

```
$('#my-div').toggle('fold',{size: 50});
```

» highlight: Highlights the background of an element. Use the color property to specify the highlight color as an RGB triplet (the default is #ffff99).

```
$('#my-div').effect('highlight',{color: 'ffd700'});
```

» puff: Hides or shows an element by scaling the element larger or smaller while simultaneously fading the element out or in. Add the percent property to set the maximum scale percentage (the default is 150).

```
$('#my-div').toggle('puff',{percent: 200});
```

» pulsate: Pulsates an element by quickly oscillating its opacity between 0 and 1. Use the times property to set the number of oscillations (the default is 5).

```
$('#my-div').effect('pulsate',{times: 10});
```

» scale: Grows or shrinks an element. For options, you can set the direction property to horizontal, vertical, or both (the default); you can use the origin property to set the vanishing point as an array of the form ['*h*','*v*'], where *h* is top, middle, or bottom, and *v* is left, center, or right (the default is ['middle','center']); you can use the percent property to set the scale factor; and you can set the scale property to box, content, or both (the default).

```
$('#my-div').effect('scale',{percent: 25, origin:
    ['top','left']});
```

» shake: Shakes an element horizontally or vertically. As options, you can set the direction property to either left (the default) or right for a horizontal shake, or to up or down for a vertical shake; you can use the distance property to set the shake displacement, in pixels (the default is 20); and you can set the times property to set the number of shakes (the default is 3).

```
$('#my-div').effect('shake',
    {
        distance: 10,
        times: 10
    },
    1000
);
```

Getting to Know jQuery UI

- `size`: Changes the dimensions of an element to a specified width and height. You set the new dimensions by adding the `to` property as an option and setting it to an object literal that specifies the `width` and `height`, in pixels. You can also use the `origin` property to set the resize fixed point as an array of the form `['h','v']`, where *h* is `top`, `middle`, or `bottom`, and *v* is `left`, `center`, or `right` (the default is `['top','left']`); and you can set the `scale` property to `box`, `content`, or `both` (the default).

  ```
  $('#my-div').effect('size',{to: {width: 200, height:
     100}});
  ```

- `slide`: Hides or shows an element by sliding it out of or into the viewport. For options, you can use the `direction` property to set the direction of the slide to `left` (the default), `right`, `up`, or `down`; you can use the `distance` property to set the length of the slide, in pixels (the default is the width of the element if `direction` is `left` or `right`, or the height of the element if `direction` is `up` or `down`).

  ```
  $('#my-div').toggle('slide',{direction: 'up'});
  ```

Taking a Look at jQuery UI Interactions

To round out this look at the main jQuery UI components, I spend the rest of this chapter looking at the jQuery UI interactions category. An *interaction* is a widget that enables page visitors to use a mouse (or trackpad or touchscreen) to control, modify, or in some other way mess with a web page element. For example, on my Web Design Playground site (see `webdesignplayground.io`), I use one of the jQuery UI interactions to enable coders to use a mouse to resize the width and height of the editors and other windows.

Applying an interaction

Before I describe the available interactions, take a look at the general syntax you use to apply one to an element:

```
$(selector).interaction(options|events);
```

- *`selector`*: A jQuery selector that specifies the web page element you want to work with.

» *interaction:* A string that specifies the name of the jQuery UI interaction you want to apply to the element.

» *options|events:* An object literal that includes one or more property-value pairs that specify the interaction options you want to use, and one or more interaction events you want to handle. Both the available options and the available events vary depending on the interaction.

For example, the following statement applies jQuery UI's `resizable` widget with two options that specify the element's minimum width and minimum height, as well as a handler for the widget's `resize` event, which fires when the element gets resized:

```
$('#my-div').resizable(
    {
        minWidth: 40,
        minHeight: 50,
        resize: function(event, ui) {
            console.log(ui.size.width);
        }
    }
);
```

In the event handler, the `event` argument refers to the event itself, whereas the `ui` argument refers to user interface object that the page visitor is interacting with. Most of the interaction widgets offer both `start` and `stop` events, which fire when the interaction begins and ends, respectively.

Getting to Know jQuery UI

Trying out the interactions

Here's a quick look at the available interactions offered by jQuery UI:

» `draggable`: Enables the user to move an element using a mouse. You can constrain the dragging to a particular direction by setting the `axis` property to either `x` (horizontal dragging only) or `y` (vertical dragging only). You can also set the transparency of the element while it's being dragged by setting the `opacity` property to a number between `0` (invisible) and `1` (fully visible). To run code while the element is dragged, create a handler for the `drag` event.

```
$('#my-div').draggable(
    {
        axis: 'x',
        opacity: .5,
```

```
            drag: function(event, ui) {
                console.log(ui.position.left);
            }
        }
    );
```

- droppable: Sets up an element as the target of a drag-and-drop operation. That is, if you apply the draggable widget to element A and the droppable widget to element B, the user can drag element A and drop it on element B. You can specify how much of the draggable element must overlap the droppable element before it is considered "dropped" by using the tolerance property set to one of the following: fit (complete overlap is required; this is the default); intersect (50 percent overlap required); pointer (the mouse pointer must be inside the droppable; or touch (any overlap will do). To run code when the element is dropped, create a handler for the drop event.

```
$('#my-div').droppable(
        {
            tolerance: 'intersect',
            drop: function(event, ui) {
                console.log('Dropped it!');
            }
        }
    );
```

- resizable: Enables the user to resize an element using a mouse. You can specify which directions the user can resize the element by adding the handles property, which is a comma-separated string consisting of one or more of the following directions: n, e, s, w, ne, se, sw, nw, and all. You can set limits on the element's dimensions (in pixels) by using the maxHeight, minHeight, maxWidth, and minWidth properties. To run code while the element is resized, create a handler for the resize event.

```
$('#my-div').resizable(
        {
            handles: 'e, se, s',
            minWidth: 50,
            minHeight: 25,
            resize: function(event, ui) {
                console.log(ui.size.width + ' ' ui.size.
    height);
            }
        }
    );
```

» `selectable`: Enables the user to select elements using a mouse. The user can either "lasso" the elements by using the mouse to drag a box around them, or the user can hold down either Ctrl (Windows) or ⌘ (Mac) and then click each element. You can specify how much of the lasso must overlap an element before it is considered "selected" by using the `tolerance` property set to either of the following: `fit` (complete overlap is required; this is the default), or `touch` (any overlap will do). To run code after each element is selected, create a handler for the `selecting` event.

```
$('#my-div').selectable(
    {
        tolerance: 'touch',
        selecting: function(event, ui) {
            console.log(ui.selecting.innerText);
        }
    }
);
```

» `sortable`: Enables the user to change the order of elements using a mouse. You can constrain the sort movement to a particular direction by setting the `axis` property to either `x` (horizontal sorting only) or `y` (vertical sorting only). You can also set the transparency of the element while it's being sorted by setting the `opacity` property to a number between `0` (invisible) and `1` (fully visible). To run code while an element is being sorted, create a handler for the `sort` event.

```
$('#my-div').sortable(
    {
        axis: 'y',
        opacity: .5,
        sort: function(event, ui) {
            console.log(ui.item[0].innerText);
        }
    }
);
```

5

Coding the Back End: PHP and MySQL

Contents at a Glance

» Building PHP expressions

» Controlling PHP code

» Figuring out functions and objects

» Debugging PHP

Chapter 1
Learning PHP Coding Basics

In the end, what I think set PHP apart in the early days, and still does today, is that it always tries to find the shortest path to solving the Web problem . . . When you need something up and working by Friday so you don't have to spend all weekend leafing through 800-page manuals, PHP starts to look pretty good.

— RASMUS LERDORF, CREATOR OF PHP

You code the front end of a web project using tools such as HTML and CSS (see Book 2), JavaScript (see Book 3), and jQuery (see Book 4). You can build really awesome web pages using just those front-end tools, but if you want to build pages that are dynamic and applike, then you need to bring in the back end and use it to harness the power of the web server. For web projects, the back end most often means storing data in a MySQL database and accessing that data using the PHP programming language. I cover all that in Chapters 2 and 3 of this minibook. For now, you need some background in PHP coding. In this chapter, you explore PHP from a web developer's perspective, and by the time you're done you'll know everything you need to know about PHP variables, expressions, arrays, loops, functions, and objects. In short, you'll be ready to join the web coding big leagues by bringing together the front end and the back end to create truly spectacular and useful web pages and apps.

Understanding How PHP Scripts Work

PHP is a *server-side* programming language, which means that PHP code executes only on the web server, not in the web browser. Most web servers today come with a piece of software called a *PHP processor*, and it's the job of the PHP processor to run any PHP code that's sent its way. That PHP code can come in two different packages:

- **A pure PHP file:** This is a file on the web server, usually one with a filename that uses the .php extension. When I call this a "pure" PHP file, I mean that the file contains nothing but PHP code. Such files are rarely loaded directly into the web browser. Instead, pure PHP files are usually called by JavaScript or jQuery code, most often either to process form input or to ask for data from a MySQL database.
- **As part of an HTML file:** This is a regular HTML file, but with one or more chunks of PHP code embedded in the file. On most web servers, this file requires the .php extension to enable the server to execute the PHP statements.

Whatever the package, the PHP code is processed as follows:

1. A web browser requests the PHP or HTML file.
2. When the web server sees that the file contains PHP code, it passes that code along to the PHP processor.
3. The PHP processor parses and executes the PHP code.
4. If the PHP code contains any statements that output text and/or HTML tags, the PHP processor returns that output to the web server.
5. The web server sends the output from Step 4 to the web browser.

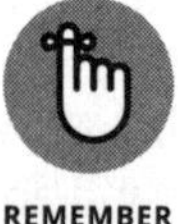
REMEMBER

It's important to understand that in the end no PHP code is ever sent to the web browser. All the browser gets is the output of the PHP code. Yes, it's possible to run PHP scripts that don't output anything, but in web development the main job of most of your PHP code will be to return some data to the browser.

Learning the Basic Syntax of PHP Scripts

You tell the web server that you want to run some PHP code by surrounding that code with the PHP tags:

```
<?php
    Your PHP statements go here
?>
```

For example, PHP's basic output mechanism is the echo *output* command, where *output* is a string containing text and/or HTML tags:

```
<?php
    echo "<h1>Hello PHP World!</h1>";
?>
```

REMEMBER

Notice that the echo statement ends with a semicolon. All PHP statements require a semicolon at the end.

If you place just the above code in a .php file and load that file into a web browser, you see the output shown in Figure 1-1.

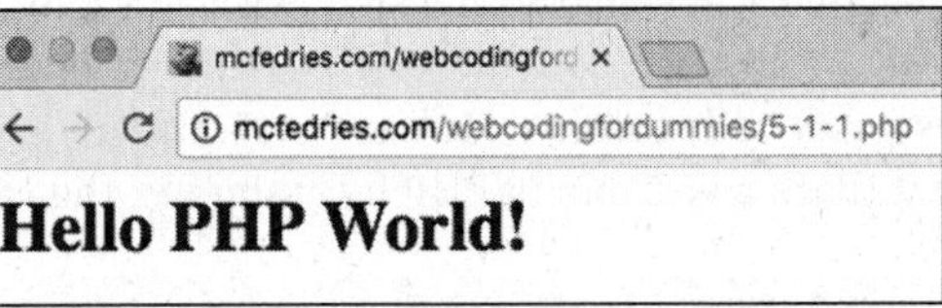

FIGURE 1-1: The output of PHP's echo command.

Alternatively, you can embed the PHP code in an HTML file, as shown in the following example:

```
<!DOCTYPE html>
<html lang="en">
    <head>
        <meta charset="UTF-8">
        <title>Book 5, Chapter 1, Example 2</title>
    </head>
    <body>
        <p>
            Here's the output of the PHP script:
        </p>
        <?php
            echo "<h1>Hello PHP World!</h1>";
        ?>
    </body>
</html>
```

Figure 1-2 shows the result.

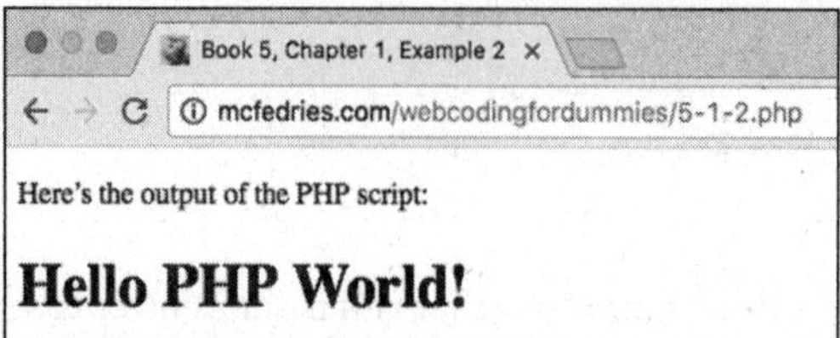

FIGURE 1-2: You can also embed PHP output within an HTML file.

Declaring PHP Variables

As with JavaScript (see Book 3, Chapter 2), PHP uses variables for storing data to use in expressions and functions, and PHP supports the standard literal data types: integers (such as `5` or `-17`), floating-point numbers (such as `2.4` or `3.14159`), strings (such as `"Hello"` or `'World'`), and Booleans (`TRUE` or `FALSE`).

PHP variable names must begin with a dollar sign (`$`), followed by a letter or underscore, then any combination of letters, numbers, or underscores. Note that PHP variable names are case-sensitive, so `$str` isn't the same variable as `$STR`.

You don't need any special keyword (such as JavaScript's `var`) to declare a variable. Instead, you declare a variable in PHP by assigning the variable a value:

```
$str = "Hello World!";
$interest_rate = 0.03;
$app_loaded = FALSE;
```

Building PHP Expressions

When you build a PHP expression — that is, a collection of symbols, words, and numbers that performs a calculation and produces a result — you can use mostly the same operators as in JavaScript (see Book 3, Chapter 3):

- **Arithmetic:** Addition (+), Subtraction (–), Multiplication (*), Division (/), Modulus (%), and Exponentiation (**).
- **Incrementing and decrementing:** Post-increment (`$var++`), Pre-increment (`++$var`), Post-decrement (`$var--`), and Pre-decrement (`--$var`).

- **Comparison:** Equal (=), Not Equal (!=), Greater Than (>), Less Than (<), Greater Than or Equal (>=), Less Than or Equal (<=), Identity (===), and Non-Identity (!==). In PHP you can also use <> as the Not Equal operator.
- **Logical:** And (&&), Or (||), and Not (!). In PHP you can also use and as the And operator and or as the Or operator.

Where PHP differs from JavaScript is with the string concatenation operator, which in PHP is the dot (.) symbol rather than JavaScript's plus (+) symbol. Here's an example, and Figure 1-3 shows the result.

```
<?php
    $str1 = "<h2>Concatenate ";
    $str2 = "Me!</h2>";
    echo $str1 . $str2;
?>
```

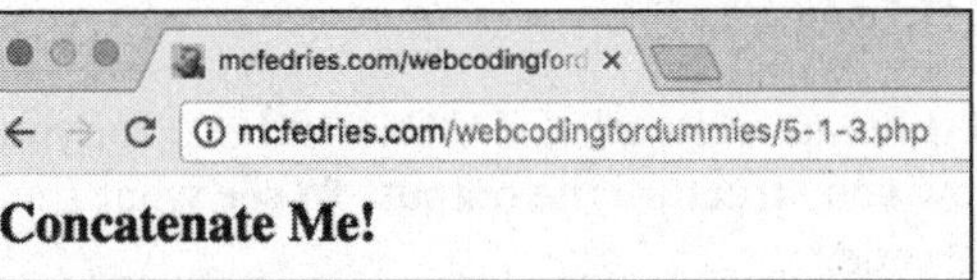

FIGURE 1-3: In PHP, you use the dot (.) operator to concatenate two strings.

Outputting Text and Tags

Your back-end PHP scripts pass data to your web app's front end (HTML and JavaScript) not by using some complex communications link, but simply by outputting the data. I talk about this in more detail in Book 5, Chapter 3, but for now let's look at the mechanisms PHP offers for outputting data.

PHP's simplest output tool is the `print` command:

```
print output;
```

- *output:* A string — which could be a string literal, string variable, string property value, or the string result of a function — that you want to output. You can include HTML tags in the output string.

```
<?php
    print "<h1>Hello World!</h1>";
?>
```

Learning PHP Coding Basics

To output more than one item, you need to use PHP's echo command:

```
echo output;
```

- **»** *output:* One or more strings — which could be string literals, string variables, string property values, or the string results of a function — that you want to output. If you include two or more output items, separate each one with a comma. You can include HTML tags in any of the output strings.

```
<?php
    $str1 = "<h2>Concatenate ";
    $str2 = "Me!</h2>";
    echo $str1, $str2;
?>
```

Adding line breaks

If you use PHP to generate quite a lot of HTML and text for your page, you need to be a bit careful how you structure the output. To see what I mean, first check out the following PHP code:

```
<?php
    $str1 = "<div>What does PHP stand for?</div>";
    $str2 = "<div>It's a <i>recursive acronym</i>:</div>";
    $str3 = "<div>PHP: Hypertext Preprocessor</div>";
    echo $str1, $str2, $str3;
?>
```

This code declares three strings — all div elements with text — and uses echo to output them. Figure 1-4 shows two browser windows. In the upper window, you can see that the output from the preceding code looks fine. However, the lower window shows the source code for the page and, as you can see, all the output text and tags appear on a single line.

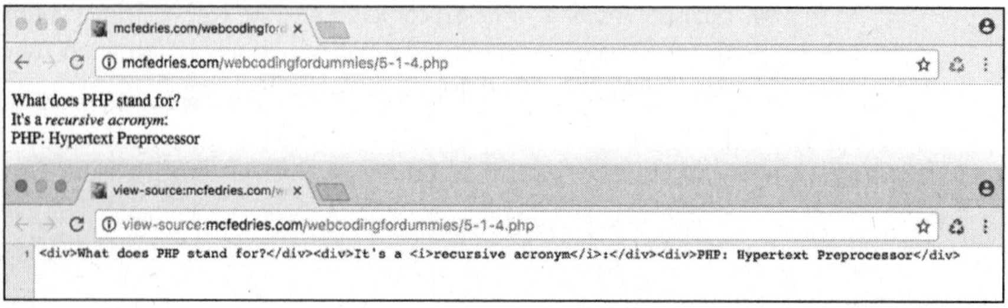

FIGURE 1-4: When you output tags and text using PHP, the strings run together in a single line in the web page source code.

To make the source code text easier to read, you should add line breaks to your PHP output strings. You insert a line break using the *newline* character `\n` (which doesn't appear on the web page). Here's the revised code (with `\n` added to the end of the `$str1` and `$str2` variables), and Figure 1-5 shows that the source code now appears on multiple lines:

```
<?php
    $str1 = "<div>What does PHP stand for?</div>\n";
    $str2 = "<div>It's a <i>recursive acronym</i>:</div>\n";
    $str3 = "<div>PHP: Hypertext Preprocessor</div>";
    echo $str1, $str2, $str3;
?>
```

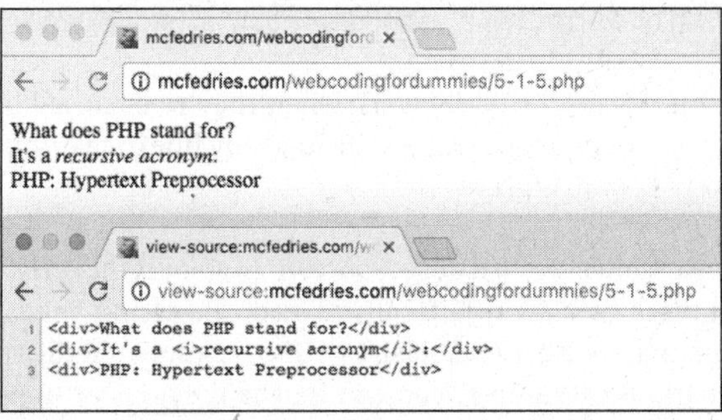

FIGURE 1-5: With newlines added to the output strings, the web page source code now appears on separate lines, making it much easier to read.

WARNING

The `\n` newline code only works in a string that uses double quotation marks. If you use single quotation marks, PHP outputs the characters `\n` instead of creating a newline. For example:

```
echo 'Ready\nSet\nGo!';
```

The output of this statement is

```
Ready\nSet\nGo!
```

Mixing and escaping quotation marks

You can enclose PHP string literals in either double quotation marks or single quotation marks, but not both:

```
$order = "Double espresso";        // This is legal
$book = 'A Singular Man';          // So's this
$weather = 'Mixed precipitation"; // This is not legal
```

However, mixing quotation mark types is sometimes necessary. Consider this:

```
$tag = "<a href="https://wordspy.com">";
```

That statement will cough up an error because PHP thinks the string ends after the second double quotation mark, so it doesn't know what to do with the rest of the statement. To solve this problem, swap the outer double quotation marks for singles:

```
$tag = '<a href="https://wordspy.com/">';
```

That works fine. However, what if you want to add some line breaks, as I describe in the previous section:

```
$tag = '<a href="https://wordspy.com/">\nWord Spy\n</a>';
```

Nice try, but newlines (`\n`) only work when they're enclosed by double quotation marks. The statement above will not include any line breaks and will show the link text as `\nWord Spy\n`. Sigh.

All is not lost, however, because you can convince the PHP processor to treat a quotation mark as a string literal (instead of a string delimiter), by preceding the quotation mark with a backslash (\). This is known in the trade as *escaping* the quotation mark. For example, you can fix the previous example by enclosing the entire string in double quotation marks (to get the newlines to work) and escaping the double quotation marks used for the `<a>` tag's `href` value:

```
$tag = "<a href=\"https://wordspy.com/\">\nWord Spy\n</a>";
```

Outputting variables in strings

One very useful feature of PHP strings is that you can insert a variable name into a string and the PHP processor will handily replace the variable name with its current value. Here's an example:

```
<?php
    $title = "Inflatable Dartboard Landing Page";
    $tag = "<title>$title</title>";
    echo $tag;
?>
```

The output of this code is

```
<title>Inflatable Dartboard Landing Page</title>
```

Some folks call this *interpolating* the variable, but we'll have none of that here.

Alas, variable value substitution only works with strings enclosed by double quotation marks. If you use single quotation marks, PHP outputs the variable name instead of its value. For example, this

```
<?php
    $title = "Inflatable Dartboard Landing Page";
    $tag = '<title>$title</title>';
    echo $tag;
?>
```

outputs this:

```
<title>$title</title>
```

Outputting long strings

If you have a long string to output, one way to do it would be to break up the string into multiple variables, add newlines at the end of each, if needed, and output each variable.

That works, but PHP offers a shortcut method where you output everything as a single string, but span the string across multiple lines. For example, I can take the final code from the "Adding line breaks" section and achieve the same result by rewriting it as follows:

```
<?php
$str1 = "<div>What does PHP stand for?</div>
<div>It's a <i>recursive acronym</i>:</div>
<div>PHP: Hypertext Preprocessor</div>";
echo $str1;
?>
```

The implied newlines at the end of the second and third lines are written to the page, so the page source code will look exactly the same as it does in Figure 1-5.

Outputting really long strings

For a super-long string, you can use PHP's *here document* (or *heredoc*) syntax:

```
<<<terminator
Super-long string goes here
terminator;
```

» `terminator`: This is a label that marks the beginning and end of the string. The label at the end must appear on a line by itself (except for the closing semicolon), with no whitespace before or after the label.

This syntax also supports variable names, so if you include a variable in the string, PHP will substitute the current value of that variable when it outputs the string.

Here's an example:

```
<?php
    $author = "Rasmus Lerdorf";
    $str = <<<END_OF_STRING
    <blockquote>
    In the end, what I think set PHP apart in the early
    days, and still does today, is that it always tries
    to find the shortest path to solving the Web
    problem. It does not try to be a general-purpose
    scripting language and anybody who's looking to
    solve a Web problem will usually find a very direct
    solution through PHP. Many of the alternatives that
    claim to solve the Web problem are just too complex.
    When you need something up and working by Friday so
    you don't have to spend all weekend leafing through
    800-page manuals, PHP starts to look pretty good.
    &mdash;$author
    </blockquote>
END_OF_STRING;
    echo $str;
?>
```

Notice that I declared a variable named `$author`, and then I included that variable name in the string (it's on the second-last line of the string). PHP treats a heredoc string as though it was enclosed by double quotation marks, so it substitutes the variable value in the output. Figure 1-6 shows the result.

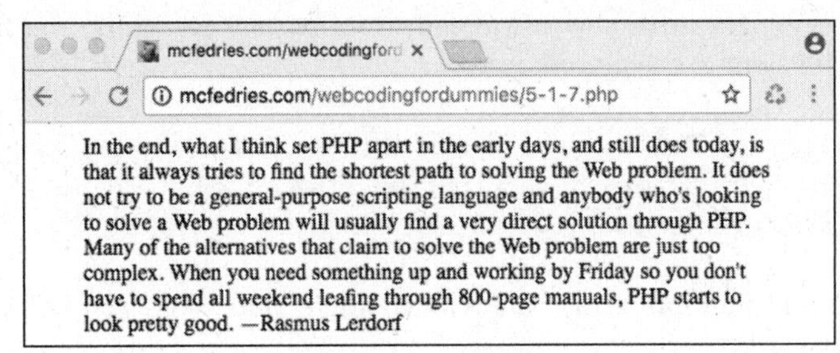

FIGURE 1-6: The really long string output to the web browser. Note that the value of the `$author` variable — `Rasmus Lerdorf` — appears instead of the variable name.

Working with PHP Arrays

Let's take a quick look at arrays in PHP. I'm going to skip lightly over arrays here because I already talk about them in detail in Book 3, Chapter 7.

Declaring arrays

PHP gives you a bunch of ways to declare and populate arrays. Probably the most straightforward method is to assign values to explicit index numbers:

```
$array_name[index] = value;
```

- *$array_name:* The name of the array variable
- *index:* The optional array index number you want to work with
- *value:* The value you want to assign to the array index number

For example, the following statements assign string values to the first three elements (that is, the elements at array indexes 0, 1, and 2) of an array named `$team_nicknames`:

```
$team_nicknames[0] = 'Banana Slugs';
$team_nicknames[1] = 'Fighting Okra';
$team_nicknames[2] = 'Golden Flashes';
```

Notice in the syntax that I said the *index* parameter was optional. If you leave it out, PHP assigns the index numbers automatically. So, as long as the variable

$team_nicknames doesn't already contain any elements, the following code is equivalent to the preceding code:

```
$team_nicknames[] = 'Banana Slugs';
$team_nicknames[] = 'Fighting Okra';
$team_nicknames[] = 'Golden Flashes';
```

To add multiple array values in a single statement, you can use PHP's array keyword:

```
$array_name = array(value1, value1, etc.);
```

- *$array_name*: The name of the array variable
- *value1*, *value2*, etc.: The values you want to assign to the array

Here's an example:

```
<?php
    $team_nicknames = array('Banana Slugs', 'Fighting Okra',
   'Golden Flashes');
    echo $team_nicknames[0];
?>
```

The output of this code is

```
Banana Slugs
```

Giving associative arrays a look

Most PHP arrays use numeric index values, but in web development work it's often handy to work with string index values, which are called *keys*. An array that uses keys instead of a numeric index is called an *associative array*, because you're associating each key with a value to create an array of key/value pairs.

Here's an example:

```
<?php
    $team_nicknames['Santa Cruz'] = 'Banana Slugs';
    $team_nicknames['Delta State'] = 'Fighting Okra';
    $team_nicknames['Kent State'] = 'Golden Flashes';
    echo $team_nicknames['Delta State'];
?>
```

The output of this code is

```
Fighting Okra
```

To create an associative array using the `array` keyword, you assign each key/value pair using the `=>` operator, as in this example:

```
<?php
    $team_nicknames = array('Santa Cruz' => 'Banana Slugs',
  'Delta State' => 'Fighting Okra', 'Kent State' => 'Golden
  Flashes');
    echo $team_nicknames['Kent State'];
?>
```

The output of this code is

```
Golden Flashes
```

Outputting array values

You can use the `echo` or `print` keyword to output individual array values. However, what if you want to see all the values stored in an array? Rather than, say, looping through the array, PHP offers the `print_r()` function, which outputs the current value of a variable:

```
print_r($variable);
```

» `$variable`: The name of the variable you want to output

If you use an array as the `print_r()` parameter, PHP outputs the contents of the array as key/value pairs. For example, the following code

```
<pre>
<?php
    $team_nicknames = array('Banana Slugs', 'Fighting Okra',
  'Golden Flashes');
    print_r($team_nicknames);
?>
</pre>
```

outputs the following:

```
Array
(
    [0] => Banana Slugs
    [1] => Fighting Okra
    [2] => Golden Flashes
)
```

TIP

Note that I surrounded the PHP code with the <pre> tag to get the output on multiple lines rather than a single hard-to-read line.

Sorting arrays

If you need your array values sorted alphanumerically, PHP offers a handful of functions that will get the job done. The function you use depends on the type of sort you want (ascending or descending) and whether your array uses numeric indexes or string keys (that is, an associative array).

For numeric indexes, you can use the `sort()` function to sort the values in ascending order (0 to 9, then A to Z, then a to z), or the `rsort()` function to sort the values in descending order (z to a, then Z to A, then 9 to 0):

```
sort($array);
rsort($array);
```

» *$array:* The name of the array you want to sort

Here's an example:

```
<pre>
<?php
    $oxymorons = array('Pretty ugly', 'Jumbo shrimp', 'Act
  naturally', 'Original copy');
    sort($oxymorons);
    print_r($oxymorons);
?>
</pre>
```

Here's the output:

```
Array
(
    [0] => Act naturally
    [1] => Jumbo shrimp
    [2] => Original copy
    [3] => Pretty ugly
)
```

For associative arrays, you can use the `asort()` function to sort the values in ascending order (0 to 9, then A to Z, then a to z), or the `arsort()` function to sort the values in descending order (z to a, then Z to A, then 9 to 0):

```
asort($array);
arsort($array);
```

» *$array*: The name of the associative array you want to sort

Here's an example:

```
<pre>
<?php
    $team_nicknames = array('Santa Cruz' => 'Banana Slugs',
  'Delta State' => 'Fighting Okra', 'Kent State' => 'Golden
  Flashes');
    arsort($team_nicknames);
    print_r($team_nicknames);
?>
</pre>
```

Here's the output:

```
Array
(
    [Kent State] => Golden Flashes
    [Delta State] => Fighting Okra
    [Santa Cruz] => Banana Slugs
)
```

Looping through array values

PHP offers a special loop called foreach() that you can use to loop through an array's values. Here's the syntax:

```
foreach($array as $key => $value) {
    Loop statements go here
}
```

- » *$array:* The name of the array you want to loop through
- » *$key:* An optional variable name that PHP uses to store the key of the current array item
- » *$value:* A variable name that PHP uses to store the value of the current array item

Here's an example:

```
<?php
    $team_nicknames = array('Santa Cruz' => 'Banana Slugs',
  'Delta State' => 'Fighting Okra', 'Kent State' => 'Golden
  Flashes');
    foreach($team_nicknames as $school => $nickname) {
        echo "The team nickname for $school is $nickname.<br>";
    }
?>
```

Here's the output:

```
The team nickname for Santa Cruz is Banana Slugs.
The team nickname for Delta State is Fighting Okra.
The team nickname for Kent State is Golden Flashes.
```

Creating multidimensional arrays

A *multidimensional array* is one where two or more values are stored within each array element. In a one-dimensional array, the *value* is usually a string, number, or Boolean. Now imagine, instead, that *value* is an array literal. For a two-dimensional array, the general syntax for assigning an array to an array element looks like this:

```
arrayName[index] = Array(value1, value2);
```

As an example, say you want to store an array of background and foreground colors. Here's how you might declare and populate such an array:

```
<?php
    $colorArray[0] = Array('white', 'black');
    $colorArray[1] = Array('aliceblue', 'midnightblue');
    $colorArray[2] = Array('honeydew', 'darkgreen');
    echo $colorArray[1][1];
?>
```

Here's the output:

```
midnightblue
```

Alternatively, you can declare and populate an associative array:

```
<?php
    $colorArray['scheme1'] = Array('foreground' => 'white',
  'background' => 'black');
    $colorArray['scheme2'] = Array('foreground' => 'aliceblue',
  'background' => 'midnightblue');
    $colorArray['scheme3'] = Array('foreground' => 'honeydew',
  'background' => 'darkgreen');
    echo $colorArray['scheme2']['foreground'];
?>
```

Here's the output:

```
aliceblue
```

Controlling the Flow of Your PHP Code

I go through a detailed discussion of controlling code with decisions and loops in Book 3, Chapter 4. That chapter focuses on JavaScript code, but the structures for making decisions and looping are identical in both JavaScript and PHP. Therefore, I just quickly summarize the available statements here, and refer you to Book 3, Chapter 4 to fill in the details.

Making decisions with if()

You make simple true/false decisions in PHP using the `if()` statement:

```
if (expression) {
    statements-if-true
}
```

- *`expression`:* A comparison or logical expression that returns `true` or `false`.
- *`statements-if-true`:* The statement or statements to run if *`expression`* returns `true`. If *`expression`* returns `false`, PHP skips over the statements.

Here's an example:

```
if ($original_amount !== 0) {
    $percent_increase = 100 * (($new_amount - $original_amount) /
  $original_amount);
}
```

To run one group of statements if the condition returns `true` and a different group if the result is `false`, use an `if()...else` statement:

```
if (expression) {
   statements-if-true
} else {
   statements-if-false
}
```

- *`expression`:* A comparison or logical expression that returns `true` or `false`
- *`statements-if-true`:* The block of statements you want PHP to run if *`expression`* returns `true`
- *`statements-if-false`:* The block of statements you want executed if *`expression`* returns `false`

Here's an example:

```
<?php
    if ($currentHour < 12) {
        $greeting = "Good morning!";
    } else {
```

```
        $greeting = "Good day!";
    }
    echo $greeting;
?>
```

There is a third syntax for the `if()...else` statement that lets you string together as many logical tests as you need:

```
if (expression1) {
   statements-if-expression1-true
} elseif (expression2) {
   statements-if-expression2-true
}
etc.
else {
   statements-if-false
}
```

REMEMBER

This syntax represents a rare instance where PHP and JavaScript control structures are different (however slightly): You use the keywords `else if` in JavaScript, but the single keyword `elseif` in PHP.

The following code shows a script that uses a nested `if()` statement.

```
<?php
    if ($currentHour < 12) {
        $greeting = "Good morning!";
    } elseif ($currentHour < 18) {
        $greeting = "Good afternoon!";
    } else {
        $greeting = "Good evening!";
    }
    echo $greeting;
?>
```

Making decisions with switch()

For situations where you need to make a whole bunch of tests (say, four or more), PHP offers the `switch()` statement. Here's the syntax:

```
switch(expression) {
    case case1:
        case1 statements
        break;
```

```
    case case2:
        case2 statements
        break;
    etc.
    default:
        default statements
}
```

The *expression* is evaluated at the beginning of the structure. It must return a value (numeric, string, or Boolean). *case1*, *case2*, and so on are possible values for *expression*. PHP examines each case value to see whether one matches the result of *expression* and, if it does, executes the block associated with that case; the `break` statement tells PHP to stop processing the rest of the `switch()` statement.

Here's an example:

```
switch($season) {
    case 'winter':
        $footwear = 'snowshoes';
        break;
    case 'spring':
        $footwear = 'galoshes';
        break;
    case 'summer':
        $footwear = 'flip-flops';
        break;
    case 'fall':
        $footwear = 'hiking boots';
        break;
}
```

Looping with while()

PHP's `while()` loop uses the following syntax:

```
while (expression) {
    statements
}
```

Here, *expression* is a comparison or logical expression that determines how many times the loop gets executed, and *statements* represents a block of statements to execute each time through the loop.

Here's an example:

```
<?php
    $counter = 1;
    while ($counter <= 12) {
        // Generate a random number between 1 and 100
        $randoms[$counter - 1] = rand(1, 100);
        $counter++;
    }
    print_r($randoms);
?>
```

Looping with for()

The structure of a PHP `for()` loop looks like this:

```
for ($counter = start; expression; $counter++) {
    statements
}
```

- *$counter:* A numeric variable used as a loop counter
- *start:* The initial value of *$counter*
- *expression:* A comparison or logical expression that determines the number of times through the loop
- *$counter++:* The increment operator applied to the *$counter* variable
- *statements:* The statements to execute each time through the loop

Here's an example:

```
<?php
    for ($counter = 0; $counter < 12; $counter++) {
        // Generate a random number between 1 and 100
        $randoms[$counter] = rand(1, 100);
    }
    print_r($randoms);
?>
```

Looping with do. . .while()

PHP's `do. . .while()` loop uses the following syntax:

```
do {
    statements
}
while (expression);
```

Here, *statements* represents a block of statements to execute each time through the loop, and *expression* is a comparison or logical expression that determines how many times PHP runs through the loop.

Here's an example:

```
<?php
    $counter = 0;
    do {
        // Generate a random number between 1 and 100
        $randoms[$counter] = rand(1, 100);
        $counter++;
    }
    while ($counter < 12);
    print_r($randoms);
?>
```

Working with PHP Functions

I talk about functions until I'm blue in the face in Book 3, Chapter 5. PHP and JavaScript handle functions in the same way, so here I just give you a quick overview from the PHP side of things.

The basic structure of a function looks like this:

```
function function_name(arguments) {
    statements
}
```

Here's a summary of the various parts of a function:

- `function`: Identifies the block of code that follows it as a function
- *`function_name`:* A unique name for the function
- *`arguments`:* One or more optional values that are passed to the function and that act as variables within the function
- *`statements`:* The code that performs the function's tasks or calculations

Here's an example:

```
function display_header() {
    echo "<header>\n";
    echo "<img src=\"/images/notw.png\" alt=\"News of the Word logo\">\n";
    echo "<h1>News of the Word</h1>\n";
    echo "<h3>Language news you won't find anywhere else (for good reason!)</h3>\n";
    echo "</header>";
}
```

To call the function, include in your script a statement consisting of the function name, followed by parentheses:

```
display_header();
```

Passing values to functions

An *argument* is a value that is "sent" — or *passed*, in programming terms — to the function. The argument acts just like a variable, and it automatically stores whatever value is sent. Here's an example:

```
display_header('notw.png');

function display_header($img_file) {
    echo "<header>\n";
    echo "<img src=\"/images/$img_file\" alt=\"News of the Word logo\">\n";
    echo "<h1>News of the Word</h1>\n";
    echo "<h3>Language news you won't find anywhere else (for good reason!)</h3>\n";
    echo "</header>";
}
```

Returning a value from a function

If your function calculates a result, you can send that result back to the statement that called the function by using a `return` statement:

```
return result;
```

As an example, I'll construct a function that calculates and then returns the tip on a restaurant bill:

```
$preTipTotal = 100.00;
$tipPercentage = 0.15;

function calculate_tip($preTip, $tipPercent) {
    $tipResult = $preTip * $tipPercent;
    return $tipResult;
}
$tipCost = calculate_tip($preTipTotal, $tipPercentage);
$totalBill = $preTipTotal + $tipCost;
echo "Your total bill is \$$totalBill";
```

Working with PHP Objects

I discuss objects from a JavaScript point of view in Book 3, Chapter 6, so here I just recall that an *object* is a programmable element that has two key characteristics:

- » You can make changes to the object's *properties*.
- » You can make the object perform a task by activating a *method* associated with the object.

I use objects extensively in Book 5, Chapter 3 when I talk about using PHP to access a MySQL database, so the next few sections provide some necessary background.

Rolling your own objects

Let's take a quick look at creating custom objects in PHP. In the object-oriented world, a *class* acts as a sort of object "template." A cookie cutter provides a good analogy. The cookie cutter isn't a cookie, but, when you use it, the cookie cutter creates an actual cookie that has a predefined shape. A class is the same way. It's not an object, but using it (or *instancing* it, to use the vernacular) creates an object that uses the class characteristics. These characteristics are governed by the *members* of the class, which are its properties and methods.

Creating a custom class

You define a custom class by using the `class` keyword:

```
class Name {
    Class properties and methods go here
}
```

» *Name:* The name you want to assign to your class. Class names traditionally begin with an uppercase letter.

Here's an example:

```
class Invoice {
}
```

I'll use this class to create customer invoice objects.

Adding properties to the class

The next step is to define the class properties, which are PHP variables preceded by the keyword `public`, which makes them available to code outside the class. Let's add a few properties to the `Invoice` class:

```
class Invoice {
    public $customer_id;
    public $subtotal;
    public $tax_rate;
}
```

A bit later I show you how to create an object from a class. In most cases you want to initialize some or all of the properties when you create the object, and to do that you must add a special `__construct()` function to the class definition. Here's the general syntax:

```
public function __construct($Arg1, $Arg2, ...) {
    $this->prop1 = $Arg1;
    $this->prop2 = $Arg2;
    etc.
}
```

» *$Arg1*, *$Arg2*, etc.: The initial values of the object properties.

» `$this->`: Refers to the object in which the code is running; the `->` character pair is called the *object operator* and you use it to access an object's properties and methods.

» *prop1*, *prop2*, etc.: References to the class properties, minus the $.

To extend the example:

```
class Invoice {
    public $customer_id;
    public $subtotal;
    public $tax_rate;

    public function __construct($Customer_ID, $Subtotal,
  $Tax_Rate) {
        $this->customer_id = $Customer_ID;
        $this->subtotal = $Subtotal;
        $this->tax_rate = $Tax_Rate;
    }
}
```

Adding methods to the class

The last step in creating your custom class is to add one or more functions that will be used as the class methods. Here's the general syntax:

```
public function method() {
    Method code goes here
}
```

» *method:* The name of the method

To complete our example class, add a method that calculates the invoice total and rounds it to two decimal places:

```
class Invoice {
    public $customer_id;
    public $subtotal;
    public $tax_rate;

    public function __construct($Customer_ID, $Subtotal,
  $Tax_Rate) {
```

```
        $this->customer_id = $Customer_ID;
        $this->subtotal = $Subtotal;
        $this->tax_rate = $Tax_Rate;
    }

    public function calculate_total() {
        $total = $this->subtotal * (1 + $this->tax_rate);
        return round($total, 2);
    }
}
```

Creating an object

Given a class — whether it's a built-in PHP class or a class that you've created yourself — you can create an object from the class, which is known as an *instance* of the class. Here's the general format to use:

```
$object = new Class(value1, value2, ...);
```

- *`$object`:* The variable name of the object
- *`Class`:* The name of the class on which to base the object
- *`value1`*, *`value2`*, etc.: The optional initial values you want to assign to the object's properties

Here's a statement that creates an instance of the `Invoice` class from the previous section:

```
$inv = new Invoice('BONAP', 59.85, .07);
```

Working with object properties

You refer to an object property by using the object operator (->):

```
object->property
```

- *`object`:* The object that has the property
- *`property`:* The name of the property you want to work with

Learning PHP Coding Basics

Here's an example that creates an object instance and then references the object's customer_id property:

```
$inv = new Invoice('BONAP', 59.85, .07);
$current_customer = $inv->customer_id;
```

To change the value of a property, use the following generic syntax:

```
object->property = value;
```

- *object*: The object that has the property
- *property*: The name of the property you want to change
- *value*: A literal value (such as a string or number) or an expression that returns the value to which you want to set the property

Here's an example:

```
$inv->subtotal = 99.95;
```

Working with object methods

To run a method, you use the following syntax:

```
object->method(arg1, arg2, ...)
```

- *object*: The object that has the method you want to work with
- *method*: The name of the method you want to execute
- *arg1*, *arg2*, etc.: The arguments required by the method, if any

Here's an example:

```
$inv = new Invoice('BONAP', 59.85, .07);
$invoice_total = $inv->calculate_total();
```

Debugging PHP

JavaScript code runs inside the browser, so debugging that code is straightforward because, in a sense, the code runs right before your eyes. This lets you set up breakpoints, watches, and the other debugging tools that I talk about in Book 3, Chapter 9. PHP code, however, runs on the server, which means that by the time it gets to you (that is, to the browser), the code is done and all you see is the output. That makes PHP code harder to debug, but, thankfully, not impossible to debug. The next few sections take you through a few PHP debugging techniques.

Configuring php.ini for debugging

Your first step in setting up PHP for debugging is the `php.ini` file, which is the PHP configuration file. In the XAMPP web development environment that I discuss in Book 1, Chapter 2, here are the default locations of `php.ini`:

- **Windows:** `C:\xampp\php\php.ini`
- **Mac:** `/Applications/XAMPP/xamppfiles/etc/php.ini`

If you can't locate the file, make sure your Apache web server is running, open the XAMPP Dashboard (`http://localhost/dashboard`), and click PHPInfo. Look for the Loaded Configuration File setting, as shown in Figure 1-7.

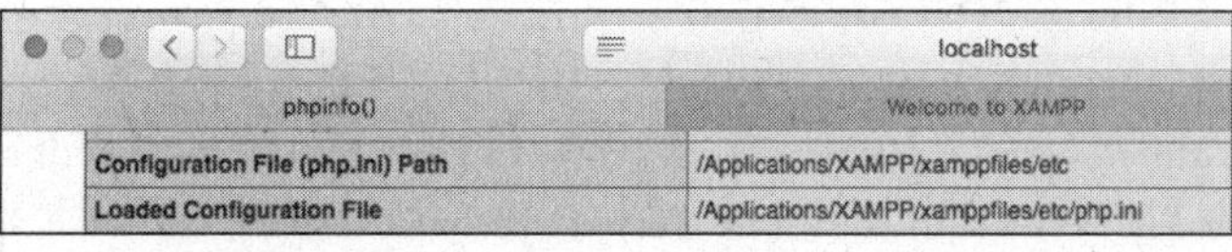

FIGURE 1-7: Examine the Loaded Configuration File setting to determine the location of php.i.

Open `php.ini` in your favorite text editor, then modify the following settings (`php.ini` is a long document, so you should search for each setting to save time):

- `display_errors`: Determines whether PHP outputs its error messages to the web browser. In a production environment, you want `display_errors` set to `Off` because you don't want site visitors seeing ugly PHP error messages. However, in a development environment, you definitely want `display_errors` set to On so you can see where your code went wrong:

```
display_errors=On
```

Learning PHP Coding Basics

» error_reporting: Specifies which types of errors PHP flags. The constant E_ALL flags all errors, and the constant E_STRICT flags code that doesn't meet recommended PHP standards. You don't need E_STRICT in a production environment, but it's useful in a development environment:

```
error_reporting=E_ALL | E_STRICT
```

With display_errors set to On, you'll now see error messages in the browser window. For example, take a look at the following statement:

```
display_header('notw.png';
```

Can you spot the error? Yep: the display_header function call is missing its closing parenthesis. Figure 1-8 shows how PHP flags this error. Notice that the message includes not only the error, but also the location of the file and, crucially, the line number of the statement that generated the error.

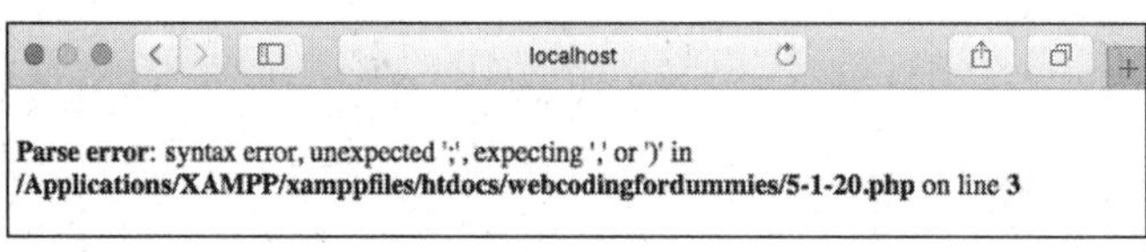

FIGURE 1-8: A typical PHP error message, showing the error, file path and name, and line number.

Accessing the PHP error log

Setting display_errors to On is very useful in your development environment, but the PHP default is to set display_errors to Off in a production environment. This prevents your visitors from seeing error messages, and it also boosts security because you don't want those visitors seeing sensitive information such as the location of your PHP script.

So what happens when PHP generates an error with display_errors set to Off? It depends on the error, but in most cases you either see a blank web page, or a server error message such as 500 - Internal server error. Neither is particularly helpful, but all is not lost because PHP still records the error message to the PHP error log.

That's nice, but where is this error log stored on the server? That depends on the server, but you can find out by running the following script:

```
<?php
    phpinfo();
?>
```

This displays the PHP configuration data, which includes an `error_log` setting that tells you where the PHP error log is stored.

In some cases, you see just the name of a file — usually `error_log` — and that means the server generates the error log in the same directory as the PHP file that caused the error. So, if you store all your PHP scripts in a php subdirectory, your error log will appear in that subdirectory.

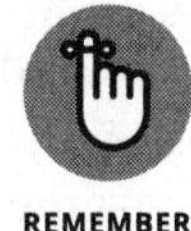

REMEMBER

Error messages appear in the error log with the oldest messages at the top, so to see the most recent error, you need to scroll to the bottom of the file.

Debugging with echo statements

You can't set up watch expressions on PHP code, but you can do the next best thing by strategically adding echo (or `print`) statements that output the current value of whatever variable or function result you want to watch.

For example, here's a loop that generates a dozen random numbers between 1 and 100. To watch the random values as they're generated, I included an echo statement within the loop:

```
<?php
    for ($i = 0; $i < 12; $i++) {
        $randoms[$i] = rand(1, 100);
        echo $randoms[$i] . '<br>';
    }
?>
```

Alternatively, you could wait until the loop completes and then run `print_r($random)` to output the entire array.

Another good use of echo statements for debugging is when your PHP code fails, but you don't get an error message. Now you have no idea where the problem lies, so what's a web developer to do? You can gradually narrow down where the error occurs by adding an echo statement to your code that outputs a message like `Made it this far!`. If you see that message, then you move the echo statement a little farther down the code, repeating this procedure until you don't see the message, meaning the code failed before getting to the echo statement.

Alternatively, you can sprinkle several echo statements throughout your code. You can either give each one a different output message, or you can take advantage of one of PHP's so-called *magic constants:* __LINE__. This constant tells you the current line of the code that's being executed, so you could add the following echo statement throughout your code:

```
echo 'Made it to line #' . __LINE__;
```

Debugging with var_dump() statements

PHP features such as echo and print_r make it easy to see values associated with variables and arrays, but sometimes your debugging efforts require a bit more information. For example, you might want to know the data type of a variable. You can get both the data type and the current value of a variable or expression by using PHP's var_dump() function:

```
var_dump(expression(s));
```

- *expression(s):* One or more variable names or expressions

Here's an update to the random number generator that dumps the value of the $randoms array after the loop:

```
<?php
    for ($i = 0; $i < 12; $i++) {
        $randoms[$i] = rand(1, 100);
    }
    var_dump($randoms);
?>
```

Here's an example of the output:

```
array(12) { [0]=> int(44) [1]=> int(92) [2]=> int(61) [3]=>
  int(61) [4]=> int(12) [5]=> int(60) [6]=> int(14) [7]=>
  int(46) [8]=> int(73) [9]=> int(29) [10]=> int(8) [11]=>
  int(71) }
```

» Building MySQL databases and tables

» Getting your head around SQL

» Selecting data with queries

» Modifying data with queries

Chapter 2

Building and Querying MySQL Databases

MySQL is a fast and powerful, yet easy-to-use, database system that offers just about anything a website would need in order to find and serve up data to browsers.

— ROBIN NIXON

One of the central themes of this book is that today's web is all about dynamic content. Sure, if you have (or your client has) just one or two web pages to show the world, then the standard front-end web development tools — HTML, CSS, and JavaScript — are more than enough to get the job done. However, it's much more likely that a modern website will consist of dozens, perhaps even hundreds of pages, with new content getting added regularly. Believe me, as the developer and/or administrator of such a site, you don't want to hand-code all those pages as static HTML and CSS. Life's too short! Fortunately, you don't have to hand-assemble all those pages if you get the back end of the web development world doing the hard work for you. The key is the database software that stores your site info on the server, and that's what this chapter is all about. Here you discover the MySQL database program and learn all that it can do to help you build and maintain dynamic, robust, and fast websites of any size.

What Is MySQL?

In simplest terms, a *database* is a collection of information with some sort of underlying structure and organization. MySQL (pronounced "my ess-kew-ell," or sometimes "my sequel") is a *database management system* (DBMS) that runs on the server. This means that MySQL will not only store the data you want to use as the source for some (or perhaps even all) of the data you want to display on your web page, but it will also supply you with the means to manage this data (by sorting, searching, extracting, and so on).

The official description of MySQL is that it's a *relational* database management system (RDBMS). The "relational" part means that you can set up relations between various parts of a database. For example, most businesses assign some sort of account number for each of their customers. So a database of customer information would include a column for this account number (as well as the name, address, credit limit, and so on). Similarly, you could also include the account number column in a collection of accounts receivable invoices (along with the invoice date, amount, and so on). This lets you relate each invoice to the appropriate customer information. (So, for example, you could easily look up phone numbers and call those deadbeat customers whose invoices are more than 90 days past due!)

MySQL is a massive piece of software that can do incredibly complicated things. Fortunately, as web developers we only need to use a small subset of MySQL's features, and we don't have to get into anything mind-blowingly complex. To get started on developing dynamic web pages, in fact, you only need to know about two pieces of the MySQL puzzle: tables and queries.

Tables: Containers for your data

In MySQL databases, you store your information in an object called a *table*. Tables are essentially a grid, where each vertical segment represents a *column* (a specific category of information) and each horizontal segment represents a *row* (a single record in the table).

Figure 2-1 shows a table of customer data. Notice how the table includes separate columns for each logical grouping of the data (company name, contact name, and so on).

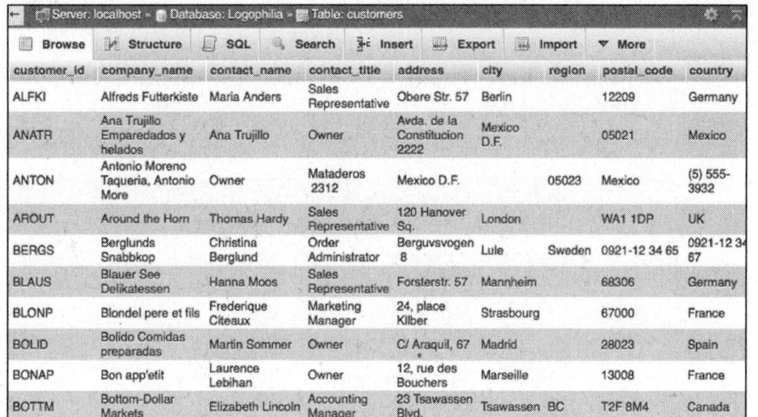

customer_id	company_name	contact_name	contact_title	address	city	region	postal_code	country
ALFKI	Alfreds Futterkiste	Maria Anders	Sales Representative	Obere Str. 57	Berlin		12209	Germany
ANATR	Ana Trujillo Emparedados y helados	Ana Trujillo	Owner	Avda. de la Constitucion 2222	Mexico D.F.		05021	Mexico
ANTON	Antonio Moreno Taqueria, Antonio More	Owner	Mataderos 2312	Mexico D.F.		05023	Mexico	(5) 555-3932
AROUT	Around the Horn	Thomas Hardy	Sales Representative	120 Hanover Sq.	London		WA1 1DP	UK
BERGS	Berglunds Snabbkop	Christina Berglund	Order Administrator	Berguvsvogen 8	Lule	Sweden	0921-12 34 65	0921-12 34 67
BLAUS	Blauer See Delikatessen	Hanna Moos	Sales Representative	Forsterstr. 57	Mannheim		68306	Germany
BLONP	Blondel pere et fils	Frederique Citeaux	Marketing Manager	24, place Kliber	Strasbourg		67000	France
BOLID	Bolido Comidas preparadas	Martin Sommer	Owner	C/ Araquil, 67	Madrid		28023	Spain
BONAP	Bon app'etit	Laurence Lebihan	Owner	12, rue des Bouchers	Marseille		13008	France
BOTTM	Bottom-Dollar Markets	Elizabeth Lincoln	Accounting Manager	23 Tsawassen Blvd.	Tsawassen	BC	T2F 8M4	Canada

FIGURE 2-1: In MySQL databases, tables store the raw data.

REMEMBER

In web development, you use MySQL tables to store the data that will appear in your pages. To get that data from the server to the web page requires five steps:

1. On the web page, some JavaScript code launches a PHP script on the server.
2. That PHP script asks a MySQL database for the data required by the web page.
3. The PHP script configures the data into a format that JavaScript can understand.
4. PHP sends the data back to the web page.
5. The JavaScript code accepts the data and displays it on the page.

I go through these steps in glorious detail in Book 5, Chapter 3 and in Book 6, Chapter 1.

Queries: Asking questions of your data

By far the most common concern expressed by new database users (and many old-timers, as well) is how to extract the information they need from all that data. What if, for example, you have a database of accounts receivable invoices and your boss wants a web page that tells her how many invoices are more than 150 days past due? You can't hand-code such a page because, for a large database, your page would be out of date before you were done. The better way would be to ask MySQL to do the work for you by creating another type of database object: a *query*. Queries are, literally, questions you ask of your data. In this case, you could ask MySQL to display a list of all invoices more than 150 days past due.

Queries let you extract from one or more tables a subset of the data. For example, in a table of customer names and addresses, what if I wanted to see a list of firms that are located in France? No problem. I'd just set up a query that asks, in effect, "Which rows have `'France'` in the `country` column?" The answer to this question is shown in Figure 2-2.

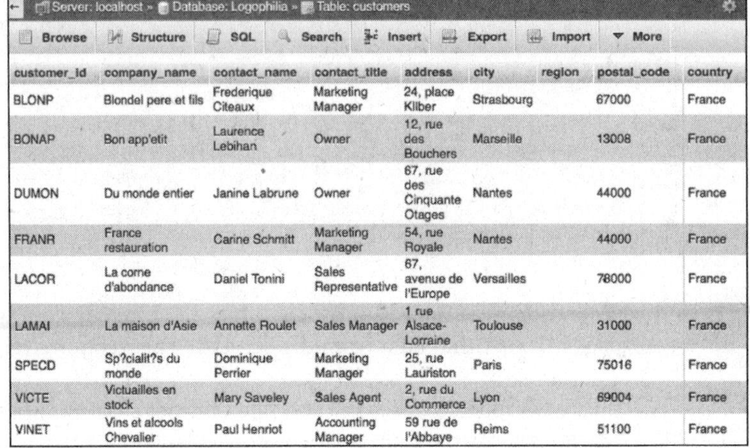

customer_id	company_name	contact_name	contact_title	address	city	region	postal_code	country
BLONP	Blondel pere et fils	Frederique Citeaux	Marketing Manager	24, place Kliber	Strasbourg		67000	France
BONAP	Bon app'etit	Laurence Lebihan	Owner	12, rue des Bouchers	Marseille		13008	France
DUMON	Du monde entier	Janine Labrune	Owner	67, rue des Cinquante Otages	Nantes		44000	France
FRANR	France restauration	Carine Schmitt	Marketing Manager	54, rue Royale	Nantes		44000	France
LACOR	La corne d'abondance	Daniel Tonini	Sales Representative	67, avenue de l'Europe	Versailles		78000	France
LAMAI	La maison d'Asie	Annette Roulet	Sales Manager	1 rue Alsace-Lorraine	Toulouse		31000	France
SPECD	Sp?cialit?s du monde	Dominique Perrier	Marketing Manager	25, rue Lauriston	Paris		75016	France
VICTE	Victuailles en stock	Mary Saveley	Sales Agent	2, rue du Commerce	Lyon		69004	France
VINET	Vins et alcools Chevalier	Paul Henriot	Accounting Manager	59 rue de l'Abbaye	Reims		51100	France

FIGURE 2-2: You use MySQL queries to extract a subset of the data from one or more tables.

The actual querying process is performed using a technology called Structured Query Language (or SQL, pronounced "ess-kew-ell"). In the five-step procedure I mention in the previous section, the SQL portion takes place in Step 2.

Introducing phpMyAdmin

To work with MySQL — whether it's creating a database, importing or exporting data, adding a table, inserting and editing data, or testing SQL statements to use in your PHP code — almost all web hosts offer a web application called phpMyAdmin. (It's an odd name, I know: It means, more or less, "PHP-based MySQL Administration.")

In the XAMPP web development environment that I discuss in Book 1, Chapter 2, you have two ways to get phpMyAdmin on the job (make sure you have the Apache web server running):

- **Dashboard:** From the XAMPP Dashboard page (`http://localhost/dashboard`), click the `phpMyAdmin` link in the header.
- **Direct:** Use a web browser to surf to `http://localhost/phpmyadmin`.

Figure 2-3 shows the default phpMyAdmin page.

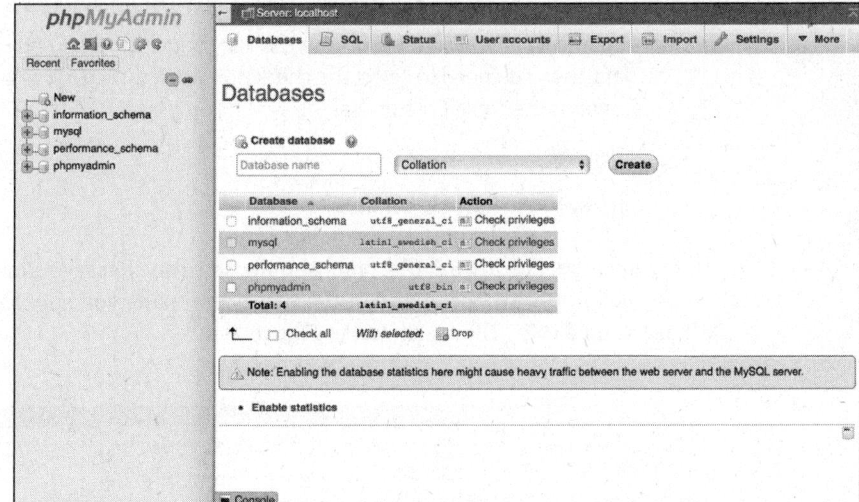

FIGURE 2-3: From the XAMPP Dashboard, click `phpMyAdmin` to open the phpMyAdmin web app.

The navigation pane on the left shows the default databases that come with phpMyAdmin (don't mess with these!), while the tabs across the top — Databases, SQL, and so on — take you to different parts of the application.

Importing data into MySQL

Before I talk about building a database from scratch, let me first go through the procedure for getting some existing data into MySQL. phpMyAdmin supports several import formats, but you'll most likely want to use a comma-separated values (`.csv`) file, where the column data in each row is separated by commas. Another possibility is a SQL (`.sql`) file, which is a backup file for a MySQL database.

1. **In phpMyAdmin, click the Import tab.**

   If you don't see the Import tab, click More, then click Import.

2. **In the File to Import section, click Browse (Windows) or Choose File (Mac).**

   Your operating system's file chooser dialog appears.

3. **Click the file that contains the data you want to import and then click Open (Windows) or Choose (Mac).**

4. **In the Format section, make sure the list shows the correct format for the file you chose.**

   If you're importing a CSV file, the list should have CSV selected; if you're importing a SQL backup file, the list should have SQL selected.

5. **If you're importing a CSV file, use the Format-Specific Options section to tell phpMyAdmin the structure of the file.**

In particular, if the first line of your CSV file contains the column names of your data, then you need to select the check box labeled The First Line of the File Contains the Table Column Names.

6. **Click Go.**

   phpMyAdmin imports the data.

If you imported a CSV file, you should see the message `Import has been successfully finished` and in the navigation pane you should see a new database named CSV_DB, as shown in Figure 2-4.

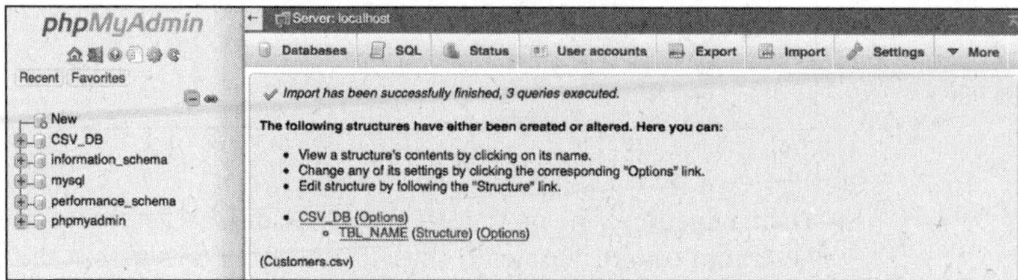

FIGURE 2-4: Importing a CSV file creates the CSV_DB database.

Here are the steps to follow to rename the database and the table that contains the imported data:

1. **In the navigation pane, click CSV_DB.**

   phpMyAdmin opens the database. Notice that you now see a table named TBL_NAME. That's the table that contains the imported CSV data. I show you how to rename it beginning with Step 6.

2. **Click the Operations tab.**

   If you don't see the Operations tab, click More, then click Operations.

3. **In the Rename Database To section, type the new database name in the text box provided.**

4. **Click Go.**

   phpMyAdmin asks you to confirm.

5. **Click OK.**

   phpMyAdmin changes the database name.

6. **In the navigation pane, click TBL_NAME.**

7. **Click the Operations tab.**

   If you don't see the Operations tab, click More, then click Operations.

8. **In the Table Options section, use the Rename Table To text box to type the new table.**
9. **Click Go.**

   phpMyAdmin changes the table name.

Backing up MySQL data

As you work with phpMyAdmin, you should run periodic backups to make sure your data is safe. Here are the steps to follow:

1. **In phpMyAdmin, click the Export tab.**

   If you don't see the Export tab, click More, then click Export.
2. **In the Format section, use the list to select SQL (although this is the default format).**
3. **Click Go.**

   phpMyAdmin exports the data, which your web browser then downloads to your computer.

Creating a MySQL Database and Its Tables

If you don't import your data, then you need to create your own MySQL databases and populate them with the tables that will hold the actual data.

Creating a MySQL database

The first question you need to ask yourself is: Do I need just a single database or do I need multiple databases? As a web developer, you'll almost always need multiple databases. Here's why:

- » You need a separate database for each website you build.
- » You need a separate database for each web app you build.
- » You need a separate database for each client you have.

If you're just building a single website or app, and you have no clients, then one database is fine, but know that MySQL is ready and willing to accommodate almost any number of databases you care to throw at it.

Here are the steps to follow to create a database using phpMyAdmin:

1. **In the navigation pane, click New that appears at the top of the navigation tree.**
2. **In the Create Database section, use the Database Name text box to type the name you want to use.**
3. **In the Collation list, select utf8_general_ci.**

   Collation refers to how MySQL compares characters (for example, when sorting data). In this case, you're telling MySQL to use a standard, case-insensitive (for example, a equals A) collation on the UTF-8 character set.
4. **Click Create.**

   phpMyAdmin creates the database for you.

Designing your table

You need to plan your table design before you create it. By asking yourself a few questions in advance, you can save yourself the trouble of redesigning your table later. For simple tables, you need to ask yourself three basic questions:

- Does the table belong in the current database?
- What type of data should I store in each table?
- What columns should I use to store the data?

The next few sections examine these questions in more detail.

Does the table belong in the current database?

Each database you create should be set up for a specific purpose: a website, a web app, a client, and so on. Once you know the purpose of the database, you can then decide if the table you want to create fits in with the database theme.

For example, if the purpose of the database is to store a client's data, it would be inappropriate to include a table that stores your personal blog posts. Similarly, it wouldn't make sense to include a table of a web app's user accounts in a database that belongs to an entirely different website.

What type of data should I store in each table?

The most important step in creating a table is determining the information you want it to contain. In theory, MySQL tables can be quite large: up to 4,096 columns and many millions (even billions) of rows. In practice, however, you should strive to keep your tables as small as possible. This saves memory and makes managing the data easier. Ideally, you should aim to set up all your tables with only essential information.

Suppose you want to store user information in a database. You have to decide whether you want all your users in a single table, or whether it would be better to create separate tables for each type of user. For example, a table of customers would include detailed information such as each person's first and last names, postal address, phone number, payment preference, and more. By contrast, a table of people who have opted-in to receive your newsletters might store each person's email address, the newsletters she wants to receive, the subscription type (full or digest), and more. There's not a lot of overlap between these two types of customers, so it probably makes sense to create two separate tables.

When you've decided on the tables you want to use, you then need to think about how much data you want to store in each table. In your customers table, for example, would you also want to include information on each person's site customizations, account creation date, date of last visit, and product preferences? This might all be crucial information for you, but you need to remember that the more data you store, the longer it will take to query and sort the data.

What columns should I use to store the data?

Now you're almost ready for action. The last thing you need to figure out is the specific columns to include in the database. For the most part, the columns are determined by the data itself. For example, a database of business contacts would certainly include columns for name, address, and phone number. But should you split the name into two columns — one for the first name and one for the last name? If you think you'll need to sort the table by last name, then, yes, you probably should. What about the address? You'll probably need individual columns for the city, state, and ZIP code.

Here are two general rules to follow when deciding how many columns to include in your tables:

- Ask yourself whether you really need the data for a particular column (or if you might need it in the near future). For example, if you think your table of contact names might someday be used to create form letters, a column to record titles (Ms., Mr., Dr., and so on) would come in handy. When in doubt, err on the side of too many columns rather than too few.
- Always split your data into the smallest columns that make sense. Splitting first and last names is common practice, but creating a separate column for, say, the phone number area code would probably be overkill.

REMEMBER

Don't sweat the design process too much. It's easy to make changes down the road (by adding or deleting columns), so you're never stuck with a bad design.

Deciding which column to use for a primary key

When you create a table, you need to decide which column to use as the *primary key*. The primary key is a column that uses a unique number or character sequence to identify each row in the table. Keys are used constantly in the real world. Your Social Security number is a key that identifies you in government records. Most machines and appliances have unique serial numbers. This book (like most books) has a 13-digit ISBN — International Standard Book Number (which you can see on the back cover).

Why are primary keys necessary? Well, for one thing, MySQL creates an *index* for the primary key column. You can perform searches on indexed data much more quickly than on regular data; therefore, many MySQL operations perform faster if a primary key is present. Keys also make it easy to find rows in a table because the key entries are unique (things such as last names and addresses can have multiple spellings, which makes them hard to find). Finally, once a table has a primary key, MySQL adds its data editing tools, which enable you to modify, copy, and delete table data.

You can configure the table so that MySQL sets and maintains the primary key for you, or you can do it yourself. Which one do you choose? Here are some guidelines:

- If your data contains a number or character sequence that uniquely defines each row, you can set the key yourself. For example, invoices usually have unique numbers that are perfect for a primary key. Other columns that can serve as primary keys are employee IDs, customer account numbers, and purchase order numbers.
- If your data has no such unique identifier, let MySQL create a key for you. This means that MySQL will set up an AUTO_INCREMENT column that will automatically assign a unique number to each row (the first row will be 1, the second 2, and so on).

Relating tables

MySQL is a *relational* database system, which means that you can establish relationships between multiple tables. As an example, suppose you have a database that contains (at least) two tables:

- `orders`: This table holds data on orders placed by your customers, including the customer name, the date of the order, and so on. It also includes an `order_id` column as the primary key, as shown in Figure 2-5.

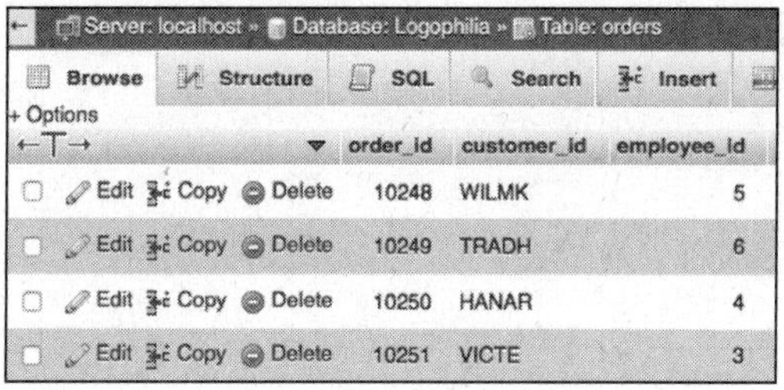

Server: localhost » Database: Logophilia » Table: orders

Browse | Structure | SQL | Search | Insert

+ Options

←T→	order_id	customer_id	employee_id
Edit Copy Delete	10248	WILMK	5
Edit Copy Delete	10249	TRADH	6
Edit Copy Delete	10250	HANAR	4
Edit Copy Delete	10251	VICTE	3

FIGURE 2-5: The `orders` table includes a column named `order_id`.

- **`order_details`:** This table holds data on the specific products that comprise each order: the product name, the unit price, the quantity ordered. It also includes an `order_id` field, as shown in Figure 2-6.

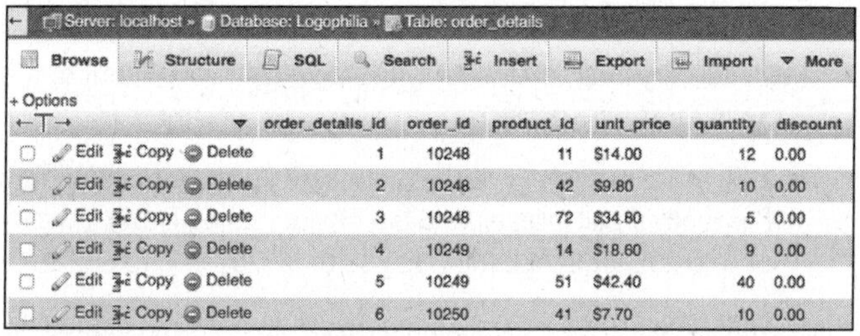

Server: localhost » Database: Logophilia » Table: order_details

Browse | Structure | SQL | Search | Insert | Export | Import | More

+ Options

←T→	order_details_id	order_id	product_id	unit_price	quantity	discount
Edit Copy Delete	1	10248	11	$14.00	12	0.00
Edit Copy Delete	2	10248	42	$9.80	10	0.00
Edit Copy Delete	3	10248	72	$34.80	5	0.00
Edit Copy Delete	4	10249	14	$18.60	9	0.00
Edit Copy Delete	5	10249	51	$42.40	40	0.00
Edit Copy Delete	6	10250	41	$7.70	10	0.00

FIGURE 2-6: The `order_details` table also includes a column named `order_id`.

Why not lump both tables into a single table? Well, that would mean that, for each product ordered, you'd have to include the name of the customer, the order date, and so on. If the customer purchased ten different products, this information would be repeated ten times. To avoid such waste, the data is kept in separate tables, and the two tables are *related* on the common column called `order_id`.

For example, notice in Figure 2-5 that the first row in the `orders` table has an `order_id` value of 10248. Now check out Figure 2-6, where you see that the first three rows of the `order_details` table also have an `order_id` value of 10248. This means that when you join these tables on the related `order_id` field, MySQL combines the data, as shown in Figure 2-7. For example, notice that the first three rows still have an `order_id` value of 10248, but they now also include the `customer_id` column from the `orders` table.

Creating a MySQL table

Here are the steps to follow to create a table in a MySQL database:

1. **In the navigation pane, click the database in which you want to add the table.**

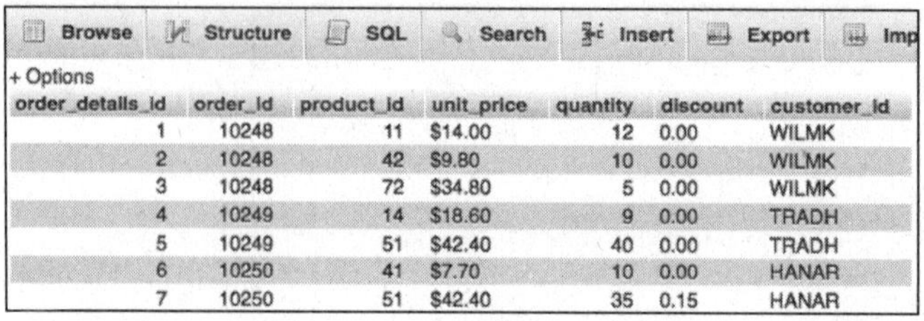

Browse Structure SQL Search Insert Export Imp

+ Options

order_details_id	order_id	product_id	unit_price	quantity	discount	customer_id
1	10248	11	$14.00	12	0.00	WILMK
2	10248	42	$9.80	10	0.00	WILMK
3	10248	72	$34.80	5	0.00	WILMK
4	10249	14	$18.60	9	0.00	TRADH
5	10249	51	$42.40	40	0.00	TRADH
6	10250	41	$7.70	10	0.00	HANAR
7	10250	51	$42.40	35	0.15	HANAR

FIGURE 2-7: The `order_details` and `orders` tables joined on the common column named `order_id`.

2. **In the Structure tab, use the Create Table section to type a name for the table, select the number of columns you want, and then click Go.**

   If you're not sure how many columns you need, just make your best guess for now. You can always add more later on.

3. **Type a name for the column.**

4. **In the Type list, select the data type you want to use for the data.**

   There's a very long list of data types to wade through, but only a few make sense in most web projects:

   - **`INT`:** Stores an integer value between -2,147,483,648 and 2,147,483,648. For really small integer values, consider using either `TINYINT` (-128 to 127 or 0 to 255) or `SMALLINT` (-32,768 to 32,767 or 0 to 65,535).
   - **`VARCHAR`:** Stores a variable-length string between 0 and 65,535 characters long. If you need to store super-long chunks of text, consider `MEDIUMTEXT` (up to 16,777,215 characters) instead.
   - **`DATE`:** Stores a date and time value.

5. **If you selected `VARCHAR` in Step 4, you can use the Length/Values field to enter a maximum size for the column.**

6. **Use the Default list to specify a default value that MySQL will enter automatically into the column when you create a new row.**

   If you want the current date and time in a `DATE` column, select `CURRENT_TIMESTAMP`. Otherwise, select `As Defined`, then enter a value in the text box that appears.

7. **In the Collation list, select `utf8_general_ci`.**

8. **To allow MySQL to enter no value into the column, select the Null check box.**

   If you leave Null deselected, then be sure you always specify a value for the column.

9. **If you want MySQL to index the column, use the Index list to select the type of index you want.**

In most cases you should choose the all-purpose `INDEX` type; if the column values are all different, select the `UNIQUE` type; for a text-heavy field, select the `FULLTEXT` type.

Don't index every column. Instead, you only need to index those columns that you'll be using for sorting and querying.

10. **Repeat Steps 3 through 9 until you've defined all your columns.**
11. **Click Save.**

Adding data to a table

Ideally, most of your table data will get inserted automatically, either by importing data or by having your page users fill in an HTML form (see Book 6, Chapters 2 and 3). If you do need to enter table data by hand, here's how it's done:

1. **In the navigation pane, click the table in which you want the data added.**
2. **Click the Insert tab.**

   phpMyAdmin displays empty text boxes for each column in the table. If you see two sets of text boxes, scroll down to the bottom of the Insert tab and change Continue Insertion with 2 Rows to Continue Insertion with 1 Row.
3. **Use the Value fields to add a value for each column.**

   If a column accepts null values (that is, if the column's Null check box is selected), then it's okay to leave that column's Value field blank.
4. **If you want to add multiple rows, use the two lists near the bottom of the page to select Insert as New Row and then Insert Another New Row.**
5. **Click Go to insert the data.**

Creating a primary key

When you import a table, MySQL doesn't automatically create a primary key, so you need to follow these steps to create the primary key yourself:

1. **In the navigation pane, click the table you want to work with.**
2. **Click the Structure tab.**
3. **Click the check box that appears to the left of the column you want to use as the primary key.**

   Make sure you select a column that contains only unique values.

4. **Click Primary.**

   MySQL configures the column as the table's primary key.

What happens if none of your table's fields contain unique items? In that case, you need to create a column to use as the primary key. Here's how:

1. **In the navigation pane, click the table you want to work with.**
2. **Click the Structure tab.**
3. **Leave the Add 1 Columns as is, but select At Beginning of Table in the list, then click Go.**
4. **Type a name for the primary key field.**

   If you're not sure what name to use, something like `table_id` would work, where *`table`* is the name of the table.
5. **Select the A_I (AUTO_INCREMENT) check box.**

   MySQL displays the Add Index dialog.
6. **Leave the default settings as they are, and then click Go.**
7. **Click Save.**

   MySQL adds the field and automatically populates it with unique integer values.

Querying MySQL Data

It's all well and good having a bunch of data hunkered down in a MySQL database, but as a web developer, your real concern is getting that data from the server to the web page. That complete journey is the subject of both Book 5, Chapter 3 and Book 6, Chapter 1, but I'm going to tackle the first leg of the trip here and show you how to specify the data that will eventually get sent to the page. The technique I'm going to show you is called *querying* the data, and the tool of choice is Structured Query Language, or SQL.

What is SQL?

SQL is a collection of commands that interrogate or modify — *query*, in the SQL vernacular — MySQL data in some way. SQL is huge, but as a web developer you really only need to know about four query types:

- **SELECT:** Returns a subset of a table's data
- **INSERT:** Adds a new row to a table
- **UPDATE:** Modifies a table's existing data
- **DELETE:** Removes one or more rows from a table

In the case of the SELECT, UPDATE, and DELETE query types, you target the specific rows you want to work with by specifying *criteria*, which are extra parameters that define one or more conditions the rows must meet. For example, you might want to run a `SELECT` query that returns only those customers where the `country` column is equal to `France`. Similarly, you might want to run a `DELETE` query only on those items in the `products` table where the `discontinued` column has the value `TRUE`.

Creating a SELECT query

The most common type of query is the SELECT query that returns rows from one or more tables based on the columns you choose and the criteria you apply to those columns. It's called a *SELECT* query not only because you use it to select certain rows, but also because it's based on the SQL language's `SELECT` statement. `SELECT` is the SQL "verb" that you'll see and work with most often, and it's used to create a subset based on the table, columns, criteria, and other clauses specified in the statement. Here's a simplified syntax for the `SELECT` verb:

```
SELECT select_columns
    FROM table_name
    WHERE criteria
    ORDER BY sort_columns [DESC]
```

- `SELECT` *`select_columns`*: Specifies the names of the columns you want in your subset. If you want all the columns, use `*` instead.
- `FROM` *`table_name`*: The name of table that contains the data.
- `WHERE` *`criteria`*: Filters the data to give you only those rows that match the specified *`criteria`*.
- `ORDER BY` *`sort_columns`*: Sorts the results in ascending order based on the data in the columns specified by *`sort_columns`* (separated by commas, if you have more than one). Use the optional `DESC` keyword to sort the rows in descending order.

The most basic SELECT query is one that returns all the rows from a table. For example, the following SELECT statement returns all the rows from the customers table:

```
SELECT *
    FROM customers
```

In the following example, only the company_name, city, and country columns are returned in the results:

```
SELECT company_name, city, country
    FROM customers
```

Here's another example that sorts the rows based on the values in the company_name column:

```
SELECT *
    FROM customers
    ORDER BY company_name
```

Understanding query criteria

The heart of any query is its criteria. They are a set of expressions that determine the rows that are included in the query results. All query expressions have the same general structure. They contain one or more *operands* — which can be literal values (such as 123 or "USA" or 2018-08-23), *identifiers* (names of MySQL objects, such as tables), or functions — separated by one or more *operators* — the symbols that combine the operands in some way, such as the plus sign (+) and the greater than sign (>).

Most criteria expressions are logical formulas that, when applied to each row in the table, return TRUE or FALSE. The subset contains only those rows for which the expression returns TRUE.

Comparison operators

You use comparison operators to compare field values to a literal, a function result, or to a value in another field. Table 2-1 lists MySQL's comparison operators.

TABLE 2-1 **Comparison Operators for Criteria Expressions**

Operator	General Form	Matches Rows Where . . .
=	= *Value*	The column value is equal to *Value*.
<>	<> *Value*	The column value is not equal to *Value*.
>	> *Value*	The column value is greater than *Value*.
>=	>= *Value*	The column value is greater than or equal to *Value*.
<	< *Value*	The column value is less than *Value*.
<=	<= *Value*	The column value is less than or equal to *Value*.

For example, suppose you have a `products` table with a `units_in_stock` column. If you want a SELECT query to return just those products that are out of stock, you'd use the following SQL statement:

```
SELECT *
    FROM products
    WHERE units_in_stock = 0
```

The LIKE operator

If you need to allow for multiple spellings in a text column, or if you're not sure how to spell a word you want to use, the *wildcard characters* can help. There are two wildcards: the underscore (_) substitutes for a single character, and the percent sign (%) substitutes for a group of characters. You use them in combination with the `LIKE` operator, as shown in Table 2-3.

TABLE 2-3 **The LIKE Operator for Criteria Expressions**

Example	Matches Rows Where . . .
`LIKE 'Re_d'`	The column value is `Reid`, `Read`, `reed`, and so on.
`LIKE 'M_'`	The column value is `MA`, `MD`, `ME`, and so on.
`LIKE 'R%'`	The column value begins with `R`.
`LIKE '%office%'`	The column value contains the word `office`.
`LIKE '2017-12-%'`	The column value is any date in December 2017.

The BETWEEN. . .AND operator

If you need to select rows where a column value lies between two other values, use the BETWEEN. . .AND operator. For example, suppose you want to see all the rows in the order_details table where the quantity value is between (and includes) 50 and 100. Here's a SELECT statement that does the job:

```
SELECT *
    FROM order_details
    WHERE quantity BETWEEN 50 AND 100
```

You can use this operator for numbers, dates, and even text.

The IN operator

You use the IN operator to match rows where the specified column value is one of a set of values. For example, suppose you want to return a subset of the customers table that contains only those rows where the region column equals NY, CA, TX, IN, or ME. Here's the SELECT statement to use:

```
SELECT *
    FROM customers
    WHERE region IN('NY','CA','TX','IN','ME')
```

The IS NULL operator

What do you do if you want to select rows where a certain column is empty? For example, a table of invoices might have a date_paid column where, if this column is empty, it means the invoice hasn't been paid yet. For these challenges, MySQL provides the IS NULL operator. Applying this operator to a column selects only those rows whereby the column is empty. Here's an example:

```
SELECT *
    FROM invoices
    WHERE date_paid IS NULL
```

To select rows when a particular column is *not* empty, use the IS NOT NULL operator.

Compound criteria and the logical operators

For many criteria, a single expression just doesn't do the job. For more sophisticated needs, you can set up *compound criteria* where you enter either multiple expressions for the same column or multiple expressions for different columns. You use the logical operators to combine or modify expressions. Table 2-4 summarizes MySQL's logical operators.

TABLE 2-4 Logical Operators for Criteria Expressions

Operator	General Form	Matches Rows When . . .
AND	*Expr1* And *Expr2*	Both *Expr1* and *Expr2* are TRUE.
OR	*Expr1* Or *Expr2*	At least one of *Expr1* and *Expr2* is TRUE.
NOT	Not *Expr*	*Expr* is not TRUE.
XOR	*Expr1* Xor *Expr2*	Only one of *Expr1* and *Expr2* is TRUE (XOR is short for *exclusive or*).

The AND and OR operators let you create compound criteria using a single expression. For example, suppose you want to match all the rows in your products table where the units_in_stock column is either 0 or greater than or equal to 100. The following SELECT statement does the job:

```
SELECT *
    FROM products
    WHERE units_in_stock = 0 OR units_in_stock >= 100
```

The NOT operator looks for rows that *don't* match a particular logical expression. In a table of customer data, for example, if you want to find all non-North American customers, you filter out the customers using the country column, like so:

```
SELECT *
    FROM customers
    WHERE NOT country = 'USA' AND
          NOT country = 'Canada' AND
          NOT country 'Mexico'
```

Querying multiple tables

Although most of your MySQL queries will use just a single table, some of the most useful and powerful queries involve two (or more) tables. The type of multiple-table query you'll see and use most often is called an *inner join* because it joins two tables based on a common column.

To create an inner join on two tables, use the following version of the FROM clause:

```
FROM table1
    INNER JOIN table2
    ON table1.column = table2.column
```

Here, *table1* and *table2* are the names of the two tables you want to join, and *table1.column* and *table2.column* are the common columns in each table. Note that the column names don't have to be the same.

For example, suppose you have two tables: orders and order_details, and they each have a column named order_id that stores a value that is unique for each order. The following SELECT statement sets up an inner join on these tables:

```
SELECT *
    FROM orders
    INNER JOIN order_details
    ON orders.order_id = order_details.order_id
```

If you only want certain columns from both tables in the results, specify the column names after the SELECT command using the *table.column* syntax, as in this example:

```
SELECT orders.order_id, orders.customer_id,
  order_details.quantity
    FROM orders
    INNER JOIN order_details
    ON orders.order_id = order_details.order_id
```

INNER JOINS? OUTER JOINS? WHAT'S THE DIFFERENCE?

TECHNICAL STUFF

Besides inner joins, MySQL also supports a variation on the multiple-table query theme called an *outer join*. To understand the difference between these two join types, let's run through some examples using the sample data in the following table.

The novelties table has two columns: name and supplier, and the suppliers table has a single column: supplier. Here are three things to note about these tables:

- The two tables have the supplier column in common.
- The novelties table includes several rows that use Internal as the supplier value, but Internal is not listed in the suppliers table.
- The suppliers table includes one row — Nov-L-T Industries — that is not used anywhere in the novelties table.

The `novelties` Table		The `suppliers` Table
name	**supplier**	**supplier**
Inflatable Dartboard	Facepalm LLC	Facepalm LLC
Banana Peel Welcome Mat	Facepalm LLC	RUSerious, Ltd.
Non-Reflective Mirror	Facepalm LLC	Silly Stuff, Inc.
Fireproof Firewood	Internal	Nov-L-T Industries
Donut Holes	Internal	
No-String Guitar	Internal	
Helium Paperweight	RUSerious, Ltd.	
Sandpaper Bathroom Tissue	RUSerious, Ltd.	
All-Stick Frying Pan	Silly Stuff, Inc.	
Water-Resistant Sponge	Silly Stuff, Inc.	

An inner join only returns the overlapping data between two tables. To visualize this, consider the following Venn diagram.

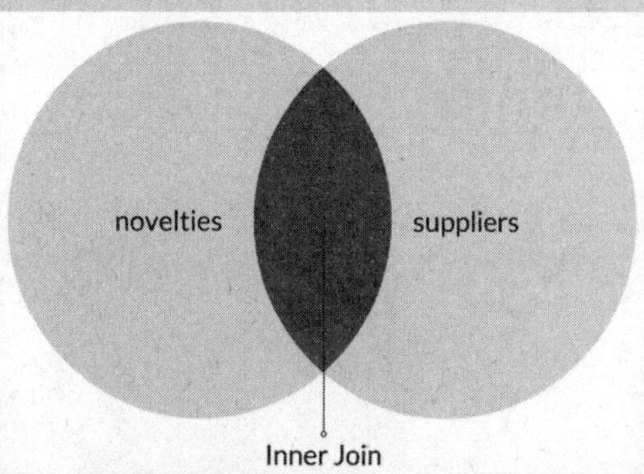

Here's a SELECT statement that runs an inner join on the `novelties` and `suppliers` tables:

```
SELECT novelties.name, suppliers.supplier
    FROM novelties
```

(continued)

(continued)

```
INNER JOIN suppliers
ON novelties.supplier = suppliers.supplier
```

Here are the results:

novelties.name	**suppliers.supplier**
Inflatable Dartboard	Facepalm LLC
Banana Peel Welcome Mat	Facepalm LLC
Non-Reflective Mirror	Facepalm LLC
Helium Paperweight	RUSerious, Ltd.
Sandpaper Bathroom Tissue	RUSerious, Ltd.
All-Stick Frying Pan	Silly Stuff, Inc.
Water-Resistant Sponge	Silly Stuff, Inc.

Notice that from the `novelties` table we don't see any of the rows that had `Internal` as the `supplier` value because that value doesn't appear in the `suppliers` table. Similarly, we don't see the `Nov-L-T Industries` supplier because that value doesn't appear in the `novelties` table.

However, suppose we want all the novelties to appear in the results. That's called a *left outer join*, and to see why, take a look at the following Venn diagram. This join includes all the `novelties` rows, plus the overlapping data from the `suppliers` table.

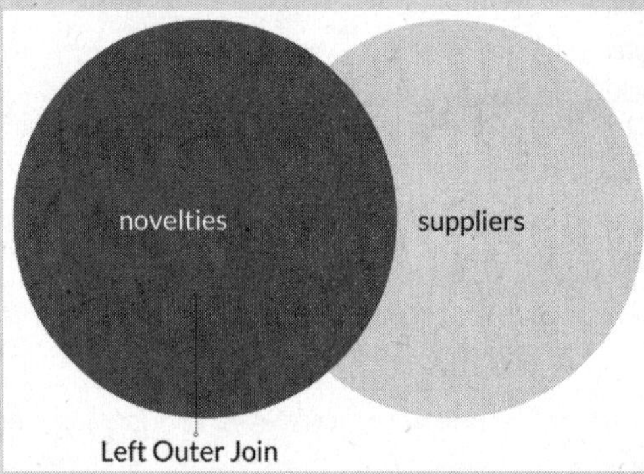

Here's a `SELECT` statement that runs a left outer join on the `novelties` and `suppliers` tables:

```
SELECT novelties.name, suppliers.supplier
    FROM novelties
    LEFT OUTER JOIN suppliers
    ON novelties.supplier = suppliers.supplier
```

Here are the results:

name	**supplier**
Inflatable Dartboard	Facepalm LLC
Banana Peel Welcome Mat	Facepalm LLC
Non-Reflective Mirror	Facepalm LLC
Fireproof Firewood	NULL
Donut Holes	NULL
No-String Guitar	NULL
Helium Paperweight	RUSerious, Ltd.
Sandpaper Bathroom Tissue	RUSerious, Ltd.
All-Stick Frying Pan	Silly Stuff, Inc.
Water-Resistant Sponge	Silly Stuff, Inc.

Notice that for those novelties that don't have a corresponding `supplier` value in the `suppliers` table, MySQL returns `NULL`.

Finally, you might want all the suppliers to appear in the results. That's called a *right outer join,* and you can see why by taking a peek at the following Venn diagram. This join includes all the `suppliers` rows, plus the overlapping data from the `novelties` table.

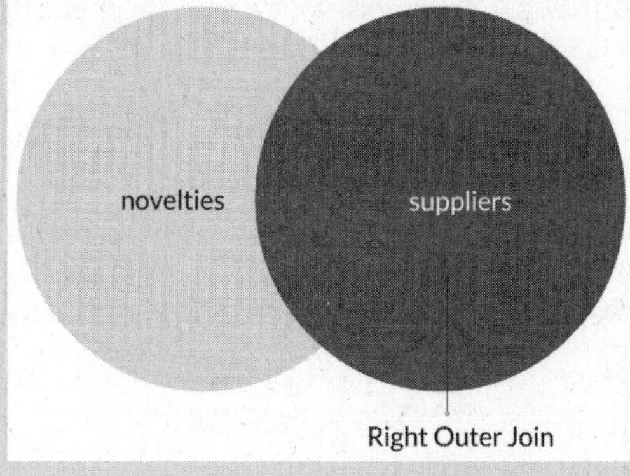

(continued)

(continued)

Here's a SELECT statement that runs a right outer join on the novelties and suppliers tables:

```
SELECT novelties.name, suppliers.supplier
    FROM novelties
    RIGHT OUTER JOIN suppliers
    ON novelties.supplier = suppliers.supplier
```

Here are the results:

name	supplier
Inflatable Dartboard	Facepalm LLC
Banana Peel Welcome Mat	Facepalm LLC
Non-Reflective Mirror	Facepalm LLC
NULL	Nov-L-T Industries
Helium Paperweight	RUSerious, Ltd.
Sandpaper Bathroom Tissue	RUSerious, Ltd.
All-Stick Frying Pan	Silly Stuff, Inc.
Water-Resistant Sponge	Silly Stuff, Inc.

Notice that for those suppliers that don't have a corresponding `supplier` value in the `novelties` table, MySQL returns NULL.

Adding table data with an INSERT query

An INSERT query adds a new row to an existing table. In MySQL, you build an INSERT query using the `INSERT` verb:

```
INSERT
    INTO table (columns)
    VALUES (values)
```

- *table:* The name of the table into which you want the row appended.
- *columns:* A comma-separated list of column names from *table*. The values you specify will be added to these columns.

» *values:* A comma-separated list of values that you want to add. The order of these values must correspond with the order of the column names in the *columns* parameter.

For example, suppose we have a table named categories that includes three fields: category_id, category_name, and description. First, assume that category_id is the table's primary key and its value is generated automatically by an AUTO_INCREMENT function, which means you can ignore it when building your INSERT query. Therefore, you can use the following SQL statement to add a new row:

```
INSERT
    INTO categories (category_name, description)
    VALUES ('Breads', 'Multi-grain, rye, and other
   deliciousness')
```

Modifying table data with an UPDATE query

An UPDATE query modifies the values in one or more columns and optionally restricts the scope of the updating to those rows that satisfy some criteria. In MySQL, you build an UPDATE query by using the UPDATE verb to construct a statement with the following syntax:

```
UPDATE table
    SET column1=value1,column2=value2,...
    WHERE criteria
```

» *table:* The table that contains the data you want to update

» *column1=value1,column2=value2,* etc.: The new values you want to assign to the specified columns

» *criteria:* The criteria that define which rows will be updated

For example, suppose you have products table and want to increase the values in the unit_price column by 5 percent for the Beverages category (category_id = 1). This is the same as multiplying the current unit_price values by 1.05, so the UPDATE statement looks like this:

```
UPDATE products
    SET unit_price = unit_price*1.05
    WHERE CategoryID = 1
```

Removing table data with a DELETE query

A DELETE query removes rows from a table and optionally restricts the scope of the deletion to those rows that satisfy some criteria. If you don't include criteria, MySQL deletes every row in the specified table.

In MySQL, you build a delete query by using the `DELETE` verb to construct a statement with the following syntax:

```
DELETE
    FROM table
    WHERE criteria
```

- *`table`:* The table that contains the rows you want to delete
- *`criteria`:* The criteria that defines which rows will be deleted

For example, if you want to delete those rows in the `products` table where the `supplier_id` value is 1, you use the following SQL statement:

```
DELETE
    FROM products
    WHERE supplier_id = 1
```

marriage

- Connecting to a MySQL database with PHP
- Using PHP to access MySQL data with a SELECT query
- Processing the SELECT query results
- Using PHP to run INSERT, UPDATE, and DELETE queries

Chapter 3

Using PHP to Access MySQL Data

PHP and MySQL work together to provide powerful, flexible components that can keep up with the expanding database driven development needs of virtually any organization, large or small.

— ISAAC DUNLAP

Run a Google search on the text `PHP MySQL "Match made in heaven"` and you get more than a few results. I'm not surprised one bit because it seems as though these two technologies were meant to be together; a case of love at first byte, as it were. What's the secret of their success as a couple? First, it helps that they're both free (not the usual prerequisite for marriage success, I know), which ensures that they're both widely available and widely supported. Second, both PHP and MySQL reward a little bit of learning effort up front with a lot of flexibility and power right off the bat. Although both are complex, sophisticated pieces of technology, you need to learn only a few basics to take your web development skills to a whole new level. I cover the first two parts of those basics in Chapters 1 and 2 of this minibook. In this chapter, I bring everything together by showing you how to combine PHP and MySQL to create the foundation you need to build truly dynamic and powerful web applications.

Understanding the Role of PHP and MySQL in Your Web App

Before getting to the trees of actual PHP code, I want to take a moment to look out over the forest of the server back end, so you're comfortable and familiar with the process. Specifically, I want to look at how PHP and MySQL team up to deliver the back-end portion of a web app. Rather than getting bogged down in an abstract discussion of what happens when a user requests a page that requires some data from the server, I'll use a concrete example. The following steps take you through the back-end process that happens when the web app I built to display this book's sample code gets a request for a specific example:

1. **A reader (perhaps even you!) requests the web page of a specific book sample page. Here's a for instance:**

   ```
   http://mcfedries.com/webcodingfordummies/example.php?book=
      4&chapter=1&example=2
   ```

   The PHP script file is `example.php` and the request data — known to the cognoscenti as a *query string* — is everything after the question mark (?): `book=4&chapter=1&example=2`. This string is requesting the second example from Book 4, Chapter 1.

2. **The web server retrieves `example.php` and sends it to the PHP processor.**
3. **The PHP script parses the query string to determine which sample the user is requesting.**

   For the query string shown in Step 1, the script would extract the book number as 4, the chapter number as 1, and the example number as 2.

4. **The script connects to the database that stores the code samples.**
5. **The script uses the query string data to create and run a SELECT query that returns the sample code.**

   The `SELECT` statement looks something like this:

   ```
   SELECT *
       FROM code_samples
       WHERE book_num=4 AND chapter_num=1 AND example_num=2
   ```

6. **The script massages the SELECT results into a format readable by the browser.**

   This format is usually just HTML, but another popular format is JSON (JavaScript Object Notation), which you learn about in Book 6, Chapter 1.

7. **The web server sends the formatted data to the web browser, which displays the code sample.**

The rest of this chapter expands on Steps 3 through 6.

Using PHP to Access MySQL Data

When used as the back end of a web app, PHP's main job is to interact with MySQL to retrieve the data requested by the app and then format that data so that it's usable by the app for display in the browser. To do all that, PHP runs through five steps:

1. Get the request parameters from the URL query string.
2. Connect to the MySQL database.
3. Create and run a SELECT query to extract the requested data.
4. Get the data ready to be sent to the browser.
5. Output the data for the web browser.

I talk about INSERT, UPDATE, and DELETE queries later in this chapter, but the next few sections take you through the details of this five-step procedure from the point of view of a SELECT query.

WARNING

In the sections that follow, I don't discuss security techniques for blocking malicious hacking attempts. That's a crucial topic, however, so I devote a big chunk of Book 7, Chapter 1 to the all-important details, which you should read before deploying any dynamic web apps.

Parsing the query string

Many PHP scripts don't require any information from the web app to get the data that the app needs. For example, if the script's job is to return every record from a table, or to return a predetermined subset of a table, then your app just needs to call the script.

However, it's more common for a web app to decide on-the-fly (say, based on user input or some other event) what data it requires, and in such cases it needs to let the server know what to send. To get your web app to request data from the web server, you send a query string to the server. You can send a query string using two different methods:

- **GET:** Specifies the data by adding the query string to the URL of the request. This is the method I talk about in this chapter.
- **POST:** Specifies the data by adding it to the HTTP header of the request. This method is associated with HTML forms and some AJAX requests, which I cover in Book 6.

In the GET case, the query string is a series of name-value pairs that use the following general form:

```
name1=value1&name2=value2&...
```

Here's an example:

```
book=4&chapter=1&example=2
```

In the case of a GET request, you build the request by taking the URL of the PHP script that will handle the request, adding a question mark (?) to designate the boundary between the script address and the query string, and then adding the query string itself. Here's an example:

```
http://mcfedries.com/webcodingfordummies/example.php?book=
   4&chapter=1&example=2
```

Now your PHP script has something to work with, and you access the query string data by using PHP's `$_GET` variable, which is an associative array created from the query string's name-value pairs. Specifically, the array's keys are the query string's names, and the array's values are the corresponding query string values. For example, the preceding URL creates the following `$_GET` array:

```
$_GET['book'] => 4
$_GET['chapter'] => 1
$_GET['example'] => 2
```

Note, however, that it's good programming practice to not assume that the `$_GET` array is populated successfully every time. You should check each element of the array by using PHP's `isset()` function, which returns `true` if a variable exists and has a value other than `null`. Here's some PHP code that checks that each element of the preceding `$_GET` array exists and isn't `null`:

```
if (isset($_GET['book'])) {
    $book_num = $_GET['book'];
} else {
    echo 'The "book" parameter is missing!<br>';
    echo 'We are done here, sorry.';
    exit(0);
}
if (isset($_GET['chapter'])) {
    $chapter_num = $_GET['chapter'];
} else {
    echo 'The "chapter" parameter is missing!<br>';
    echo 'Sorry it didn\'t work out.';
    exit(0);
}
if (isset($_GET['example'])) {
    $example_num = $_GET['example'];
} else {
    echo 'The "example" parameter is missing!<br>';
    echo 'You had <em>one</em> job!';
    exit(0);
}
```

This code checks each element of the `$_GET` array:

- If the element exists and isn't `null`, the code assigns the array value to a variable.
- If the element either doesn't exist or is `null`, the code outputs a message specifying the missing parameter and then stops the code by running the `exit(0)` function (the `0` just means that you're terminating the script in the standard way).

Connecting to the MySQL database

You give PHP access to MySQL through an object called `MySQLi` (short for *MySQL Improved*). There are actually several ways to bring PHP and MySQL together, but MySQLi is both modern and straightforward, so it's the one I cover in this book.

You connect to a MySQL database by creating an instance of the `MySQLi` object. Here's the general format to use:

```
$var = new MySQLi(hostname, username, password, database);
```

» `$var`: The variable that stores the new `MySQLi` object.

» `hostname`: The name of the server that's running MySQL. If the server is on the same computer as your script (which is usually the case), then you can use `localhost` as the `hostname`.

» `username`: The account name of a user who has access to the MySQL database.

» `password`: The password associated with the `username` account.

» `database`: The name of the MySQL database.

Here's a script that sets up the connection parameters using four variables, and then creates the new `MySQLi` object:

```
<?php
    $host = 'localhost';
    $user = 'logophil_reader';
    $password = 'webcodingfordummies';
    $database = 'logophil_webcodingfordummies';

    $mysqli = new MySQLi($host, $user, $password, $database);
?>
```

However, you shouldn't connect to a database without also checking that the connection was successful. Fortunately, the `MySQLi` object makes this easy by setting two properties when an error occurs:

» `connect_errno`: The error number

» `connect_error`: The error message

These properties are `null` by default, so your code can use an `if()` test to check if either `connect_error` or `connect_errno` has been set:

```
if($mysqli->connect_error) {
    echo 'Connection Failed!
          Error #' . $mysqli->connect_errno
             . ': ' . $mysqli->connect_error;
    exit(0);
}
```

If an error occurs, the code displays a message like the one shown in Figure 3-1 and then runs `exit(0)` to stop execution of the script.

FIGURE 3-1: An example of an error number and message generated by the MySQLi object.

Connection Failed! Error #1045: Access denied for user 'logophil_reader'@'localhost' (using password: YES)

Before moving on to querying the database, there are two quick housekeeping chores you need to add to your code. First, tell your MySQLi object to use the UTF-8 character set:

```
$mysqli->set_charset('utf8');
```

Second, use the MySQLi object's close() method to close the database connection by adding the following statement at the end of your script (that is, just before the ?> closing tag):

```
$mysqli->close();
```

Using PHP to Access MySQL Data

Creating and running the SELECT query

To run a SELECT query on the database, you need to create a string variable to hold the SELECT statement and then use that string to run the MySQLi object's query() method. Here's an example:

```
$sql = 'SELECT category_name, description
        FROM categories';
$result = $mysqli->query($sql);

// Check for a query error
if (!$result) {
    echo 'Query Failed!
          Error: ' . $mysqli->error;
    exit(0);
}
```

The result of the query is stored in the $result variable. You might think that this variable now holds all the data, but that's not the case. Instead, $result is an object that contains information about the data, not the data itself. You make use of that information in the next section, but for now notice that you can use the result object to check for an error in the query. That is, if $result is null, the query failed, so display the error message (using the MySQLi object's error property) and exit the script.

TIP

If you want to know how many rows the SELECT query returned, you can reference the result object's `num_rows` property:

```
$result->num_rows
```

Storing the query results in an array

The object returned by the `query()` method is really just a pointer to the actual data, but you can use the object to retrieve the SELECT query's rows. There are various ways to do this, but I'll go the associative array route, which uses the result object's `fetch_all(MYSQLI_ASSOC)` method to return all the rows as an associative array. (If you prefer to work with a numeric array, replace the `MYSQLI_ASSOC` constant with `MYSQLI_NUM`):

```
$array = $mysqli_result->fetch_all(MYSQLI_ASSOC);
```

- *$array*: The name of the associative array you want to use to hold the query rows
- *$mysqli_result*: The result object returned by MySQLi's `query()` method

Note that this is a two-dimensional array, which makes sense because table data is two-dimensional (that is, it consists of one or more rows and one or more columns).

I'll make this more concrete by extending the example:

```
$sql = 'SELECT category_name, description
        FROM categories';
$result = $mysqli->query($sql);

// Check for a query error
if (!$result) {
    echo 'Query Failed!
          Error: ' . $mysqli->error;
    exit(0);
}

// Get the query rows as an associative array
$rows = $result->fetch_all(MYSQLI_ASSOC);

// Get the total number of rows
$total_rows = count($rows);

echo "Returned $total_rows categories:<br>";
```

Here, `fetch_all()` stores the query result as an array named `$rows`. The code then uses `count()` to get the total number of rows in the array.

Looping through the query results

By storing the query results in an array, you make it easy to process the data by looping through the array using a `foreach()` loop:

```
// Get the query rows as an associative array
$rows = $result->fetch_all(MYSQLI_ASSOC);

// Loop through the rows
foreach($rows as $row) {
    echo $row['category_name'] . ': ' .
         $row['description'] . '<br>';
}
```

Here's what's happening in the `foreach()` loop:

- Each item in the `$rows` array is referenced using the `$row` variable.
- Each `$row` item is itself an associative array, where the key-value pairs are the column names and their values.
- Because the keys of the `$row` array are the column names, the code can refer to the values using the `$row['`*`column`*`']` syntax.

Incorporating query string values in the query

I talk earlier in this chapter about how you can use `$_GET` to parse a URL's query string, so now I show you an example that uses a query string value in a SELECT query. First, here's the code:

```
<body>
<?php
    // Parse the query string
    if (isset($_GET['category'])) {
        $category_num = $_GET['category'];
    } else {
```

Using PHP to Access MySQL Data

```
        echo 'The "category" parameter is missing!<br>';
        echo 'We are done here, sorry.';
        exit(0);
    }

    // Store the database connection parameters
    $host = 'localhost';
    $user = 'logophil_reader';
    $password = 'webcodingfordummies';
    $database = 'logophil_webcodingfordummies';

    // Create a new MySQLi object with the
    // database connection parameters
    $mysqli = new MySQLi($host, $user, $password, $database);

    // Create and run a SELECT query
    // This is an INNER JOIN of the products and
    // categories tables, based on the category_id
    // value that was in the query string
    $sql = "SELECT products.product_name,
                   products.unit_price,
                   products.units_in_stock,
                   categories.category_name
                FROM products
                INNER JOIN categories
                ON products.category_id = categories.category_id
                WHERE products.category_id = $category_num";
    $result = $mysqli->query($sql);

    // Get the query rows as an associative array
    $rows = $result->fetch_all(MYSQLI_ASSOC);

    // Get the category name
    $category = $rows[0]['category_name'];

    echo "<h2>$category</h2>";
    echo '<table>';
    echo '<tr>';
    echo '<th>Product</th>';
    echo '<th>Price</th>';
    echo '<th>In Stock</th>';
    echo '</tr>';

    // Loop through the rows
    foreach($rows as $row) {
```

```
            echo '<tr>';
            echo '<td>' . $row['product_name']. '</td>
                  <td>' . $row['unit_price'] . '</td>
                  <td>' . $row['units_in_stock'] . '</td>';
            echo '</tr>';
        }
        echo '</table>>';

        // That's it for now
        $mysqli->close();
?>
</body>
```


First, note that to keep the code shorter, I removed the error checking code. There's quite a bit going on here, so I'll go through it piece by piece:

- The script resides within an HTML file, and you'd load the file using a URL that looks something like this:

  ```
  http://mcfedries.com/webcodingfordummies/5-3-4.
     php?category=1
  ```

- The first part of the script uses `$_GET['category']` to get the category number from the query string, and that value is stored in the `$category_num` variable.
- The script then builds a SQL `SELECT` statement, which is an inner join on the `products` and `categories` tables. The `WHERE` clause restricts the results to just those products that have the category value from the query string:

  ```
  WHERE products.category_id = $category_num
  ```

- The `query()` method runs the SELECT query and stores the result in the `$result` object.
- The `fetch_all(MYSQLI_ASSOC)` method stores the returned row in an associative array named `$rows`.
- Each element in the `$rows` array includes the category name in the `category_name` column, so the script arbitrarily uses `$rows[0]['category_name']` to get the category name and store it in the `$category` variable.
- The script then outputs an `<h2>` heading for the category name, as well as some HTML table tags.
- A `foreach()` loop runs through the query rows. During each pass, the code outputs an HTML table row (`<tr>`) and a table cell (`<td>`) for each value.

» Finally, the code outputs the closing `</table>` tag and closes the `MySQLi` connection.

Figure 3-2 shows the result.

Beverages		
Product	**Price**	**In Stock**
Chai	$18.00	39
Chang	$19.00	17
Guaran Fantastica	$4.50	20
Sasquatch Ale	$14.00	111
Steeleye Stout	$18.00	20
Cote de Blaye	$263.50	17
Chartreuse verte	$18.00	69
Ipoh Coffee	$46.00	17
Laughing Lumberjack Lager	$14.00	52
Outback Lager	$15.00	15
Rhonbreu Klosterbier	$7.75	125
Lakkalikiri	$18.00	57

FIGURE 3-2: The output of the script, which lays out the query data in an HTML table.

Creating and Running Insert, Update, and Delete Queries

Performing INSERT, UPDATE, and DELETE queries in PHP is much simpler than performing SELECT queries because once your code has checked whether the query completed successfully, you're done. Here's an example that runs an INSERT query:

```
<?php

    // Store the database connection parameters
    $host = 'localhost';
    $user = 'logophil_reader';
    $password = 'webcodingfordummies';
    $database = 'logophil_webcodingfordummies';

    // Create a new MySQLi object with the
    // database connection parameters
    $mysqli = new MySQLi($host, $user, $password, $database);

    // Check for a connection error
    if($mysqli->connect_error) {
        echo 'Connection Failed!
```

```
            Error #' . $mysqli->connect_errno
                . ': ' . $mysqli->connect_error;
        exit(0);
    }

    // Create and run an INSERT query
    $sql = "INSERT
            INTO categories (category_name, description)
            VALUES ('Breads', 'Multi-grain, rye, and other
  deliciousness')";
    $result = $mysqli->query($sql);

    // Check for a query error
    if (!$result) {
        echo 'Query Failed!
            Error: ' . $mysqli->error;
        exit(0);
    }
?>
```


When given an `INSERT`, `UPDATE`, or `DELETE` statement, MySQLi's `query()` method returns `true` if the query executed successfully, or `false` if the query failed.

Separating Your MySQL Login Credentials

When you're building a web app or some other medium-to-large web project that requires a back end, you'll soon notice that your PHP scripts that access the project's MySQL data begin to multiply in a rabbitlike fashion. Before you know it, you've got 10 or 20 such scripts lying around. What do these scripts all have in common? They all include the same code for connecting to the project's MySQL database. It's not a big deal to just copy and paste that code into each new script, but it can be a huge deal if one day you have to change your login credentials. For example, for security reasons you might decide to change the password. That means you now have to wade through every single one of your scripts and make that change. Annoying!

A better way to go is to make use of PHP's `require` statement, which enables you to insert the contents of a specified PHP file into the current PHP file:

```
require php_file;
```

- ***php_file*:** The path and filename of the PHP file you want to insert

So what you do is take your MySQL database credentials code and paste it into a separate PHP file:

```
<?php
    $host = 'localhost';
    $user = 'logophil_reader';
    $password = 'webcodingfordummies';
    $database = 'logophil_webcodingfordummies';
?>
```

Say this file is named `credentials.php`. If it resides in the same directory as your scripts, then you'd replace the credentials code in your PHP scripts with the following statement:

```
require 'credentials.php';
```

If the credentials file resides in a subdirectory, then you need to include the full path to the file:

```
require '/includes/credentials.php';
```

Note that if PHP can't find or load this file for some reason, the script will halt with an error.

6 Coding Dynamic Web Pages

Contents at a Glance

IN THIS CHAPTER

» Loading server data into a page element

» Sending data to and receiving data from the server

» Getting to know JSON

» Using JSON to work with complex data from the server

Chapter 1
Melding PHP and JavaScript with Ajax and JSON

Basically, what "Ajax" means is "JavaScript now works." And that in turn means that web-based applications can now be made to work much more like desktop ones.

— PAUL GRAHAM

When coding web pages, it feels like there's a great divide between the browser front end and the server back end. When you're working on the front end, you can use HTML tags, CSS properties, and JavaScript code to build, style, and animate your pages. When you're working on the back end, you can use MySQL and PHP code to define, access, and manipulate data. That all works, but front-end code without back-end data produces a lifeless page, whereas back-end data without front-end code produces useless information. To create a truly dynamic web page, you need to cross this divide. You need to give your web page a mechanism to interact with the server to ask for and receive server data, and you need to give the server a mechanism to return that data in a format the page can understand and manipulate.

In this chapter, you investigate two such mechanisms: Ajax for sending data back and forth between the web page and the server, and JSON for putting that data into a format that's easily read by your web page code.

What Is Ajax?

Back in the early days of the web, the only way to see new data in a web page was to reload the entire page from the server. It didn't matter if just a single word or a single color had been changed, you still needed to grab everything from the server and refresh the entire page. This was back in the days when broadband Internet access wasn't as widespread as it is now (at least in some places), so that page reload could take quite a long time, depending on the size of your Internet tubes.

The sheer inefficiency of this process led some very smart people to wonder if there was a better way. Would it be possible, they asked, to somehow get the web browser to set up a communications channel with the web server that would enable the browser to request new data from the server without requiring a complete page reload?

Thankfully for modern web developers such as you and I, the answer to that question was a resounding "Yes!" The result was a new technology with the decidedly unlovely name of *Asynchronous JavaScript and XML*, which nowadays we shorten, with gratitude in our hearts, to *Ajax*.

TECHNICAL STUFF

Ajax is a mind-bogglingly complicated technology under the hood, but we won't be opening that hood even a tiny bit. Instead, I only go so far as to say that what Ajax does is insert a layer — called the *Ajax engine* — between the web page and the web server. With that idea in mind, let me give you a quickie explanation of what the Ajax name means:

- *Asynchronous:* The web page doesn't have to wait for the server to resend the entire page when the page changes. Instead, requests are handled by the Ajax engine, which uses an object called `XMLHttpRequest` (XHR, for short) to ask the server for the data while also keeping the page displayed so the user can still interact with it.
- *JavaScript:* The language used by the Ajax engine and also the language used to send requests to the server and to handle the response. A pure JavaScript approach is quite complicated, however, so in this book I use jQuery to greatly simplify the interaction.

» *XML:* The eXtensible Markup Language, which is the data format that the Ajax engine uses to send data to the server and to receive data from the server. Fortunately, you don't have to worry about this because jQuery makes it easy to send the data, and JSON (discussed later) makes it easy to process the received data.

Making Ajax Calls with jQuery

In Book 4, I talk a lot about how jQuery makes many everyday JavaScript coding tasks easier and faster. That's certainly the case with Ajax, because the jQuery programmers put a lot of effort into making Ajax calls as painless as possible. As I hope to show in this section, I believe they succeeded admirably.

To begin, understand that jQuery's Ajax support isn't limited to a single technique; far from it. There are actually quite a few Ajax-related features in the jQuery library, but for this book I'm going to focus on just the four easiest ones:

» `.load()`: Enables you to load the data returned by the server into a specified web page element

» `.get()`: Sends a GET request to the server, which is suitable for sending a relatively small amount of data

» `.post()`: Sends a POST request to the server, which is suitable for sending a relatively large amount of data

» `.getJSON()`: Sends a GET request to the server, and accepts data from the server in the JSON format

The rest of this section covers `.load()`, `.get()`, and `.post()` in more detail. I tackle `.getJSON()` a bit later when I talk about JSON stuff.

Learning more about GET and POST requests

REMEMBER

When you're working with Ajax calls to the server, one of the decisions you have to make is what request method to use: GET or POST. How on Earth are you supposed to do that? Fortunately, it really only comes down to one thing: the length of the data. GET requests are meant to be used when the data you send to the server is relatively short. The actual limit depends on the web server, but the most common ceiling is 2,048 characters. Anything longer than that and the server might cough up a `414 Request URI Too Long` error. If you're sending long data (such as a blog entry), use a POST request.

Some folks will tell you that POST is more secure than GET, but is that true? From an Ajax perspective, no, there's not much difference. Normal GET requests operate by adding a query string to the end of the URL, which is easily seen by the user. In an Ajax GET call, the page URL doesn't change, but the URL used for the Ajax request does change to include the query string. This URL is easily seen by opening the browser's web development tools. In Chrome, for example, select the Network tab, as shown in Figure 1-1. If that query string contains sensitive data, a savvy user can find it without too much trouble.

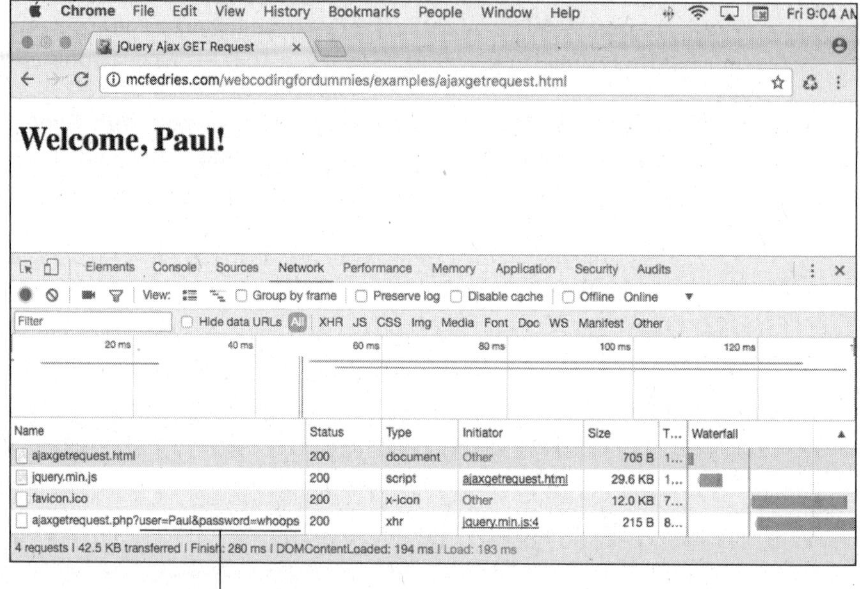

FIGURE 1-1: The Ajax GET request query string is easily visible in the browser's development tools.

Alas, POST request data is also readily seen by a sophisticated user. In Chrome's dev tools, for example, click the Network tab, click the Ajax request (it's the one that shows `xhr`, short for the `XMLHttpRequest` object used by Ajax) in the Type column, click the Headers tab, then scroll down to the Form Data section, as shown in Figure 1-2.

TIP

If you only ever send relatively small amounts of data to the server, you can certainly stick with using just GET requests. However, some developers use both, even when sending small amounts of data, as a way of making their code more readable:

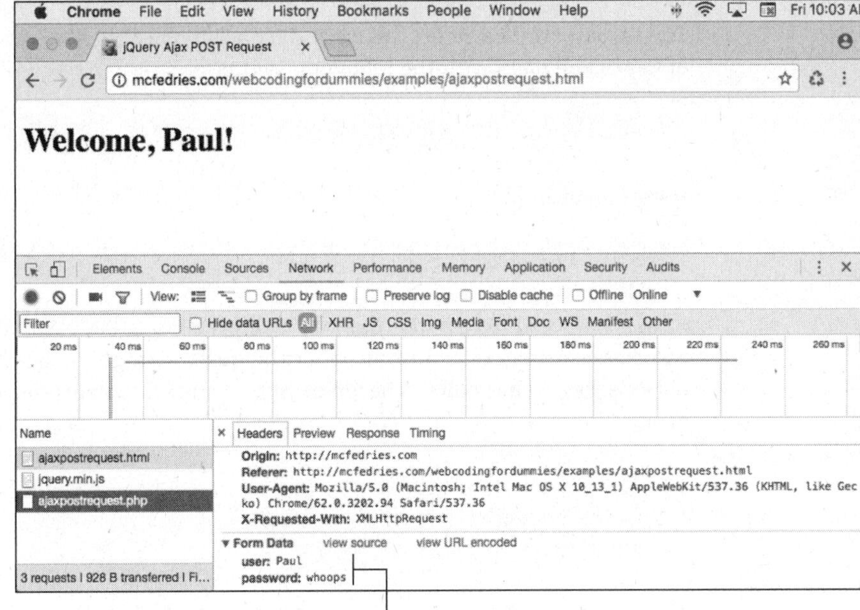

FIGURE 1-2: The Ajax POST request data is only slightly harder to find in the browser's development tools.

- Use a GET request when you want to retrieve data from the server without modifying the server data in any way.
- Use a POST request when you want to modify — that is, add, update, or delete — server data.

Handling POST requests in PHP

I cover handling GET requests in PHP code in Book 5, Chapter 3. Handling POST requests is very similar, so here I just take a quick look at how you handle them in PHP.

POST requests can be sent in two ways. The first method is as a query string consisting of a series of name-value pairs that use the following general form:

```
name1=value1&name2=value2&...
```

Here's an example:

```
book=4&chapter=1&example=2
```

The second method sends the POST data as an object literal consisting of a series of key-value pairs with the following syntax:

```
{key1: value1,key2: value2,...}
```

Here's an example:

```
{book: 4,chapter: 1,example: 2}
```

Either way, you access the data by using PHP's `$_POST` variable, which is an associative array created from either the query string's name-value pairs or the object's key-value pairs. The preceding examples create the following `$_POST` array:

```
$_POST['book'] => 4
$_POST['chapter'] => 1
$_POST['example'] => 2
```

As with the `$_GET` array, your code should check that each of the expected elements of the `$_POST` array exist by using PHP's `isset()` function, which returns `true` if a variable exists and has a value other than `null`. Here's an example:

```
if (isset($_POST['book'])) {
    $book_num = $_POST['book'];
} else {
    echo 'The "book" parameter is missing!<br>';
    echo 'We are done here, sorry.';
    exit(0);
}
```

Using .load() to update an element with server data

One of the most common and most useful Ajax techniques is to update just a single element on the page with data from the server. All the other elements on the page stay the same, so the user's experience isn't disrupted by a jarring and annoying page reload.

jQuery makes this technique very straightforward by offering the `.load()` method. How you use this method depends on what you want to load, whether you want to send data to the server, and whether you want to run some code when the load is done. The next few sections take you through the possibilities.

Loading an HTML file

The most common use of `.load()` is to populate a page element with the contents of an HTML file. Here's the general syntax to use:

```
$(element).load(HTMLFile);
```

- » *element:* A jQuery selector that specifies the element into which the HTML will be loaded.
- » *HTMLFile:* The name of the file that contains the HTML code you want loaded into *element*. If the file resides in a directory that's different than the current file's directory, you need to include the path info, as well.

For example, here's an `<h1>` tag that represents the entire contents of a file named `helloajaxworld.html`:

```
<h1>Hello Ajax World!</h1>
```

Now consider the following HTML code:

```
<script>
    $(document).ready(function() {
        $('#target').load('helloajaxworld.html');
    });
</script>
<body>
    <div id="target">
    </div>
</body>
```

The `<body>` tag includes a `div` element that uses an `id` value of `target`. When the page is loaded (that is, when the `document` object's `ready` event fires), the script runs the following statement:

```
$('#target').load('helloajaxworld.html');
```

This statement tells the browser to use an Ajax call to grab the contents of `helloajaxworld.html` from the server and then insert that content into the element that uses the `id` value of `target` (that is, the page's `<div>` tag). Figure 1-3 shows the result.

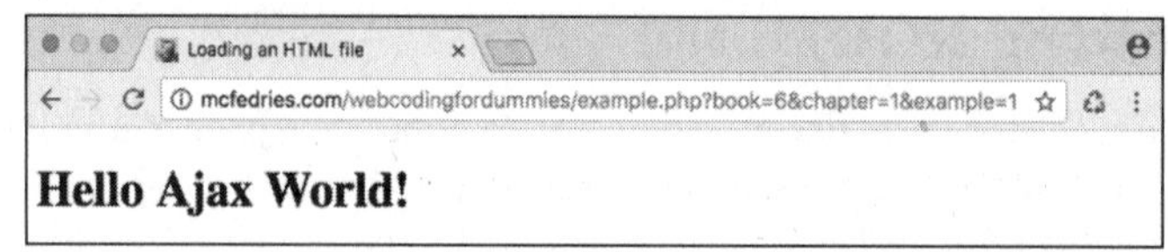

FIGURE 1-3: Using jQuery's `.load()` method to load the contents of an HTML file into a page element.

WARNING

There's a built-in browser security restriction called the *same-origin policy*, which only allows a script to access data from another file if both files have the same *origin*, meaning the following must be the same for both:

- **Protocol:** This usually means both files must use `http` or both must use `https`. If one file uses `http` and the other uses `https`, the Ajax call will fail.
- **Host name:** The two files can't be on different subdomains. If one file uses `mydomain.com` and the other uses `www.mydomain.com`, the Ajax call will fail.
- **Port number:** The two files must use the same port number. The standard HTTP port is 80, but if you call the script with, say, port 88 (that is, `http://mydomain.com:88/`), the Ajax call will fail.

Therefore, make sure that the HTML file you request has the same origin as the file that contains the `.load()` statement.

Loading a common header and footer

TIP

Why not just put the HTML file's content into the page by hand? You should definitely do that if you'll only be using that content once. However, it's very common in web development to have content that is repeated over multiple pages. For example, a particular web project might use the same header and the same footer on every page. Adding the header and footer code by hand is easy as pie if the project consists of just one or two pages. But what if it contains a dozen pages, or two dozen? Yep, you can copy and paste the code no problem, but if you have to change anything in the header or footer, then have fun updating a couple of dozen files.

Forget all that. Instead, put your header code in a separate file (called, say, `header.html`), your footer code in another file (called, you guessed it, `footer.html`), and then store them in a separate directory (called, say, `includes`). Then use `.load()` to insert that content. That is, all your pages would include code similar to the following:

```
<script>
    $(document).ready(function() {
        $('header').load('includes/header.html');
        $('footer').load('includes/footer.html');
    });
```

```
</script>
<body>
    <header></header>
    The rest of the page stuff goes here
    <footer></footer>
</body>
```

Loading output from a PHP script

If you have a PHP script that uses `echo` or `print` to output HTML tags and text, you can use `.load()` to insert that output into a page element. The general syntax is nearly identical to the one for loading an HTML file:

```
$(element).load(PHPFile);
```

- *`element`:* A jQuery selector that specifies the element into which the PHP output will be loaded.
- *`PHPFile`:* The name of the file that contains the PHP code. If the PHP file sits in a directory other than the current file's directory, include the path info.

For example, here's a PHP file named `get-server-time.php`:

```
<?php
    $current_time = date('H:m:s');
    echo "The time on the server is $current_time.";
?>
```

The script gets the current time on the server and then outputs a message displaying the time. Now consider the following HTML code:

```
<script>
    $(document).ready(function() {
        $('#target').load('get-server-time.php');
    });
</script>
<body>
    <h2 id="target">
    </h2>
</body>
```

When the page is ready, the `.load()` method calls `get-server-time.php` and loads the output into the `<h2>` tag, as shown in Figure 1-4.

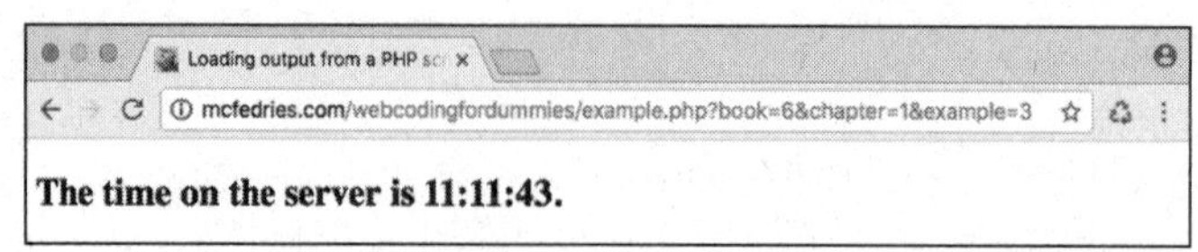

FIGURE 1-4: Using jQuery's `.load()` method to load the output of a PHP script into a page element.

WARNING

The same-origin policy that I mention earlier for HTML files is also in effect for PHP files. That is, the PHP script you request must have the same origin as the file that contains the `.load()` statement.

Loading a page fragment

Most of the time you'll use `.load()` to insert the entire contents of an HTML file or PHP output into a page element. However, jQuery also offers a mechanism to insert just a fragment of the page or output. Here's the syntax:

```
$(element).load(file fragment);
```

- *`element`:* A jQuery selector that specifies the element into which the HTML tags and text will be loaded
- *`file`:* The name of the file (plus its directory path, if needed) that contains either the HTML code or PHP output you want loaded into *`element`*
- *`fragment`:* A jQuery selector that specifies the portion of *`file`* that gets loaded into *`element`*

For example, suppose you want to set up a summary page that lists the titles and first paragraphs from a collection of longer posts. Here's the partial code from one of those posts:

```
<header>
    <h1>It's Official: Teen Instant Messages Nothing But
   Gibberish</h1>
</header>
<main>
    <article>
        <section class="first-paragraph">
            In a scathing report released today, communications
   experts have declared that the instant messages teenagers
   exchange with each other are in reality nothing but gibberish.
   U.S. Chatmaster General Todd Dood, with technical help from
   the National Security Agency, examined thousands of instant
   messages.
```

```
        </section>
        The rest of the post's sections go here
    </article>
</main>
```

Notice two things in this code:.

- The title of the post is inside an `<h1>` tag.
- The first paragraph of the post is assigned the class `first-paragraph`.

Given these two tidbits, and assuming this page is located in `posts/post1.html`, you can use a couple of `.load()` statements to add the title and first paragraph to the summary page (see Figure 1-5 for the results):

```
<script>
    $(document).ready(function() {
        $('#title1').load('posts/post1.html h1');
        $('#intro1').load('posts/post1.html .first-paragraph');
    });
</script>
<body>
    <header id="title1">
    </header>
    <article id="intro1">
    </article>
    <div>
        <a href="posts/post1.html">Read the rest of the
  post&hellip;</a>
    </div>
</body>
```

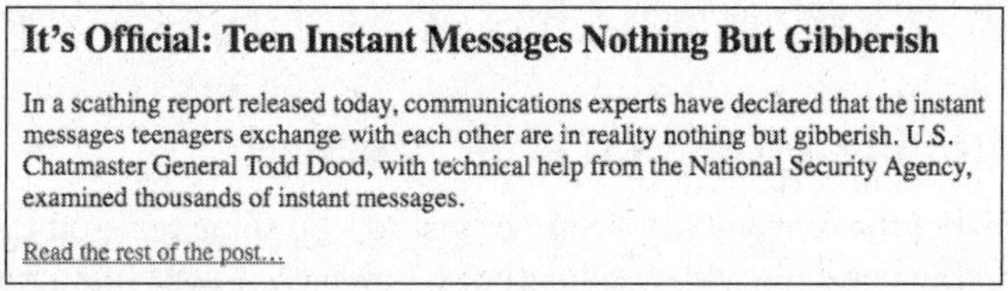

It's Official: Teen Instant Messages Nothing But Gibberish

In a scathing report released today, communications experts have declared that the instant messages teenagers exchange with each other are in reality nothing but gibberish. U.S. Chatmaster General Todd Dood, with technical help from the National Security Agency, examined thousands of instant messages.

Read the rest of the post...

FIGURE 1-5: Using jQuery's `.load()` method to load the title and first paragraph from another page.

Sending data to the server

If you want to load the output from a PHP script, sometimes you might want to pass along to the script some parameters that specify or limit the data sent back by the script. For example, you might ask for the data from a particular user account, the customers from a specified region, or the ten most recent blog posts.

Here's the variation of the `.load()` syntax that enables you to send data to the server:

```
$(element).load(PHPfile, data);
```

- *element:* A jQuery selector that specifies the element into which the PHP output will be loaded.
- *PHPfile:* The name of the PHP file (plus its directory path, if needed) that creates the PHP output you want loaded into *element*.
- *data:* The data to send to the server. This can be string or object literal:
  - **String:** A query string that specifies a set of name-value pairs using the following format:

    ```
    'name1=value1&name2=value2,...'
    ```

    jQuery sends the query string as a GET request.
  - **Object:** An object literal that specifies a set of key-value pairs using the following format:

    ```
    {key1: value1, key2: value2,...}
    ```

    jQuery sends the object as a POST request.

For example, suppose you have a PHP file named `get-category.php` that uses `$_POST` to look for a category number in an object literal and then returns data about that category. Here's how you'd load the PHP script's output into a page element with `id` value of `category-output`:

```
$('#category-output').load('get-category.php', {category: 1});
```

Running a function after the load

Most of the time you'll be content just to load some text and tags into an element and then be done with it. Sometimes, however, it's useful to run some code post-load. You can do that by adding a callback function to the `.load()` method:

```
$(element).load(file, data, function() {
    Code to run after the load finishes goes here
});
```

For example, you might want to search the loaded data for a particular value. Similarly, you might want to adjust the data's CSS based on some criteria.

As an example of the latter, suppose you have a `<nav>` tag and you use `.load()` to populate the element with your site's main navigation links. In most cases, you'd put that code in an external JavaScript file and then include the file in each page so that all your pages load the same navigation links. That's fine, but it's useful for site visitors if you mark up each of the main navigation links in some way when a visitor is viewing one of those pages. For example, if you have a "What's New" page, your `What's New` link should appear different from the other navigation links when someone is viewing that page.

You can do that by adding a callback function that examines the filename of the current page. If it matches the filename of a navigation link, it applies a class to that link. Here's some code that does this:

CSS:

```
.current-nav-link {
    background-color: black;
    color: white;
}
```

HTML (nav.html):

```
<a href="/index.html" id="home">Home</a>
<a href="/whatsnew.html" id="whatsnew">What's New</a>
<a href="/pages/whatsold.html" id="whatsold">What's Old</a>
<a href="/whatswhat.html" id="whatswhat">What's What</a>
```

jQuery:

```
$('nav').load('nav.html', function() {
    var current_page = window.location.pathname.split('/').
  pop();
    switch (current_page) {
        case 'whatsnew.html':
            $('#whatsnew').addClass('current-nav-link');
            break;

        case 'whatsold.html':
            $('#whatsold').addClass('current-nav-link');
            break;
```

```
        case 'whatswhat.html':
            $('#whatswhat').addClass('current-nav-link');
            break;

        default:
            $('#home').addClass('current-nav-link');
    }
});
```

The CSS defines a class named `current-nav-link` that switches the background to black and the text color to white. The HTML shows `nav.html`, the file that holds the navigation links. The jQuery code uses `.load()` to load `nav.html` into the `<nav>` tag (not shown in the code), and then a callback function does two things:

- It determines the filename of the current page by taking the URL's path (given by `window.location.pathname`), splitting it into an array with the backslash (/) as the separator, and then running the `pop()` method to get the last item in the array (that is, the filename).
- It uses a `switch()` statement to check whether the current filename is equal to the filename used by one of the main navigation links. If so, then the code uses jQuery's `addClass()` method to add the `current-nav-link` class to the link element.

Figure 1-6 shows an example of this code at work.

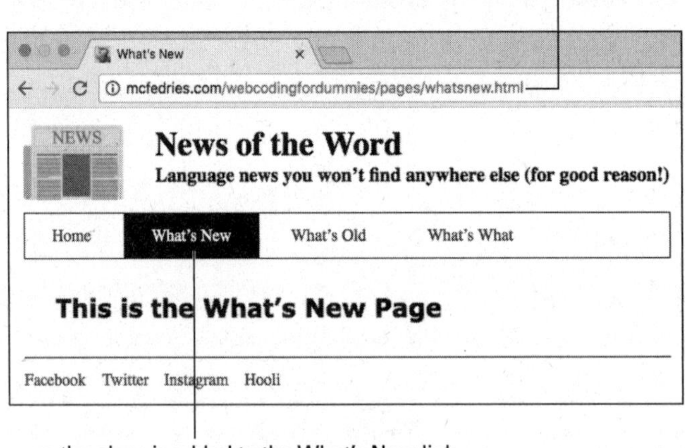

FIGURE 1-6: The `.load()` callback function determines the current page's filename. If that filename is the same as the filename of a navigation link, the code adds a class to that link.

Using .get() or .post() to communicate with the server

If you want to communicate with the server via Ajax without that communication being tied to a specific page element, use the `.get()` or `.post()` functions, which send GET and POST requests, respectively. These functions use the same general syntax:

```
$.get(script, data-to-send, function(returned-data) {
    Code to run if the operation is successful
});
$.post(script, data-to-send, function(returned-data) {
    Code to run if the operation is successful
});
```

- *`script`*: The name of the PHP file (plus its directory path, if needed) that you want to run.
- *`data-to-send`*: Specifies the data to send to the server. This can be string or object literal:
  - **String:** A query string that specifies a set of name-value pairs using the following format:

    ```
    'name1=value1&name2=value2,...'
    ```

  - **Object:** An object literal that specifies a set of key-value pairs using the following format:

    ```
    {key1: value1, key2: value2,...}
    ```

- `function(`*`returned-data`*`)`: A function that jQuery runs if the GET or POST operation was success. The data returned by the server is stored in the *`returned-data`* parameter.

Note, first, that the syntax is slightly unusual in that you don't specify an element after the `$()` method.

These are extremely versatile functions that you can use in a number of different ways:

- **Run a script:** If all you want to do is execute a server script, run either method with just the *`script`* parameter. For example:

  ```
  $.get('php/update-rss-feeds.php');
  ```

- **Run a script with data:** If you want to run a server script and also supply that script with some data, run either method with both the `script` and *data-to-send* parameters. For example:

```
$.get('php/update-rss-feeds.php', 'feedID=2');
```

- **Retrieve data:** If you want to run a server script and process the data that the script sends back, run either method with the `script` parameter and the `function(returned-data)` callback function. For example:

```
$.post('total-inventory.php', function(data) {
    console.log('Total inventory: ' + data);
});
```

- **Send and retrieve data:** If you want to run a server script, supply that script with some data, and process the data that the script sends back, run either method with all the parameters. For example:

```
$.post('total-inventory.php', 'category=1', function(data) {
    console.log('Total Beverage inventory: ' + data);
});
```

For example, suppose you want to know the total value of the inventory (that is, the units in stock multiplied by the price of each unit) for a particular category. Here's a partial PHP script named `total-inventory.php` that does the job:

```
// Parse the query string
$category_num = $_POST['category'];

// Create and run a SELECT query
$sql = "SELECT unit_price, units_in_stock
        FROM products
        WHERE category_id = $category_num";
$result = $mysqli->query($sql);

// Get the query rows as an associative array
$rows = $result->fetch_all(MYSQLI_ASSOC);
$inventory_total = 0;

// Loop through the rows
foreach($rows as $row) {
    $inventory_total += $row['unit_price'] * $row['units_in_
    stock'];
}
echo $inventory_total;
```

This script (which has many parts not shown, such as the MySQL connection statements), takes a category value via POST and runs a SELECT query that returns the unit_price and units_in_stock for that category. The code then loops through the returned rows, adding to the inventory_total variable each time by multiplying unit_price and units_in_stock. The script finishes by echoing the final value of inventory_total.

Now consider the front-end code:

CSS:

```
div {
    color: green;
    font-size: 1.25rem;
}
.warning {
    color: red;
    font-weight: bold;
}
```

HTML:

```
<h1>Inventory Report</h1>
<div></div>
```

JavaScript/jQuery:

```
$(document).ready(function() {
    $.post('total-inventory.php', 'category=1', function(data) {
        var msg = 'The total inventory is $' + data;
        if (data >= 10000) {
            msg = 'WARNING! Total inventory is $' + data;
            $('div').addClass('warning');
        }
        $('div').html(msg);
    });
});
```

The jQuery .post() function calls total-inventory.php and sends category=1 as the data. The callback function stores the PHP output (that is, the $inventory_total value) in the data parameter, sets up a default message, and checks to see if data is over 10000. If it is, the code changes the message and adds the warning class to the div element. Finally, the code displays the message in the div. Figure 1-7 shows an example result.

FIGURE 1-7: A warning message displayed by the `.post()` callback function.

Inventory Report

WARNING! Total inventory is $12480.25

Introducing JSON

As I show over and over in this chapter, when the PHP script is ready to send data back to the front end, it uses one or more `echo` (or `print`) statements to output the data. That process works fine if all your web page needs from the server is some relatively simple output, such as HTML tags, text, or a single value (such as a number or string).

However, with a web app, it's common to require more sophisticated data, usually some subset of a table or a join of two or more tables. You can't send pure MySQL data back to the web browser because there are no front-end tools that can work with data in that format. Instead, what you need to do is convert the server data into a special format called *JavaScript Object Notation*, or *JSON* (pronounced like the name Jason), for short.

Learning the JSON syntax

I talk about JavaScript object literals in several places in this book, and if you know about object literals, then JSON objects will look very familiar. Here's the general syntax:

```
{
    "property1": value1,
    "property2": value2,
    ...
    "propertyN": valueN
}
```

JSON data looks like an object, but it's really just text that consists of one or more property-value pairs with the following characteristics:

- Each property name is surrounded by double quotation marks (").
- Each value can be one of the following:
  - A number
  - A string (in which case the value must be surrounded by double quotation marks)

- A Boolean (`true` or `false`)
- `null` (that is, no value)
- A JavaScript array literal (comma-separated values surrounded by square brackets — [and])
- A JavaScript object literal (comma-separated *property*: *value* pairs surrounded by braces — { and })

» The property-value pairs are separated by commas.

» The block of property-value pairs is surrounded by braces ({ and }).

Here's an example:

```
{
    "account": 853,
    "name": "Alfreds Futterkiste",
    "supplier": false,
    "recentOrders": [28394,29539,30014],
    "contact": {
        "name": "Maria Anders",
        "phone": "030-0074321",
        "email": "m.anders@futterkiste.com"
    }
}
```

Declaring and using JSON variables

In the next section, I talk about how useful JSON is for getting complex data — especially database records — from the server to your web page. However, you can also use JSON data in your non-Ajax code. You begin by declaring a JSON variable:

```
var customer = {
    "account": 853,
    "name": "Alfreds Futterkiste",
    "supplier": false,
    "recentOrders": [28394,29539,30014],
    "contact": {
        "name": "Maria Anders",
        "phone": "030-0074321",
        "email": "anders@futterkiste.com"
    }
}
```

You can then refer to any property in the JSON data by using the *variable.property* syntax. Here are some examples:

```
customer.account           // Returns 853
customer.name              // Returns "Alfreds Futterkiste"
customer.recentOrders[1] // Returns 29539
customer.contact.email     // Returns "anders@futterkiste.com"
```

TIP

The JSON syntax can be a bit tricky, so it's a good idea to check that your data is valid before using it in your code. The easiest way to do that is to use the JSONLint (`https://jsonlint.com`) validation tool. Copy your JSON code, paste it into the JSONLint text area, then click Validate JSON.

Returning Ajax Data as JSON Text

The real power of JSON becomes clear during Ajax calls when you want to return a complex set of data to the web page. This usually means an array of database records. Sure, you can use your PHP code to loop through the array and output the data along with some HTML tags and text. However, most web apps don't want to merely display the data; they want to process the data in some way, and that means handling the data using a callback function. That still leaves the rather large problem of getting the server data to the web page, but that's where JSON comes in. Because JSON data is just text, it's easy to transfer that data between the server and the web page.

Converting server data to the JSON format

You might be shaking in your boots imagining the complexity of the code required to convert an array of database records into the JSON format. Shake no more, because, amazingly, it takes but a single line of PHP code to do the job! That's because PHP comes with a handy and powerful function called `json_encode()` that can take any value and automagically turn it into a JSON object. Here's the syntax:

```
json_encode(value, options)
```

» *`value`:* The value you want to convert to JSON. For most of your Ajax calls, this will be an array of MySQL table rows returned by the `fetch_all()` method.

» *options*: An optional series of constants, separated by the OR operator (|). These constants determine how the function encodes special characters such as quotation marks. Here are four you'll use most often:

- JSON_HEX_TAG: Encodes less than (<) and greater than (>) as \u003C and \u003E, respectively
- JSON_HEX_AMP: Encodes ampersands (&) as \u0026
- JSON_HEX_APOS: Encodes single quotation marks (') as \u0027
- JSON_HEX_QUOT: Encodes double quotation marks (") as \u0022

The usual procedure is to store the output of `json_encode()` in a variable, then `echo` or `print` that variable. Here's an example (where it's assumed that the variable `$rows` contains an array of MySQL rows):

```
$JSON_data = json_encode($rows, JSON_HEX_APOS | JSON_HEX_QUOT);
echo $JSON_data;
```

Here's a longer example that assumes you've already used PHP to connect to a MySQL database, and the resulting `MySQLi` object is stored in the `$mysqli` variable:

```
// Create and run a SELECT query
$sql = "SELECT company_name, contact_name, contact_title,
  contact_email
          FROM suppliers";
$result = $mysqli->query($sql);

// Get the query rows as an associative array
$rows = $result->fetch_all(MYSQLI_ASSOC);

// Convert the array to JSON, then output it
$JSON_data = json_encode($rows, JSON_HEX_APOS | JSON_HEX_QUOT);
echo $JSON_data;
```

Here's a partial listing of what gets stored in `$JSON_data`:


```
[{
    "company_name": "Exotic Liquids",
    "contact_name": "Charlotte Cooper",
    "contact_title": "Purchasing Manager",
    "contact_email": "charlottec@exoticliquids.com"
}, {
    "company_name": "New Orleans Cajun Delights",
    "contact_name": "Shelley Burke",
```

```
    "contact_title": "Order Administrator",
    "contact_email": "sburke@neworleanscajundelights.com"
}, {
    "company_name": "Grandma Kelly\u0027s Homestead",
    "contact_name": "Regina Murphy",
    "contact_title": "Sales Representative",
    "contact_email": "regina.murphy@grandmakellyshomestead.com"
},
etc.
]
```

Notice that this is an array of JSON strings, each of which represents a row from the data returned by the MySQL SELECT query. Note, too, that I've formatted this with newlines and spaces to make it easier to read. That actual data stored in the variable contains no whitespace.

Handling JSON data returned by the server

By far the easiest way to process JSON data returned by a PHP script is to use jQuery's `.getJSON()` function to initiate the Ajax call. Here's the syntax:

```
$.getJSON(script, data-to-send, function(JSON-array) {
    Code to run if the operation is successful
});
```

- *`script`:* The name of the PHP file (plus its directory path, if needed) that you want to run.
- *`data-to-send`:* The data to send to the server, which can be a string or an object literal.
- `function(`*`JSON-array`*`)`: A function that jQuery runs if the operation was successful. The data returned by the server is stored in the *`JSON-array`* parameter.

Because the PHP script returns an array of JSON strings, the `.getJSON()` callback function will usually use a `.each()` loop to run through the array:

```
$.each(JSON-array, function(index, JSON-string) {
    Code to handle each JSON string goes here
});
```

- *JSON-array:* The JSON array returned by the server
- *index:* The current index value of the array
- *JSON-string:* The current array item, which is a JSON string

Here's some code that processes the PHP output from the previous section:

HTML:

```
<h1>Supplier Contacts</h1>
<main></main>
```

JavaScript/jQuery:

```
$.getJSON('php/get-supplier-contacts.php',function(data) {
    $.each(data, function(index, contact) {
        $('main').append('<section id="contact' + index +
    '"/>');
        $('#contact' + index).append('<div>Company: ' + contact.
    company_name + '</div>');
        $('#contact' + index).append('<div>Contact: ' + contact.
    contact_name + '</div>');
        $('#contact' + index).append('<div>Title: ' + contact.
    contact_title + '</div>');
        $('#contact' + index).append('<div>Email: ' + contact.
    contact_email + '</div>');
    });
});
```

The code uses `.each()` to loop through the array of supplier contacts:

- A new `<section>` with an `id` set to `"contact"+index` is appended to `main`.
- A `<div>` tag for each of the four pieces of contact data (company_name, contact_name, `contact_title`, and `contact_email`) is appended to the new `<section>` tag.

Figure 1-8 shows part of the resulting page.

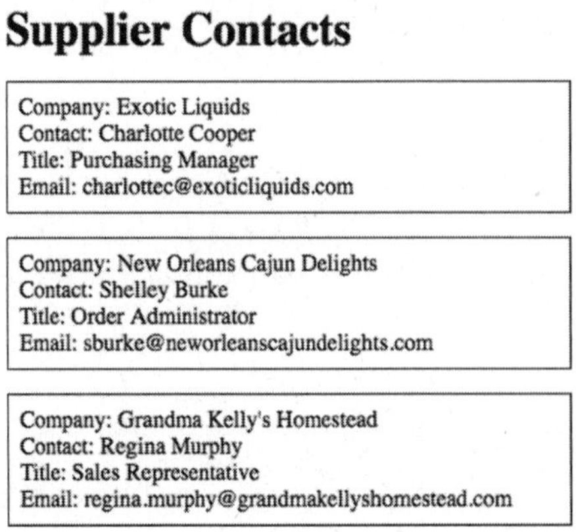

Supplier Contacts

Company: Exotic Liquids
Contact: Charlotte Cooper
Title: Purchasing Manager
Email: charlottec@exoticliquids.com

Company: New Orleans Cajun Delights
Contact: Shelley Burke
Title: Order Administrator
Email: sburke@neworleanscajundelights.com

Company: Grandma Kelly's Homestead
Contact: Regina Murphy
Title: Sales Representative
Email: regina.murphy@grandmakellyshomestead.com

FIGURE 1-8: The callback loops through the JSON array, appending each object to the `<main>` tag.

The `.getJSON()` function sends the data to the server using a GET request. What if you want to use a POST request, instead? Alas, jQuery doesn't offer a function such as `.postJSON()`. Instead, you use the `.post()` function, but when you get the JSON data back from the server, you turn it into a JavaScript object by using the `JSON.parse()` function:

```
JSON.parse(data)
```

- *data*: The JSON data returned by the server

Here's an example:

```
$.post('php/get-supplier-contacts.php',function(data) {

    // Convert the JSON text to a JavaScript object
    var obj = JSON.parse(data);

    $.each(obj, function(index, contact) {
        $('main').append('<section id="contact' + index +
  '"/>');
        $('#contact' + index).append('<div>Company: ' + contact.
  company_name + '</div>');
        $('#contact' + index).append('<div>Contact: ' + contact.
  contact_name + '</div>');
        $('#contact' + index).append('<div>Title: ' + contact.
  contact_title + '</div>');
        $('#contact' + index).append('<div>Email: ' + contact.
  contact_email + '</div>');
    });
});
```

IN THIS CHAPTER

» Understanding web form basics

» Coding text boxes, checkboxes, and radio buttons

» Programming lists, labels, and buttons

» Monitoring and triggering form events

» Getting the form data to the server

Chapter 2

Building and Processing Web Forms

From humble beginnings, forms in HTML5 are now tremendously flexible and powerful, providing natively much of the functionality that we as developers have been adding in with JavaScript over the years.

— PETER GASSTON

A dynamic web page is one that interacts with the user and responds in some way to that interaction. However, when I use the word "interaction" here, I don't mean (or I don't just mean) users scrolling through your content and clicking a link here and there. A dynamic web page solicits feedback from the user and then responds to that feedback in an appropriate way (whatever "appropriate" might mean in that context). Sure, you can pester your page visitors for info by tossing them a `confirm` or `prompt` box or two, but these are mere toys in the land of web interactivity. The real tools for soliciting feedback and then acting on it — that is, for making your pages truly dynamic — are web forms.

In this chapter, you explore all that web forms have to offer. After mastering the basics, you investigate the amazing new features offered by HTML5 web forms, unearth the power of form events, and learn how to dress up your form data and send it off to the web server. It's a veritable forms smorgasbord, so belly up!

What Is a Web Form?

Most modern programs toss a dialog box in your face if they need to extract some information from you. For example, selecting a program's Print command most likely results in some kind of Print dialog box showing up. The purpose of this dialog box is to ask for info such as the number of copies you want, the pages you want to print, the printer you want to use, and so on.

A form is essentially the web page equivalent of a dialog box. It's a page section populated with text boxes, lists, checkboxes, command buttons, and other controls to get information from the user. For example, Figure 2-1 shows a form from my website. This is a form that people can use to send me a message. The form includes a text box for the person's name, another for her email address, a larger text area for the message, and a command button to send the data to my server.

Contact Me

FILL IN THE FORM FIELDS AND CLICK SEND

Name Your name (optional)

Email† Email address (optional)

Message

Send

†Your email address is safe with me. I promise never to sell it, rent it, trade it, or give it away.

FIGURE 2-1: A typical web form.

Contact forms are very common, but there are lots of other uses for forms:

- If you put out a newsletter, you can use a form to sign up subscribers.
- If your website includes pages with restricted access, you can use a form to get a person's username and password for verification.
- If you have information in a database, you can use a form to have people specify what information they want to access.
- If your site has a search feature, you can use a form to get the search text and offer options for filtering and sorting the search results.

Understanding How Web Forms Work

A web form is a little data-gathering machine. What kinds of data can it gather? You name it:

- » Text, from a single word up to a long post
- » Numbers, dates, and times
- » Which item is (or items are) selected in a list
- » Whether a checkbox is selected
- » Which one of a group of radio buttons is selected

What happens to that data after you've gathered it? There are two roads the data can travel: Server Street and Local Lane.

The Server Street route means that your web server gets in on the action. Here are the basic steps that occur:

1. The user clicks a button to submit the form.
2. Your JavaScript/jQuery code gathers and readies the form data for sending.
3. The code uses an Ajax call to send the form data to a PHP script on the server.
4. The PHP script extracts the form data.
5. PHP uses some or all of the form data to build and execute a MySQL query.
6. PHP outputs either the requested data or some kind of code that indicates the result of the operation.
7. Your JavaScript/jQuery code processes the data returned by the server and updates the web page accordingly.

The Local Lane route doesn't get the web server involved at all:

1. The user changes the form data in some way.
2. Your JavaScript/jQuery code detects the changed data.
3. The event handler for the changed form field updates the web page based on the changed data.

In this chapter, I show you how to build a form and then how to handle form events, which will enable you to stroll down Local Lane as much as you want. I also cover submitting data at the end of the chapter, which gives you everything you need to know for getting to Server Street.

Building an HTML5 Web Form

You build web forms with your bare hands using special HTML tags. The latest version of HTML — HTML5 — includes many new form goodies, most of which now have great browser support, so I show you both the oldie-but-goodie and the latest-and-greatest in the form world over the next few sections.

Setting up the form

To get your form started, you wrap everything inside the `<form>` tag:

```
<form>
</form>
```

In this book, you create forms that either update the page locally or submit data to the server via Ajax. All that front-end interaction is controlled by JavaScript and jQuery code, so you don't need any special attributes in the `<form>` tag.

However, I'd be remiss if I didn't mention the version of the `<form>` tag you need to use if you want your form data submitted directly to a script on the server:

```
<form action="script" method="method">
```

- *script*: The URL of the server script you want to use to process the form data.
- *method*: The method you want to use to send the data: `get` or `post`. (I talk about the difference between these two methods in Book 6, Chapter 1.)

Here's an example:

```
<form
action="http://mcfedries.com/webcodingfordummies/php/get-
  supplier-contacts.php"
method="post">
```

WARNING

If you're just using the form to add local interaction to the web page and you won't be submitting any form data to the server, then technically you don't need the `<form>` tag at all. However, you should use one anyway most of the time because including the `<form>` tag enables the user to submit the form by pressing Enter or Return, and it also gets you a submit button (such as Go) in mobile browsers.

Adding a form button

Most forms include a button that the user clicks when he's completed the form and wants to initiate the form's underlying action. This is known as *submitting* the form, and that term has traditionally meant sending the form data to a server-side script for processing. These days, however, and certainly in this book, "submitting" the form can also mean:

- Updating something on the web page without sending anything to the server. For example, clicking a button might set the page's background color.
- Running a function that gathers the form data and uses an Ajax call to send the data to the server and process what the server sends back. For example, if the form asks for the person's username and password, clicking the form button would launch the login process.

The old style of submitting a form is to use an `<input>` where the `type` attribute is set to `submit`:

```
<input type="submit" value="buttonText">
```

- *buttonText:* The text that appears on the button face

For example:

```
<input type="submit" value="Submit Me!">
```

This style is rarely used in modern web development because it's a bit tricky to style such a button. For that reason, most web developers use the `<button>` tag, instead:

```
<button type="submit">buttonText</button>
```

- *buttonText:* The text that appears on the button face

For example:

```
<button type="submit">Ship It</button>
```

TIP

For better-looking buttons, use CSS to style the following:

- **Rounded corners:** To control the roundness of the button corners, use the `border-radius` property set to either a measurement (in, say, pixels) or a percentage. For example:

```
button {
    border-radius: 15px;
}
```

- **Drop shadow:** To add a drop shadow to a button, apply the `box-shadow` *x y blur color* property, where *x* is the horizontal offset of the shadow, *y* is the vertical offset of the shadow, *blur* is amount the shadow is blurred, and *color* is the shadow color. For example:

```
button {
    box-shadow: 3px 3px 5px gray;
}
```

Working with text fields

Text-based fields are the most commonly used form elements, and most of them use the `<input>` tag:

```
<input type="textType" name="textName" value="textValue" placeho
    lder="textPrompt">
```

- *textType:* The kind of text field you want to use in your form.
- *textName:* The name you assign to the field. If you'll be submitting the form data via Ajax, you must include a `name` value for each field.
- *textValue:* The initial value of the field, if any.
- *textPrompt:* Text that appears temporarily in the field when the page first loads and is used to prompt the user about the required input. The placeholder text disappears as soon as the user starts typing in the field.

Here's a list of the available text-based types you can use for the `type` attribute:

» `text`: Displays a text box into which the user types a line of text. Add the `size` attribute to specify the width of the field, in characters (the default is `20`). Here's an example:

```
<input type="text" name="company" size="50">
```

» `number`: Displays a text box into which the user types a numeric value. Most browsers add a spin box that enables the user to increment or decrement the number by clicking the up or down arrow, respectively. Check out this example:

```
<input type="number" name="points" value="100">
```

I should also mention the `range` type, which displays a slider control that enables the user to click and drag to choose a numeric value between a specified minimum and maximum:

```
<input type="range" name="transparency" min="0" max="100"
  value="100">
```

» `email`: Displays a text box into which the user types an email address. Add the `multiple` attribute to allow the user to type two or more addresses, separated by commas. Add the `size` attribute to specify the width of the field, in characters. An example for you:

```
<input type="email" name="user-email" placeholder="you@
  yourdomain.com">
```

» `url`: Displays a text box into which the user types a URL. Add the `size` attribute to specify the width of the field, in characters. Here's a for instance:

```
<input type="url" name="homepage" placeholder="e.g.,
  http://domain.com/">
```

» `tel`: Displays a text box into which the user types a telephone number. Use the `size` attribute to specify the width of the field, in characters. Here's an example:

```
<input type="tel" name="mobile" placeholder="(xxx)xxx-
  xxxx">
```

» `time`: Displays a text box into which the user types a time, usually hours and minutes. For example:

```
<input type="time" name="start-time">
```

- password: Displays a text box into which the user types a password. The typed characters appear as dots (•). Add the autocomplete attribute to specify whether the user's browser or password management software can automatically enter the password. Set the attribute to current-password to allow password autocompletion, or to off to disallow autocompletion. Need an example? Done:

```
<input type="password" name="userpassword"
  autocomplete="current-password">
```

- search: Displays a text box into which the user types a search term. Add the size attribute to specify the width of the field, in characters. Why, yes, I do have an example:

```
<input type="search" name="q" placeholder="Type a search
  term">
```

- hidden: Adds an input field to the form, but doesn't display the field to the user. That sounds weird, I know, but it's a handy way to store a value that you want to include in the submit, but you don't want the user to see or modify. Here's an example:

```
<input id="userSession" name="user-session" type="hidden"
  value="jwr274">
```

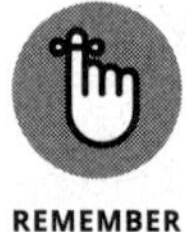

REMEMBER

Some older browsers don't get special text fields such as email and time, but you can still use them in your pages because those clueless browsers will ignore the type attribute and just display a standard text field.

That was a lot of text-related fields, but we're not done yet! There are two others you need to know about:

- <textarea>: This tag displays a text box into which the user can type multiple lines .of text. Add the rows attribute to specify how many lines of text are displayed. If you want default text to appear in the text box, add the text between the <textarea> and </textarea> tags. Here's an example:

```
<textarea name="message" rows="5">
Default text goes here.
</textarea>
```

- `<label>`: Associates a label with a form field. There are two ways to use a label:

  Method #1 — Surround the form field with `<label>` and `</label>` tags, and insert the label text before or after the field, like so:

  ```
  <label>
  Email:
  <input type="email" name="user-email" placeholder="you@
    yourdomain.com">
  </label>
  ```

  Method #2 — Add an `id` value to the field tag, set the `<label>` tag's `for` attribute to the same value, and insert the label text between the `<label>` and `</label>` tags, as I've done here:

  ```
  <label for="useremail">Email:</label>
  <input id="useremail" type="email" name="user-email"
    placeholder="you@yourdomain.com">
  ```

Figure 2-2 demonstrates each of these text fields.

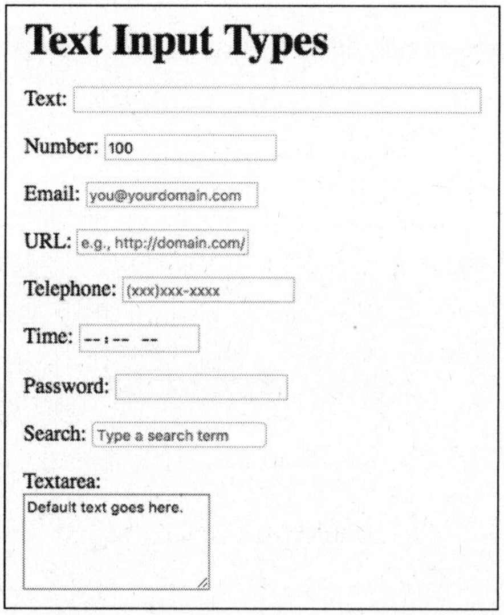

FIGURE 2-2: The various text input types you can use in your forms.

Referencing text fields by field type

One common form-scripting technique is to run an operation on every field of the same type. For example, you might want to apply a style to all the URL fields. Here's the jQuery selector to use to select all `input` elements of a given type:

```
$('input[type=fieldType]')
```

» *fieldType:* The type attribute value you want to select, such as `text` or `url`

For example, the following selector returns the set of all `input` elements that use the type `url`:

```
$('input[type=url]')
```

Getting a text field value

Your script can get the current value of any text field by using jQuery's `val()` method:

```
$(field).val()
```

» *field:* A selector that specifies the form field you want to work with

Here's an example:

HTML:

```
<label>
Search the site:
<input id="search-field" name="q" type="search">
</label>
```

jQuery:

```
var searchString = $('#search-field').val();
```

Setting a text field value

To set a text field value, use jQuery's `val()` method, but with a value:

```
$(field).val(value)
```

» *field:* A selector that specifies the form field you want to work with

» *value:* The value you want to assign to the text field

Here's an example:

HTML:

```
<label>
Type your homepage address:
<input id="homepage-field" name="homepage" type="url">
</label>
```

JavaScript/jQuery:

```
var homepageURL = $('#homepage-field').val();
$('#homepage-field').val(homepageURL.toLowerCase());
```

This code grabs a URL, converts it to all lowercase characters, then returns it to the same `url` field.

Coding checkboxes

You use a checkbox in a web form to toggle a setting on (that is, the checkbox is selected) and off (the checkbox is deselected). You create a checkbox by including in your form the following version of the `<input>` tag:

```
<input type="checkbox" name="checkName" value="checkValue"
   [checked]>
```

» *checkName:* The name you want to assign to the checkbox. If you'll be submitting the form data via Ajax, you must include both a `name` and a `value` for the checkbox.

» *checkValue:* The value you want to assign to the checkbox. Note that this is a hidden value sent to the server when the form is submitted; the user never sees it.

» `checked`: When this optional attribute is present, the checkbox is initially selected.

Here's an example:

```
<fieldset>
    <legend>
        What's your phobia? (Please check all that apply):
    </legend>
    <div>
        <label>
            <input type="checkbox" name="phobia"
  value="Ants">Myrmecophobia (Fear of ants)
        </label>
    </div>
    <div>
        <label>
            <input type="checkbox" name="phobia"
  value="Bald">Peladophobia (Fear of becoming bald)
        </label>
    </div>
    <div>
        <label>
            <input type="checkbox" name="phobia" value="Beards"
  checked>Pogonophobia (Fear of beards)
        </label>
    </div>
    <div>
        <label>
            <input type="checkbox" name="phobia"
  value="Bed">Clinophobia (Fear of going to bed)
        </label>
    </div>
    <div>
        <label>
            <input type="checkbox" name="phobia" value="Chins"
  checked>Geniophobia (Fear of chins)
        </label>
    </div>
    <div>
        <label>
            <input type="checkbox" name="phobia"
  value="Flowers">Anthophobia (Fear of flowers)
        </label>
    </div>
    <div>
```

```
        <label>
            <input type="checkbox" name="phobia"
    value="Flying">Aviatophobia (Fear of flying)
        </label>
    </div>
    <div>
        <label>
            <input type="checkbox" name="phobia"
    value="Purple">Porphyrophobia (Fear of purple)
        </label>
    </div>
    <div>
        <label>
            <input type="checkbox" name="phobia" value="Teeth"
    checked>Odontophobia (Fear of teeth)
        </label>
    </div>
    <div>
        <label>
            <input type="checkbox" name="phobia"
    value="Thinking">Phronemophobia (Fear of thinking)
        </label>
    </div>
    <div>
        <label>
            <input type="checkbox" name="phobia" value="Vegetabl
    es">Lachanophobia (Fear of vegetables)
        </label>
    </div>
    <div>
        <label>
            <input type="checkbox" name="phobia" value="Fear"
    checked>Phobophobia (Fear of fear)
        </label>
    </div>
    <div>
        <label>
            <input type="checkbox" name="phobia"
    value="Everything">Pantophobia (Fear of everything)
        </label>
    </div>
</fieldset>
```

Some notes about this code:

- You use the `<fieldset>` tag to group a collection of form fields together.
- You use the `<legend>` tag to create a caption for the parent `fieldset` element. Figure 2-3 shows how this looks in the browser.
- Because the `<input>` tags are wrapped in their respective `<label>` tags, it means the user can select or deselect each checkbox by clicking the checkbox itself or by clicking its label.

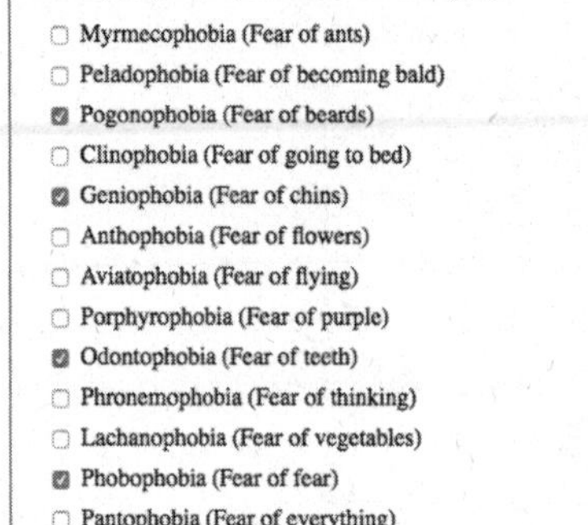

FIGURE 2-3: Some checkbox form fields, wrapped in a `fieldset` group with a `legend` element.

REMEMBER

One strange thing about a checkbox field is that it's only included in the form submission if it's selected. If the checkbox is deselected, it's not sent to the server.

Referencing checkboxes

If your code needs to reference all the checkboxes in a page, use the following jQuery selector:

```
$('input[type=checkbox]')
```

If you just want the checkboxes from a particular form, use a descendent or child selector on the form's `id` value:

```
$('#formid input[type=checkbox]')
```

Getting the checkbox state

You have to be a bit careful when discussing the "value" of a checkbox. If it's the `value` attribute you want to work with, then getting this is no different than getting the `value` property of a text field by using jQuery's `val()` method.

However, what you're more likely to be interested in is whether a checkbox is selected or deselected. This is called the checkbox *state*. In that case, you need to examine the `checked` attribute, instead:

```
$(checkbox).prop('checked')
```

» *checkbox:* A selector that specifies the checkbox you want to work with

The `checked` attribute returns `true` if the checkbox is selected, or `false` if the checkbox is deselected.

As an example, consider this code:

```
<label>
    <input id="autosave" type="checkbox" name="autosave">
    Autosave this project?
</label>
```

The following statement stores the checkbox state in a variable named `autosaveState`:

```
var autosaveState = $('#autosave').prop('checked');
```

Setting the checkbox state

To set a checkbox field to either the selected or deselected state, assign a Boolean expression to the `checked` attribute:

```
$(checkbox).prop('checked', Boolean)
```

» *checkbox:* A selector that specifies the checkbox you want to modify.

» *`Boolean`:* The Boolean value or expression you want to assign to the checkbox. Use `true` to select the checkbox; use `false` to deselect the checkbox.

For example, take a look back at the long list of phobia checkboxes (that is, the code demonstrated in Figure 2-3). Suppose you want to set up that form so that the user can select at most three checkboxes. Here's some code that does the job:

```
$('form').click(function(e) {
    // Get the checkbox that was clicked
    var clickedCheckbox = e.target.value;
```

```
    // Get the total number of selected checkboxes
    var totalSelected = $('input[type=checkbox]:checked').
  length;

    // Do we now have more than three selected checkboxes?
    if (totalSelected > 3) {

        // If so, deselect the checkbox that was just clicked
        $('input[value=' + clickedCheckbox + ']').
  prop('checked', false);
    }
});
```

This event handler runs when anything inside the `form` element is clicked. The code first saves the `value` of the clicked checkbox. Then the code uses jQuery's `:checked` selector to return the set of all `checkbox` elements that have the `checked` attribute, and the `length` property tells you how many are in the set. An `if()` test checks to see if more than three are now selected. If that's true, the code deselects the checkbox that was just clicked.

Working with radio buttons

If you want to offer your users a collection of related options, only one of which can be selected at a time, then radio buttons are the way to go. Form radio buttons congregate in groups of two or more where only one button in the group can be selected at any time. If the user clicks another button in that group, it becomes selected and the previously selected button becomes deselected.

You create a radio button using the following variation of the `<input>` tag:

```
<input type="radio" name="radioGroup" value="radioValue"
  [checked]>
```

- *`radioGroup`:* The name you want to assign to the group of radio buttons. All the radio buttons that use the same `name` value belong to that group.
- *`radioValue`:* The value you want to assign to the radio button. If this radio button is selected when the form is submitted, then this is the value sent to the server.
- `checked`: When this optional attribute is present, the radio button is initially selected.

Here's an example, and Figure 2-4 shows what happens:

```
<fieldset>
    <legend>
        Select a delivery method
    </legend>
    <div>
        <input type="radio" id="carrier-pigeon" name="delivery"
  value="pigeon" checked>
        <label for="carrier-pigeon">Carrier pigeon</label>
    </div>
    <div>
        <input type="radio" id="pony-express" name="delivery"
  value="pony">
        <label for="pony-express">Pony express</label>
    </div>
    <div>
        <input type="radio" id="snail-mail" name="delivery"
  value="postal">
        <label for="snail-mail">Snail mail</label>
    </div>
    <div>
        <input type="radio" id="some-punk" name="delivery"
  value="bikecourier">
        <label for="some-punk">Some punk on a bike</label>
    </div>
</fieldset>
```

Select a delivery method

- Carrier pigeon
- Pony express
- Snail mail
- Some punk on a bike

FIGURE 2-4: Some radio button form fields.

Referencing radio buttons

If your code needs to work with all the radio buttons in a page, use this jQuery selector:

```
$('input[type=radio]')
```

If you want the radio buttons from a particular form, use a descendent or child selector on the form's `id` value:

```
$('#formid input[type=radio]')
```

If you require just the radio buttons from a particular group, use the following jQuery selector, where *radioGroup* is the common name of the group:

```
$('input[name=radioGroup]')
```

Getting a radio button state

If your code needs to know whether a particular radio button is selected or deselected, you need to determine the radio button *state*. You do that by examining the radio button's `checked` attribute, like so:

```
$(radio).prop('checked')
```

- *radio:* A jQuery selector that specifies the radio button field you want to work with

The `checked` attribute returns `true` if the radio button is selected, or `false` if the button is deselected.

For example, given the radio buttons shown earlier, the following statement stores the state of the radio button with the `id` value of `pony-express`:

```
var ponySelected = $('#pony-express').prop('checked');
```

However, it's more likely that your code will want to know which radio button in a group is selected. You can do that by applying jQuery's `:checked` selector to the group:

```
var deliveryMethod = $('input[name=delivery]:checked');
```

TIP

To get the text of the label associated with a radio button, you can take advantage of a selector called the *sibling* selector, which uses the tilde (~) symbol. The sibling selector returns elements that have the same parent element. In the radio button code I show earlier, the `<input>` and `<label>` tags are siblings, so you can use the following expression to return the selected radio button's label text:

```
$('input[name=delivery]:checked ~ label').text();
```

Setting the radio button state

To set a radio button field to either the selected or deselected state, assign a Boolean expression to the checked attribute:

```
$(radio).prop('checked', Boolean)
```

- *radio:* A jQuery selector that specifies the radio button you want to change.
- *Boolean:* The Boolean value or expression you want to assign to the radio button. Use `true` to select the radio button; use `false` to deselect the radio button.

For example, if the initial state of the form group had the first radio button selected, you can reset the group by selecting that button. The easiest way to do this is to use jQuery's `.first()` method, which returns the first item in a set:

```
$('input[name=delivery]').first().prop('checked', true);
```

Adding selection lists

Selection lists are common sights in HTML forms because they enable the web developer to display a relatively large number of choices in a compact control that most users know how to operate. When deciding between a checkbox, radio button group, or a selection list, here are some rough guidelines to follow:

- If an option or setting has only two values that can be represented by on and off, use a checkbox.
- If the option or setting has three or four values, use a group of three or four radio buttons.
- If the option or setting has five or more values, use a selection list.

This section shows you how to create and program selection lists. As you work through this part, it'll help to remember that a selection list is really an amalgam of two types of fields: the list container and the options within that container. The former is a `select` element and the latter is a collection of `option` elements.

To create the list container, you use the `<select>` tag:

```
<select name="selectName" size="selectSize" [multiple]>
```

- *selectName*: The name you want to assign to the selection list.
- *selectSize*: The optional number of rows in the selection list box that are visible. If you omit this value, the browser displays the list as a drop-down box.
- `multiple`: When this optional attribute is present, the user is allowed to select multiple options in the list.

For each item in the list, you add an `<option>` tag between the `<select>` and `</select>` tags:

```
<option value="optionValue" [selected]>
```

- *optionValue*: The value you want to assign to the list option.
- `selected`: When this optional attribute is present, the list option is initially selected.

Here are some examples:

```
<form>
    <div>
        <label for="hair-color">Select your hair color:
   </label><br>
        <select id="hair-color" name="hair-color">
            <option value="black">Black</option>
            <option value="blonde">Blonde</option>
            <option value="brunette" selected>Brunette</option>
            <option value="red">Red</option>
            <option value="neon">Something neon</option>
            <option value="none">None</option>
        </select>
    </div>
    <div>
        <label for="hair-style">Select your hair style:
   </label><br>
        <select id="hair-style" name="hair-style" size="4">
            <option value="bouffant">Bouffant</option>
            <option value="mohawk">Mohawk</option>
            <option value="page-boy">Page Boy</option>
            <option value="permed">Permed</option>
            <option value="shag">Shag</option>
```

```
            <option value="straight" selected>Straight</option>
            <option value="none">Style? What style?</option>
        </select>
    </div>
    <div>
        <label for="hair-products">Hair products used in the
  last year:</label><br>
        <select id="hair-products" name="hair-products" size="5"
  multiple>
            <option value="gel">Gel</option>
            <option value="grecian-formula">Grecian Formula
  </option>
            <option value="mousse">Mousse</option>
            <option value="peroxide">Peroxide</option>
            <option value="shoe-black">Shoe black</option>
        </select>
    </div>
</form>
```

There are three lists here (see Figure 2-5):

- `hair-color`: This list doesn't specify a size, so the browser displays it as a drop-down list.
- `hair-style`: This list uses a `size` value of 4, so there are four options visible in the list.
- `hair-products`: This list uses a `size` value of 5, so there are five options visible in the list. Also, the `multiple` attribute is set, so you can select multiple options in the list.

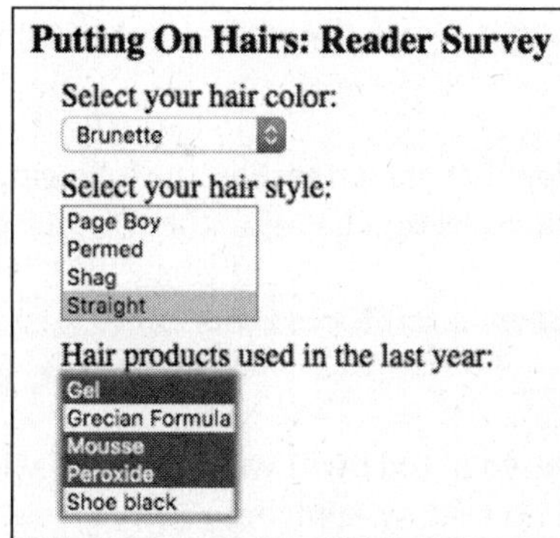

FIGURE 2-5: Some examples of selection lists.

Building and Processing Web Forms

Referencing selection lists

If your code needs to work with all the options in a selection list, use this jQuery selector, where *listid* is the id value of the select element:

```
$('#listid > option')
```

To work with a particular option within a list, use jQuery's nth-child(*n*) selector, where *n* specifies the option's position in the list (1 is the first option, 2 is the second option, and so on):

```
$('#listid > option:nth-child(2)')
```

TIP

If you want a reference to the first option in the list, you can use :first-child instead of :nth-child(1).

To get the option's text (that is, the text that the user sees in the list), run the text() method:

```
$('#listid > option:nth-child(2)').text();
```

Getting the selected list option

If your code needs to know whether a particular option in a selection list is selected or deselected, examine the option's selected attribute, like so:

```
$(option).prop('selected')
```

» *option:* A jQuery selector that specifies the option element you want to work with

The selected attribute returns true if the option is selected, or false if the option is deselected.

For example, given the selection lists shown earlier, the following statement stores the state of the first item in the selection list with the id value of hair-color:

```
var black = $('#hair-color > option:first-child').
   prop('selected');
```

However, it's more likely that your code will want to know which option in the selection list is selected. You do that by applying jQuery's :selected selector to the list's option elements:

```
var hairColor = $('#hair-color > option:selected').text();
```

If the list includes the multiple attribute, then :selected returns a set that contains all the selected elements.

Changing the selected option

To set a selection list option to either the selected or deselected state, assign a Boolean expression to the selected attribute:

```
$(option).prop('selected', Boolean)
```

- *option:* A jQuery selector that specifies the option element you want to modify.
- *Boolean:* The Boolean value or expression you want to assign to the option. Use true to select the option; use false to deselect the option.

For example, if the initial state of a multiple-selection list had no items selected, you might want to reset the list by deselecting all the options. You can do that by returning the set of all the selected options in the list, and then applying the selected attribute as false:

```
$('#hair-products > option:selected').prop('selected', false);
```

Programming pickers

HTML also offers a number of other <input> tag types that fall under a category I call "pickers," meaning that in each case the field displays a button that, when clicked, opens a control that enables the user to pick a value. Here's a quick look at the available pickers:

- color: Opens a color picker dialog that enables the user to choose a color. The color picker varies depending on the browser and operating system; Figure 2-6 shows the Microsoft Edge version. Set the value attribute in the #rrggbb format to specify an initial color (the default is black: #000000). Here's an example:

  ```
  <input type="color" name="bg-color" value="#ff6347">
  ```

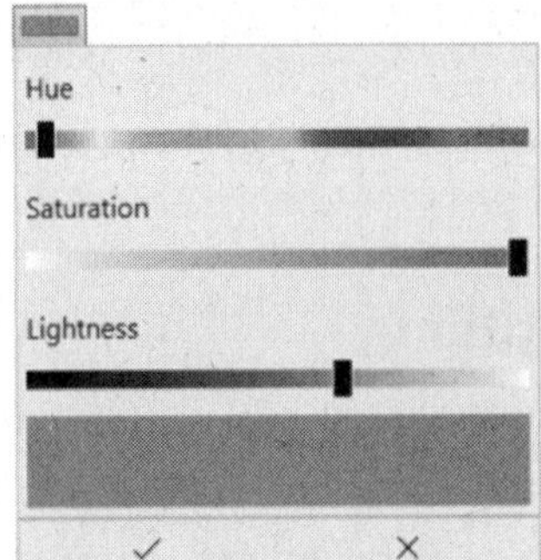

FIGURE 2-6: The color picker that appears in Microsoft Edge.

- `date`: Opens a date picker dialog so that the user can choose a date. Figure 2-7 shows the Chrome version. Set the `value` attribute in the yyyy-mm-dd format to specify an initial date. Note that the date the user sees might use a different format (such as mm/dd/yyyy, as seen in Figure 2-7), but the value returned by the element is always in the yyyy-mm-dd format. Here's an example:

```
<input type="date" name="appt-date" value="2018-08-23">
```

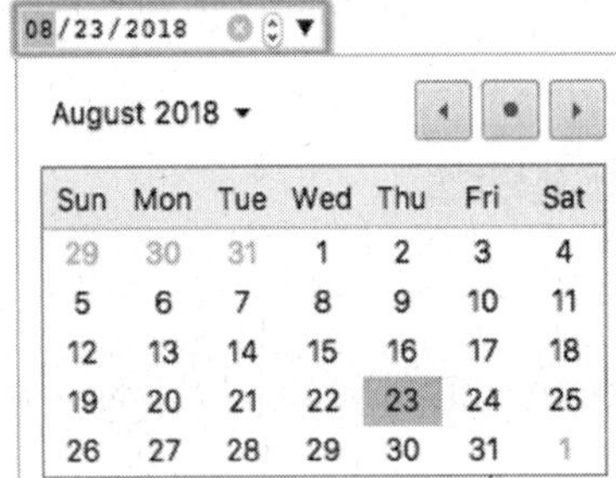

FIGURE 2-7: The date picker that appears in Google Chrome for Mac.

- `file`: Opens the user's operating system's file picker dialog so that the user can select a file. You can add the `multiple` attribute to enable the user to select more than one file. Here's an example:

```
<input type="file" name="user-photo">
```

- month: Opens a month picker dialog to enable the user to choose a month and year. Set the value attribute in the yyyy-mm format to specify an initial month and year. The value the user sees might be in a different format (such as August 2018), but the value returned by the element is always in the yyyy-mm format. Here's an example:

```
<input type="month" name="birthday-month" value="2018-08">
```

- week: Opens a week picker dialog for the user to select a week and year. To specify an initial year and month, set the value attribute in the yyyy-W*nn* format, where *nn* is the two-digit week number. The value shown to the user might be in another format (such as Week 34, 2018), but the value returned by the element is always in the yyyy-W*nn* format. Here's an example:

```
<input type="week" name="vacation-week" value="2018-W34">
```

Handling and Triggering Form Events

With all the clicking, typing, tabbing, and dragging that goes on, web forms are veritable event factories. Fortunately, you can let most of these events pass you by, but there are a few that come in handy, both in running code when the event occurs, and in triggering the events yourself.

Most form events are clicks, so you can handle them by setting click event handlers using jQuery's .click() method (which I cover in Book 4, Chapter 2). Here's an example:

HTML:

```
<form>
    <div>
        <label for="user">Username:</label>
        <input id="user" type="text" name="username">
    </div>
    <div>
        <label for="pwd">Password:</label>
        <input id="pwd" type="password" name="password">
    </div>
</form>
```

Building and Processing Web Forms

jQuery:

```
$('form').click(function() {
    console.log('Thanks for clicking the form!');
});
```

This example listens for clicks on the entire `form` element, but you can also create `click` event handlers for buttons, `input` elements, checkboxes, radio buttons, and more.

Setting the focus

One simple feature that can improve the user experience on your form pages is to set the focus on the first form field when your page loads. This saves the user from having to make that annoying click inside the first field.

To get this done, run jQuery's `focus()` method on the element you want to have the focus at startup:

```
$(field).focus();
```

» *field*: A selector that specifies the form field you want to have the focus

Here's an example that sets the focus on the text field with `id` equal to `user` at startup:

HTML:

```
<form>
    <div>
        <label for="user">Username:</label>
        <input id="user" type="text" name="username">
    </div>
    <div>
        <label for="pwd">Password:</label>
        <input id="pwd" type="password" name="password">
    </div>
</form>
```

jQuery:

```
$(document).ready(function() {
    $('#user').focus();
});
```

Monitoring the focus event

Rather than setting the focus, you might want to monitor when a particular field gets the focus (for example, by the user clicking or tabbing into the field). You can do that by setting up a `focus()` event handler on the field:

```
$(field).focus(function() {
    Focus code goes here
});
```

» *field:* A selector that specifies the form field you want to monitor for the focus event

Here's an example:

```
$('#user').focus(function() {
    console.log('The username field has the focus!');
});
```

Blurring an element

One of the more annoying browser interface quirks is the focus ring that appears around certain elements — especially buttons — when you click them. This focus ring is not only ugly, but also slightly dangerous because it means the user can "click" the button again just by pressing the spacebar. You can work around this by applying jQuery's `blur()` method on the element, which causes it to lose focus:

```
$(field).blur();
```

» *field:* A selector that specifies the form field you no longer want to have the focus

Here's an example that uses a `button` element's `click` event handler to blur the button (in the handler, the expression `$(this)` refers to the element that was clicked, in this case the button):

HTML:

```
<button id="reset-products" type="button">
    Reset Products
</button>
```

jQuery:

```
$('#reset-products').click(function() {
    // Deselect everything
    $('#hair-products > option:selected').prop('selected',
   false);

    // Blur the button
    $(this).blur();
});
```

Monitoring the blur event

Rather than blurring an element, you might want to run some code when a particular element is blurred (for example, by the user clicking or tabbing out of the field). You can do that by setting up a `blur()` event handler:

```
$(field).blur(function() {
    Blur code goes here
});
```

- *`field`*: A selector that specifies the form field you want to monitor for the `blur` event.

Here's an example:

```
$('#user').blur(function() {
    console.log('The username field no longer has the focus!');
});
```

Listening for element changes

One of the most useful form events is the change event, which fires when the value or state of a field is modified in some way. When this event fires depends on the element type:

- For a `textarea` element and the various text-related `input` elements, the change event fires when the element loses the focus.
- For checkboxes, radio buttons, selection lists, and pickers, the change event fires as soon as the user clicks the element to modify the selection or value.

You listen for a field's change events by setting up a change() event handler:

```
$(field).change(function() {
    Change code goes here
});
```

» *field*: A selector that specifies the form field you want to monitor for the change event

Here's an example:

HTML:

```
<div>
    <label for="bgcolor">Select a background color</label>
    <input id="bgcolor" type="color" name="bg-color"
  value="#ffffff">
</div>
```

jQuery:

```
$('#bgcolor').change(function() {
    var bgColor = $(this).val();
    $('body').css('background-color', bgColor);
});
```

The HTML code sets up a color picker. The jQuery code applies the change event handler to the color picker. When the change event fires on the picker, the code stores the new color value in the bgColor variable, then applies that color to the body element's background-color property.

Submitting the Form

There's one form event that I didn't cover in the previous section, and it's a biggie: the submit event, which fires when the form data is to be sent to the server. Here's the general syntax:

```
$(form).submit(function(e) {
    Submit code goes here
});
```

- *form:* A selector that specifies the form you want to monitor for the `submit` event.
- e: This argument represents the `event` object.

You'll rarely, if ever, allow the `submit` event to occur directly. Instead, you'll want to intercept the submit so that you can gather the data and then send it to the server yourself using an Ajax call. Handling the `submit` event yourself gives you much more control over both what gets sent to the server and how what gets sent back from the server gets processed.

Triggering the submit event

Here's a list of the various ways that the `submit` event gets triggered:

- When the user clicks a `button` or `input` element that resides within a `<form>` tag and has its `type` attribute set to `submit`
- When the user clicks a `button` element that resides within a `<form>` tag and has no `type` attribute
- When the user presses Enter or Return while a form element has the focus, and either a `button` or `input` element resides within the `<form>` tag and has its `type` attribute set to `submit`, or a `button` element resides within the `<form>` tag and has no `type` attribute
- When your code runs jQuery's `.submit()` method:

  ```
  $(form).submit();
  ```

  - *form:* A selector that specifies the form you want to submit

Preventing the default form submission

You control the form submission yourself by sending the data to the server with an Ajax call. The `submit` event doesn't know that, however, and it will try to submit the form data anyway. That's a no-no, so you need to prevent the default form submission by using the `event` object's `preventDefault()` method:

```
$('form').submit(function(e) {
    e.preventDefault();
});
```

Preparing the data for submission

Before you can submit your form data, you need to convert it to a format that your server's PHP script can work with. The format depends on the Ajax request method you want to use:

- **»** GET: This format requires a string of *name=value* pairs, separated by ampersands (&). To convert your form data to this format, use jQuery's `serialize()` function:

  ```
  $(form).serialize();
  ```

  - *form:* A selector that specifies the form you want to work with

- **»** POST: This format requires an array of *key: value* pairs, separated by commas (`,`). To convert your form data to this format, use jQuery's `serializeArray()` function:

  ```
  $(form).serializeArray();
  ```

  - *form:* A selector that specifies the form you want to work with

For example:

```
var formData = $('form').serialize();
```

Most commonly, your code stores the result of the `serialize()` or `serializeArray()` function in a variable, and that variable gets submitted to the server.

Submitting the form data

Now you're almost ready to submit the data. As an example, here's some HTML code for a form and `div` that I'll use to output the form results:

```
<form>
    <div>
        <label for="first">First name:</label>
        <input id="first" type="text" name="first-name">
    </div>
    <div>
        <label for="last">Last name:</label>
        <input id="last" type="text" name="last-name">
    </div>
    <div>
        <label for="nick">Nickname:</label>
        <input id="nick" type="text" name="nickname">
```

```
    </div>
    <button type="submit">Submit</button>
</form>

<div class="output">
</div>
```

Now here's the JavaScript/jQuery code that submits the form (using `.get()` in this case) and processes the result (which just echoes back the form data, as shown in Figure 2-8):

```
$('form').submit(function(e) {
    // Prevent the default form submission
    e.preventDefault();

    // Convert the data to GET format
    var formData = $(this).serialize();

    // Submit the data using an Ajax GET request
    $.get('php/echo-form-fields-get.php', formData,
   function(data) {
        // Show the data returned by the server
        $('.output').html(data);
    });
});
```

First name: Peter

Last name: Viscus

Nickname: Slippery Pete

Submit

Here are your form values

Field	Value
first-name	Peter
last-name	Viscus
nickname	Slippery Pete

FIGURE 2-8: An example form submission.

WARNING

We're missing one very important stop on our road to dynamic web pages: We haven't validated the form data! Form validation is so important, in fact, that I devote an entire chapter to it: Book 6, Chapter 3. Don't miss it!

IN THIS CHAPTER

» Validating data in the browser and on the server

» Making a field mandatory

» Setting restrictions on form fields

» Practicing good data hygiene

Chapter 3

Validating Form Data

Garbage in, garbage out. Or rather more felicitously: The tree of nonsense is watered with error, and from its branches swing the pumpkins of disaster.

— NICK HARKAWAY

In the old computing axiom of *garbage in, garbage out* (*GIGO*), or if in your genes or heart you're British, *rubbish in, rubbish out* (yes, *RIRO*), lies a cautionary tale. If the data that goes into a system is inaccurate, incomplete, incompatible, or in some other way invalid, the information that comes out of that system will be outdated, outlandish, outrageous, or just outright wrong. What does this have to do with you as a web developer? Plenty, because it's your job to make sure that the data the user enters into a form is accurate, complete, and compatible with your system. In a word, you have to make sure the data is valid. If that sounds like a lot of work, then I've got some happy news for you: HTML5 has data validation baked in, so you can just piggyback on the hard work of some real nerds. In this chapter, you explore these HTML5 validation techniques. Ah, but your work isn't over yet, friend. You also have to validate the same data once again on the server. Crazy? Like a fox. But there's more good news on the server side of things, because PHP has a few ready-to-run tools that take most of the pain out of validation. In this chapter, you also dive deep into those tools. Sleeves rolled up? Then let's begin.

Validating Form Data in the Browser

Before JavaScript came along, web servers would spend inordinate amounts of processing time checking the data submitted from a form and, all too often, returning the data back to the user to fill in an empty field or fix some invalid entry. Someone eventually realized that machines costing tens of thousands of dollars (which was the cost of the average server machine when the web was in swaddling clothes) ought to have better things to do with their time than chastising users for not entering their email address correctly (or whatever). Wouldn't it make infinitely more sense for the validation of a form's data to first occur within the browser *before* the form was even submitted?

The answer to that is an unqualified "Duh!" And once JavaScript took hold with its browser-based scripting, using it to do form validation on the browser became the new language's most important and useful feature. Alas, data validation is a complex business, so it didn't take long for everyone's JavaScript validation code to run to hundreds or even thousands of lines. Plus there was no standardization, meaning that every web project had to create its own validation code from scratch, pretty much guaranteeing it wouldn't work like any other web project's validation code. Isn't there a better way?

Give me another "Duh!" Perhaps that's why the big brains who were in charge of making HTML5 a reality decided to do something about the situation. Several types of form validation are part of HTML5, which means now you can get the web browser to handle your validation chores.

WARNING

HTML5 validation has huge browser support, so no major worries there. However, there's still a tiny minority of older browsers that will scoff at your browser validation efforts. Not to worry, though: You'll get them on the server side!

Making a form field mandatory

It's common for a form to contain at least one field that the user must fill in. For example, if your form is for a login, then you certainly need both the username and password fields to be mandatory, meaning you want to set up the form so that the submission won't go through unless both fields are filled in.

Here are a few things you can do to encourage users to fill in mandatory fields:

- Make it clear which fields are mandatory. Many sites place an asterisk before or after a field and include a note such as `Fields marked with * are required` at the top of the form.

- For a radio button group, always set up your form so that one of the `<input>` tags includes the checked attribute. This ensures that one option will always be selected.
- For a selection list, make sure that one of the `<option>` tags includes the `selected` attribute.

Outside of these techniques, you can make any field mandatory by adding the `required` attribute to the form field tag. Here's an example:

```
<form>
    <div>
        <label for="fave-beatle">Favorite Beatle:</label>
        <input id="fave-beatle" type="text" required>
        <button type="submit">Submit</button>
    </div>
</form>
```

The `<input>` tag has the `required` attribute. If you leave this field blank and try to submit the form, the browser prevents the submission and displays a message telling you to fill in the field. This message is slightly different, depending on the web browser. Figure 3-1 shows the message that Chrome displays.

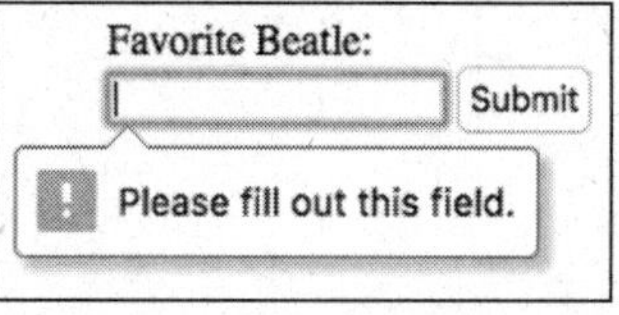

FIGURE 3-1: Add the `required` attribute to a form field to ensure it gets filled in.

Restricting the length of a text field

Another useful built-in HTML5 validation technique is setting restrictions on the length of the value entered into a text field. For example, you might want a password value to have a minimum length, and you might want a username to have a maximum length. Easier done than said:

- To add a minimum length restriction, set the `minlength` attribute to the least number of characters the user must enter.
- To add a maximum length restriction, set the `maxlength` attribute to the most number of characters the user can enter.

Take a look at an example:

```
<form>
    <div>
        <label for="acct-handle">Account handle (6-12
    chars):</label>
        <input id="acct-handle"
               type="text"
               placeholder="Enter 6-12 characters"
               minlength="6"
               maxlength="12">
        <button type="submit">Submit</button>
    </div>
</form>
```

The `<input>` tag asks for a value no less than 6 and no more than 12 characters long. If the user enters a value shorter or longer and tries to submit the form, the browser prevents the submission and displays a message asking for more or fewer characters. Figure 3-2 shows the version of the message that Firefox displays.

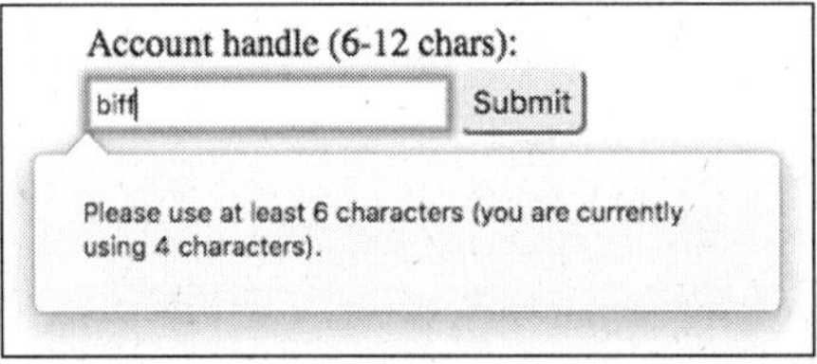

FIGURE 3-2: Use the `minlength` and/or `maxlength` attributes to restrict a field's length.

Setting maximum and minimum values on a numeric field

HTML5 can also validate a numeric field based on a specified minimum or maximum value for the field. Here are the attributes to use:

- `min`: To add a minimum value restriction, set the `min` attribute to the smallest allowable value the user can enter.
- `max`: To add a maximum value restriction, set the `max` attribute to the largest allowable value the user can enter.

Here's an example:

```
<form>
    <div>
```

```
        <label for="loan-term">Loan term (years):</label>
        <input id="loan-term"
               type="number"
               placeholder="3-25"
               min="3"
               max="25">
        <button type="submit">Submit</button>
    </div>
</form>
```

The number <input> tag asks for a value between 3 and 25. If the user enters a value outside of this range and tries to submit the form, the browser prevents the submission and displays a message to reenter a value that's either less than or equal to the maximum (as shown in Figure 3-3) or greater than or equal to the minimum.

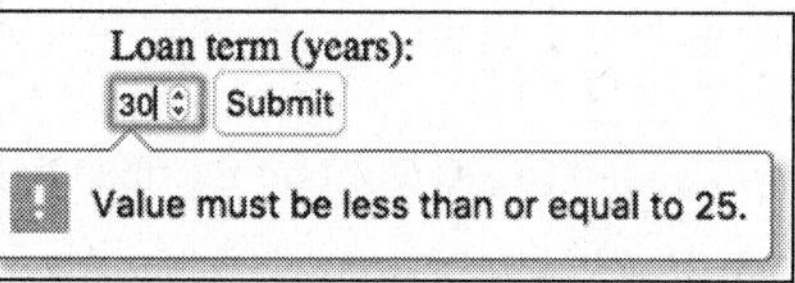

FIGURE 3-3: Use the min and/or max attributes to accept values within a specified range.

Validating email fields

Generic field validation attributes such as required, minlength, and max are very useful, but some form fields need a more targeted validation technique. In a field that accepts an email address, for example, any entered value should look something like username@domain. If that sounds like a daunting challenge, you're right, it is. Fortunately, that challenge has already been taken up by some of the best coders on the planet. The result? Built-in HTML5 validation for email addresses. And when I say "built-in," I mean built-in, because once you specify type="email" in the <input> tag, modern web browsers will automatically validate the field input to make sure it looks like an email address when the form is submitted, as shown in Figure 3-4.

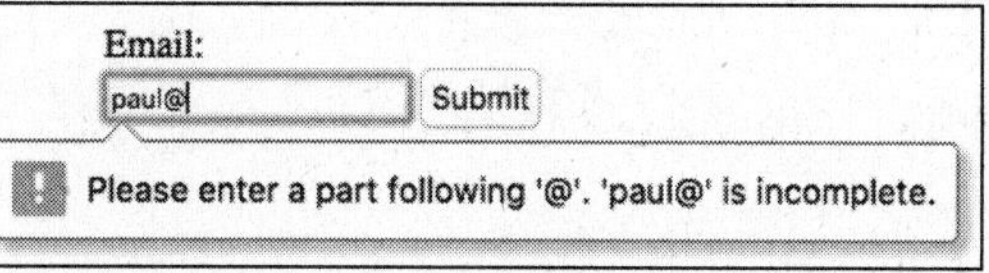

FIGURE 3-4: Modern browsers automatically validate email fields.

Making field values conform to a pattern

One of the most powerful and flexible HTML5 validation techniques is *pattern matching*, where you specify a pattern of letters, numbers, and other symbols that the field input must match. You add pattern matching validation to a `text`, `email`, `url`, `tel`, `search`, or `password` field by adding the `pattern` attribute:

```
pattern="regular_expression"
```

» *`regular_expression`:* A type of expression called a *regular expression* that uses special symbols to define the pattern you want to apply to the field

For example, suppose you want to set up a pattern for a ten-digit North American telephone number that includes dashes, such as 555-123-4567 or 888-987-6543. In a regular expression, the symbol `\d` represents any digit from 0 to 9, so your regular expression would look like this:

```
\d\d\d-\d\d\d-\d\d\d\d
```

Here's the regular expression added to a telephone number field:

```
<input id="user-phone"
       type="tel"
       pattern="\d\d\d-\d\d\d-\d\d\d\d"
       placeholder="e.g., 123-456-7890"
       title="Enter a 10-digit number in the format 123-456-
  7890">
```

TIP

It's a good idea to add the `title` attribute and use it to describe the pattern you want to user to enter. Also, you can find all kinds of useful, ready-made patterns at the HTML5 Pattern site: `http://html5pattern.com`.

Table 3-1 summarizes the most useful regular expression symbols to use with the `pattern` attribute. See "Regular Expressions Reference," later in this chapter, for a more detailed look at this powerful tool.

From this table, you can see that an alternative way to write the 10-digit telephone regular expression would be the following:

```
[0-9]{3}-[0-9]{3}-[0-9]{4}
```

TABLE 3-1 The Most Useful Regular Expression Symbols

Symbol	Matches
\d	Any digit from 0 through 9
\D	Any character that is not a digit from 0 through 9
.	Any character
\s	Any whitespace character, such as the space, tab (\t), newline (\n), and carriage return (\r)
\S	Any non-whitespace character
[]	Whatever characters are listed between the square brackets
[*c1*-*c2*]	Anything in the range of letters or digits from *c1* to *c2*
[^]	Everything except whatever characters are listed between the square brackets
[^*c1*-*c2*]	Everything except the characters in the range of letters or digits from *c1* to *c2*
?	If the character preceding it appears just once or not at all
*	If the character preceding it is missing or if it appears one or more times
+	If the character preceding it appears one or more times
{*n*}	If the character preceding it appears exactly *n* times
{*n*,}	If the character preceding it appears at least *n* times
{*n*,*m*}	If the character preceding it appears at least *n* times and no more than *m* times
p1|*p2*	Pattern *p1* or pattern *p2*

Styling invalid fields

One useful thing you can do as a web developer is make it obvious for the user when a form field contains invalid data. Sure, the browser will display its little tooltip to alert the user when she submits the form, but that tooltip only stays onscreen for a few seconds. It would be better to style the invalid field in some way so the user always knows it needs fixing.

One straightforward way to do that is to take advantage of the CSS `:invalid` pseudo-selector, which enables you to apply a CSS rule to any invalid field.

For example, here's a rule that adds a red highlight around any `<input>` tag that is invalid:

```
input:invalid {
    border-color: rgba(255, 0, 0, .5);
    box-shadow: 0 0 10px 2px rgba(255, 0, 0, .8);
}
```

The problem, however, is that the web browser checks for invalid fields as soon as it loads the page. So, for example, if you have fields with the `required` attribute that are initially empty when the page loads, the browser will flag those as invalid and apply the `invalid` styling. Your users will be saying, "Gimme a break, I just got here!"

One way to work around this problem is to display an initial message (such as `required`) beside each required field, then replace that message with something positive (such as a check mark) when the field is filled in.

Here's some code that does that:

CSS:

```
input:invalid+span::after {
    content:'(required)';
    color: red;
}
input:valid+span::after {
    content:'\2713';
    color: green;
}
```

HTML:

```
<form>
    <div>
        <label for="user-name">Name:</label>
        <input id="user-name"
               type="text"
               placeholder="Optional"
               required>
        <span></span>
    </div>
    <div>
        <label for="user-email">Email:</label>
        <input id="user-email"
```

```
                 type="email"
                 placeholder="e.g., you@domain.com"
                 required>
          <span></span>
      </div>
      <button type="submit">Submit</button>
  </form>
```

Notice in the HTML that both fields have the `required` attribute and both fields also have an empty `span` element right after them. Those `span` elements are where you'll put your messages, and that's what the CSS code is doing:

- The first CSS rule looks for any invalid `input` field, then uses the adjacent sibling select (+) to select the `span` that comes immediately after the field. The `::after` pseudo-element adds the content `(required)` to the `span` and colors it `red`.
- The second CSS rule is very similar, except that it looks for any valid `input` field, then adds a green check mark (given by Unicode character `2713`) to the `span`.

Figure 3-5 shows these rules in action, where the `Name` field is valid and the `Email` field is invalid.

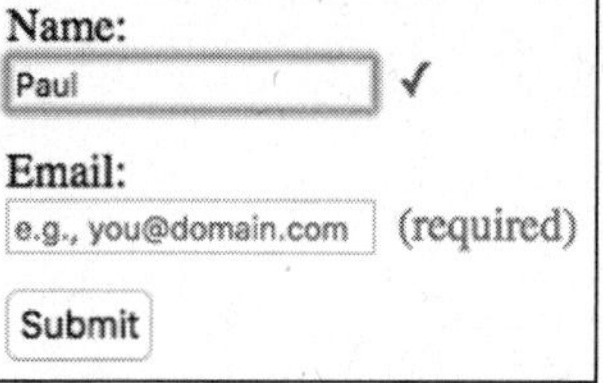

FIGURE 3-5: The CSS rules add a green check mark to valid fields, and the red text `(required)` to invalid fields.

Another approach is to use jQuery to listen for the `invalid` event firing on any `input` element. The `invalid` event fires when the user tries to submit the form and one or more fields contain invalid data. In your event handler, you could then apply a predefined class to the invalid field. Here's some code that does just that:

CSS:

```
.error {
    border-color: rgba(255, 0, 0, .5);
    box-shadow: 0 0 10px 2px rgba(255, 0, 0, .8);
}
```

```
input:valid {
    border-color: lightgray;
    box-shadow: none;
}
```

HTML:

```
<form>
    <div>
        <label for="user-name">Name:</label>
        <input id="user-name"
               type="text"
               placeholder="Your name"
               required>
    </div>
    <div>
        <label for="user-email">Email:</label>
        <input id="user-email"
               type="email"
               placeholder="e.g., you@domain.com"
               required>
    </div>
    <button type="submit">Submit</button>
</form>
```

jQuery:

```
$("input").on("invalid", function() {
    $(this).addClass('error');
});
```

The HTML is the same as in the previous example, minus the extra `<span>` tags. The CSS code defines a rule for the `error` class that uses `border-color` and `box-shadow` to add a red-tinged highlight to an element. The `input:valid` selector removes the border and box shadow when the field becomes valid. The jQuery code listens for the `invalid` event on any `input` element. When it fires, the event handler adds the `error` class to the element.

Validating Form Data on the Server

You might have looked at the title of this section and cried, "The server! But we just went through validating form data in the browser! Surely we don't have to validate on the server, as well!?" First of all, calm down. Second, yep, it would be nice if we lived in a world where validating form data in the web browser was good enough. Alas, that Shangri-La doesn't exist. The problem, you see, is that there are still a few folks surfing with very old web browsers that wouldn't know HTML5 from Maroon 5, and so don't support either `<input>` tag types such as `number`, `email`, and `date`, or browser-based validation. It's also possible that someone might, innocently or maliciously, bypass your form and send data directly to the server (say, by using a URL query string).

Either way, you can't be certain that the data that shows up on the server's doorstep has been validated, so it's up to your server script to ensure the data is legit before processing it. Happily, as you see in the next few sections, PHP is loaded with features that make validating data straightforward and painless.

Checking for required fields

If one or more fields in your form are mandatory, you can check those fields on the server by using PHP's `empty()` function:

```
empty(expression)
```

» *expression:* The literal, variable, expression, or function result that you want to test

The `empty()` function returns `FALSE` if the expression exists and has a non-empty, non-zero value; it returns `TRUE`, otherwise.

I'll go through a complete example that shows one way to handle validation errors on the server. First, here's some HTML:

```
<form>
    <div>
        <label for="user-name">Name</label>
        <input id="user-name"
               type="text"
               name="user-name">
    </div>
    <div>
        <label for="user-email">Email</label>
        <input id="user-email"
               type="email"
               name="user-email">
    </div>
    <button type="submit">Submit</button>
```

```
</form>
<article class="output"></article>
```

The form has two text fields, and there's also an `<article>` tag that you'll use a bit later to output the server results.

On the server, I created a PHP file named `validate-required-fields.php`:

```
<?php
    // Store the default status
    $server_results['status'] = 'success';

    // Check the user-name field
    if(isset($_GET['user-name'])) {
        $user_name = $_GET['user-name'];
        // Is it empty?
        if(empty($user_name)) {
            // If so, update the status and add an error
    message for the field
            $server_results['status'] = 'error';
            $server_results['user-name'] = 'Missing user name';
        }
    }
    // Check the user-email field
    if(isset($_GET['user-email'])) {
        $user_email = $_GET['user-email'];
        // Is it empty?
        if(empty($user_email)) {
            // If so, update the status and add an error
    message for the field
            $server_results['status'] = 'error';
            $server_results['user-email'] = 'Missing email
  address';
        }
    }
    // If status is still "success", add the success message
    if($server_results['status'] === 'success') {
        $output = "Success! Thanks for submitting the form,
  $user_name.";
        $server_results['output'] = $output;
    }
    // Create and then output the JSON data
    $JSON_data = json_encode($server_results, JSON_HEX_APOS |
    JSON_HEX_QUOT);
```

```
    echo $JSON_data;
?>
```

This script uses the `$server_results` associative array to store the data that gets sent back to the browser. At first the array's `status` key is set to `success`. Then the script checks the `user-name` field from the `$_GET` array: If the field is empty, the array's `status` key is set to `error` and an array item is added that sets an error message for the field. The same process is then used for the `user-email` field. If after those checks the array's `status` key is still set to `success` (meaning there were no validation errors), then the array is updated with a success message. Finally, the array is converted to JSON and outputted.

Back on the client, the `form` element's `submit` event handler converts and submits the form data, and then processes the result:

```
$('form').submit(function(e) {

    // Prevent the default form submission
    e.preventDefault();

    // Convert the data to a query string
    var formData = $(this).serialize();

    // Send the data to the server
    $.getJSON('php/validate-required-fields.php', formData,
    function(data) {

        // Display the output element
        $('.output').css('display', 'block');

        // Check the validation status
        if(data.status === 'success') {
            // Output the success result
            $('.output').html(data.output);
        } else {
            // Output the validation error(s)
            $('.output').html('<section>Whoops! There were
    errors:</section>');
            $.each(data, function(key, error) {
                if(key !== 'status') {
                    // Get the label text
                    var label = $('label[for=' + key +
    ']').text();
                    $('.output').append('<section>Error in ' +
    label + ' field: ' + error + '</section>');
```

```
                    }
                });
            }
        });
});
```

Note, in particular, the `.getJSON()` callback function checks the value of `data.status`: If it equals `success`, the script's success message is displayed. Otherwise, the `.each()` loop adds each error message to the output element. Figure 3-6 shows an example.

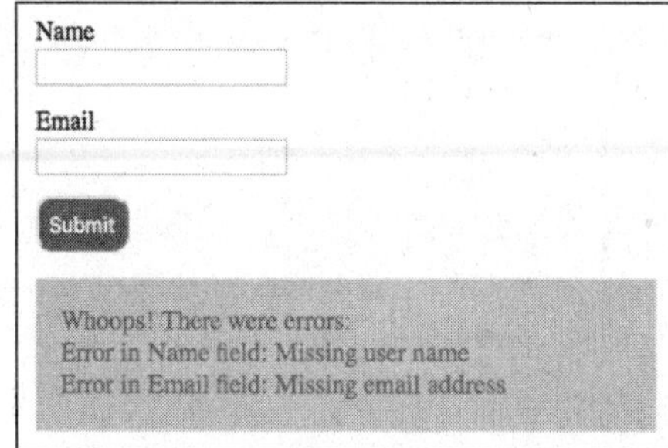

FIGURE 3-6: Some example validation error messages returned from the server script.

Validating text data

Besides validating that a text field exists, you might also want to perform two other validation checks on a text field:

- **The field contains alphabetic characters only.** To ensure the field contains only lowercase or uppercase letters, use the `ctype_alpha()` function:

  ```
  ctype_alpha(text)
  ```

  - *`text`:* Your form field's text data

  The `ctype_alpha()` function returns `TRUE` if the field contains only letters, `FALSE` otherwise.

- **The field length is greater than some minimum and/or less than some maximum value.** To check the length of the field, use the `strlen()` function:

  ```
  strlen(text)
  ```

  - *`text`:* Your form field's text data

  The `strlen()` function returns the number of characters in the field.

Here's some PHP code that performs these checks on a form field called `user-name`:

```
<?php
    // Store the default status
    $server_results['status'] = 'success';

    // Check the user-name field
    if(isset($_GET['user-name'])) {
        $user_name = $_GET['user-name'];
        // Is it empty?
        if(empty($user_name)) {
            // If so, update the status and add an error
  message for the field
            $server_results['status'] = 'error';
            $server_results['user-name'] = 'Missing user name';
        } else {
            // Does it contain non-alphabetic characters?
            if(!ctype_alpha($user_name)){
                // If so, update the status and add an error
  message for the field
                $server_results['status'] = 'error';
                $server_results['user-name'] = 'User name must
  be text';
            } else {
                // Does the user name contains less than 3 or
  more than 12 characters?
                if(strlen($user_name) < 3 || strlen($user_name)
  > 12) {
                    // If so, update the status and add an error
  message for the field
                    $server_results['status'] = 'error';
                    $server_results['user-name'] = 'User name
  must be 3 to 12 characters long';
                }
            }
        }
    }
    // If status is still "success", add the success message
    if($server_results['status'] === 'success') {
        $output = "Success! Thanks for submitting the form,
  $user_name.";
        $server_results['output'] = $output;
    }
```

```
    // Create and then output the JSON data
    $JSON_data = json_encode($server_results, JSON_HEX_APOS |
  JSON_HEX_QUOT);
    echo $JSON_data;
?>
```

Validating a field based on the data type

If you want to ensure the value of a field is a particular data type, PHP offers a powerful function called `filter_var()` that can help:

```
filter_var(var, filter, options)
```

- *var:* The variable, expression, or function result you want to check.
- *filter:* An optional constant value that determines the data type you want to check. Here are some useful filters:
  - `FILTER_VALIDATE_BOOLEAN`: Checks for a Boolean value.
  - `FILTER_VALIDATE_EMAIL`: Checks for a valid email address.
  - `FILTER_VALIDATE_FLOAT`: Checks for a floating point value.
  - `FILTER_VALIDATE_INT`: Checks for an integer value.
  - `FILTER_VALIDATE_URL`: Checks for a valid URL.
- *options:* An optional array that sets one or more options for the *filter*. For example, `FILTER_VALIDATE_INT` accepts the options `min_range` and `max_range`, which set the minimum and maximum allowable integers. Here's the setup for a minimum of 0 and a maximum of 100:

  ```
  array('options' => array('min_range' => 0, 'max_range' =>
    100))
  ```

The `filter_var()` function returns the data if it's valid according to the specified filter; if the data isn't valid, the function returns `FALSE` (or `NULL`, if you're using `FILTER_VALIDATE_BOOLEAN`).

Here's an example script that checks for integer values within an allowable range:

```
<?php
    // Store the default status
    $server_results['status'] = 'success';
```

```
    // Check the user-age field
    if(isset($_GET['user-age'])) {
        $user_age = $_GET['user-age'];
        // Is it empty?
        if(empty($user_age)) {
            // Add an error message for the field
            $server_results['status'] = 'error';
            $server_results['user-age'] = 'Missing age value';
        } else {
            // Is the field not an integer?
            if(!filter_var($user_age, FILTER_VALIDATE_INT)){
                // Add an error message for the field
                $server_results['status'] = 'error';
                $server_results['user-age'] = 'Age must be an
integer';
            } else {
                // Is the age not between 14 and 114?
                $options = array('options' => array('min_range'
=> 14, 'max_range' => 114));
                if(!filter_var($user_age, FILTER_VALIDATE_INT,
$options)) {
                    // Add an error message for the field
                    $server_results['status'] = 'error';
                    $server_results['user-age'] = 'Age must be
between 14 and 114';
                }
            }
        }
    }
    // If status is "success", add the success message
    if($server_results['status'] === 'success') {
        $output = "Success! You don't look a day over " .
intval($user_age - 1) . ".";
        $server_results['output'] = $output;
    }
    // Create and then output the JSON data
    $JSON_data = json_encode($server_results, JSON_HEX_APOS |
JSON_HEX_QUOT);
    echo $JSON_data;
?>
```

The script uses `filter_var($user_age, FILTER_VALIDATE_INT)` twice: first without and then with the *`options`* parameter. The first instance just checks for an integer value, whereas the second checks for an integer between 14 and 114. The integer check is redundant here, but I added both so you could get a feel for how `filter_var()` works.

Validating against a pattern

If you want to use a regular expression to validate a field value, PHP says "No problem!" by offering you the `preg_match()` function. Here's the simplified syntax:

```
preg_match(pattern, string)
```

- *pattern:* The regular expression, which you enter as a string. Note, too, that the regular expression must be surrounded by slashes (/).
- *string:* The string (such as a form field value) that you want to match against the regular expression.

The `preg_match()` function returns `TRUE` if `string` matches `pattern`, and `FALSE`, otherwise.

For example, suppose you want to check an account number to ensure that it uses the pattern AA-12345 — that is, two uppercase letters, a hyphen, then five numbers. Assuming the value is stored in a variable named `$account_number`, here's a `preg_match()` function that will validate the variable:

```
preg_match('/[A-Z]{2}-[0-9]{5}/', $account_number)
```

Regular Expressions Reference

TECHNICAL STUFF

You can validate form data using regular expressions either in the web browser by adding a `pattern` attribute to the field, or on the server by using PHP's `preg_match()` function. To help you get the most out of these powerful techniques, the rest of this chapter takes you through some examples that show you how to use the regular expression symbols. In the examples that follow, remember to surround the regular expression with slashes (/) when you use it in the `preg_match()` function; you don't need the slashes when you use the regular expression as a `pattern` attribute value.

Here are the symbols you can use in your regular expressions:

- \d: Matches any digit from 0 through 9:

Regular Expression	String	Match?
\d\d\d	"123"	Yes
\d\d\d\d	"123"	No

Regular Expression	String	Match?
\d\d\d	"12C"	No
\d\d\d-\d\d\d-\d\d\d\d	"123-555-6789"	Yes

- \D: Matches any character that's not a digit from 0 through 9:

Regular Expression	String	Match?
/\D\D\D/	"AB!"	Yes
/\D\D\D/	"A1B"	No
/\D-\D\D\D\D/	"A-BCDE"	Yes

- \w: Matches any character that's a letter, a digit, or an underscore (_):

Regular Expression	String	Match?
\w\w\w	"F1"	Yes
\w\w\w	"F+1"	No
A\w\	"A"	Yes
A\w\	"A!"	No

- \W: Matches any character that's not a letter, a digit, or an underscore (_):

Regular Expression	String	Match?
\W\W\W\W	"<!--"	Yes
\W\W\W	"<a>"	No
1\W\	"10"	No
1\W\	"1!"	Yes

- . (dot): Matches any character that's not a newline:

Regular Expression	String	Match?
`....`	"ABCD"	Yes
`....`	"123"	No
`A..`	"A@B"	Yes

- \s: Matches any whitespace character, such as the space, tab (\t), newline (\n), and carriage return (\r):

Regular Expression	String	Match?
`\d\d\d\s\d\d\d\d`	"123 4567"	Yes
`\d\d\d\s\d\d\d\d`	"123-4567"	No
`\d\d\d\s\d\d\d\d`	"123 4567"	No

- \S: Matches any non-whitespace character:

Regular Expression	String	Match?
`\d\d\d\S\d\d\d\d`	"123 4567"	No
`\d\d\d\S\d\d\d\d`	"123-4567"	Yes
A\SB	"A+B"	Yes

- [ ]: Matches whatever characters are listed between the square brackets. The [ ] symbol also accepts a range of letters and/or digits:

Regular Expression	String	Match?
`[+-]\d\d\d`	"+123"	Yes
`[+-]\d\d\d`	"$123"	No
[2468]-A	"2-A"	Yes
[2468]-A	"1-A"	No
[(]\d\d\d[)]\d\d\d-\d\d\d\d	"(123)555-6789"	Yes

Regular Expression	String	Match?
[A-Z]\d\d\d	"A123"	Yes
[A-Z]\d\d\d	"a123"	No
[A-Za-z]\d\d\d	"a123"	Yes
[0-5]A	"3A"	Yes
[0-5]A	"6A"	No
[0-59]A	"9A"	Yes

REMEMBER

Remember that the range [0-59] matches the digits 0 to 5 or 9 and *not* the range 0 to 59.

» [^]: Matches everything but whatever characters are listed between the square brackets. As with the [] symbol, you can use letter or digit ranges.

Regular Expression	String	Match?
[^+-]\d\d\d	"+123"	No
[^+-]\d\d\d	"123"	Yes
[^2468]-A	"2-A"	No
[^2468]-A	"1-A"	Yes
[^A-Z]\d\d\d	"A123"	No
[^A-Z]\d\d\d	"a123"	Yes
[^A-Za-z]\d\d\d	"#123"	Yes
[^0-5]A	"3A"	No
[^0-5]A	"6A"	Yes
[^0-59]A	"9A"	No

» \b: Matches one or more characters if they appear on a word boundary (that is, at the beginning or the end of a word). If you place \b before the characters, it matches if they appear at the beginning of a word; if you place \b after the characters, it matches if they appear at the end of a word.

Regular Expression	String	Match?
\bode	"odeon"	Yes
\bode	"code"	No
ode\b	"code"	Yes
ode\b	"odeon"	No
\bode\b	"ode"	Yes

- \B: Matches one or more characters if they don't appear on a word boundary (the beginning or the end of a word). If you place \B before the characters, it matches if they don't appear at the beginning of a word; if you place \B after the characters, it matches if they don't appear at the end of a word.

Regular Expression	String	Match?
/\Bode/	"odeon"	No
/\Bode/	"code"	Yes
/ode\B/	"code"	No
/ode\B/	"odeon"	Yes
/\Bode\B/	"code"	No
/\Bode\B/	"coder"	Yes

- ?: Matches if the character preceding it appears just once or not at all:

Regular Expression	String	Match?
e-?mail	"email"	Yes
e-?mail	"e-mail"	Yes
e-?mail	"e--mail"	No
e-?mail	"e:mail"	No

- *: Matches if the character preceding it is missing or if it appears one or more times:

Regular Expression	String	Match?
`e-*mail`	"email"	Yes
`e-*mail`	"e-mail"	Yes
`e-*mail`	"e--mail"	Yes
`e-*mail`	"e:mail"	No

» +: Matches if the character preceding it appears one or more times:

Regular Expression	String	Match?
`e-+mail`	"email"	No
`e-+mail`	"e-mail"	Yes
`e-+mail`	"e--mail"	Yes
`e-+mail`	"e:mail"	No

» {*n*}: Matches if the character preceding it appears exactly *n* times:

Regular Expression	String	Match?
`lo{2}p`	"loop"	Yes
`lo{2}p`	"lop"	No
`\d{5}`	"12345"	Yes
`\d{5}-\d{4}`	"12345-6789"	Yes

» {*n*,}: Matches if the character preceding it appears at least *n* times:

Regular Expression	String	Match?
`lo{2,}p`	"loop"	Yes
`lo{2,}p`	"lop"	No
`lo{2,}p`	"looop"	Yes
`\d{5,}`	"12345"	Yes

Regular Expression	String	Match?
`\d{5,}`	"123456"	Yes
`\d{5,}`	"1234"	No

» `{n,m}`: Matches if the character preceding it appears at least *n* times and no more than *m* times:

Regular Expression	String	Match?
`lo{1,2}p`	"loop"	Yes
`lo{1,2}p`	"lop"	Yes
`lo{1,2}p`	"looop"	No
`\d{1,5}`	"12345"	Yes
`\d{1,5}`	"123456"	No
`\d{1,5}`	"1234"	Yes

» ^: Matches if the characters that come after it appear at the beginning of the string:

Regular Expression	String	Match?
^Java	"JavaScript"	Yes
^Java	"HotJava"	No
^[^+-]?\d\d\d	"123"	Yes
^[^+-]?\d\d\d	"+123"	No

» $: Matches if the characters that come after it appear at the end of the string:

Regular Expression	String	Match?
Java$	"JavaScript"	No
Java$	"HotJava"	Yes

Regular Expression	String	Match?
\d\d\.\d%$	"12.3%"	Yes
\d\d\.\d%$	"12.30%"	No

TIP

If you need to include one of the characters from a regular expression symbol as a literal in your expression, escape the character by preceding it with a backslash (\). For example, suppose you want to see if a string ends with `.com`. The following regular expression won't work:

```
.com$
```

That's because the dot (`.`) symbol represents any character except a newline. To force the regular expression to match only a literal dot, escape the dot, like this:

```
\.com$
```

» `|`: Place this symbol between two patterns, and the regular expression matches if the string matches one pattern or the other. (Don't confuse this symbol with JavaScript's OR operator: `||`.)

Regular Expression	String	Match?
`^(\d{5}|\d{5}-\d{4})$`	"12345"	Yes
`^(\d{5}|\d{5}-\d{4})$`	"12345-6789"	Yes
`^(\d{5}|\d{5}-\d{4})$`	"123456789"	No

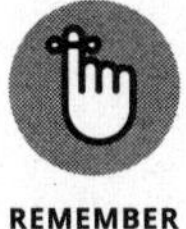

REMEMBER

The preceding examples use parentheses to group the two patterns together. With regular expressions, you can use parentheses to group items and set precedence, just as you can with JavaScript expressions. A regular expression of the form `^(`*`pattern`*`)$` means that the pattern defines the entire string, not just some of the characters in the string.

7 Coding Web Apps

Contents at a Glance

IN THIS CHAPTER

» Learning about web apps

» Planning your app's data, workflow, and interface

» Planning a responsive web app

» Planning an accessible web app

» Becoming familiar with web app security issues

Chapter 1
Planning a Web App

What you can do, or dream you can, begin it,

Boldness has genius, power, and magic in it.

— JOHANN WOLFGANG VON GOETHE

There are many reasons to get and stay interested in web coding and development. Here are a just a few: the challenge of learning something new; the confidence that comes from figuring out hard or complex problems; the satisfactions that inhere from getting code to work; the desire to get a job in web development; the feeling that you're operating right at the leading edge of the modern world. These are all great and motivating reasons to code for the web, but there's another reason to dive deep into CSS and JavaScript and all the rest: as an outlet for your creative side. Sure, anybody who learns a bit of HTML and a few CSS properties can put up pages of information, but as a full-stack web developer who also knows JavaScript, jQuery, MySQL, and PHP, you've got all the tools you need to create bold and beautiful apps for the web. That's where the real creativity lies: having a vision of something cool, interesting, and fun and then using code to realize that vision for other people to see and use. This minibook helps you unleash the right side of your brain and make your creative vision a reality by showing you how to use all your web coding and development skills and know-how to build web apps. First up: the all-important planning process.

What Is a Web App?

If you go to the web home for a company called Alphabet (`https://abc.xyz`), you get a general introduction to the company, plus some information for investors, news releases, links to corporate documents such as the company bylaws, and so on. But Alphabet is also the parent company for some of the web's most iconic spots:

- **Google (`www.google.com`):** Search the web.
- **Gmail (`https://mail.google.com`):** Send and receive email messages.
- **Google Maps (`https://maps.google.com`):** Locate and get directions to places using maps.
- **YouTube (`www.youtube.com`):** Play and upload videos.

What's the difference between the parent Alphabet site and these other sites? Lots, of course, but there are two differences that I think are most important:

- Each of the other sites is focused on a single task or topic: searching, emailing, maps, or videos.
- Each of the other sites offers an interface that enables the user to "operate" the site in some way. For example, Google has a simple search form, whereas Gmail looks like an email Inbox and offers commands such as Compose and Reply.

REMEMBER

In other words, the Alphabet home is a basic website that's really just a collection of documents you can navigate, whereas the likes of Google, Gmail, Google Maps, and YouTube are more like the applications you use on your computer. They are, in short, *web apps*, because although they reside on the web and are built using web technologies such as HTML, CSS, JavaScript, MySQL, and PHP, they enable you to perform tasks and create things just like a computer application.

Fortunately, you don't have to have an idea for the next YouTube or Gmail to get started coding web apps. (Although, hey, if you do, I say go for it!) Web apps can be anything you want, as long as they enable you or your users to do something. If that something happens to be fun, creative, interesting, or useful, then congratulations: You've made the world a better place.

Planning Your Web App: The Basics

If you're like me, when you come up with an exciting idea for a web app, the first thing you want to do is open your trusty text editor and start bashing out some code. That's a satisfying way to go, but, believe me, that satisfaction dissipates awfully fast when you're forced to go back and redo a bunch of code or completely restructure your database because, in your haste, you took a wrong turn and ended up at a dead end or too far from your goal.

I plea, then, for just a bit of restraint so that you can spend the first hour or two of your project thinking about what you want to build and laying out the steps required to get there. Think of it like planning a car trip. You know your destination, but it's unlikely you'll want to just get in the car and start driving in the general direction of your goal. You need to plan your route, load up with supplies such as gas, water, and food, gather tools such as a GPS, and so on. To figure out the web-development equivalents of such things, it helps to ask yourself five questions:

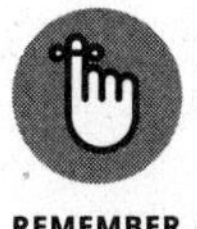

REMEMBER

- What is my app's functionality?
- What are my app's data requirements?
- How will my app work?
- How many pages will my app require?
- What will my app's pages look like?

The next few sections go through these questions both in a general way and more specifically with the app I'm going to build. It's called FootPower! and it's a simple app for logging and viewing foot-propelled activities such as walking, running, and cycling.

What is my app's functionality?

The first stage in planning any web app is understanding what you want the app to do. You can break this down into two categories:

- **User functions:** These are the tasks that the user performs when she operates whatever controls your app provides. The standard four tasks are given by the unfortunately named CRUD acronym: creating, reading, updating, and deleting.
- **App functions:** These are tasks that your app performs outside of the interface controls. Examples are creating user accounts, signing users in and out, handling forgotten passwords, and backing up data.

For FootPower!, here's a list of the user functions I want to implement:

- Creating new activities, each of which records activity details such as the type of activity, and the activity date, distance, and duration
- Viewing previous activities, with the capability to filter the activities by date and type
- Editing an existing activity
- Deleting an activity

Here are the app functions I want to implement:

- Creating new users
- Verifying new users by sending a verification email
- Signing existing users in and out
- Maintaining a user's app settings
- Handling forgotten passwords
- Deleting a user account

What are my app's data requirements?

Web apps don't necessarily have to use a back end. If your web app is a calculator, for example, then you'd only need to present the front-end interface to the user; no back-end database or Ajax calls are required. (I talk about how to build an app that doesn't require a back end in Book 8.) But if your app requires persistent data — which might be data you supply or data that's created by each user — then you need to store that data in a MySQL database and use Ajax calls to transfer that data between the browser and the server.

REMEMBER

Before you load up phpMyAdmin, however, you need to sit down and figure out what you want to store in your database. Web app data generally falls into three categories:

- **User data:** If your app has user accounts, then you need to store account data such as the username or email address, password, profile settings, and site preferences.
- **User-generated data:** If your app enables users to create things, then you need to save that data so that it can be restored to the user the next time he signs in.

- **App data:** If your app presents data to users, then you need to store that data in MySQL. You might also want to store behind-the-app-scenes data such as analytics and visitor statistics.

My FootPower! app's data requirements fall into two segments:

- The app will have user accounts, so I need a MySQL table to store each account's email address, password, verification status, and a few site preferences.
- Users will be recording their foot-propelled movements, so I need two tables to store this data:
  - Each user is creating a log of his activities, so I need a table to record the data for each of these logs, basically just a unique log ID, the ID of the user who owns the log, and the date the log was created.
  - Within each user's log will be the activities themselves, which I'll store in a separate table that includes a unique ID for each activity, the user's log ID, and fields for each chunk of activity data: type, date, distance, and duration.

How will my app work?

REMEMBER

Once you know what you want your app to do and what data your app requires, you're ready to tackle how your app works. This is called the app's *workflow* and it covers at a high level what the app does and the order in which it does those things. A simple flowchart is usually the way to go here: Just map out what happens from the time users type in your app URL to the time they leave the page.

Figure 1-1 shows the workflow I envision for my FootPower! app.

How many pages will my app require?

Your app's workflow should tell you fairly specifically how many pages your app needs. Most web apps are focused on a single set of related tasks, so your users will spend most of their time on the page that provides the app's main interface, usually the home page. However, your app will need other pages to handle tasks such as registering users, signing in users, and displaying account options. Record every page you need, which will act as an overall to-do list for the front end.

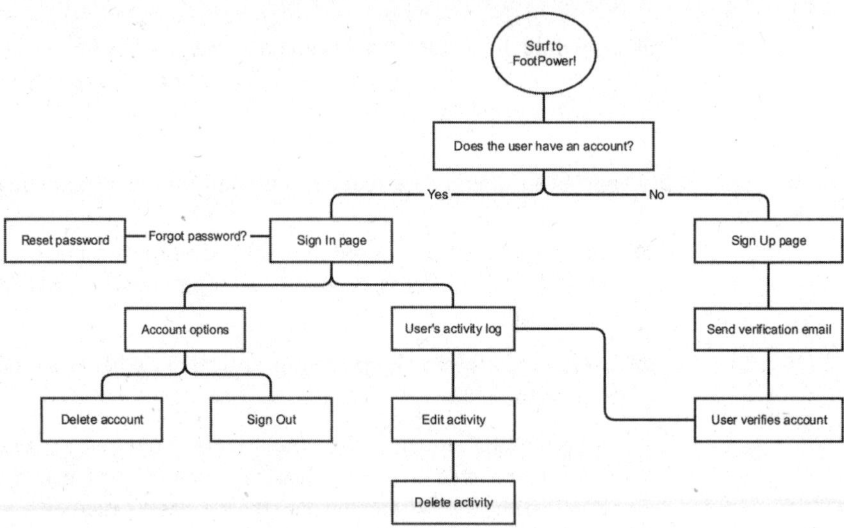

FIGURE 1-1: The workflow for my Foot-Power! app.

Here's my list for the FootPower! app:

- The home page, which will require two versions:
  - The unregistered or signed-out version of the home page, which will serve as a kind of ad for the app
  - The signed-in version, which will show the user's activity log and enable log-based tasks such as creating, filtering, editing, and deleting activities
- A page that enables new users to register
- A page letting new users know that a verification email has been sent
- A sign-in page
- A page that enables the user to edit and delete activities
- A password reset page
- An account options page
- An account delete page

What will my app's pages look like?

Before you start laying down your HTML and CSS code, you need to have a decent sense of what you want your app's pages to look like. Sure, all of that might be in your head, but it really pays in the long run to get those images down on paper with a sketch or two. These sketches don't have to be fancy in the least. Just take a pen, pencil, or your favorite Crayola color and rough out the overall structure. Simple forms (such as those for signing in or resetting a password) don't require much effort, but for more elaborate pages, such as your app's home page, you need to flesh out the design a bit: header, navigation, main content, sidebar, footer, and so on.

Figure 1-2 shows my sketch for the home page that a signed-in user will see.

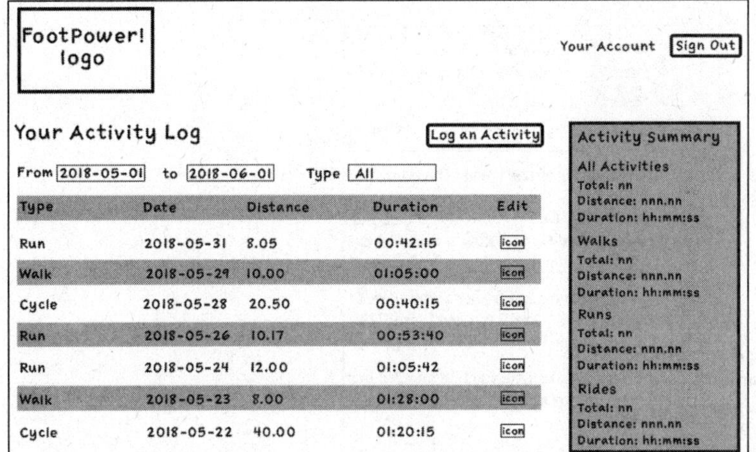

FIGURE 1-2: A sketch of the signed-in user's home page for the FootPower! app.

Planning Your Web App: Responsiveness

A web app is something like the online equivalent of a desktop program, but that doesn't mean you should build your web app to look good and work properly only on desktop-sized screens. Why not? For the simple reason that your app's visitors will be using a wide range of device sizes, from PCs with gigantic displays several feet wide, all the way down to smartphones with screens just a few inches wide. On the modern web, one size definitely does not fit all, so you need to plan your app so that its *user experience* (*UX*, to the cognoscenti) — that is, what visitors see and interact with — is positive for everyone.

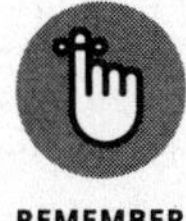

REMEMBER

To make your web app look good and operate well on any size screen, you need to plan your app with *responsiveness* in mind. A responsive web app is one that changes its layout, styling, and often also its content to ensure that the app works on whatever screen the reader is using.

To see why you need to code responsively from the start of your web app, consider the two main non-responsive layouts you could otherwise use:

- **Fixed-width:** A layout where the width of the content is set to a fixed size. In this case, if the fixed-width is greater than the width of the screen, most of the time the user has to scroll horizontally to see all the content, as shown in Figure 1-3.

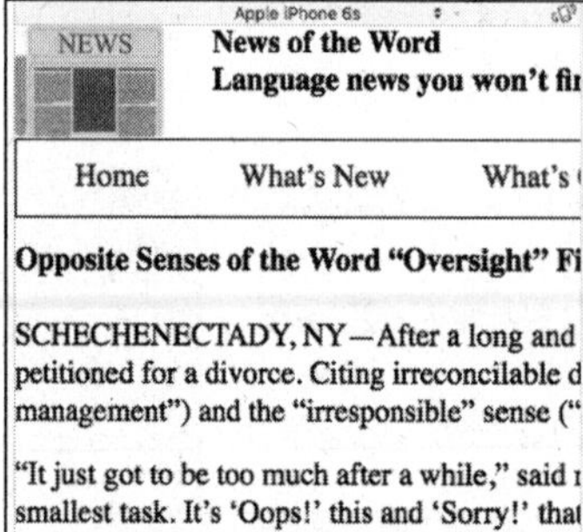

FIGURE 1-3: When a page has a fixed width, users with small screens have to scroll horizontally to see all the content.

- **No-width:** A layout where the width of the content has no set width. You might think having no width would enable the text and images to wrap nicely on a small screen, and you'd be right. However, the problem is on larger screens, where your text lines expand to fill the browser width and, as you can see in Figure 1-4, those lines can become ridiculously long, to the point where scanning the lines becomes just about impossible.

FIGURE 1-4: When a page has no maximum width, the lines of text become too long for comfortable reading.

To work around these problems and to ensure your web app looks good on any screen size, you need to implement the following responsive techniques:

- **Set the viewport:** To ensure that your layout works well in smaller screens, use the following `<meta>` tag to tell the browser to set the viewport width to the width of the current device's screen, and to set the viewport's zoom level to 1 (that is, not zoomed in or zoomed out).

```
<meta name="viewport" content="width=device-width,
   initial-scale=1.0">
```

- **Liquid layout:** A layout in which the overall width is set to a maximum (so that text lines never get too long to read), but the page elements have their widths set in percentages (or a similar relative measure such as viewport width: `vw`). Since even really old web browsers support percentages, this is a good fallback layout to use. For example:

  CSS:

```
body {
    max-width: 800px;
}
article {
    width: 67%;
}
aside {
    width: 33%;
}
```

  HTML:

```
<body>
    <main>
        <article>
        </article>
        <aside>
        </aside>
    </main>
</body>
```

» **Flexible layout:** A layout that uses flexbox to automatically wrap items when the browser window is too narrow to contain them. You set the container's `flex-wrap` property to `wrap`, as shown in the following example:

CSS:

```
body {
    max-width: 800px;
}
main {
    display: flex;
    flex-wrap: wrap;
}
article {
    flex-grow: 2;
    flex-shrink: 0;
    flex-basis: 300px;
}
aside {
    flex-grow: 1;
    flex-shrink: 0;
    flex-basis: 150px;
}
```

HTML:

```
<body>
    <main>
        <article>
        </article>
        <aside>
        </aside>
    </main>
</body>
```

Note, too, that I've set `flex-shrink` to `0` and added `flex-basis` values, which combine to create a minimum width for each element.

» **Adaptive layout:** A layout that changes depending on the current value of certain screen features, such as width. An adaptive layout uses a CSS feature called a *media query,* which is an expression accompanied by a code block consisting of one or more style rules. The expression interrogates some feature of the screen, usually its width. If that expression is true for the current device, then the browser applies the media query's style rules; if the expression is false, the browser ignores the media query's rules. Here's the syntax:

```
@media (expression) {
    Style rules go here
}
```

Here's an example that applies two style rules whenever the current screen width is less than or equal to `767px`:

```
@media (max-width: 767px) {
    header {
        height: 48px;
    }
    .site-title {
        font-size: 24px;
    }
}
```

Figures 1-5 through 1-7 demonstrate a more advanced example, where the layout of the page changes, depending on the screen width.

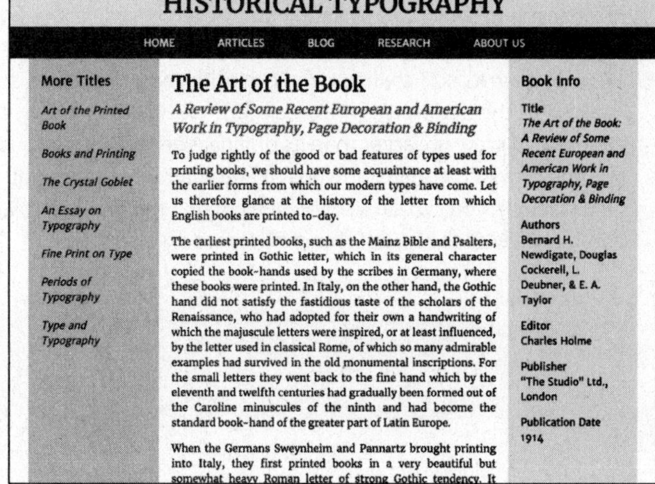

FIGURE 1-5: A typical page with header, navigation, an article, and two sidebars. On a desktop screen, the article is flanked by the sidebars.

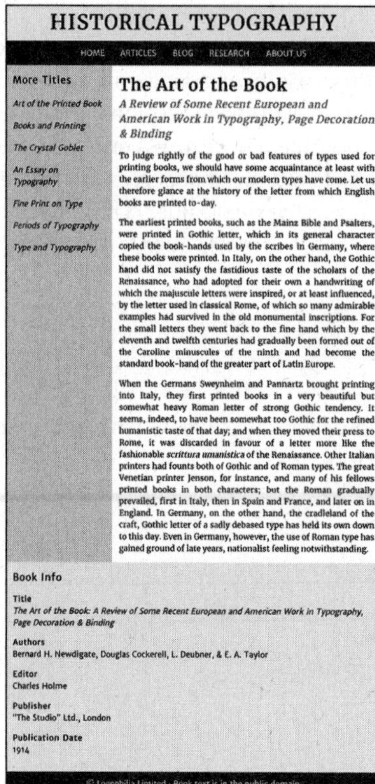

FIGURE 1-6: On a narrower tablet-sized screen, the right sidebar wraps below the left sidebar and the article.

REMEMBER

- **Responsive images:** Renders an image fluidly so that its size adjusts to different screen sizes. Ideally, you want the image to scale no larger than its original size to avoid ugly pixilation and jagged edges, and you want the width and height to maintain the original aspect ratio so that the image doesn't look skewed when its size changes. You can achieve both goals by styling the image with the declarations `max-height: 100%`, which allows the image to scale but to grow no larger than its original size, and `height: auto`, which tells the browser to adjust the height automatically as the width changes. (Alternatively, you can set `width: auto` to get the browser to adjust the width automatically as the height changes). Here's an example:

```
.aside-img {
    max-height: 100%;
    height: auto;
}
```

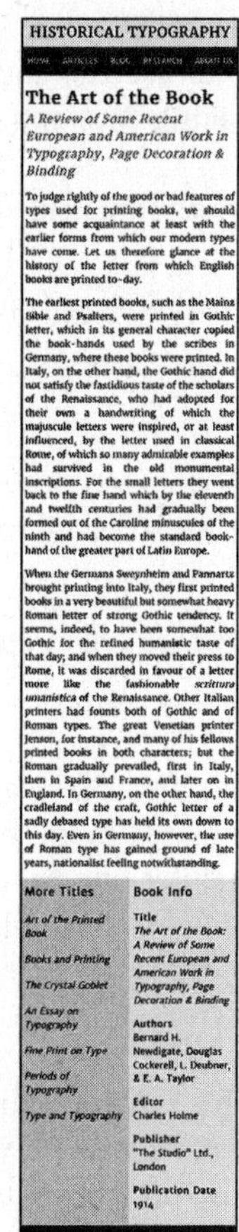

FIGURE 1-7: On an even narrower smartphone-sized screen, both sidebars appear below the article.

- **Responsive typography:** Renders font sizes and vertical measures (such as `height` and `margin-top`) with the relative units `em` or `rem` rather than fixed-size pixels (`px`); renders horizontal measures (such as `width` and `padding-right`) in percentages (`%`) instead of pixels (`px`). Using relative measurement units enables the page typography to flow seamlessly as the screen size changes.

Planning Your Web App: Accessibility

When planning a web app, the thoughtful developer remains aware at all times that the people who visit and use the app come with different abilities. When planning a web app, the ethical developer understands that, even though every person is different, they all have an equal right to use the app. When you give everyone equal access to your web app, you're making your app *accessible*.

REMEMBER

Planning for accessibility means taking the following impairments into account:

- **Visual:** Includes full or partial blindness, color-blindness, and reduced vision.
- **Auditory:** Includes full or partial deafness, difficulty hearing, the inability to hear sounds at certain frequencies, and tinnitus.
- **Motor:** Includes the inability to use a pointing device such as a mouse, restricted movement, lack of fine motor control, excessive trembling or shaking, and slow reflexes or response times.
- **Cognitive:** Includes learning disabilities, focusing problems, impaired memory, and extreme distractibility.

An accessible design is the right choice ethically, but it's also the right choice practically because a significant percentage (estimates range from 5 to 20 percent) of the people who use your web app will exhibit one or more of the above disabilities in varying degrees. Fortunately, as long as you build your app with equal access in mind from the get-go, adding accessible features takes very little effort on your part.

TIP

Before you get started, it's a good idea to crank up a screen reading application so that you can test out how your web app works when "heard." If you use Windows, start up the Narrator utility; if you're on a Mac, fire up the VoiceOver utility.

Web app accessibility is a massive topic, but for our purposes you can boil it down to implementing the following techniques:

- **Include alternative text for all images.** For the visually impaired, a screen reader reads aloud the value of every `<img>` tag's `alt` attribute, so important or structural images should include a brief description as the `alt` value:

  ```
  <img src="twitter.png" alt="Icon for link to Twitter">
  ```

  You don't need to add an `alt` value for purely decorative images, but you must include the `alt` tag (set to an empty string: `alt=""`) or your HTML code won't validate.

- **Add an ARIA label to all form fields.** ARIA stands for Accessible Rich Internet Applications, and it's a technology for adding accessibility to web apps. When you add the `aria-label` attribute to an `<input>`, `<select>`, or `<textarea>` tag, the screen reader reads that attribute's text:

```
<input type="radio"
       id="pony-express"
       name="delivery"
       value="pony"
       aria-label="Pony express delivery option">
```

- **Add a label for all form fields.** Adding the `<label>` tag — either by using the `for` attribute to reference the `id` of the corresponding field, or by surrounding the field with `<label>` and `</label>` tags — enables the user to select the field by also clicking the label. This increases the target area for clicking, which helps users with unsteady hands. Be sure to add a label for every `<input>` tag, as well as each `<select>` and `<textarea>` tag:

```
<label for="user-email">Email address</label>
<input id="user-email" type="email">
```

- **Use headings hierarchically.** All page headings should use `<h1>` through `<h6>` tags, where that order reflects the hierarchy of the heading structure: `<h1>` is the top-level heading in a section of the page, `<h2>` is the second-level heading in that section, and so on. Don't skip heading levels (say, by jumping from `<h2>` to `<h4>`).

- **Use semantic HTML5 page tags.** These include `<header>`, `<nav>`, `<main>`, `<article>`, `<section>`, `<aside>`, and `<footer>`. These so-called *landmarks* help assistive technologies make sense of your web app. You should also add ARIA `role` attributes to these tags, as follows:

```
<header role="banner">
<nav role="navigation">
<main role="main">
<article role="contentinfo">
<section role="contentinfo">
<aside role="complementary">
<aside role="note">
<footer role="contentinfo">
```

  Wait: two `role` possibilities for the `<aside>` tag? Yep: Choose the `role` value that best fits the content of the sidebar.

» **Add ARIA roles to non-semantic elements.** If your app uses non-semantic elements, such as a jQuery UI or jQuery Mobile widget, you can alert assistive technologies to what the widget does by adding the `role` attribute and setting it equal to the widget's function in the app. Some example `role` values are `dialog`, `menu`, `menubar`, `progressbar`, `scrollbar`, `slider`, `tab`, `tablist`, `tabpanel`, and `toolbar`. For example, here's how you'd add the various tab-related roles to jQuery UI's Tabs widget:

```
<div id="my-tabs">
    <ul role="tablist">
        <li><a href="#my-tab-1" role="tab">This</a></li>
        <li><a href="#my-tab-2" role="tab">That</a></li>
        <li><a href="#my-tab-3" role="tab">The Other
  </a></li>
    </ul>
    <div id="my-tab-1" role="tabpanel">
        This is the first tab's content.
    </div>
    <div id="my-tab-2" role="tabpanel">
        This is the second tab's content.
    </div>
    <div id="my-tab-3" role="tabpanel">
        Yep, this is the third tab's content.
    </div>
</div>
```

See Mozilla Developer Network's Using ARIA page at `https://developer.mozilla.org/en-US/docs/Web/Accessibility/ARIA/ARIA_Techniques` to see a complete list of ARIA roles.

» **Ensure your app's colors have sufficient contrast.** If text colors too closely match the background color, the text will be hard to decipher, particularly for the visually impaired.

Once your app is on the web, you can check its accessibility by heading over to the Web Accessibility Evaluation Tool (WAVE) at `http://wave.webaim.org`. Paste your web app's address into the text box and press Enter/Return to see a report.

Planning Your Web App: Security

Like it or not (and I suspect not), we live in a world populated by a small but determined band of miscreants who spend all their time and energy trying to deface, destroy, or exploit web apps just like the one you're about to build. And make no mistake: If you put an unprotected web app online, it will be found by one (or more) of these rapscallions and bad things will ensue.

So you need to take a piece of paper, write the word "SECURITY" in bold letters, and tape it to your cat's forehead as a constant reminder that building a web app really means building a secure web app. And I don't mean building your app and then bolting on some security features at the very end — no, you need to bake in the security goodness right from the start.

As important as web app security is, you might be surprised to hear that I can summarize it with just two axioms:

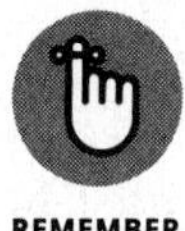
REMEMBER

- **Never trust data sent to the server.** For example, if you have a form with a text field, an attacker can insert a specially constructed text string that forces MySQL to perform unwanted actions, such as deleting data. Alternatively, it's possible for an attacker to submit data to the server without using your form at all.
- **Always control data sent from the server.** When you send data back to the web page, you need to be sure that you're not sending anything dangerous. For example, if an attacker uses a form's text field to submit a `<script>` tag with malicious JavaScript code, and you then redisplay the form's values without checking them, that script will execute. Similarly, if you use the server to store sensitive data such as sign-in passwords and private information, you need to install safeguards so that this data doesn't fall into the wrong hands.

Understanding the dangers

There are, it often seems, almost as many security exploits as there are low-lifes trying to compromise our apps. However, the most common security dangers fall into four main categories: SQL injection, cross-site scripting, insecure file uploads, and unauthorized access.

SQL injection

WARNING

Probably the most common exploit, *SQL injection* involves inserting some malicious code into an ordinary SQL command, such as a `SELECT` or `DELETE` statement. Consider the following sign-in form:

```
<form>
    <label for="username">User name:</label>
    <input id="username" type="text" name="user">
```

```
    <label for="password">Password:</label>
    <input id="password" type="password" name="pass">
</form>
```

When this form is submitted, a PHP script to sign in the user might look, in part, like this:

```
<?php
    $user = $_POST['user'];
    $pass = $_POST['pass'];
    $sql = "SELECT *
            FROM users
            WHERE username='$user' AND password='$pass'";
?>
```

That works fine as long as the user types a legit username and password, but what happens if some scoundrel types `admin' #` in the user field and nothing at all in the password field? Here's the resulting value of the `$sql` variable:

```
SELECT * FROM users WHERE username='admin' #' AND password=''
```

The key here is the hash symbol (`#`), which marks the beginning of a comment in an SQL command, meaning that the rest of the line is ignored. (Just so you know, MySQL also uses `--` to mark the start of a comment.) That is, the actual SQL command that gets processed is this:

```
SELECT * FROM users WHERE username='admin'
```

Congratulations, some criminal has just signed in as the administrator!

As another example, suppose your web app has a button that, when clicked, deletes an item from the current user's data. Your Ajax call might pass along a `user-id` and an `item-id`, meaning that your PHP script would do something like the following to remove the specified item:

```
<?php
    $user_id = $_POST['user-id'];
    $item_id = $_POST['item-id'];
    $sql = "DELETE
            FROM items
            WHERE userid='$user_id' AND itemid='$item_id'";
?>
```

Looks fine from here, but suppose some fiend passes the following as the `user-id` value: `whatever' OR 1=1 #`. Assuming the `item-id` value is blank, here's the resulting `$sql` variable value:

```
DELETE FROM items WHERE userid='whatever' OR 1=1 #' AND
   itemid=''
```

Taking the comment symbol (`#`) into account, the actual command looks like this:

```
DELETE FROM items WHERE userid='whatever' OR 1=1
```

The `1=1` part always returns `TRUE`, so the result is that the command deletes everything from the `items` table!

Cross-site scripting (XSS)

WARNING

Cross-site scripting (usually shortened to *XSS*) is a way of surreptitiously forcing an innocent user to launch an attacker's malicious script. This most often happens when the malefactor uses a phishing email or similar ruse to trick the user into visiting a page that spoofs a form used on a legitimate site.

For example, suppose the form asks the user to enter her credit card number and password. If this was a normal form submission and the user entered either the wrong credit card number of the wrong password, the PHP script on the server might redisplay the form to ask the user to try again:

```
<?php
    $cc = $_POST['credit-card'];
    $pw = $_POST['password'];

    // Code that checks these inputs goes here

    // If one or both inputs are invalid:
    echo '<input type="text" name="credit-card" value="' .
  $cc . '">';
    echo '<input type="password" name="password">';
?>
```

Notice, in particular, that this "helpful" script redisplays the credit card value (stored in the `$cc` variable) in the text field. Imagine, then, that our attacker's spoofed form actually sends the following text instead of the credit card number:

```
"><script>alert('Ha ha!');</script><a href="
```

Here's the resulting HTML (which I've tidied up a bit so you can see what's going on):

```
<input type="text" name="credit-card" value="">
<script>
    alert('Ha ha!');
</script>
<a href="">
<input type="password" name="password" value="">
```

What happens here? That's right: The JavaScript code between the `<script>` and `</script>` tags executes and, believe me, in the real world it's unlikely to just display an innocuous alert box.

Insecure file uploads

If your web app allows users to upload files — for example, you might want to allow each user to upload a small image to use as a profile avatar — then you open up a new can of security worms because a malicious user can:

- Upload huge files, which tax the server's resources.
- Upload a nasty script instead of, say, an image.
- Overwrite existing server files.

Unauthorized access

If your web app requires users to sign in with a username (or email address) and password, then keeping those passwords secure is of paramount importance. Otherwise, an unauthorized interloper could sign in as a legitimate user and either destroy or tamper with that user's data, post messages or other content under that user's name, and even delete the user's account.

Defending your web app

There's an alarming number of potential exploits that a villainous user can use to wreak havoc on your web app. Fortunately, if you implement multiple lines of defense — a strategy sometimes called *defense in depth* — you can inoculate your app against all but the most determined attacks.

Sanitizing incoming data

Defending your web app begins with *sanitizing* any data sent to the server. There are four main ways to sanitize data:

» **Converting:** Encoding an input's characters to harmless equivalents. The most useful PHP function for this is htmlentities(), which takes a string input and converts any special characters to either an HTML entity code, if one exists, or to an HTML character code. In particular, htmlentities() changes < to <, > to >, " to ", and & to &. For example, htmlentities ('<script>alert("Take that!")</script>') returns the following (now harmless) string:

```
&lt;script&gt;alert(&quot;Take that!&quot;)&lt;/script&gt;
```

» **Filtering:** Removing unwanted characters from an input. Use PHP's filter_var() function and specify one or more of the function's sanitizing filters:

```
filter_var(input, filter)
```

- *input*: The input value you want to sanitize.
- *filter*: An constant value that determines the characters you want to remove from *input*. Here are some useful filters:
  - FILTER_SANITIZE_EMAIL: Removes all characters except letters, numbers, and the following: !#$%&'*+-=?^_`{|}~@.[]
  - FILTER_SANITIZE_NUMBER_FLOAT: Removes all characters except numbers, plus (+), and minus (–). To allow decimals, add the FILTER_FLAG_ALLOW_FRACTION flag:

```
filter_var($val, FILTER_SANITIZE_NUMBER_FLOAT,
FILTER_FLAG_ALLOW_FRACTION)
```

  - FILTER_SANITIZE_STRING: Removes all HTML tags. For example:

```
filter_var('<script>alert("Take that!")</script>',
FILTER_SANITIZE_STRING)
```

Returns:

```
alert("Take that!");
```

  - FILTER_SANITIZE_URL: Removes all characters except letters, numbers, and the following: $-_.+!*'(),{}|\\^~[]`<>#%";/?:@&=

» **Data type checking:** Testing the data type of an input to ensure that it matches what's expected. PHP calls this *character type checking,* and it offers the following functions:

- ctype_alnum(*input*) — Returns TRUE if *input* contains only letters and/or numbers

- `ctype_alpha(input)` — Returns TRUE if *input* contains only letters
- `ctype_digit(input)` — Returns TRUE if *input* contains only numbers
- `ctype_lower(input)` — Returns TRUE if *input* contains only lowercase letters
- `ctype_upper(input)` — Returns TRUE if *input* contains only uppercase letters

» **Whitelisting:** Allowing only certain values in an input. For example, suppose the input is an account number of the form 12-3456; that is, two numbers, a dash (–), then four numbers. You can't use `ctype_digit()` on this value directly because of the dash, but you can temporarily remove the dash and then check the resulting value:

```
$acct_num = $_POST['account-number'];
$allowed = '-';
$new_input = str_replace($allowed, '', $acct_num);
if(ctype_digit($new_input) === false) {
    exit(0);
}
```

TIP

This code uses the `str_replace()` function to replace dashes with the empty string (which removes them) and then runs `ctype_digit()` on the result. If your input has multiple acceptable characters, you can whitelist them all by setting the `$allowed` variable to an array:

```
$allowed = array(',', '.', '$');
```

Using prepared statements

As I show earlier in this chapter, the nastiness that is SQL injection works by tricking an innocent SQL statement into running malevolent code. You can (and should) try to prevent that by sanitizing your form inputs, but MySQL also offers a powerful technique that gives you exquisite control over the type of data that gets included in an SQL statement. The technique is called *prepared statements* (or sometimes *parameterized statements* or *parameterized queries*), and it means you no longer send an SQL statement directly to the database server. Instead, the query now proceeds in three separate stages:

1. **The preparation stage.**

   This stage involves running an SQL-like statement through MySQLi's `prepare()` method. Most importantly, you replace each external value (that is, each value received from a web form) with a question mark (?), which acts as a placeholder for the value. The statement you've thus prepared acts as a kind of template that MySQLi will use to run the query.

2. **The binding stage.**

   This stage involves using MySQLi's `bind_param()` method to define each external value as a parameter, and then bind that parameter to the prepared statement. Specifically, MySQLi replaces each ? placeholder with a parameter. The binding specifies a data type (such as a string or integer) for each parameter.

3. **The execution stage.**

   The final stage runs MySQLi's `execute()` method on the prepared statement. This hands off the actual running of the SQL command to the server, which uses the combination of the prepared statement template and the bound parameters to run the SQL operation.

Because the server knows what data types to except for the external values, it can't run injected SQL code as actual code. Instead, it treats the injection as text (or whatever data type you specify), and the SQL operation runs in complete safety.

Here's an example:

```
<?php
    // Assume these external values came from a
    // form submission and have been sanitized
    $customer = 'ALFKI';
    $employee = 1;

    // Declare a string for the query template
    // Use ? to add a placeholder for each external value
    $sql = "SELECT *
            FROM orders
            INNER JOIN customers
            ON orders.customer_id = customers.customer_id
            WHERE orders.customer_id = ?
            AND orders.employee_id = ?";

    // Prepare the statement template
    $stmt = $mysqli->prepare($sql);

    // Bind the parameters (one string, one integer)
    $stmt->bind_param("si", $customer, $employee);

    // Execute the prepared statement
    $stmt->execute();

    // Get the results
    $result = $stmt->get_result();
?>
```

To save space, the code declares two variables — `$customer` and `$employee` — that are assumed to be external values that came from a form and have been sanitized. The code then declares the string `$sql` to the SQL text, but with `?` placeholders used instead of the actual external values. The code runs the `prepare($sql)` method to create the prepared statement, which is stored in the `$stmt` variable. Now the code runs `bind_param()` to bind the external values:

```
bind_param(types, parameter(s))
```

- *types:* A string that specifies, in order, the data type of each parameter. The four possible values are `s` (string), `i` (integer), `d` (double; that is, a floating-point value), and `b` (blob; that is, a binary object, such as an image).
- *parameter(s):* The parameters you want to bind, separated by commas.

Finally, the code runs the `execute()` method to run the prepared statement, and then uses `get_result()` to get the result of the SQL operation.

Escaping outgoing data

Before you send data back to the web page, you need to ensure that you're not sending back anything that could produce unexpected or even malicious results. That means converting problematic characters such as ampersands (`&`), less than (`<`), greater than (`>`), and double quotation marks (`"`) to HTML entities or character codes. This is called *escaping* the data.

How you do this depends on how you're returning the data:

- **If you're returning strings via `echo` (or `print`):** Apply the `htmlentities()` function to each string that might contain data that needs to be escaped:

  ```
  echo htmlentities($user_bio);
  ```

- **If you're returning JSON via `echo` (or `print`):** Apply the `json_encode()` function to the data and specify one or more flags (separated by `|`) that specify which values you want encoded: `JSON_HEX_AMP` (ampersands), `JSON_HEX_APOS` (single quotations), `JSON_HEX_QUOT` (double quotations), or `JSON_HEX_TAG` (less than and greater than). Here's an example:

  ```
  $JSON_text = json_encode($rows, JSON_HEX_APOS |
    JSON_HEX_QUOT | JSON_HEX_TAG);
  echo $JSON_text;
  ```

Securing file uploads

Here are a few suggestions to beef up security when allowing users to upload files:

- **Restrict the maximum file upload size.** If you have access to `php.ini`, change the `upload_max_filesize` setting to some relatively small value, depending on what types of uploads you're allowing. For example, if users can upload avatar images, you might set this value to `2MB`.
- **Verify the file type.** Run some checks on the uploaded file to make sure its file type conforms to what your web app is expecting. For example, check the file extension to make sure it matches the type (or types) of file you allow. If you're expecting a binary file such as an image, run PHP's `is_binary()` function on the uploaded file; if this function returns `FALSE`, then you can reject the upload because it might be a script (which is text).
- **Use PHP's FTP functions to handle the upload.** If you have access to an FTP server, then PHP's built-in FTP functions are a secure way to handle the file upload:
  - `ftp_connect()`: Sets up a connection to the FTP server
  - `ftp_login()`: Sends your login credentials to the FTP server
  - `ftp_put()`: Transfers a file from the user's PC to the server
  - `ftp_close()`: Disconnects from the FTP server

Planning a Web App

Securing passwords

If your web app has registered users who must sign in with a password, it's essential that you do everything you can to enable users to create strong passwords and to store those passwords on the server is a secure way.

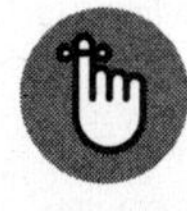

REMEMBER

Letting users create strong passwords means following these guidelines:

- Don't place any restrictions on the character types (lowercase letters, uppercase letters, numbers, and symbols) that can be used to build a password.
- Do require that users form their passwords using at least one character from three or, ideally, all four character types.
- Don't set a maximum length on the password. Longer passwords are always more secure than shorter ones.
- Do set a minimum length on the password. Eight characters is probably reasonable.

Here are some suggestions for storing and handling passwords securely:

- **Don't transfer passwords in a URL query string.** Query strings are visible in the browser window and get added to the server logs, so any passwords are exposed.
- **Don't store passwords in plain text.** If you do, and your system gets compromised, the attacker will have an easy time wreaking havoc on your user's accounts.
- **Do store passwords encrypted.** You encrypt each password using a *hash,* which is a function that scrambles the password by performing a mathematical function that's easy to run, but extremely difficult to reverse. PHP makes it easy to hash a password by offering the `password_hash()` function.
- **Do salt your passwords.** A *salt* is random data added to the password before it gets hashed, which makes it even harder to decrypt. Salting is handled automatically by the `password_hash()` function.
- **Do allow users to change their passwords.** It's good (though seldom followed) practice to change your password regularly, so you should offer this capability to your users.
- **Don't send a password over email.** Email is sent as plain text, so it's easy for a malicious user to intercept the password.

I go through a detailed example of registering user accounts, storing passwords securely, handling sign-ins, and offering password change and recovery features in Chapter 4 of this minibook.

IN THIS CHAPTER

» Getting your directory structure set up

» Creating the app database and adding the required tables

» Understanding PHP sessions

» Creating your app's startup files

» Making your coding life easier by taking a modular approach

Chapter 2
Laying the Foundation

Every great developer you know got there by solving problems they were unqualified to solve until they actually did it.

— PATRICK MCKENZIE

A well-built web app begins with a solid foundation. Sure, when you've got a great idea for a web app, it's always tempting to work on the visible front end first, even if it's just cobbling together a quick proof-of-concept page. However, party pooper that I am, I'm going to gently suggest that it's a good idea to nail down at least some of the more fundamental work off the top. Not only does that give you some major items to check off your app to-do list, but having a solid foundation under your feet will help you immeasurably when it comes time to code the rest of your app.

This chapter is all about laying down that solid foundation. First I show you how to figure out your app's directory structure. I then talk about constructing the database and tables. From there, I crank up the text editor and talk about some useful PHP techniques such as defining constants, setting up and securing sessions, and including code from one PHP file in another. Finally, I show you how to code the startup files your app needs for both its back end and its front end. Along the way, you see a practical example of every technique as I build out the foundation code for my own FootPower! app.

Setting Up the Directory Structure

Start by opening the "Employees Only" door and heading into the back room of the web app. Your back-end work begins by setting up some directories and subdirectories to store your app's files. Doing this now offers two benefits:

REMEMBER

- **Organization:** Even a small app can end up with quite a few files, from PHP scripts to HTML code to external CSS and JavaScript files. If you add your directories on-the-fly as they're needed, it's a certainty they'll end up a bit of a mess, with files scattered hither and thither (as my old grandmother used to say). It's better to come up with a sensible directory structure now and stick with it throughout the development cycle.
- **Security:** A smart back-end developer divides her files between those files that users need to view and operate the web app and those files that only do work behind the scenes. The former should be accessible to the public, but it's best to configure things so that the latter aren't accessible to anyone but you.

Okay, I hear you saying, "Organization I can get on board with, but what's all this about security?" Good question. Here's the answer:

WARNING

When your app is on the web, it's stored in a directory that the web server makes publicly available to anyone who comes along. This public accessibility means that it's at least technically possible for someone to gain direct access to the files stored in that directory. That access isn't a big thing for your HTML, CSS, and JavaScript files, which anyone can easily view. However, it's a huge deal for your PHP files, which can contain sensitive information such as your database credentials.

REMEMBER

To see how you prevent such unauthorized access, you need to understand that every web app has a top-level directory, which is known as either the *web root* or the *document root*. The web root is the directory that the server makes accessible to the public, which means that anything outside of the web root is inaccessible to remote users (while still being available to your web app).

So your directory structure begins by creating one directory and two subdirectories:

- The directory is the overall storage location for your app. You can name this whatever you want, but it's probably best to use the name of the app.
- One subdirectory will be the web root. I'm going to name my web root `public` to reinforce that only files that should be publicly accessible go in this subdirectory.

- The other subdirectory will contain the PHP files that you don't want remote users to be able to access. I'm going to name this subdirectory `private` to remind me that this is where I put files that should not have public access.

Setting up the public subdirectory

After you've created the `public` subdirectory, you need to tell the web server that this location is the new web root. If you set up the XAMPP web development environment as I describe in Book 1, Chapter 2, then you change the web root by editing a document named `httpd.conf`, the location of which depends on your operating system:

- **Windows:** Look for `httpd.conf` in the following folder:

  ```
  c:/xampp/apache/conf
  ```

- **Mac:** Look for `httpd.conf` here:

  ```
  /Applications/XAMPP/xamppfiles/etc
  ```

Open `httpd.conf` in a text editor and then scroll to or search for the line that begins with `DocumentRoot`. For example, here's the Mac version of the line:

```
DocumentRoot: "/Applications/XAMPP/xamppfiles/htdocs"
```

Edit this line to point to your app's web root subdirectory. For example, if you added your main app folder to `htdocs`, add a slash (/), the app folder name, and then `/public`. Here's the web root path that I'm using for my FootPower! app:

```
DocumentRoot:
   "/Applications/XAMPP/xamppfiles/htdocs/footpower/public"
```

By default, the web server denies permission to the entire server filesystem, with one exception: the web root. Therefore, you must now tell the server that it's okay for remote users to access the new web root. To do that, first look for the line in `httpd.conf` that begins with `<Directory`, followed by the path to the old web root. For example, here's the Mac version of the line:

```
<Directory "/Applications/XAMPP/xamppfiles/htdocs">
```

Edit this line to point to your app's web root, as in this example:

```
<Directory
   "/Applications/XAMPP/xamppfiles/htdocs/footpower/public">
```

Laying the Foundation

Save the file and restart the web server to put the new configuration into effect.

TIP

To make sure your web root is working properly, create a new PHP file in the `public` directory, give it the name `index.php`, and then add an `echo` statement, something like this:

```
<?php
    echo "Hello World from the web root!";
?>
```

Now surf to `localhost` and make sure you see the correct output, as shown in Figure 2-1.

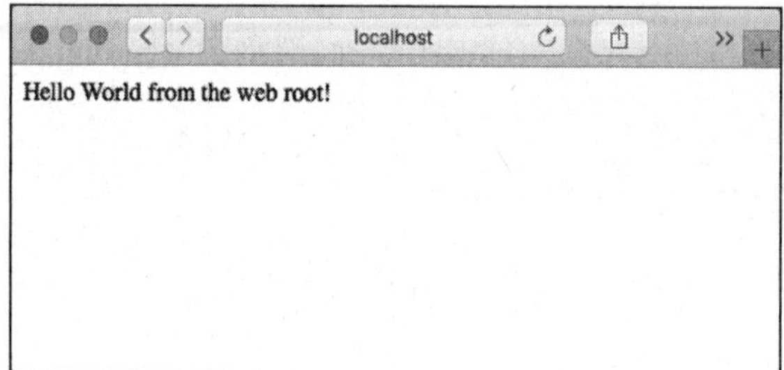

FIGURE 2-1: The new web root, ready for action.

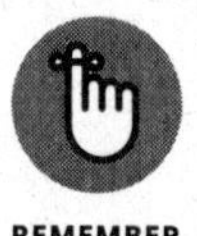

REMEMBER

It's unlikely you'll have access to `http.conf` when you put your web app online. However, your web host will offer some sort of mechanism for specifying a particular directory as the web root, so check the host's Help or Support documentation.

Your final chore for setting up the `public` directory is to add the subdirectories you'll use to store various file types. Here are my suggestions:

Subdirectory	What It Stores
`/common`	Files that are used in all your web app's pages, including the top part of each page (the opening tags and the head section) and common page elements such as a header, sidebar, and footer
`/css`	Your web app's CSS files
`/handlers`	Files that handle Ajax requests from the front end
`/images`	Image files used in your web app
`/js`	Your web app's JavaScript files

To give you a kind of road map to where we're going, Figure 2-2 shows the final file structure of my FootPower! app's `public` directory.

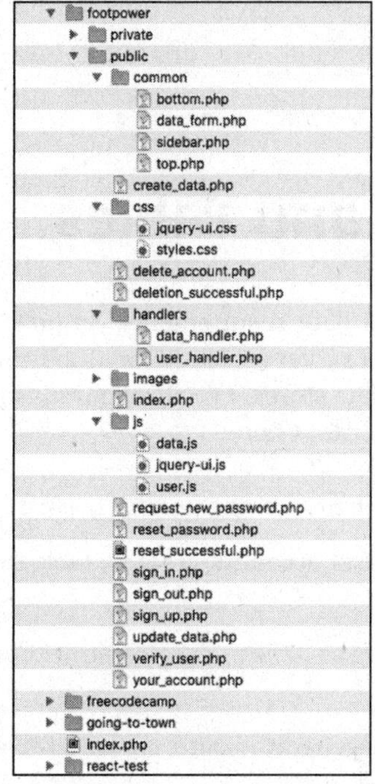

FIGURE 2-2: All the `public` files and directories I use in the final version of my FootPower! app.

Setting up the private subdirectory

Getting the `private` subdirectory configured is much easier because you only have to create the subdirectories you need to organize your app's back-end files. Here are my suggestions:

Subdirectory	What It Stores
`/classes`	Files that contain the code for your web app's classes
`/common`	Files that are used in other back-end files
`/logs`	Log files, such as the error log

Figure 2-3 shows the final file structure of my FootPower! app's `private` directory.

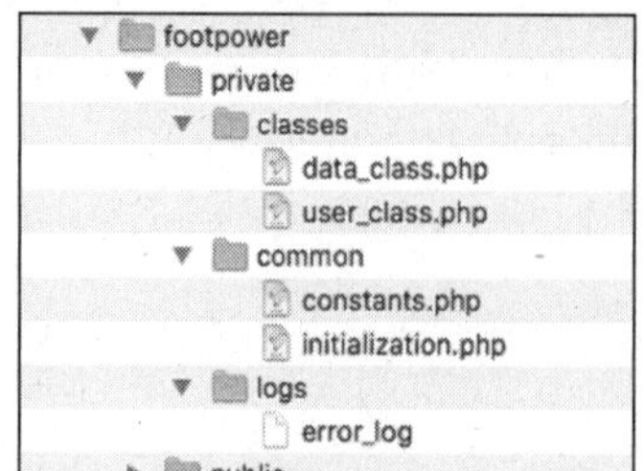

FIGURE 2-3: The `private` files and directories in the final version of my FootPower! app.

Creating the Database and Tables

You already know your web app's data requirements, so now it's time to load phpMyAdmin on your development server (`http://localhost/phpMyAdmin`), and then use it to create your MySQL data stores. I go through this in detail in Book 5, Chapter 2, so I only list the general steps here:

1. **Create a database for your web app using the `utf8_general_ci` collation.**
2. **If your app needs to support user accounts, create a table to hold the account data.**

   At a minimum, this table will have an ID field, a username field, and a password field.
3. **If your app needs to save user-generated data, create a table to hold the data.**

   This table should have an ID field as well as user ID field that, for each user, contains the same ID from the user table you created in Step 2.
4. **If your app is configured so that the user creates one main item and then many subitems, create a table to hold the subitems.**

   To be clear, the table you created in Step 3 holds each user's main item, and this new table holds the subitems. This table should have an ID field, a field that points to the ID of the main item, and a field for each tidbit of data you want to store.

An example might make this clearer, so I'll go through the data structures for my FootPower! app. First, here's the `users` table:

Field Name	Type	Other Settings
user_id	INT	PRIMARY KEY, AUTO_INCREMENT
username	VARCHAR(150)	UNIQUE, NOT NULL
password	VARCHAR(255)	NOT NULL

Field Name	Type	Other Settings
distance_unit	VARCHAR(10)	DEFAULT 'miles'
verification_code	VARCHAR(32)	NOT NULL
verified	TINYINT	DEFAULT 0
creation_date	TIMESTAMP	DEFAULT CURRENT_TIMESTAMP

Each registered user gets an activity log in which to record her activities, so next up is the `logs` table:

Field Name	Type	Other Settings
log_id	INT	PRIMARY KEY, AUTO_INCREMENT
user_id	INT	NOT NULL
creation_date	TIMESTAMP	DEFAULT CURRENT_TIMESTAMP

Note that both the `users` and `logs` tables have a common `user_id` field. This enables me to link each log to the user who owns it.

For now, go ahead and add one record to this table, where `user_id` equals `1` and `creation_date` is today's date (in YYYY-MM-DD format).

Finally, each log records the user's foot-propelled activities, so I'll store this data in the `activities` table:

Field Name	Type	Other Settings
activity_id	INT	PRIMARY KEY, AUTO_INCREMENT
log_id	INT	NOT NULL
type	VARCHAR(25)	NOT NULL
date	DATE	NOT NULL
distance	DECIMAL(10,6)	
duration	TIME	

Note that both the `logs` and `activities` tables have a common `log_id` field. This will enable me to link each activity to the log in which it belongs.

Getting Some Back-End Code Ready

The back end of a web app consists of both the MySQL data and the PHP code that manipulates that data and returns information to the app's front end. You can get some of the PHP code written now, and you can add the rest as you build the app.

Defining PHP constants

It's a rare web app that doesn't have one or more variables that are used throughout the back-end code, but where the value of those variables must never change. For example, when you're managing server data, your PHP files are constantly logging into the MySQL database, which requires credentials such as a username and password. That username and password are the same throughout your code, but your code will fail if, somehow, these values get changed.

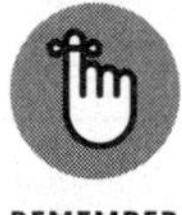

REMEMBER

A variable that never changes value sounds almost like an oxymoron, so perhaps that's why programmers of yore came up with the idea of the *constant*, a special kind of variable that, once defined with a value, can't be changed. You set up a constant in PHP by using the `define()` function:

```
define(name, value)
```

- *name:* The name of the constant. By convention, constant names are all uppercase and don't begin with a dollar sign ($).
- *value:* The value of the constant. The value must be an integer, floating point number, string, or Boolean.

Here's an example:

```
define("GREETING", "Hello Constant World!")
```

It's good web app practice to gather all your constants and put them in a separate file, which you can then include in any other PHP file that requires one or more of the constants. (I talk about how you include a PHP file in another PHP file later in this chapter.) For example, here's a PHP file that defines the database credentials for my FootPower! app:

```
<?php
    define('HOST', 'localhost');
    define('USER', 'root');
    define('PASSWORD', '');
    define('DATABASE', 'footpower');
?>
```

I've named this file `constants.php` and added it to the app's `private/common/` directory.

Understanding PHP sessions

One of the biggest web app challenges is keeping track of certain bits of information as the user moves from page to page within the app. For example, when someone first surfs to the app's home page, your PHP code might store the current date and time in a variable, with the goal of, say, tracking how long that person spends using the app. A worthy goal, to be sure, but when the user moves on to another page in the app, your saved date and time gets destroyed.

Similarly, suppose the user's first name is stored in the database and you use the first name to personalize each page. Does that mean every time the user accesses a different page in your app, your code must query the database just to get the name?

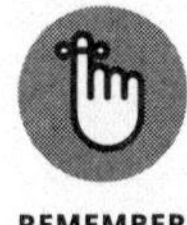

REMEMBER

The first scenario is ineffective and the second is inefficient, so is there a better way? You bet there is: PHP sessions. In the PHP world, a *session* is the period that a user spends interacting with a web app, no matter how many different app pages she navigates.

You start a session by invoking the `session_start()` function:

```
session_start();
```

Once you've done that, the session remains active until the user closes the browser window. Your web server also specifies a maximum lifetime for a session, usually 1,440 seconds (24 minutes). You can check this by running `echo phpinfo()` and looking for the `session.gc_maxlifetime` value. You can work around this timeout in one of two ways:

- By adding the `session_start()` function to each page, which refreshes the session.
- By running PHP's `session_status()` function, which returns the constant `PHP_SESSION_NONE` if the user doesn't have a current session.

How does a session help you keep track of information about a user? By offering an array called `$_SESSION`, which you can populate with whatever values you want to track:

```
$_SESSION['start_time'] = time();
$_SESSION['user_first_name'] = 'Biff';
$_SESSION['logged_in'] = 1;
```

Securing a PHP session

A PHP session is a vital link between your users and your app because it enables you to store data that make each user's experience easier, more efficient, and more seamless. However, because sessions are such a powerful tool, the world's dark-side hackers have come up with a number of ingenious ways to hijack user sessions and thereby gain access to session data.

A full tutorial on protecting your users from would-be session-stealers would require an entire book, but there's a relatively simple technique you can use to thwart all but the most tenacious villains. The technique involves a value called a *token*, which is a random collection of numbers and letters, usually 32 characters long. How does a token serve to keep a session secure? It's a three-step process:

1. When the session begins, generate a new token and store it in the `$_SESSION` array.
2. In each form used by your web app, include a hidden `input` field (that is, an `<input>` tag where the `type` attribute is set to `hidden`) and set the `value` of that field to the session's token value.
3. In your PHP script that processes the form data, compare the value of the form's hidden field with the token value stored in the `$_SESSION` array. If they're identical, it means the form submission is secure (that is, the form was submitted by the session user) and you can safely proceed; if they're different, however, it almost certainly means that an attacker was trying to pull a fast one and your code should stop processing the form data.

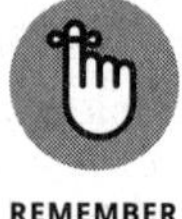

REMEMBER

There are a bunch of ways to create some random data in PHP, but a good one for our purposes is `openssl_random_pseudo_bytes()`:

```
openssl_random_pseudo_bytes(length)
```

» *`length`:* An integer that specifies the number of random bytes you want returned

The `openssl_random_pseudo_bytes()` function returns a string of random bytes, but byte values aren't much good to us. We need to convert the binary string to a hexadecimal string, and that's the job of PHP's `bin2hex()` function:

```
bin2hex(str)
```

» *`str`:* The binary string you want to convert

For example, 16 bytes will convert to 32 hex characters, so you can use something like the following expression to generate a token:

```
bin2hex(openssl_random_pseudo_bytes(16));
```

This creates a value similar to the following:

```
387f90ce4b3d8f9bd7e4b38068c9fce3
```

For your session, you'd store the result in the `$_SESSION` array, like so:

```
$_SESSION['token'] = bin2hex(openssl_random_pseudo_bytes(16));
```

It's also good practice to generate a fresh token after a certain period of time has elapsed, say 15 minutes. To handle this, when the session starts you use the `$_SESSION` array to store the current time plus the expiration time:

```
$_SESSION['token_expires'] = time() + 900;
```

PHP's `time()` function returns the number of seconds since January 1, 1970, so adding `900` sets the expiration time to 15 minutes in the future. Your web app would then use each session refresh to check whether the token has expired:

```
if (time() > $_SESSION['token_expires']){
    $_SESSION['token'] = bin2hex(openssl_random_pseudo_bytes(16));
    $_SESSION['token_expires'] = time() + 900;
}
```


Including code from another PHP file

Most web apps are multi-page affairs, which means your app consists of multiple PHP files, each of which performs a specific task, such as creating data, retrieving data, or logging in a user. Depending on the structure of your app, each of these PHP files will include some or all of the following:

- Constants used throughout the project
- Database login credentials
- Database connection code

- Classes, functions, and other code used on each page
- Common interface elements such as the header, app navigation, sidebar, and footer

You don't want to copy and paste all this code into each PHP file because if the code changes, then you have to update every instance of the code. Instead, place each chunk of common code in its own PHP file and save those files in a subdirectory. Earlier in this chapter, I explain that you should create two `common` subdirectories for such files, one in the `public` directory and one in the `private` directory. To get a common file's code into another PHP file, use PHP's `include_once` statement:

```
include_once file;
```

- *`file`*: The path and name of the file with the code you want to include

For example, here's a PHP file that defines some constants that hold the database credentials for my FootPower! app:

```
<?php
    define('HOST', 'localhost');
    define('USER', 'root');
    define('PASSWORD', '');
    define('DATABASE', 'footpower');
?>
```

I've stored this code in a file named `constants.php` in the `private/common/` subdirectory, so I'd use the following statement to include it from the web root folder:

```
include_once '../private/common/constants.php';
```

The double dots (`..`) stand for "go up one directory," so here they take the script up to the app's filesystem root, and from there the statement adds the path to `constants.php`.

Creating the App Startup Files

All web apps perform a number of chores at the beginning of any task. On the back end, these initialization chores include starting a user session and connecting to the database, and on the front end the startup includes outputting the app's common HTML (especially the <head> section) and including the app's common components, such as a header and footer.

Rather than repeating the code for these startup chores in every file, you should create two files — one for the back end initialization and one for the front end's common code — and then include the files as you begin each web app task. The next two sections provide the details.

Creating the back-end initialization file

When performing any task, a typical web app must first run through a number of back-end chores, including the following:

- Setting the error reporting level
- Starting a session for the current user, if one hasn't been started already
- Creating a token for the session
- Including common files, such as a file of constants used throughout the app
- Connecting to the database, if the app uses server data

You should store this file in your web app's `private/common/` directory. For FootPower!, I created an initialization file named `/private/common/initialization.php`:

```
<?php
    // Make sure we see all the errors and warnings
    error_reporting(E_ALL | E_STRICT);

    // Start a session
    session_start();

    // Have we not created a token for this session,
    // or has the token expired?
    if (!isset($_SESSION['token']) ||  time() >
  $_SESSION['token_expires']){
        $_SESSION['token'] =
  bin2hex(openssl_random_pseudo_bytes(16));
        $_SESSION['token_expires'] = time() + 900;
        $_SESSION['log_id'] = 1;
    }
```

Laying the Foundation

```
    // Include the app constants
    include_once 'constants.php';

    // Connect to the database
    $mysqli = new MySQLi(HOST, USER, PASSWORD, DATABASE);

    // Check for an error
    if($mysqli->connect_error) {
        echo 'Connection Failed!
              Error #' . $mysqli->connect_errno
                . ': ' . $mysqli->connect_error;
        exit(0);
    }
?>
```

This code cranks up the error reporting to 11 for the purposes of debugging, starts a new session, creates a session token (if needed), includes the constants file (which contains the database credentials), and then connects to the database and creates a `MySQLi` object. Note, too, that I set `$_SESSION['log_id']` to `1`, but this is temporary. In Book 7, Chapter 4, you see that this value gets set to the user's log ID value when the user signs in to the app.

WARNING

You want to use `error_reporting(E_ALL | E_STRICT)` when you're developing your web app because you want the PHP processor to let you know when something's amiss, either as an error (`E_ALL`) or as non-standard PHP code (`E_STRICT`). However, you certainly don't want your app's users to see these errors or warnings, so when you're ready for your web app to go live, edit `initialization.php` to follow this statement:

```
error_reporting(E_ALL | E_STRICT)
```

with these statements:

```
ini_set('display_errors', 0);
ini_set('log_errors', 1);
ini_set('error_log', '../private/logs/error_log');
```

These statements configure PHP to not display errors onscreen, but to log them to a file, the name and path of which is specified in the final statement.

Creating the front-end common files

Each page of your web app has a common structure. For example, the top part of each page includes the following elements:

- » The DOCTYPE and the <html> tag
- » The head element, including the <meta> tags, page title, CSS <link> tags, and JavaScript <script> tags
- » An event handler for jQuery's ready event
- » The <body> tag
- » Common page elements, such as the <header>, <nav>, and <main> tags

Here's an example, which I'm going to name public/common/top.php:

```
<!DOCTYPE html>
<html lang="en">
<head>
    <meta charset="utf-8">
    <meta name="viewport" content="width=device-width, initial-
  scale=1.0">
    <title>FootPower! | <?php echo $page_title ?></title>
    <link href="css/styles.css" rel="stylesheet">
    <script src="https://ajax.googleapis.com/ajax/libs/
  jquery/3.2.1/jquery.min.js"></script>
    <script>
        $(document).ready(function() {

        });
    </script>
</head>
<body>
    <header role="banner">
    </header>
    <main role="main">
        <article role="contentinfo">
            <header class="article-header" role="banner">
                <div class="header-title">
                    <h1><?php echo $page_title ?></h1>
                </div>
            </header>
```

In this code, note that the page title is given by the following inline PHP:

```
<?php echo $page_title ?>
```

TIP

The idea here is that each page will set the `$page_title` variable just before including `top.php`, which enables you to define a custom title for each page. For example, the home page might do this:

```
<?php
    $page_title = 'Home';
    include_once 'common/top.php';
?>
```

Note that this same title also gets inserted in the page `header` element, within the `<h1>` tag.

Most web apps also include a sidebar — defined by an `<aside>` tag — that includes info common to all pages, such as a description of the app, instructions for using the app, the latest app news, or a newsletter sign-up form. For this sidebar, create a separate file called, say, `public\common\sidebar.php` and include your code:

```
<aside role="complementary">
    Your sidebar text and tags go here
</aside>
```

Finally, you need a file to handle the common elements that appear at the bottom of each page, including the `</main>` closing tag, a footer, and the `</body>` and `</html>` closing tags. For this code, create a separate file called, say, `public\common\bottom.php` and add your code:

```
    </main>
    <footer role="contentinfo">
        Copyright <?php echo date('Y'); ?> Your Name
    </footer>
    <script src="js/data.js"></script>
    <script src="js/user.js"></script>
</body>
</html>
```

TIP

The footer uses the PHP statement `echo date('Y')` to output the current year for the Copyright notice. This file also adds references to the app's two external JavaScript files: `data.js` and `user.js`. Adding these at the bottom of the page (instead of the usual place in the page's head section) ensures that your JavaScript code can work with the elements added to the page on the fly.

Building the app home page

With the initialization files in place, it's time to build the skeleton for the app's home page. At the moment, this page is nothing but PHP:

```
<?php
    include_once '../private/common/initialization.php';
    $page_title = 'Home';
    include_once 'common/top.php';
?>
Main app content goes here
<?php
    include_once 'common/sidebar.php';
    include_once 'common/bottom.php';
?>
```

Save this file as `index.php` in the web root directory.

IN THIS CHAPTER

» Setting up your app's data class

» Creating a script to handle the app's Ajax data requests

» Creating new data items

» Reading, updating, and deleting data

» Handling data robustly and securely

Chapter 3 Managing Data

Talk is cheap. Show me the code.

— LINUS TORVALDS

Some web apps are relatively simple and don't require a back-end database. Such apps are all front end, with maybe a bit of data stored in the user's browser. Front-end-only apps are very common and can be amazingly useful, a claim I hope to live up to when I talk about building just such an app in Book 8.

The rest of the web app world is a sophisticated and powerful marriage of both front-end interface and back-end infrastructure, and a big part of that server scaffolding is the data stored in a database such as MySQL. One of hats you must wear as a web developer is writing the code that enables data to pass robustly and securely between the front and back ends, and that code is the main topic of this chapter. First, I show you how to set up the PHP classes and functions. With that done, it's time to explore the unglamorous but necessary world of creating, reading, updating, and deleting data. Along the way, you see a practical example of every technique as I build out the data-handling code for my own FootPower! app.

Handling Data the CRUD Way

Most web apps that deal with back-end data need to implement at least four common tasks:

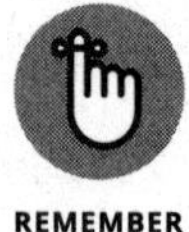
REMEMBER

- **Create new data:** Enables the user or the app itself (or both) to add new data items
- **Read data:** Retrieves some or all of the items in the database and displays them in a web page
- **Update data:** Enables the user or the app (or, again, both) to edit an existing item and have those changes written back to the database
- **Delete data:** Enables the user or the app (or, yep, both) to remove an item from the database

As you can deduce from the first letters of each of these tasks, this data model is known affectionately in the web development trade as CRUD. I devote the rest of this chapter to showing you a method for building CRUD into your web app. Before getting to all of that, here's the big picture view of what I'll be up to in the next few pages:

1. Build a class for handling data interactions. That class includes one method for each of the CRUD verbs: create, read, update, and delete.
2. Provide the user with an interface for initiating any of the CRUD actions. For example, you might build a form to enable the user to create a new data item.
3. To start processing a CRUD verb, set up an event handler for each CRUD interface element. If you're using a form, for example, then you might set up a `submit` event handler for that form.
4. Use each CRUD event handler to send the form data to a single PHP script via Ajax. Importantly, that form data includes the value of a hidden field that specifies the type of task being performed (create, update, and so on).
5. In the PHP script, create a new object from the class of Step 1, check the CRUD type sent by the Ajax call, and then call the corresponding class method. For example, if the event is creating a new data item, the script would call the class method that handles creating new items.

The next couple of sections cover setting up the first part of the data class and building the PHP script that handles the Ajax form submissions.

Starting the web app's data class

In most cases, web app data forms a one-to-many relationship, where one item in a table is related to many items in another table. Some examples:

- One blog can contain many posts.
- One shopping cart can contain many products.
- For my FootPower! app, one activity log can contain many activities.

The idea is to create a class for the "one" side of the relationship, which is often called the *master* table. The master class for your web app's data needs to do the following three things, at a minimum:

- Accept a parameter that references the current `MySQLi` object.
- Define a method for each of the four CRUD verbs.
- Define any helper functions required by the CRUD verbs.

With these goals in mind, here's the skeleton class file:

```
<?php
class Data {

    // Holds the app's current MySQLi object
    private $_mysqli;

    // Use the class constructor to store the passed MySQLi
   object
    public function __construct($mysqli=NULL) {
        $this->_mysqli = $mysqli;
    }

    // Here comes the CRUD
    public function createData() {

    }
    public function readAllData() {

    }
    public function readDataItem() {

    }
```

Managing Data

```
    public function updateData() {

    }
    public function deleteData() {

    }
}
?>
```

The class declares the private property `$_mysqli`, which it uses to store the current instance of the `MySQLi` object (created earlier in the `initialization.php` script). The class then declares functions for each CRUD verb, including two for the read task: one to read all the data and one to read a single data item. Store this file in `private/classes/data_class.php`.

To create an instance of this class, you'd use a statement similar to the following:

```
$log = new Data($mysqli);
```

Creating a data handler script

All the CRUD verbs — create, read, update, and delete — will be initiated via Ajax calls to a single PHP script. The Ajax call needs to specify the CRUD verb required, and the PHP code routes the request to the corresponding method in the `Data` class.

Here's the PHP script, saved as `public/handlers/data_handler.php`:

```
<?php

    // Initialize the app
    include_once '../../private/common/initialization.php';

    // Include the Data class
    include_once '../../private/classes/data_class.php';

    // Initialize the results
    $server_results['status'] = 'success';
    $server_results['message'] = '';

    // Make sure a log ID was passed
    if (!isset($_POST['log-id'])) {
```

```
      $server_results['status'] = 'error';
      $server_results['message'] = 'Error: No log ID
specified!';
  }
  // Make sure a data verb was passed
  elseif (!isset($_POST['data-verb'])) {
      $server_results['status'] = 'error';
      $server_results['message'] = 'Error: No data verb
specified!';
  }
  // Make sure a token value was passed
  elseif (!isset($_POST['token'])) {
      $server_results['status'] = 'error';
      $server_results['message'] = 'Error: Invalid action!';
  }
  // Make sure the token is legit
  elseif ($_SESSION['token'] !== $_POST['token']) {
      $server_results['status'] = 'error';
      $server_results['message'] = 'Timeout Error!<p>Please
refresh the page and try again.';
  }
  // If we get this far, all is well, so go for it
  else {

      // Create a new Data object
      $data = new Data($mysqli);

      // Pass the data verb to the appropriate method
      switch ($_POST['data-verb']) {

          // Create a new data item
          case 'create':
              $server_results = json_decode($data-
>createData());
              break;

          // Read all the data items
          case 'read-all-data':
              $server_results = json_decode($data-
>readAllData());
              break;

          // Read one data item
          case 'read-data-item':
```

Managing Data

```
                $server_results = json_decode($data-
>readDataItem());
                break;
            // Update a data item
            case 'update':
                $server_results = json_decode($data-
>updateData());
                break;

            // Delete a new data item
            case 'delete':
                $server_results = json_decode($data-
>deleteData());
                break;

            default:
                $server_results['status'] = 'error';
                $server_results['message'] = 'Error: Unknown
data verb!';
        }
    }
    // Create and then output the JSON data
    $JSON_data = json_encode($server_results, JSON_HEX_APOS |
JSON_HEX_QUOT);
    echo $JSON_data;
?>
```

After initializing the app by including `initialization.php`, the code also includes the `Data` class file. The code then sets up an array named `$server_results`, which holds the results that the script sends back to the front end:

- `$server_results['status']` will be either `success` or `error`.
- `$server_results['message']` holds the success or error message to display.

The code next runs through a series of checks: making sure there's a reference to the database item you want to work with (`log-id`, in the preceding example); making sure a CRUD verb was passed; making sure a token value was passed; and comparing that token value with the session token. If the code gets past those tests, a `switch()` statement runs through the possible values for `$_POST['data-verb']` — `create`, `read-all-data`, `read-data-item`, `update`, or `delete` — and calls the corresponding `Data` method.

In the rest of this chapter, I fill in the details for the various `Data` methods and the front-end interfaces that support them.

Creating New Data

If your web app enables users to work with data items, then you won't be able to display anything to the user until she has created an item or three, which means setting up the "create" portion of your CRUD system should be your first order of business. To enable users to create data, you need to do three things:

REMEMBER

1. Build a form to capture the data.
2. Create a `submit` event handler that uses an Ajax call to send the form data to the server.
3. Validate and sanitize the form data, then insert the new info into the database.

Building the form

In most CRUD-based web apps, the forms used to create and edit items are identical. In such cases, rather than creating two separate forms that merely repeat the same the HTML code, it's best to use a single form. That is, go ahead and create separate pages for the create and edit tasks, but place the form code in a separate file and then include that file in each page. When you load each page, you add JavaScript code that adjusts the form controls accordingly:

- » When the user wants to create a new data item, reset the form controls to blank or default values.
- » When the user wants to edit an existing data item, populate the form controls with the existing data.

I go through the specifics of building HTML forms in Book 6, Chapter 2, so I won't go into the details again here. Instead, I'll just show you the form code I'm using for my FootPower! app (which I've stored as `public/common/data_form.php`):

```
<form id="data-form">
    <div class="form-wrapper">
        <div class="form-row">
            <div class="control-wrapper">
                <label for="activity-type">Activity type</label>
                <select id="activity-type" name="activity-type"
  size="1" aria-label="Select the type of activity">
                    <option value="Walk">Walk</option>
                    <option value="Run">Run</option>
                    <option value="Cycle">Cycle</option>
                </select>
            </div>
```

Managing Data

```
            <div class="control-wrapper">
                <label for="activity-date">Activity date</label>
                <input id="activity-date" type="date"
name="activity-date" aria-label="The date of the activity"
required>
            </div>
        </div>
        <div class="form-row">
            <div class="control-wrapper">
                <label for="activity-distance">Distance</label>
                <input id="activity-distance" type="number"
name="activity-distance" min="0" max="999" step=".01" data-
distance="0" aria-label="The distance of the activity">
                <span><?php echo $_SESSION['distance_unit'] ?>
(<a href="your_account.php">change</a>)</span>
            </div>
            <div class="control-wrapper" id="activity-duration">
                <label for="activity-duration">Duration
(hh:mm:ss)</label>
                <input id="activity-duration-hours"
type="number" name="activity-duration-hours" min="0" max="999"
placeholder="hh" aria-label="The number of hours the activity
required"> :
                <input id="activity-duration-minutes"
type="number" name="activity-duration-minutes"
min="0" max="59" placeholder="mm" aria-label="The number of
minutes the activity required"> :
                <input id="activity-duration-seconds"
type="number" name="activity-duration-seconds"
min="0" max="59" placeholder="ss" aria-label="The number of
seconds the activity required">
            </div>
        </div>
        <div class="form-row">
            <div class="control-wrapper">
                <div>
                    <button id="data-save-button" class="btn
data-save-button" type="submit" role="button">Save</button>
                </div>
                <div>
                    <button id="data-cancel-button" class="btn
btn-plain data-cancel-button" role="button">Cancel</button>
                    <span id="result" class="result-text"></span>
                </div>
            </div>
```

```
            <div class="control-wrapper">
                <div>
                    <button id="data-delete-button" class="btn
    data-delete-button" type="button" role="button">Delete this
    Activity</button>
                </div>
            </div>
        </div>
    </div>
    <span id="form-error" class="error error-message
    form-error-message"></span>
    <span id="form-message" class="form-message"></span>
    <input type="hidden" id="log-id" name="log-id" value="<?php
    echo $_SESSION['log_id']; ?>">
    <input type="hidden" id="activity-id" name="activity-id">
    <input type="hidden" id="data-verb" name="data-verb">
    <input type="hidden" id="token" name="token" value="<?php
    echo $_SESSION['token']; ?>">
</form>
```

This form gathers four bits of info from the user: the activity type, the activity date, the distance (which can be expressed in either kilometers or miles; see Book 7, Chapter 4), and the duration (given by separate fields for the hours, minutes, and seconds). Note, too, the four hidden fields:

- **»** `log-id`: The ID of the log to which the new item will be added, as given by PHP's `$_SESSION['log_id']` variable. As I mention in Book 7, Chapter 2, this is set to 1 now because I assume at this point that the app has only a single user. However, when I add users in Book 7, Chapter 4, the value of the `log-id` field will reflect the log ID value of the currently logged-in user.
- **»** `activity-id`: During an update task, the ID of the activity the user is currently editing.
- **»** `data-verb`: The type of CRUD verb the form is for (such as `create` or `update`).
- **»** `token`: The current session token, as given by PHP's `$_SESSION['token']` variable.

To use this form, I include it in the `create_data.php` file, which is stored in the web root:

```
<?php
    include_once '../private/common/initialization.php';
    $page_title = 'Add an Activity';
```

```
    include_once 'common/top.php';
    include_once 'common/data_form.php';
    include_once 'common/sidebar.php';
    include_once 'common/bottom.php';
?>
```

Figure 3-1 shows the resulting form. (To save space, I haven't shown the CSS behind the form, but you can see it online at `https://mcfedries.com/webcodingfordummies`.)

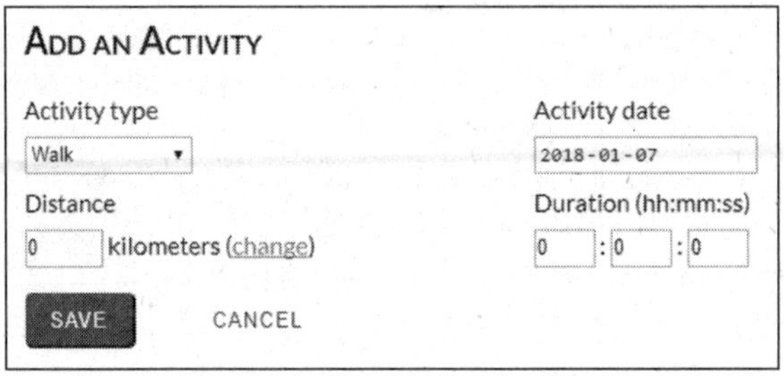

FIGURE 3-1: The FootPower! form that enables a user to create a new activity.

How does the form get its default values? In the common page startup file — `top.php`, which I talk about in Book 7, Chapter 2, I added the following code:

```
$(document).ready(function() {

    // Get the current filename and run code for that file
    var currentURL = window.location.pathname;
    var currentFile =
  currentURL.substr(currentURL.lastIndexOf('/') + 1);
    switch (currentFile) {

        // Display the signed-in user's Activity Log
        case 'index.php':
            readActivities();
            break;

        // Set up the Create Data form
        case 'create_data.php':
            initializeCreateDataForm();
            break;

        // Set up the Edit Data form
        case 'update_data.php':
```

```
            initializeUpdateDataForm();
            break;
    }
});
```

The code extracts the filename for the current URL, and then uses a `switch()` statement to call a function depending on the result. For the `create_data.php` file, the code calls the `initializeCreateDataForm()` function:

```
function initializeCreateDataForm() {

    // Hide the Delete button
    $('#data-delete-button').hide();

    // Set the data verb to 'create'
    $('#data-verb').val('create');

    // Populate the form
    $('#activity-type').val('Walk');
    var d = new Date();
    var todaysDate = d.getFullYear() + '-' + Number(d.getMonth()
  + 1).padWithZeros(2, 'left') + '-' + d.getDate().
  padWithZeros(2, 'left');
    $('#activity-date').val(todaysDate);
    $('#activity-distance').val(0);
    $('#activity-duration-hours').val(0);
    $('#activity-duration-minutes').val(0);
    $('#activity-duration-seconds').val(0);
}
```

This function does three things:

- Hides the form's Delete button.
- Sets the value of the form's `data-verb` field to `create`.
- Resets the form fields. In particular, it sets the `date` field to today's date and the numeric fields to `0`.

To store this code, the code for the other CRUD event handlers, as well as any helper code required for data interactions, I created an external JavaScript file and saved it to `public/js/data.js`.

Sending the form data to the server

To process the form, you need to set up a handler for the form's `submit` event. Here's the one I'm using for the FootPower! app:

```
$('#data-form').submit(function(e) {

    // Prevent the default submission
    e.preventDefault();

    // Disable the Save button to prevent double submissions
    $('#data-save-button').prop('disabled', true);

    // Convert the data to POST format
    var formData = $(this).serializeArray();

    // Submit the data to the handler
    $.post('/handlers/data_handler.php', formData,
  function(data) {

        // Convert the JSON string to a JavaScript object
        var result = JSON.parse(data);

        if(result.status === 'error') {

            // Display the error
            $('#form-error').html(result.message).css('display',
  'inline-block');

            // Enable the Save button
            $('#data-save-button').prop('disabled', false);

        } else {

            // Display the success message
            $('#form-message').html(result.message).
  css('display', 'inline-block');

            // Return to the home page after 3 seconds
            window.setTimeout("window.location='index.php'",
  3000);
        }
    });
});
```

This code prevents the default form submission, disables the Save button, converts the form data to the POST format, then uses jQuery's `.post()` method to send the data to the `data_handler.php` script on the server. The callback function runs JavaScript's `JSON.parse()` method on the returned JSON string to convert it into a JavaScript object, and then outputs the result. If the data gets inserted successfully, the user is sent back to the home page.

Adding the data item

When the server script receives the data via the Ajax call, it must validate and sanitize the data; then, assuming everything checks out, run a prepared SQL `INSERT` statement to add a new record to the table. All this happens in the `Data` class's `createData()` method. Here's the code from my FootPower! app:

```
public function createData() {

    // Store the default status
    $server_results['status'] = 'success';
    $server_results['control'] = 'form';

    // Check the log-id field
    $log_id = $_POST['log-id'];
    if(empty($log_id)) {
        $server_results['status'] = 'error';
        $server_results['message'] = 'Error: Missing log ID';
    } else {
        // Sanitize it to an integer
        $log_id = filter_var($log_id,
  FILTER_SANITIZE_NUMBER_FLOAT);
        if (!$log_id) {
            $server_results['status'] = 'error';
            $server_results['message'] = 'Error: Invalid
  log ID';
        } else {
            // Check the activity-type field (required)
            if(isset($_POST['activity-type'])) {
                $activity_type = $_POST['activity-type'];
                if(empty($activity_type)) {
                    $server_results['status'] = 'error';
                    $server_results['message'] = 'Error:
  Missing activity type';
                } else {
```

Managing Data

```
                // Sanitize it by accepting only one of
three values: 'Walk', 'Run', or 'Cycle'
                if ($activity_type !== 'Walk' AND
$activity_type !== 'Run' AND $activity_type !== 'Cycle') {
                    $server_results['status'] = 'error';
                    $server_results['message'] = 'Error:
Invalid activity type';
                } else {
                    // Check the activity-date field
(required)
                    if(isset($_POST['activity-date'])) {
                        $activity_date = $_POST[
'activity-date'];
                        if(empty($activity_date)) {
                            $server_results['status'] =
'error';
                            $server_results['message'] =
'Error: Missing activity date';
                        } else {
                            // Check for a valid date (that
is, one that uses the pattern YYYY-MM-DD)
                            if(!preg_match('/^[0-9]{4}-
(0[1-9]|1[0-2])-(0[1-9]|1[0-9]|2[0-9]|3[0-1])$/',
$activity_date)) {
                                $server_results['status'] =
'error';
                                $server_results['message'] =
'Error: Invalid activity date';
                            }
                        }
                    }
                }
            }
        }
    }
  }
  // Check the activity-distance field
  $activity_distance = 0;
  if(isset($_POST['activity-distance'])) {
      $activity_distance = $_POST['activity-distance'];

      // Sanitize it to a floating-point value
      $activity_distance = filter_var($activity_distance,
FILTER_SANITIZE_NUMBER_FLOAT, FILTER_FLAG_ALLOW_FRACTION);
```

```
    }
    // Check the activity-duration-hours field
    $activity_hours = 0;
    if(isset($_POST['activity-duration-hours'])) {
        $activity_hours = $_POST['activity-duration-hours'];
        $activity_hours = filter_var($activity_hours,
  FILTER_SANITIZE_NUMBER_FLOAT);
    }
    // Check the activity-duration-minutes field
    $activity_minutes = 0;
    if(isset($_POST['activity-duration-minutes'])) {
        $activity_minutes = $_POST['activity-duration-minutes'];
        $activity_minutes = filter_var($activity_minutes,
  FILTER_SANITIZE_NUMBER_FLOAT);
    }
    // Check the activity-duration-seconds field
    $activity_seconds = 0;
    if(isset($_POST['activity-duration-seconds'])) {
        $activity_seconds = $_POST['activity-duration-seconds'];
        $activity_seconds = filter_var($activity_seconds,
  FILTER_SANITIZE_NUMBER_FLOAT);
    }
    $activity_duration = $activity_hours . ':' .
  $activity_minutes . ':' . $activity_seconds;

    if($server_results['status'] === 'success') {

        // Create the SQL template
        $sql = "INSERT INTO activities
                        (log_id, type, date, distance, duration)
                VALUES (?, ?, ?, ?, ?)";

        // Prepare the statement template
        $stmt = $this->_mysqli->prepare($sql);

        // Bind the parameters
        $stmt->bind_param("issds", $log_id, $activity_type,
  $activity_date, $activity_distance, $activity_duration);

        // Execute the prepared statement
        $stmt->execute();

        // Get the results
        $result = $stmt->get_result();
```

Managing Data

```
        if($this->_mysqli->errno === 0) {
            $server_results['message'] = 'Activity saved
successfully! Sending you back to the activity log...';
        } else {
            $server_results['status'] = 'error';
            $server_results['message'] = 'MySQLi error #: ' .
$this->_mysqli->errno . ': ' . $this->_mysqli->error;
        }
    }
    // Create and then output the JSON data
    $JSON_data = json_encode($server_results, JSON_HEX_APOS |
JSON_HEX_QUOT);
    return $JSON_data;
}
```

This code runs through each of the form fields, checking for valid values and sanitizing as needed. Along the way, the results are stored in the `$server_results` array, where `$server_results['status']` is either `success` or `error`, and `$server_results['message']` is the message that gets displayed to the user.

Reading and Displaying Data

Once your database has at least one item stored, then it's time to handle the "R" in CRUD: reading the data and displaying it to the user. I handle this in five stages:

- » Getting the home page's HTML ready to receive data
- » Writing the code for the Ajax call that requests the data
- » Updating the `Data` class file to handle the read task
- » Displaying the returned data
- » Wiring up the controls that filter the data

Getting the home page ready for data

Right now the home page (`index.php`) file is a skeleton with an empty `main` element. Your job now is to fill that `main` element with the app's data, as well as some controls for operating the app. Here an example from my FootPower! app:

```
<div class="activity-log-toolbar" role="toolbar">
    <label for="activity-filter-date-from">From </label>
    <input id="activity-filter-date-from" class="activity-
  filter" type="date" value="<?php echo date('Y-m-d',
  strtotime('-30 days')) ?>">
    <label for="activity-filter-date-to"> to </label>
    <input id="activity-filter-date-to" class="activity-filter"
  type="date" value="<?php echo date('Y-m-d') ?>">
    <label for="activity-filter-type">Type</label>
    <select id="activity-filter-type" class="activity-filter">
        <option id="activity-filter-type-all">All</option>
        <option id="activity-filter-type-walk">Walk</option>
        <option id="activity-filter-type-run">Run</option>
        <option id="activity-filter-type-cycle">Cycle</option>
    </select>
    <button id="data-create-button" class="btn"
  role="button">Add New</button>
</div>

<!-- The Activity Log appears here -->
<section id="activity-log" class="activity-log">
</section>

<!-- This hidden form contains the values we need to read the
  data: log-id, data-verb, and token -->
 <form id="data-read-form" class="hidden">
    <input type="hidden" id="log-id" name="log-id" value="<?php
  echo $_SESSION['log_id']; ?>">
    <input type="hidden" id="data-verb" name="data-verb"
  value="read-all-data">
    <input type="hidden" id="token" name="token" value="<?php
  echo $_SESSION['token']; ?>">
</form>

<!-- If there's an error reading the data, the error message
  appears inside this span -->
<span id="read-error" class="error error-message"></span>
```

Here are the components you see in this code:

- A `div` element, which is a toolbar that includes the controls for filtering the data by date or by activity type. Note the bits of inline PHP that set the "to" date to the current date and the "From" date to 30 days earlier.
- An empty `section` element, which is where the data will appear.

- A form element that includes three hidden fields: log-id, data-verb (set to read-all-data), and token.
- A span element that will be used to display an error messages that crop up.

Earlier in this chapter, I show that jQuery's ready() method called different functions depending on the file being opened. For index.php, that function is readActivities(), which initiates the read task and which I discuss shortly. For now, if I comment out that function call, Figure 3-2 shows you what the home page looks like before things go any further.

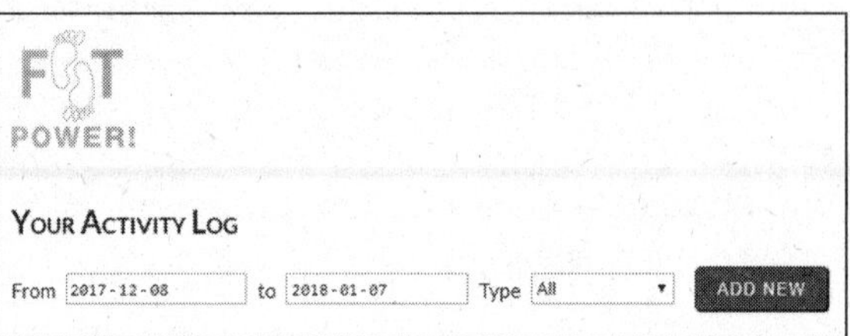

FIGURE 3-2: The FootPower! home page, ready to receive the activity log data.

Making an Ajax request for the data

Once you've got your home page HTML set up, you're ready to initiate the read process, which gathers the hidden form data and then makes the Ajax request to the data handler script on the server.

For my FootPower! app, I initiate the Ajax request by calling the readActivities() function:

```
function readActivities() {

    // Get the form data and convert it to POST
    formData = $('#data-read-form').serializeArray();

    // Submit the data to the handler
    $.post('/handlers/data_handler.php', formData,
   function(data) {
        Code to handle the data returned from the server will
   go here
}
```

The function grabs the data from the hidden form, converts it to POST format, and then sends it to the server's data_handler.php script.

Reading the data

As I discuss earlier, the main job of the `data_handler.php` script is to route the Ajax request depending on the value of the CRUD verb. For the `read-all-data` value, the handler calls the data class's `readAllData()` method. This method takes the ID of the `Data` object, validates and sanitizes it, then uses it to create a `SELECT` statement that grabs the master object's data items.

Here's the code for the FootPower! version of the `readAllData()` method:

```
public function readAllData() {

    // Store the default status
    $server_results['status'] = 'success';

    // Check the log-id field
    $log_id = $_POST['log-id'];
    if(empty($log_id)) {
        $server_results['status'] = 'error';
        $server_results['message'] = 'Error: Missing log ID';
    } else {
        // Sanitize it to an integer
        $log_id = filter_var($log_id, FILTER_SANITIZE_NUMBER_
  FLOAT);
       if (!$log_id) {
            $server_results['status'] = 'error';
            $server_results['message'] = 'Error: Invalid
  log ID';
        }
    }
    if($server_results['status'] === 'success') {

        // Create the SQL template
        $sql = "SELECT * FROM activities
                    WHERE log_id=?
                    ORDER BY date DESC";

        // Prepare the statement template
        $stmt = $this->_mysqli->prepare($sql);

        // Bind the parameter
        $stmt->bind_param("i", $log_id);

        // Execute the prepared statement
        $stmt->execute();
```

Managing Data

```
        // Get the results
        $result = $stmt->get_result();

        if($this->_mysqli->errno === 0) {
            // Get the query rows as an associative array
            $rows = $result->fetch_all(MYSQLI_ASSOC);

            // Convert the array to JSON, then output it
            $JSON_data = json_encode($rows, JSON_HEX_APOS |
    JSON_HEX_QUOT);
            return $JSON_data;
        } else {
            $server_results['status'] = 'error';
            $server_results['message'] = 'MySQLi error #: ' .
    $this->_mysqli->errno . ': ' . $this->_mysqli->error;
        }

    }
    if($server_results['status'] === 'error') {
        // Create and then output the JSON string
        $JSON_data = json_encode($server_results, JSON_HEX_APOS |
    JSON_HEX_QUOT);
        return $JSON_data;
    }
}
```

The code validates and sanitizes the log ID, then sets up a prepared `SELECT` statement to grab all the records from the `activities` table using the `log_id` value (sanitized and stored in the `$log_id` variable) as the filter. The results are then returned as a JSON string.

Displaying the data

The server sends back either an error message or the actual data for displaying, so your front-end code needs to allow for both possibilities.

Here's the updated version of the FootPower! app's `readActivities()` function, with the added code shown in bold:

```
function readActivities() {

    // Get the form data and convert it to POST
    formData = $('#data-read-form').serializeArray();
    // Submit the data to the handler
```

```
    $.post('/handlers/data_handler.php', formData,
function(data) {

        // Convert the JSON string to a JavaScript object
        var result = JSON.parse(data);

        // If there was an error, result.status will be defined
        if (typeof result.status !== 'undefined') {

            // If so, display the error
            $('#read-error').html(result.message).css('display',
'inline-block');

        } else {

            // Otherwise, go ahead and display the data
            activityLog = result;
            applyFilters();
        }
    });
}
```

The returned `data` is converted to a JavaScript object with `JSON.parse(data)`, and that object is stored in the `results` variable. To check for an error, the code tests whether `activityLog.status` is `undefined`. If not, the code outputs the error message; otherwise, the code stores the returned data in the `activityLog` variable, which is declared as a global variable, and then calls `applyFilters()` (which I discuss in the next section).

Filtering the data

If your app might end up presenting the user with a ton of data, you should consider implementing controls to enable the user to filter the data to see only a manageable subset of the records. For example, you could set up a couple of `<input type="date">` tags that enable the user to choose a date range. Similarly, you could create a `<select>` list that includes the unique options for a field, and when the user selects one of these options, the data is filtered to show only the records that match the selected value.

My FootPower! app implements each of these filter options:

- A `date` field that specifies the earliest activity data displayed
- A second `date` field that specifies the latest activity data displayed

» A `select` list that enables the user to choose a specific activity type: `Walk`, `Run`, or `Cycle` (or `All` to see every type)

I displayed the HTML for these controls earlier. Here's the JavaScript that handles the `change` events for these controls:

```
/*
 * Click handler for the Activity Log's Date "From" filter
 */
$('#filter-activity-date-from').change(function() {
    applyFilters();
    });
/*
 * Click handler for the Activity Log's Date "To" filter
 */
$('#filter-activity-date-to').change(function() {
    applyFilters();
});
/*
 * Click handler for the Activity Log's Type filter
 */
$('#filter-activity-type').change(function() {
    applyFilters();
});
/*
 * Applies the current Activity Log filters
 */
function applyFilters() {

    // Get the current filter values
    var earliestDateFilter = $('#filter-activity-date-from').
  val();
    var latestDateFilter = $('#filter-activity-date-to').val();
    var activityTypeFilter = $('#filter-activity-type >
  option:selected').text();

    // Filter based on the "From" date
    filteredLog = activityLog.filter(function(activity) {
        return activity.date >= earliestDateFilter;
    });
```

```
    // Filter based on the "To" date
    filteredLog = filteredLog.filter(function(activity) {
        return activity.date <= latestDateFilter;
    });

    // Filter based on the "Type" value
    if(activityTypeFilter === 'All') {
        displayActivityLog(filteredLog);
    } else {
        filteredLog = filteredLog.filter(function(activity) {
            return activity.type === activityTypeFilter;
        });
        displayActivityLog(filteredLog);
    }
}
```

All three of the event handlers do nothing else but call the `applyFilters()` function. This function first gets the current filter values and then it applies each filter in turn. In each case, the code uses JavaScript's `filter()` method to return a subset of the array. Note, however, that the first time `filter()` runs, it applies the filter on the full `activityLog` array and returns the filtered array as `filteredLog`. The second time `filter()` runs, it applies the filter to the `filteredLog` array, which makes the filter cumulative. For the Type filter, if the value is `All`, the code just outputs the filtered data by calling `displayActivityLog()` with the filtered array as a parameter. Otherwise, it applies the filter and then displays the data.

Here's the function that performs the actual displaying of the data:

```
function displayActivityLog(log) {
    $('.activity-log').html('<div id="activity-log-header"
  class="activity activity-log-header">');
    $('#activity-log-header').append('<div class="activity-
  item">Type</div>');
    $('#activity-log-header').append('<div class="activity-
  item">Date</div>');
    $('#activity-log-header').append('<div class="activity-
  item">Distance</div>');
    $('#activity-log-header').append('<div class="activity-
  item">Duration</div>');
```

```
  $('.activity-log').append('</div>');
  $.each(log, function(index, activity) {
      $('.activity-log').append('<div id="activity' + index +
'" class="activity">');
      switch (activity.type) {
          case 'Walk':
              activityIcon = '<img src="images/walk.png"
alt="Walk activity icon">';
              break;
          case 'Run':
              activityIcon = '<img src="images/run.png"
alt="Run activity icon">';
              break;
          case 'Cycle':
              activityIcon = '<img src="images/cycle.png"
alt="Cycle activity icon">';
              break;
      }
        $('#activity' + index).append('<div class=
"activity-item">' + activityIcon + activity.type + '</div>');
      $('#activity' + index).append('<div class=
"activity-item">' + activity.date + '</div>');
      $('#activity' + activity.activity_id).append
('<div class="activity-item">' + Number(activity.distance).
toFixed(2) + '</div>');
      $('#activity' + index).append('<div class=
"activity-item">' + activity.duration + '</div>');
      $('#activity' + activity.activity_id).append
('<div class="activity-item"><input id="activity-' + activity.
activity_id + '" class="data-edit-button" type="image"
src="images/pencil.png" alt="Pencil icon; click to edit this
activity"></div>');
      $('.activity-log').append('</div>');
  });
}
```

This code mostly just appends HTML to the home page's empty `<section>` tag (which I've given the class name `activity-log`). A `switch()` statement checks the activity type to output the corresponding icon image. The CSS, which I don't have room to show, configures the data with a flexbox layout that alternates the data item background to make it easier to read, as you can see in Figure 3-3.

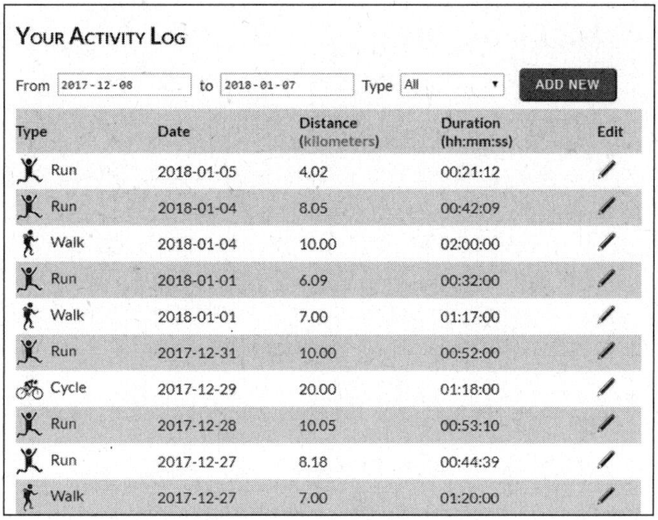

YOUR ACTIVITY LOG

From 2017-12-08 to 2018-01-07 Type All ADD NEW

Type	Date	Distance (kilometers)	Duration (hh:mm:ss)	Edit
Run	2018-01-05	4.02	00:21:12	
Run	2018-01-04	8.05	00:42:09	
Walk	2018-01-04	10.00	02:00:00	
Run	2018-01-01	6.09	00:32:00	
Walk	2018-01-01	7.00	01:17:00	
Run	2017-12-31	10.00	00:52:00	
Cycle	2017-12-29	20.00	01:18:00	
Run	2017-12-28	10.05	00:53:10	
Run	2017-12-27	8.18	00:44:39	
Walk	2017-12-27	7.00	01:20:00	

FIGURE 3-3: The FootPower! home page, now with fresh data.

Updating and Editing Data

To enable the user to update existing data items, you need to add an Edit button for each item. In most cases, clicking this button presents a form that's identical to the one used to create an item, although with the existing item's data already filled in. Submitting that form should then run an `UPDATE` query on the server to preserve the user's edits.

To handle this in my FootPower! app, I included an Edit column to the Activity Log, and for each activity I displayed a pencil icon, as shown in Figure 3-3.

Here's the jQuery code I used to add the pencil icons to each activity:

```
$('#activity' + activity.activity_id).append('<div
   class="activity-item"><input id="activity-' + activity.
   activity_id + '" class="activity-crud-update" type="image"
   src="images/pencil.png" alt="Pencil icon; click to edit this
   activity"></div>');
```

Note, in particular, that for each `<input>` tag, the `id` value is set to `activity-`*`id`*, where *`id`* is the `activity_id` value of the current activity.

Here's the `click` event handler that runs when the user clicks a pencil icon:

```
$('#activity-log').click(function(e) {
    e.preventDefault();
```

```
    // Make sure we're dealing with an edit link
    if(e.target.className === 'data-edit-button') {

        //Get the activity's ID
        var activityID = Number(e.target.id.split('-')[1]);

        // Load the Update form and send the activity ID in the
  query string
        window.location = 'update_data.php?activity-id=' +
  activityID;
    }
});
```

Here's what happening in this code:

- Since you created the edit links in code, you can't use them as jQuery selectors, so you use the closest DOM ancestor, which is the `<section id="activity-log")` tag.
- The clicked activity's ID value is extracted and stored in the `activityID` variable.
- The browser is sent to the `update_data.php` file, with the activity ID stored in the URL's query string.

First, here's the code for the `update_data.php` page:

```
<?php
    include_once '../private/common/initialization.php';
    $page_title = 'Edit Activity';
    include_once 'common/top.php';
    include_once 'common/data_form.php';
?>
            <!-- The jQuery UI dialog markup for Delete This
  Activity-->
            <div id="confirm-delete" class="activity-delete-
  dialog" title="Delete This Activity?" role="dialog">
                <p>Are you sure you want to remove this
  activity from your log?
                This action can't be undone!</p>
            </div>

<?php
    include_once 'common/sidebar.php';
    include_once 'common/bottom.php';
?>
```

REMEMBER

Note the extra markup for a jQuery UI dialog. I talk about this in the next section.

The document's `ready()` event (shown earlier) looks for this file and runs the `initializeUpdateDataForm()` function:

```
function initializeUpdateDataForm() {

    // Get the activity ID from the URL query string and save it
  to the form
    var activityID = Number(window.location.search.split('=')
  [1]);
    $('#activity-id').val(activityID);

    // Get the data for this item
    var formData = [
        {"name": "log-id", "value": $('#log-id').val()},
        {"name": "activity-id", "value": $('#activity-id').
  val()},
        {"name": "data-verb", "value": "read-data-item"},
        {"name": "token", "value": $('#token').val()}
    ];

    // Submit the data to the handler
    $.post('/handlers/data_handler.php', formData,
  function(data) {

        // Convert the JSON string to a JavaScript object
        // We know that "data" is a single-item array, so just
  take the first item
        var result = JSON.parse(data)[0];

        // If there was an error, result.status will be defined
        if (typeof result.status !== 'undefined') {

            // If so, display the error
            $('#form-error').html(result.message).css('display',
  'inline-block');

        } else {
           // Show the Delete button
            $('#data-delete-button').show();

            // Set the data verb to "update"
            $('#data-verb').val('update');
```

```
            // Store the activity values
            // We know that "result" is a single-item array,
so just take the first item
            activity = result[0];
            var activityType = activity.type;
            var activityDate = activity.date
            var activityDistance = Number(activity.distance).
toFixed(2);
            var activityDuration = activity.duration.split(':');

            // Use the activity values to populate the edit form
            $('#activity-id').val(activityID);
            $('#activity-type').val(activityType);
            $('#activity-date').val(activityDate);
            $('#activity-distance').val(activityDistance);
            $('#activity-duration-hours').
val(activityDuration[0]);
            $('#activity-duration-minutes').
val(activityDuration[1]);
            $('#activity-duration-seconds').
val(activityDuration[2]);
        }
    });
}
```

The first part of this code grabs the activity to be updated from the server. The ID of the activity is extracted from the URL's query string and then stored in the form's hidden `activity-id` field. The form's hidden field values are gathered and then sent via the `.post()` method to the `data_handler.php` script on the server. Note in particular then the `data-verb` value is set to `read-data-item`, which means the server script will call the `Data` class's `readDataItem()` method:

```
public function readDataItem() {

    // Store the default status
    $server_results['status'] = 'success';

    // Check the log-id field
    $log_id = $_POST['log-id'];
    if(empty($log_id)) {
        $server_results['status'] = 'error';
        $server_results['message'] = 'Error: Missing log ID';
    } else {
```

```
        // Sanitize it to an integer
        $log_id = filter_var($log_id, FILTER_SANITIZE_NUMBER_
FLOAT);
       if (!$log_id) {
            $server_results['status'] = 'error';
            $server_results['message'] = 'Error: Invalid
log ID';
        } else {
            // Check the activity-id field
            $activity_id = $_POST['activity-id'];
            if(empty($activity_id)) {
                $server_results['status'] = 'error';
                $server_results['message'] = 'Error: Missing
activity ID';
            } else {
                // Sanitize it to an integer
                $activity_id = filter_var($activity_id,
FILTER_SANITIZE_NUMBER_FLOAT);
               if (!$activity_id) {
                    $server_results['status'] = 'error';
                    $server_results['message'] = 'Error: Invalid
activity ID';
                }
            }
        }
    }
    // Are we good?
    if($server_results['status'] === 'success') {

        // Create the SQL template
        $sql = "SELECT * FROM activities
                    WHERE log_id=?
                    AND activity_id=?
                    LIMIT 1";

        // Prepare the statement template
        $stmt = $this->_mysqli->prepare($sql);

        // Bind the parameters
        $stmt->bind_param("ii", $log_id, $activity_id);

        // Execute the prepared statement
        $stmt->execute();
```

Managing Data

```
        // Get the results
        $result = $stmt->get_result();

        if($this->_mysqli->errno === 0) {

            // Get the query row as an associative array
            $row = $result->fetch_all(MYSQLI_ASSOC);

            // Convert the array to JSON, then return it
            $JSON_data = json_encode($row, JSON_HEX_APOS |
  JSON_HEX_QUOT);
            return $JSON_data;
        } else {
            $server_results['status'] = 'error';
            $server_results['message'] = 'MySQLi error #: ' .
  $this->_mysqli->errno . ': ' . $this->_mysqli->error;
        }
    }
    if($server_results['status'] === 'error') {
        // Create and then return the JSON string
        $JSON_data = json_encode($server_results,
  JSON_HEX_APOS | JSON_HEX_QUOT);
        return $JSON_data;
    }
}
```

Back in `initializeUpdateDataForm()`, the returned item is stored in `result` and checked for an error. If there was no error, the form's `data-verb` value is set to `update` and the hidden Delete button is displayed. Finally, the activity's values are stored in variables, and then those variable values are used to populate the form controls.

Figure 3-4 shows an example of an activity ready to be edited.

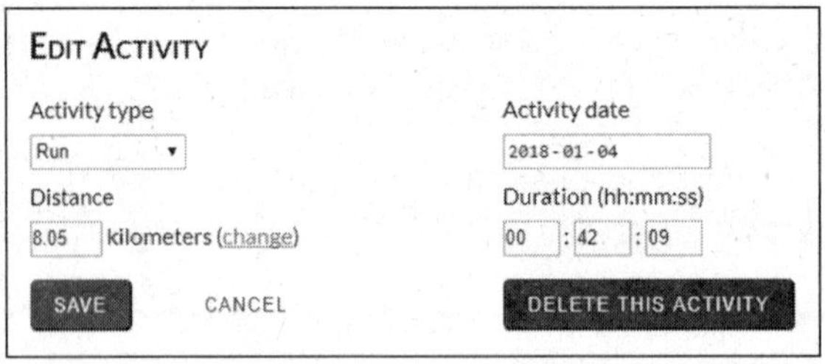

FIGURE 3-4: Clicking an activity's Edit icon displays the form populated with the activity's values.

Clicking Save runs the same event handler that I show earlier. The `data_handler.php` code on the server routes the Ajax request to the `Data` object's `updateData()` method. This method runs the same validation and sanitization code as `createData()`, shown earlier, except that `updateData()` also checks the `update` verb's `activity-id` value (which holds the ID of the activity being updated) and stores the sanitized version in the `$activity_id` variable:

```
// Check the activity-id field
$activity_id = $_POST['activity-id'];
if(empty($activity_id)) {
    $server_results['status'] = 'error';
    $server_results['activity-type'] = 'Missing activity ID';
} else {
    // Sanitize it to an integer
    $activity_id = filter_var($activity_id, FILTER_SANITIZE_
  NUMBER_FLOAT);
    if (!$activity_id) {
        $server_results['status'] = 'error';
        $server_results['message'] = 'Invalid activity ID';
    }
}
```

If everything checks out, the code prepares an SQL `UPDATE` statement to save the activity edit to the database:

```
if($server_results['status'] === 'success') {

    // Create the SQL template
    $sql = "UPDATE activities
                SET type=?, date=?, distance=?, duration=?
                WHERE log_id=? AND activity_id=?";

    // Prepare the statement template
    $stmt = $this->_mysqli->prepare($sql);

    // Bind the parameters
    $stmt->bind_param("ssdsii", $activity_type, $activity_date,
  $activity_distance, $activity_duration, $log_id,
  $activity_id);

    // Execute the prepared statement
    $stmt->execute();
```

```
    // Get the results
    $result = $stmt->get_result();

    if($this->_mysqli->errno === 0) {
        $server_results['message'] = 'Activity updated
  successfully!';
    } else {
        $server_results['status'] = 'error';
        $server_results['message'] = 'MySQLi error #: ' .
  $this->_mysqli->errno;
    }
}
// Create and then return the JSON data
$JSON_data = json_encode($server_results, JSON_HEX_APOS |
  JSON_HEX_QUOT);
return $JSON_data;
```

Deleting Data

As a final data-handling chore, your web app should provide an interface that enables the user to delete data items from the server. Careful, though: You also need some way to ask the user to confirm the deletion, to avoid accidental (and non-reversible) data loss. The usual way to confirm an action in a web app is to display a so-called *modal* dialog, which prevents the user from doing anything else on the screen until the dialog is dismissed. You could code such a dialog by hand, but why go to that trouble when our friends at jQuery UI have an awesome dialog widget that you can use with just a few lines of code?

Before I get to that, take a look back at Figure 3-4, which includes a Delete This Activity button. Clicking this button displays the confirmation dialog, so let's see how that works. Assuming you've downloaded a version of jQuery UI that contains the dialog widget (see Book 4, Chapter 3), you first add the HTML markup for the dialog:

```
<div id="confirm-delete" title="Delete This Activity?">
    <p>Are you sure you want to remove this activity from your
  log? This action can't be undone.</p>
</div>
```

The `title` attribute of the `div` element becomes the dialog title, and the text within the `div` element becomes the dialog's body text.

To configure the dialog, you add the following code:

```
$("#confirm-delete").dialog({
    autoOpen: false,
    closeOnEscape: true,
    modal: true,
    width: 400,
    buttons: [
        {
            text: 'Cancel',
            click: function() {
                $(this).dialog('close');
            }
        },
        {
            text: 'Delete',
            click: function() {
                $(this).dialog('close');
            Code to initiate the Ajax call to the server will
  go here
            }
        }
    ]
});
```

There are five options specified here (see `http://api.jqueryui.com/dialog/` for the complete list):

- `autoOpen`: Determines whether the dialog opens automatically when the page loads. The default is `true`, so use `false` to control when the dialog appears.
- `closeOnEscape`: When `true`, enables the user to close the dialog by pressing the Esc key.
- `modal`: Set to `true` to make the dialog modal.
- `width`: Specifies the width, in pixels, of the dialog.
- `buttons`: This array specifies the command buttons that appear in the dialog. Use the `text` value to set the button text and the `click` value to specify a callback function that runs when the button is clicked.

To open the modal dialog, set up a `click` event handler for the button that you want to display the dialog:

```
$('#data-delete-button').click(function(e) {

    // Take the focus off the button
    $(this).blur();

    // Open the jQuery UI dialog
    $('#confirm-delete').dialog('open');

    // Prevent the default action
    e.preventDefault();
});
```

Figure 3-5 shows the confirmation dialog I'm using for my FootPower! web app.

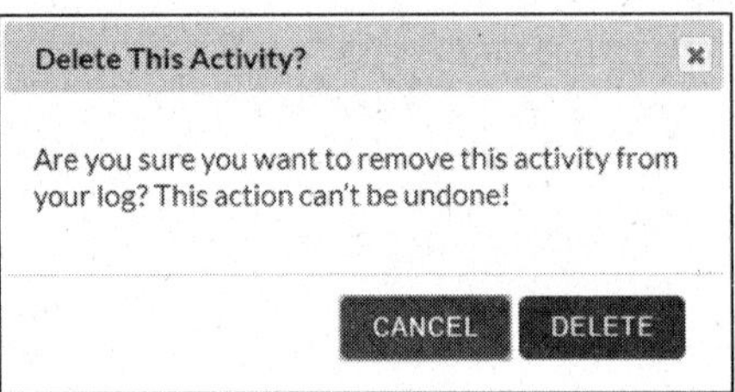

FIGURE 3-5: When the user clicks Delete This Activity, this modal confirmation dialog appears.

Clicking the `Cancel` button just closes the dialog with no further action. Clicking `Delete`, however, means the user is serious about the deletion, so you need to add some code to this button's `click` handler:

```
click: function() {

    // Close the dialog
    $(this).dialog('close');

    // Disable all the buttons
    $('#data-form button').prop('disabled', true);

    // Set the data verb to "delete"
    $('#data-verb').val('delete');

    // Get the form data and convert it to a POST-able format
    // We only need the log ID, activity ID, CRUD verb, and
   token from the form,
```

```
    // so we'll build the array by hand instead of using
   serializeArray()
    formData = [
        {"name": "log-id", "value": $('#log-id').val()},
        {"name": "activity-id", "value": $('#activity-id').
   val()},
        {"name": "data-verb", "value": $('#data-verb').val()},
        {"name": "token", "value": $('#token').val()}
    ];

    // Submit the data to the handler
    $.post('/handlers/data_handler.php', formData,
   function(data) {

        // Convert the JSON string to a JavaScript object
        var result = JSON.parse(data);

        if(result.status === 'error') {

            // Display the error
            $('#form-error').html(result.message).css('display',
   'inline-block');

            // Enable all the buttons
            $('#data-form button').prop('disabled', false);

        } else {

            // Display the success message
            $('#form-message').html(result.message).
   css('display', 'inline-block');

            // Return to the home page after 1 second
            window.setTimeout("window.location='index.php'",
   1000);
        }
    });
}
```

Here's what happening in this code:

- The form's `data-verb` value is set to `delete`.
- The form's `log-id`, `activity-id`, `crud-verb`, and `token` values are added to the POST array.

» The POST data is passed along via Ajax to the data_handler.php script on the server.

The data_handler.php script sees that the data-verb value is delete, so it routes the Ajax request to the Data object's deleteData() method. That method validates and sanitizes the log-id and activity-id values, then uses them to prepare and execute a SQL DELETE statement:

```
if($server_results['status'] === 'success') {

    // Create the SQL template
    $sql = "DELETE FROM activities WHERE log_id=? AND
  activity_id=?";

    // Prepare the statement template
    $stmt = $this->_mysqli->prepare($sql);

    // Bind the parameters
    $stmt->bind_param("ii", $log_id, $activity_id);

    // Execute the prepared statement
    $stmt->execute();

    // Get the results
    $result = $stmt->get_result();

    if($this->_mysqli->errno === 0) {
        $server_results['message'] = 'Activity deleted
  successfully! Sending you back to the activity log...';
    } else {
        $server_results['status'] = 'error';
        $server_results['message'] = 'MySQLi error #: ' .
  $this->_mysqli->errno . ': ' . $this->_mysqli->error;
    }
}
// Create and then return the JSON data
$JSON_data = json_encode($server_results, JSON_HEX_APOS |
  JSON_HEX_QUOT);
return $JSON_data;
}
```

IN THIS CHAPTER

» Setting up your app's user class

» Creating new user accounts

» Signing users in and out of the web app

» Handling forgotten passwords

» Managing user accounts flexibly and securely

Chapter 4
Managing App Users

The craft of programming begins with empathy, not formatting or languages or tools or algorithms or data structures.

— KENT BECK

If your web app enables users to create data items, then those users will come with the more than reasonable expectation that your web app will preserve that data. The simplest web apps honor that expectation by saving user data locally in the web browser, a topic that I talk about in Book 8, Chapter 1. However, your users might also come with the further expectation that their data should be available to them no matter which device or web browser they happen to be using. This level of expectation is certainly still reasonable, but it's considerably more complex because now you're in the realm of managing user accounts on the server. This means creating user accounts, securely storing passwords, verifying new accounts, managing both sign-ins and sign-outs, updating user credentials, handling forgotten passwords, and more.

Yep, it's a big job, but I have a feeling you're more than up to the task. In this chapter, you explore the fascinating world of user management and delve into all the details required to set up a bulletproof and secure user account system.

Configuring the Home Page

One of the main changes you need to make when you want to add support for user accounts is configuring the web app's home page to show a different set of tags depending on whether the user is signed in or not:

- If a user is signed in, show the user's data and a Sign Out button.
- If the visitor doesn't have an account or isn't signed in, show an introductory screen and a Sign Up button that encourages those without an account to create one, and show a Sign In button so that users with accounts can access their data.

Fortunately, you don't need to create two different home pages. Instead, you can use some inline PHP to check whether a user is signed in and display the appropriate HTML tags and text depending on the result.

TIP

To make this sort of thing easier, PHP has an alternative `if()...else` syntax that you can use to add HTML tags to a page based on one or more conditions. Here's the general structure:

```
<?php
    if(condition):
?>
    HTML tags to display if condition is TRUE
<?php
    else:
?>
    HTML tags to display if condition is FALSE
<?php
    endif;
?>
```

The *condition* in your web app will be something that returns `TRUE` if the user is signed in, and `FALSE` otherwise. There are various ways to approach this, but the easiest is to set a session variable when the user signs in. Because a username is required to sign in, it makes sense to use the username as the session variable. For example, assuming your web app has some sort of sign-in form (more on that in a bit) that includes a `username` field, then the following PHP statement would store a sanitized version of the username in a session variable named `username`:

```
$_SESSION['username'] = htmlentities($_POST['username'],
   ENT_QUOTES);
```

You can then use `isset($_SESSION['username'])` as the condition to determine what HTML tags the user sees. Here's a partial modification of the FootPower! `index.php` file:

```
<?php
    include_once '../private/common/initialization.php';
    if(isset($_SESSION['username'])) {
        $page_title = 'Your Activity Log';
    } else {
        $page_title = 'Welcome to FootPower!';
    }
    include_once 'common/top.php';

    if(isset($_SESSION['username'])):
?>
        The rest of the Activity Log code goes here (see Book 7,
  Chapter 3)
<?php
    else:
?>
        <section class="footpower-intro" role="contentinfo">
            <p>
                Are you a walker, a runner, or a cyclist? Heck,
  maybe you're all three! Either way, you know the joy and
  satisfaction of propelling yourself across the face of the
  Earth using nothing but the power of your own two feet.
            </p>
            <p>
                Have you walked, ran, or cycled recently? If so,
  we salute you! But why relegate the details of that activity
  to the dim mists of history and memory? Why not save your
  effort for posterity? Just sign up for a free FootPower!
  account and you'll never forget a walk, run, or ride again!
            </p>
            <div>
                <img src="images/walk-large.png" alt="Drawing of
  a walker.">
                <img src="images/run-large.png" alt="Drawing of
  a runner.">
                <img src="images/cycle-large.png" alt="Drawing
  of a cyclist.">
            </div>
        </section>
    </article>
```

```
<?php
    endif;
    include_once 'common/sidebar.php';
    include_once 'common/bottom.php';
?>
```

If the `username` session variable is set, the user is logged in, so display the Activity Log for that user. Otherwise, display an introductory message.

You also need conditional code that determines the buttons the user sees. Here's the modified version of the FootPower! `top.php` file:

```
<body>
    <header class="top-header" role="banner">
        <div class="top-header-logo">
            <img src="images/footpower-logo.png" alt="FootPower!
  logo">
        </div>
        <div class="top-header-user">
<?php
    if(isset($_SESSION['username'])):
?>
            <button id="show-user-account-button" class="btn-
  plain">Your Account</button>
            <button id="user-sign-out-button" class="btn">Sign
  Out</button>
<?php
    else:
?>
            <button id="show-sign-in-page-button" class="btn-
  plain">Sign In</button>
            <button id="show-sign-up-page-button"
  class="btn">Sign Up</button>
<?php
    endif;
?>
        </div>
    </header>
    <main role="main">
```

When the user is signed in, she sees the Your Account and Sign Out buttons; otherwise, she sees both a Sign In and a Sign Up button. Figure 4-1 shows the FootPower! home page when a user is not signed in.

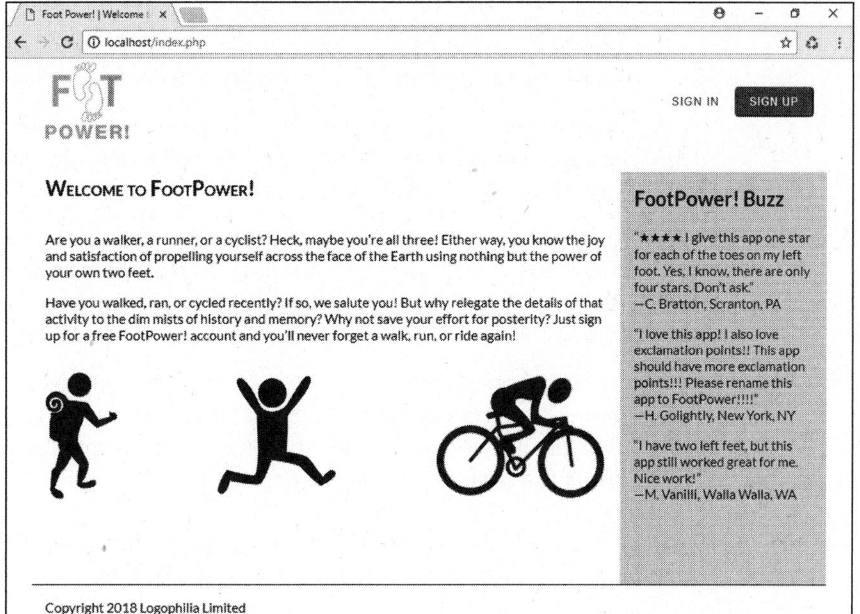

FIGURE 4-1: The FootPower! home page when a user is not signed in.

Setting Up the Back End to Handle Users

Most web apps that manage users need to implement at least the following tasks:

- **Signing up new users:** Includes not only capturing the user's email address (to use as a username) and password, but also sending out a verification email to make sure the user isn't a bot or spammer
- **Signing in users:** Enables each user to access her own data
- **Signing out users:** Prevents others from accessing a user's account when his computer is left unattended
- **Updating user data:** Enables each user to change her password and to reset a forgotten password
- **Deleting users:** Enables a user to remove his account and data from the server

The rest of this chapter shows you how to implement each of these functions. Before I get to that, here's the bird's-eye view of what I'll be doing:

1. Build a class for handling user interactions. That class includes one method for each of the preceding tasks.

2. Provide the user with an interface for signing up, signing in, signing out, modifying account data, and deleting the account.

3. To start processing a user task, set up an event handler for each account-focused interface element. If you're using a sign-in form, for example, then you might set up a `submit` event handler for that form.

4. Use each event handler to send the form data to a single PHP script via Ajax. Importantly, that form data includes the value of a hidden field that specifies the type of "user verb" being performed (sign up, sign in, reset password, and so on).

5. In the PHP script, create a new object from the class of Step 1, check the user verb sent by the Ajax call, and then call the corresponding class method. For example, if the event is signing up a new user, the script would call the class method that handles creating new user accounts.

The next couple of sections cover setting up the first part of the user class and building the PHP script that handles the Ajax requests.

Starting the web app's user class

The class for your web app's users needs to do at least the following three things:

- Accept a parameter that references the current `MySQLi` object.
- Define a method for each of the user verbs.
- Define any helper functions required by the user verbs.

With these goals in mind, here's the skeleton class file:

```
<?php
class User {

    // Holds the app's current MySQLi object
    private $_mysqli;

    // Use the class constructor to store the passed MySQLi
   object
    public function __construct($mysqli) {
        $this->_mysqli = $mysqli;
    }
```

```
    // Here are the user chores we need to handle
    public function createUser() {

    }
    public function verifyUser() {

    }
    public function signInUser() {

    }
    public function sendPasswordReset() {

    }
    public function resetPassword() {

    }
    public function getDistanceUnit() {

    }
    public function updateDistanceUnit() {

    }
    public function deleteUser() {

    }
}
?>
```

The class declares the private property `$_mysqli`, which it uses to store the current instance of the `MySQLi` object (created earlier in the `initialization.php` script). Store this file in `private/classes/user_class.php`.

To create an instance of this class, you'd use a statement similar to the following:

```
$user = new User($mysqli);
```

Creating a user handler script

The various user verbs will be initiated via Ajax calls to a single PHP script. Each Ajax call needs to specify the user verb required, and the PHP code routes the request to the corresponding method in the `User` class.

Here's the PHP script, which I'll save as `public/handlers/user_handler.php`:

```
<?php

    // Initialize the app
    include_once '../../private/common/initialization.php';

    // Include the User class
    include_once '../../private/classes/user_class.php';

    // Initialize the results
    $server_results['status'] = 'success';
    $server_results['control'] = '';
    $server_results['message'] = '';

    // Make sure a user verb was passed
    if (!isset($_POST['user-verb'])) {
        $server_results['status'] = 'error';
        $server_results['control'] = 'form';
        $server_results['message'] = 'Error: No user verb
  specified!';
    }
    // Make sure a token value was passed
    elseif (!isset($_POST['token'])) {
        $server_results['status'] = 'error';
        $server_results['control'] = 'form';
        $server_results['message'] = 'Error: Invalid user
  session!';
    }
    // Make sure the token is legit
    elseif ($_SESSION['token'] !== $_POST['token']) {
        $server_results['status'] = 'error';
        $server_results['control'] = 'form';
        $server_results['message'] = 'Timeout Error! Please
  refresh the page and try again.';
    }
    // If we get this far, all is well, so go for it
    else {

        // Create a new User object
        $user = new User($mysqli);

        // Pass the user verb to the appropriate method
        switch ($_POST['user-verb']) {
```

```
        // Sign up a new user
        case 'sign-up-user':
            $server_results = json_decode($user-
>createUser());
            break;

        // Sign in an existing user
        case 'sign-in-user':
            $server_results = json_decode($user-
>signInUser());
            break;

        // Send a request to reset a user's password
        case 'send-password-reset':
            $server_results = json_decode($user-
>sendPasswordReset());
            break;

        // Reset a user's password
        case 'reset-password':
            $server_results = json_decode($user-
>resetPassword());
            break;

        // Get the user's distance unit
        case 'get-distance-unit':
            $server_results = json_decode($user-
>getDistanceUnit());
            break;

        // Update distance unit
        case 'update-unit':
            $server_results = json_decode($user-
>updateDistanceUnit());
            break;

        // Delete a user
        case 'delete-user':
            $server_results = json_decode($user-
>deleteUser());
            break;

        default:
            $server_results['status'] = 'error';
```

```
                $server_results['control'] = 'token';
                $server_results['message'] = 'Error: Unknown
user verb!';
        }
    }
    // Create and then output the JSON data
    $JSON_data = json_encode($server_results, JSON_HEX_APOS |
JSON_HEX_QUOT);
    echo $JSON_data;
?>
```

After initializing the app by including `initialization.php`, the code also includes the `User` class file. The code then sets up an array named `$server_results`, which holds the results that the script sends back to the front end:

- `$server_results['status']` will be either `success` or `error`.
- `$server_results['message']` holds the success or error message to display.

The code next runs through a series of checks: making sure a verb was passed, making sure a token value was passed, and then comparing that token value with the session token. If the code gets past those tests, a `switch()` statement runs through the possible values for `$_POST['user-verb']` and calls the corresponding `User` method.

In the rest of this chapter, I fill in the details for the various `User` methods and the front-end interfaces that support them.

Signing Up a New User

The process of signing up a new user takes four general steps:

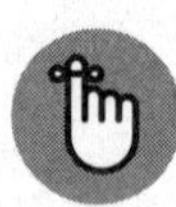

REMEMBER

1. Present the user with a form that asks for the person's username (usually just her email address) and a password.
2. Send the data to the server and provisionally add the user to the `users` table.
3. Send to the user a verification email that includes a unique link that the user must click to verify her account.
4. Verify the user.

Once the user is verified, and each subsequent time the user signs in to the app, you need to set a session variable that the app can use to check whether the user is signed in. I like to keep things simple here and just set `$_SESSION['username']` to the current account's username.

Building the form

When the user clicks the Sign Up button, he sees the `sign_up.php` page:

```
<?php
    include_once '../private/common/initialization.php';
    if(isset($_SESSION['username'])) {
        $page_title = 'You're Already Signed Up';
    } else {
        $page_title = 'Sign Up For a Free FootPower! Account';
    }
    include_once 'common/top.php';

    // Is the user already signed in?
    if(isset($_SESSION['username'])):
?>
            <section>
                <p>
                    You already have an account, so nothing to
  see here.
                </p>
                <p>
                    Did you want to <a href="create_data.
  php">log an activity</a>, instead?
                </p>
                <p>
                    Or perhaps you want to <a href="sign_out.
  php">sign out</a>?
                </p>
            </section>
<?php
    else:
?>
                                <p>Your feet will thank you.</p>
            <form id="user-sign-up-form">
                <div class="form-wrapper">
                    <div class="control-wrapper">
```

```
                    <label for="username">Email</label>
                    <input id="username" class="form-
control" name="username" type="email" aria-label="Type your
email address." required/>
                    <span id="username-error" class="error
error-message"></span>
                </div>
                <div class="control-wrapper">
                    <label for="password">Password</label>
                    <div>
                        <input id="password" class="form-
control" name="password" type="password" minlength="8"
aria-label="Type your password." required>
                        <br>
                        <input id="password-toggle"
type="checkbox"><label for="password-toggle" class="label-
horizontal">Show password</label>
                    </div>
                    <span id="password-error" class="error
error-message"></span>
                </div>
                <button id="sign-me-up-button" class="btn
btn-form" type="submit">Sign Me Up</button>
                <span id="form-error" class="error error-
message form-error-message"></span>
                <span id="form-message" class="form-
message"></span>
                <input type="hidden" id="user-verb"
name="user-verb" value="sign-up-user">
                <input type="hidden" id="token" name="token"
value="<?php echo $_SESSION['token']; ?>">
            </div>
        </form>
<?php
    endif;
    include_once 'common/sidebar.php';
    include_once 'common/bottom.php';
?>
```

This page plays it safe and checks to see if the user is already logged in, in which case it lets the user know and offers some links. Otherwise, the code displays the Sign Up form, shown in Figure 4-2.

Sign Up For a Free FootPower! Account

Your feet will thank you.

Email

Password

Show password

SIGN ME UP

FIGURE 4-2: The FootPower! form for signing up a new user.

Sending the data to the server

Clicking Sign Me Up invokes the form's `submit` event, so you need to add a handler for this:

```
$('#user-sign-up-form').submit(function(e) {

    // Prevent the default submit
    e.preventDefault();

    // Disable the Sign Me Up button to prevent double
  submissions
    $('#sign-me-up-button').prop('disabled', true);

    // Clear and hide all the message spans ($ = "ends with")
    $('span[id$="error"').html('').css('display', 'none');
    $('#form-message').html('').css('display', 'none');

    // Get the form data and convert it to a POST-able format
    formData = $(this).serializeArray();

    // Submit the data to the handler
    $.post('/handlers/user_handler.php', formData,
  function(data) {

        // Convert the JSON string to a JavaScript object
        var result = JSON.parse(data);

        if(result.status === 'error') {

            // Display the error
            $('#' + result.control + '-error').html(result.
  message).css('display', 'inline-block');
```

```
            // Enable the Sign Me Up button
            $('#sign-me-up-button').prop('disabled', false);

        } else {
            $('#form-message').html(result.message).
  css('display', 'inline-block');
        }
    });
});
```

This code prevents the default submission, disables the Sign Me Up button to prevent the user from accidentally clicking it again, clears the messages, and then sends the form data to the server. When the `user_handler.php` script sees that the `user-verb` is set to `sign-up-user`, it routes the task to the `User` object's `createUser()` method. The first part of this method validates and sanitizes the username and password:

```
public function createUser() {

    // Store the default status
    $server_results['status'] = 'success';

    // Was the username sent?
    if(empty($_POST['username'])) {
        $server_results['status'] = 'error';
        $server_results['control'] = 'username';
        $server_results['message'] = 'Um, you really do need to
  enter your email address.';
    } else {

        // Sanitize it
        //$username = htmlentities($username);
        $username = $_POST['username'];
        $username = filter_var($username, FILTER_SANITIZE_
  EMAIL);
        if (!$username) {
            $server_results['status'] = 'error';
            $server_results['control'] = 'username';
            $server_results['message'] = 'Hmmm. It looks like
  that email address isn\'t valid. Please try again.';
        } else {
```

```
            // Make sure the username doesn't already exist in
the database
            $sql = "SELECT *
                    FROM users
                    WHERE username=?";
            $stmt = $this->_mysqli->prepare($sql);
            $stmt->bind_param("s", $username);
            $stmt->execute();
            $result = $stmt->get_result();

            // If the username already exists, num_rows will be
greater than 0
            if ($result->num_rows > 0) {
                $server_results['status'] = 'error';
                $server_results['control'] = 'username';
                $server_results['message'] = 'Whoops! That email
address is already being used. Please try again.';
            }
        }
    }

    // If all is still well, check the password
    if($server_results['status'] === 'success') {

        // Was the password sent?
        if(empty($_POST['password'])) {
            $server_results['status'] = 'error';
            $server_results['control'] = 'password';
            $server_results['message'] = 'That\'s weird: the
password is missing. Please try again.';
        } else {

            // Sanitize it
            $password = $_POST['password'];
            $password = filter_var($password, FILTER_SANITIZE_
STRING);

            // Is the password still valid?
            if (!$password) {
                $server_results['status'] = 'error';
                $server_results['control'] = 'password';
                $server_results['message'] = 'Sorry, but the
password you used was invalid. Please try again.';
            }
```

```
            // Is the password long enough?
            elseif (strlen($password) < 8 ) {
                $server_results['status'] = 'error';
                $server_results['control'] = 'password';
                $server_results['message'] = 'Sorry, but the
    password must be at least 8 characters long. Please try
    again.';
            } else {

                // If all's well, hash the password
                $password = password_hash($password, PASSWORD_
    DEFAULT);
            }
        }
    }
```

For the username, the code makes sure it was entered and that it's a legit email address. It also runs a prepared SQL `SELECT` statement to make sure the user isn't already signed up. The password is checked for validity, sanitized, and checked for length (minimum eight characters). If those checks pass, the password is hashed using PHP's `password_hash()` function (see Book 7, Chapter 2).

Sending a verification email

If both the username and password check out, the next step is to send the user a verification email. The `createUser()` method continues:

```
if($server_results['status'] === 'success') {

    // Create a random, 32-character verification code
    $ver_code = bin2hex(openssl_random_pseudo_bytes(16));

    // Send the verification email
    $send_to = $username;
    $subject = 'Please verify your FootPower! account';
    $header = 'From: FootPower! <mail@mcfedries.com>' . "\r\n" .
              'Content-Type: text/plain';
    $body = <<<BODY
You have a new account at FootPower!

Your username is the email address you provided: $username

Please activate your account by clicking the link below.
```

```
https://footpower.mcfedries.com/verify_user.php?vercode=$ver_
    code&username=$username

If you did not create a FootPower! account, you can safely
    delete this message.

Thanks!

Paul
footpower.mcfedries.com
BODY;

    $mail_sent = mail($send_to, $subject, $body, $header);
```

This code uses our old friends `bin2hex()` and `openssl_random_pseudo_bytes()` to generate a random 32-character string that's used as a unique verification code for the user. The code sets up the email by specifying the recipient, subject, headers, and message body. Note, in particular, that the body includes a link that the user must click to verify her account. That link's URL includes both the verification code and the username:

```
https://footpower.mcfedries.com/verify_user.php?vercode=$ver_
    code&username=$username
```

Finally, the code runs PHP's `mail()` function to send the message.

WARNING

For the `mail()` function to work, you need a mail server installed and configured. If you're coding the app in your local development environment, you almost certainly won't have a mail server running, so the `mail()` function will fail. You can comment out the function for now, then try it after you have your code on the web.

Adding the user to the database

Now it's time to add the user to the users table. Here's the rest of the `createUser()` method:

```
if($mail_sent) {

    // Create and prepare the SQL template
    $sql = "INSERT INTO users
                (username, password, verification_code)
            VALUES (?, ?, ?)";
    $stmt = $this->_mysqli->prepare($sql);
```

```
    $stmt->bind_param("sss", $username, $password, $ver_code);
    $stmt->execute();
    $result = $stmt->get_result();

    if($this->_mysqli->errno === 0) {
        $server_results['control'] = 'form';
        $server_results['message'] = 'You\'re in! We\'ve sent
  you a verification email.<br>Be sure to click the link in that
  email to verify your account.';
    } else {
        $server_results['status'] = 'error';
        $server_results['control'] = 'form';
        $server_results['message'] = 'MySQLi error #: ' .
  $this->_mysqli->errno . ': ' . $this->_mysqli->error;
    }
} else {
    $server_results['status'] = 'error';
    $server_results['control'] = 'form';
    $server_results['message'] = 'Error! The verification email
  could not be sent, for some reason. Please try again.';
    }
}

// Create and then return the JSON data
$JSON_data = json_encode($server_results, JSON_HEX_APOS | JSON_
  HEX_QUOT);
return $JSON_data;
```

The code checks the return value of the `mail()` function: If it's `TRUE`, the code continues. (If you're coding in a local development environment that doesn't have a mail server, add `$mail_sent = TRUE` before running the `if()` statement to ensure your code adds the user successfully.) The code prepares an SQL `INSERT` statement that adds the user's username, password, and verification code. After checking for errors, the code returns the JSON data to the front end.

Verifying the user

With the verification email sent, it's now up to the user to click the link in the sent message. That links calls up the `verify_user.php` page, which includes the following code:

```
<?php

    // Initialize the results
    $server_results['status'] = 'success';
    $server_results['control'] = '';
    $server_results['message'] = '';

    // Make sure a verification code was passed
    if (!isset($_GET['vercode'])) {
        $server_results['status'] = 'error';
        $server_results['control'] = 'form';
        $server_results['message'] = 'Error: Invalid URL. Sorry
   it didn\'t work out.';
    }
    // Make sure the username was passed
    elseif (!isset($_GET['username'])) {
        $server_results['status'] = 'error';
        $server_results['control'] = 'form';
        $server_results['message'] = 'Error: Invalid user.';
    }
    // If we get this far, all is well, so go for it
    else {

        // Include the User class
        include_once '../private/classes/user_class.php';

        // Create a new User object
        $user = new User($mysqli);

        // Verify the new account
        $server_results = json_decode($user->verifyUser(),
   TRUE);
    }
    }
    include_once 'common/top.php';

    if(isset($_SESSION['username'])):
?>
```

The code initializes the usual `$server_results` array, then uses `$_GET` to check that both the verification code and the username were sent in the URL's query string. If all's well, a new `User` object is created and the `verifyUser()` method is called.

The verifyUser() method does a ton of important work in the app, so take a careful look at the code. Here's the first part:

```
public function verifyUser() {

    // Store the default status
    $server_results['status'] = 'success';

    // Get the query string parameters
    $ver_code = $_GET['vercode'];
    $username = $_GET['username'];

    // Sanitize them
    $ver_code = filter_var($ver_code, FILTER_SANITIZE_STRING);
    $username = filter_var($username, FILTER_SANITIZE_EMAIL);

    // Prepare the SQL SELECT statement
    $sql = "SELECT *
            FROM users
            WHERE verification_code=?
            AND username=?
            AND verified=0
            LIMIT 1";

    $stmt = $this->_mysqli->prepare($sql);
    $stmt->bind_param("ss", $ver_code, $username);
    $stmt->execute();
    $result = $stmt->get_result();

    // Was there an error?
    if ($this->_mysqli->errno !== 0) {
        $server_results['status'] = 'error';
        $server_results['control'] = 'form';
        $server_results['message'] = 'MySQLi error #: ' .
  $this->_mysqli->errno . ': ' . $this->_mysqli->error;
    }
```

The first part of the method sets up the standard $server_results array, then grabs and sanitizes the verification code and the username from the URL's query string using $_GET. Then the code prepares an SQL SELECT statement that queries the users table for a record that matches both the verification code and the username, and where the verified field equals 0. The code then checks for an error. If no error occurred, execution continues with the following code:

```
  // Otherwise, if a row is returned, it means the user can be
verified
  elseif ($result->num_rows === 1) {

      // Set the success message
      $server_results['message'] = 'Your account is now
verified.<p>You\'re signed in, so go ahead and <a
href="create_data.php">log a walk, run, or ride.</a>';

      // Sign in the user
      $_SESSION['username'] = $username;

      // Get the user's ID and distance unit
      $row = $result->fetch_all(MYSQLI_ASSOC);
      $user_id = $row[0]['user_id'];
      $distance_unit = $row[0]['distance_unit'];
      $_SESSION['distance_unit'] = $distance_unit;

      // Set the user's verified flag in the database
      $sql = "UPDATE users
              SET verified=1
              WHERE username=?";

      $stmt = $this->_mysqli->prepare($sql);
      $stmt->bind_param("s", $username);
      $stmt->execute();
      $result = $stmt->get_result();

      // Create a master data record (in this case, an
activity log) for the user
      $sql = "INSERT INTO logs
                     (user_id)
              VALUES (?)";
      $stmt = $this->_mysqli->prepare($sql);
      $stmt->bind_param("i", $user_id);
      $stmt->execute();
      $result = $stmt->get_result();

      // Get the user's log ID
      $sql = "SELECT *
              FROM logs
              WHERE user_id=?
              LIMIT 1";
      $stmt = $this->_mysqli->prepare($sql);
```

```
        $stmt->bind_param("i", $user_id);
        $stmt->execute();
        $result = $stmt->get_result();
        $row = $result->fetch_all(MYSQLI_ASSOC);
        $log_id = $row[0]['log_id'];
        $_SESSION['log_id'] = $log_id;
```

REMEMBER

There is a ton of important app stuff going on here, so here's a summary of what's happening:

- The `elseif` statement checks to see if a row was returned — in which case, `$result->num_rows` would be equal to `1`. If that's true, then the rest of the code executes.
- The success message is set.
- The `$_SESSION['username']` variable is set to `$username`, meaning the user is signed in to her account.
- The user's record is fetched and stored in the `$row` variable, which enables the code to then determine the user's ID and preferred unit of distance (miles or kilometers). The latter is used in other parts of the app, so it's stored in the `$_SESSION['distance_unit']` variable.
- A prepared SQL `UPDATE` statement changes the user's `verified` field value to `1`.
- A prepared SQL `INSERT` statement creates a new master data record for the user. Note that this data record is tied to the user by the common `user_id` field value.
- A prepared SQL `SELECT` statement returns the user's master data record, which enables the code to determine the ID of that record. The master data ID is used throughout the app, so it gets stored in the `$_SESSION['log_id']` variable.

Here's the rest of the `verifyUser()` method:

```
    } else {
        // Handle the case where the user is already verified
        // Prepare the SQL SELECT statement
        $sql = "SELECT username
                FROM users
                WHERE verification_code=?
                AND username=?
                AND verified=1";
```

```
        $stmt = $this->_mysqli->prepare($sql);
        $stmt->bind_param("ss", $ver_code, $username);
        $stmt->execute();
        $result = $stmt->get_result();

        // Was there an error?
        if($this->_mysqli->errno === 0) {
            $server_results['status'] = 'error';
            $server_results['control'] = 'form';
            $server_results['message'] = 'MySQLi error #: ' .
  $this->_mysqli->errno . ': ' . $this->_mysqli->error;
        }
        // Otherwise, if a row is returned, it means the user is
  already verified
        elseif ($result->num_rows > 0) {
            $server_results['status'] = 'error';
            $server_results['control'] = 'form';
            $server_results['message'] = 'Yo, you\'re already
  verified.<p>Perhaps you\'d like to <a href="create_data.
  php">log a walk, run, or ride</a>?';
        } else {
            $server_results['status'] = 'error';
            $server_results['control'] = 'form';
            $server_results['message'] = 'Yikes. A database
  error occurred. These things happen.';
        }
    }

    // Create and then return the JSON data
    $JSON_data = json_encode($server_results, JSON_HEX_APOS |
  JSON_HEX_QUOT);
    return $JSON_data;
}
```

This portion of the code handles the case where the user is already verified. For example, the user might click the verification link a second time, or reload the `verify_user.php` page.

TIP

The `users` table has a `creation_date` field that defaults to the date and time each user is added. This enables you to purge users who never verify their accounts. For example, you could run an SQL `DELETE` command that purges any records where the `creation _date` value is more than a month old.

Signing a User In and Out

The user gets signed in automatically during the verification procedure, but the user will also need to sign in manually if, say, the session token expires or the user signs out manually (discussed later in the "Signing out a user" section). To handle sign-ins, I created the `sign_in.php` page.

Checking for a signed-in user

REMEMBER

All pages that deal with user interactions need a defensive strategy:

- For a page that requires the user to be signed in, handle the case where the user accesses the page while signed out.
- For a page that requires the user to be signed out, handle the case where the user accesses the page while signed in.

For your sign-in page, the assumption is that the user is signed out, but he just might end up on the page while signed in. This means your code needs to check whether the `$_SESSION['username']` variable is set. Here's how I do this in `sign_in.php`:

```
<?php
    include_once '../private/common/initialization.php';

    // Set the page title depending on whether the user is
  signed in
    if(isset($_SESSION['username'])) {
        $page_title = 'You're Signed In to Your Account';
    } else {
        $page_title = 'Sign In to Your Account';
    }
    include_once 'common/top.php';

    // Is the user already signed in?
    if(isset($_SESSION['username'])):
?>
            <section>
                <p>
                    You're already signed in, so nothing to see
  here.
                </p>
```

```
                <p>
                    Did you want to <a href="create_data.
  php">log an activity</a>, instead?
                </p>
                <p>
                    Or perhaps you want to <a href="sign_out.
  php">sign out</a>?
                </p>
            </section>
<?php
    else:
?>
    The sign-in form code will go here
<?php
    endif;
    include_once 'common/sidebar.php';
    include_once 'common/bottom.php';
?>
```

This code actually checks the `$_SESSION['username']` variable twice:

- At the top of the script, I use the result of `isset($_SESSION['username'])` to set the `$page_title` variable accordingly.
- The second time, if `isset($_SESSION['username'])` returns `TRUE`, then I display a message to the user telling him he's already signed in and offering a couple of links to move on.

Adding the form

If the user isn't signed in, then the code from the previous section displays the sign-in form:

```
<form id="user-sign-in-form">
    <div class="form-wrapper">
        <div class="control-wrapper">
            <label for="username">Email</label>
            <input id="username" class="form-control"
  name="username" type="email" aria-label="Type your email
  address." required/>
            <span id="username-error" class="error error-
  message"></span>
        </div>
```

```
        <div class="control-wrapper">
            <label for="password">Password</label>
            <div>
                <input id="password" class="form-control"
name="password" type="password" minlength="8" aria-label="Type
your password." required>
                <br>
                <input id="password-toggle"
type="checkbox"><label for="password-toggle" class="label-
horizontal">Show password</label>
            </div>
            <span id="password-error" class="error error-
message"></span>
        </div>
        <button id="sign-me-in-button" class="btn btn-form"
type="submit">Sign Me In</button>
        <span id="form-error" class="error error-message form-
error-message"></span>
        <span id="form-message" class="form-message"></span>
        <input type="hidden" id="user-verb" name="user-verb"
value="sign-in-user">
        <input type="hidden" id="token" name="token"
value="<?php echo $_SESSION['token']; ?>">
    </div>
</form>
<div>
    <a href="request_new_password.php">Forgot your password?</a>
</div>
```

Figure 4-3 shows the form.

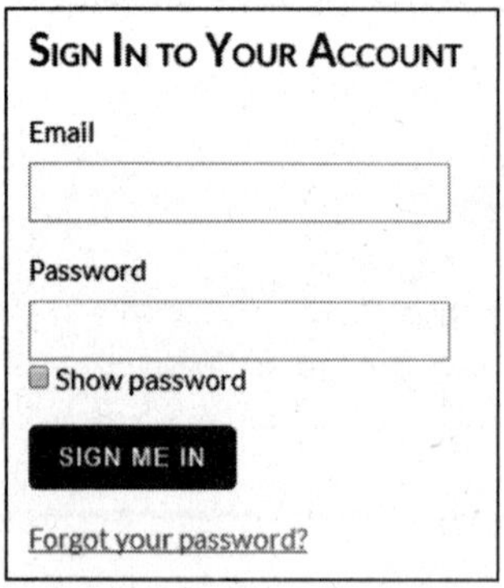

FIGURE 4-3: The FootPower! sign-in form.

The form looks quite simple, but it has a few interesting features:

- Both <input> tags are followed by <span> tags that are used to display field-specific error messages.

TIP

- The Password field is accompanied by a Show Password checkbox that, when checked, shows the password in plain text instead of dots. Enabling the user to see the password means you don't have to burden the user with having to enter the password twice as a verification. To show the password, the code changes the <input> tag's type value to text. Here's the click event handler that controls this (this code is in public/js/user.js):

```
$('#password-toggle').click(function() {

    // Is the checkbox checked?
    if($(this).prop('checked') === true) {

        // If so, change the <input> type to 'text'
        $('#password').attr('type', 'text');
        $('label[for=password-toggle').text('Hide
password');
    } else {

        // If not, change the <input> type to 'password'
        $('#password').attr('type', 'password');
        $('label[for=password-toggle').text('Show
password');
    }
});
```

- Below the <button> tag are two <span> tags used to display the form-level error and success messages.
- A hidden field sets the user-verb value to sign-in-user.
- Below the form is a Forgot your password? link, which I discuss later in this chapter.

When the user fills in the form and then clicks Sign Me In, the form's submit event fires, and that event is handled by the following code in public/js/user.js:

```
$('#user-sign-in-form').submit(function(e) {

    // Prevent the default submit
    e.preventDefault();
```

```
  // Disable the Sign Me In button to prevent double
submissions
  $('#sign-me-in-button').prop('disabled', true);

  // Clear and hide all the message spans ($ = "ends with")
  $('span[id$="error"').html('').css('display', 'none');
  $('#form-message').html('').css('display', 'none');

  // Get the form data and convert it to a POST-able format
  formData = $(this).serializeArray();

  // Submit the data to the handler
  $.post('/handlers/user_handler.php', formData,
function(data) {

      // Convert the JSON string to a JavaScript object
      var result = JSON.parse(data);

      if(result.status === 'error') {

          // Display the error
          $('#' + result.control + '-error').html(result.
message).css('display', 'inline-block');

          // Enable the Sign Me In button
          $('#sign-me-in-button').prop('disabled', false);

      } else {

          // The user is now signed in, so display the
home page
          window.location = 'index.php';
      }
  });
});
```

This code is nearly identical to the sign-up code I talk about earlier.

Checking the user's credentials

When the `user_handler.php` script gets the sign-in form data, it detects that the `user-verb` value is `sign-in-user` and routes the Ajax request to the `User` object's `signInUser()` method:

```
public function signInUser() {

    // Store the default status
    $server_results['status'] = 'success';

    // Was the username sent?
    if(empty($_POST['username'])) {
        $server_results['status'] = 'error';
        $server_results['control'] = 'username';
        $server_results['message'] = 'Doh! You need to enter
  your email address.';
    } else {

        // Sanitize it
        $username = $_POST['username'];
        $username = filter_var($username, FILTER_SANITIZE_
  EMAIL);
        if (!$username) {
            $server_results['status'] = 'error';
            $server_results['control'] = 'username';
            $server_results['message'] = 'Well, it appears that
  email address isn\'t valid. Please try again.';
        } else {

            // Make sure the username exists in the database
            $sql = "SELECT *
                    FROM users
                    WHERE username=?
                    LIMIT 1";
            $stmt = $this->_mysqli->prepare($sql);
            $stmt->bind_param("s", $username);
            $stmt->execute();
            $result = $stmt->get_result();

            // If the username doesn't exist, num_rows will be 0
            if ($result->num_rows === 0) {
                $server_results['status'] = 'error';
                $server_results['control'] = 'username';
                $server_results['message'] = 'Sorry, but that
  email address isn't associated with an account. Please try
  again.';
            } else {
```

```
            // If all is still well, check the password
            // Was the password sent?
            if(empty($_POST['password'])) {
                $server_results['status'] = 'error';
                $server_results['control'] = 'password';
                $server_results['message'] = 'That\'s weird:
the password is missing. Please try again.';
            } else {

                // Sanitize it
                $password = $_POST['password'];
                $password = filter_var($password, FILTER_
SANITIZE_STRING);

                // Is the password still valid?
                if (!$password) {
                    $server_results['status'] = 'error';
                    $server_results['control'] = 'password';
                    $server_results['message'] = 'Sorry, but
the password you used was invalid. Please try again.';
                } else {

                    // Get the user data
                    $row = $result->fetch_all(MYSQLI_ASSOC);

                    // Confirm the password
                    if(!password_verify($password, $row[0]
['password'])) {
                        $server_results['status'] = 'error';
                        $server_results['control'] =
'password';
                        $server_results['message'] = 'Sorry,
but the password you used was incorrect. Please try again.';
                    } else {

                        // Sign in the user
                        $_SESSION['username'] = $username;
                        $user_id = $row[0]['user_id'];
                        $distance_unit = $row[0]['distance_
unit'];
                        $_SESSION['distance_unit'] =
$distance_unit;

                        // Get the user's log ID
                        $sql = "SELECT *
```

```
                                FROM logs
                                WHERE user_id=?";
                        $stmt = $this->_mysqli-
>prepare($sql);
                        $stmt->bind_param("i", $user_id);
                        $stmt->execute();
                        $result = $stmt->get_result();
                        $row = $result->fetch_all(MYSQLI_
ASSOC);
                        $log_id = $row[0]['log_id'];
                        $_SESSION['log_id'] = $log_id;
                    }
                }
            }
        }
    }
}

    // Create and then return the JSON data
    $JSON_data = json_encode($server_results, JSON_HEX_APOS |
JSON_HEX_QUOT);
    return $JSON_data;
}
```

This code is a long series of validity checks and sanitization:

- For the username, the code checks that it was sent, sanitizes it as an email address, then uses a prepared SQL `SELECT` statement to check that the username exists in the `users` table. If all that checks out, the code moves on to the password.
- For the password, the code checks that it was sent, sanitizes it as a string, then fetches the user data from the `SELECT` result. The user's password is stored in the table as a hashed value, so to check the correctness of the received password you must use PHP's `password_verify()` function:

REMEMBER

```
password_verify(password, hashed_password)
```

  - *password:* The password entered by the user in the sign-in form
  - *hashed_password:* The hashed password value from the database

If both the username and password check out, then the code signs in the user by setting the `$_SESSION['username']` variable, and then sets the other session variables: `$_SESSION['distance_unit']` and `$_SESSION['log_id']`.

Signing out a user

Signing out a user means ending the user's session, so here's the full code of the sign_out.php page:

```
<?php
    session_start();

    // Free up all the session variables
    session_unset();
?>
<!-- Display the sign-in page -->
<meta http-equiv="refresh" content="0;sign_in.php">
```

PHP's session_unset() function frees up all the session variables, then the user is redirected to the sign-in page.

Resetting a Forgotten Password

The user can change her password in one of two ways:

- If the user has forgotten her password, she can click the Forgot your password? link in the sign-in form.
- If the user wants to change her password, she can click the Change Your Password link in the Your Account page (your_account.php).

Either way, the user winds up at the Request a New Password page (request_new_password.php), shown in Figure 4-4.

REQUEST A NEW PASSWORD

Enter your account email address below, and we'll send you a link with instructions for resetting your password.

Email

SEND IT

FIGURE 4-4: The FootPower! Request a New Password form.

Here's the page code:

```
<?php
    include_once '../private/common/initialization.php';
    $page_title = 'Request a New Password';
    include_once 'common/top.php';
?>
            <p>
                Enter your account email address below, and
  we'll send you a link with instructions for resetting your
  password.
            </p>
            <form id="user-send-password-reset-form">
                <div class="form-wrapper">
                    <div class="control-wrapper">
                        <label for="email">Email</label>
                        <input id="username" class="form-
  control" name="username" type="email" aria-label="Type your
  email address." required/>
                        <span id="username-error" class="error
  error-message"></span>
                    </div>
                    <button id="send-reset-password-button"
  class="btn btn-form" type="submit">Send It</button>
                    <span id="form-error" class="error error-
  message form-error-message"></span>
                    <span id="form-message" class="form-
  message"></span>
                    <input type="hidden" id="user-verb"
  name="user-verb" value="send-password-reset">
                    <input type="hidden" id="token" name="token"
  value="<?php echo $_SESSION['token']; ?>">
                </div>
            </form>
<?php
    include_once 'common/sidebar.php';
    include_once 'common/bottom.php';
?>
```

Note that the hidden `user-verb` value is `send-password-request`. The `user_handler.php` script routes this verb to the `User` object's `sendPasswordReset()` method:

```
public function sendPasswordReset() {

    // Store the default status
    $server_results['status'] = 'success';

    // Was the email address entered?
    if(empty($_POST['username'])) {
        $server_results['status'] = 'error';
        $server_results['control'] = 'username';
        $server_results['message'] = 'Um, you really do need to
  enter your email address.';
    } else {

        // Sanitize it
        $username = $_POST['username'];
        $username = filter_var($username, FILTER_SANITIZE_
  EMAIL);
        if (!$username) {
            $server_results['status'] = 'error';
            $server_results['control'] = 'username';
            $server_results['message'] = 'Hmmm. It looks like
  that email address isn\'t valid. Please try again.';
        } else {

            // Make sure the email address exists in the
  database
            $sql = "SELECT *
                    FROM users
                    WHERE username=?
                    LIMIT 1";
            $stmt = $this->_mysqli->prepare($sql);
            $stmt->bind_param("s", $username);
            $stmt->execute();
            $result = $stmt->get_result();

            // If the email doesn't exist, num_rows will be 0
            if ($result->num_rows === 0) {
                $server_results['status'] = 'error';
                $server_results['control'] = 'username';
```

```
            $server_results['message'] = 'Sorry, but that
  email address isn't associated with an account. Please try
  again.';
        } else {

            // Get the user's verification code
            $row = $result->fetch_all(MYSQLI_ASSOC);
            $ver_code = $row[0]['verification_code'];
        }
    }
}

// If we're still good, it's time to get the reset started
if($server_results['status'] === 'success') {

    // Send the password reset email
    $send_to = $username;
    $subject = 'Reset your FootPower! password';
    $header = 'From: FootPower! <mail@mcfedries.com>' .
  "\r\n" .
              'Content-Type: text/plain';
    $body = <<<BODY
You're receiving this message because you requested a password
  reset for your FootPower! account.

Please click the link below to reset your password.

https://footpower.mcfedries.com/reset_password.php?vercode=$ver_
  code&username=$username

If you do not have a FootPower! account, you can safely delete
  this message.

Thanks!

Paul
footpower.mcfedries.com
BODY;
    if(mail($send_to, $subject, $body, $header)) {

        // Unset the user's verified flag in the database
        $sql = "UPDATE users
                SET verified=0
                WHERE username=?";
```

```
            $stmt = $this->_mysqli->prepare($sql);
            $stmt->bind_param("s", $username);
            $stmt->execute();
            $result = $stmt->get_result();


            if($this->_mysqli->errno === 0) {
                $server_results['control'] = 'form';
                $server_results['message'] = 'Okay, we\'ve sent
  you the reset email.<br>Be sure to click the link in that
  email to reset your password.';
            } else {
                $server_results['status'] = 'error';
                $server_results['control'] = 'form';
                $server_results['message'] = 'MySQLi error
  #: ' . $this->_mysqli->errno . ': ' . $this->_mysqli->error;
            }
        } else {
            $server_results['status'] = 'error';
            $server_results['control'] = 'form';
            $server_results['message'] = 'Error! The reset email
  could not be sent, for some reason. Please try again.';
        }
    }
    // Create and then return the JSON data
    $JSON_data = json_encode($server_results, JSON_HEX_APOS |
  JSON_HEX_QUOT);
    return $JSON_data;
}
```

This method is very similar to the `verifyUser()` method I discuss earlier, but there are two main differences to note:

- `sendPasswordReset()` uses a prepared SQL `UPDATE` statement to set the user's `verified` field in the database to `0`.
- `sendPasswordReset()` sends an email message to the user with a link to the `reset_password.php` page, with the user's verification code and username in the query string. When the user clicks that link, she's sent to the page shown in Figure 4-5.

FIGURE 4-5: The FootPower! Reset Your Password form.

Here's the code for the `reset_password.php` page:

```
<?php
    include_once '../private/common/initialization.php';

    // Initialize the results
    $server_results['status'] = 'success';
    $server_results['control'] = '';
    $server_results['message'] = '';

    // Make sure a verification code was passed
    if (!isset($_GET['vercode'])) {
        $server_results['status'] = 'error';
        $server_results['control'] = 'form';
        $server_results['message'] = 'Error: Invalid URL. Sorry
  it didn\'t work out.';
    }
    // Make sure the email address was passed
    elseif (!isset($_GET['username'])) {
        $server_results['status'] = 'error';
        $server_results['control'] = 'form';
        $server_results['message'] = 'Error: Invalid email
  address.';
    }
    // If we get this far, all is well, so go for it
    else {

        // Get the query string parameters
        $ver_code = $_GET['vercode'];
        $username = $_GET['username'];

        // Sanitize them
        $ver_code = filter_var($ver_code, FILTER_SANITIZE_
  STRING);
```

```
        $username = filter_var($username, FILTER_SANITIZE_
    EMAIL);

    }
    $page_title = 'Reset Your Password';
    include_once 'common/top.php';

    if($server_results['status'] === 'error'):
?>
            <div class="result-message"><?php echo $server_
    results['message'] ?></div>

<?php
    else:
?>
                <p>
                    You're resetting the password for <?php echo
    $username ?>.
                </p>
                <p>
                    If this is not your FootPower! email
    address, please <a href="request_new_password.php">send a new
    password reset request</a>.
                </p>
                <form id="user-reset-password-form">
                <div class="form-wrapper">
                    <div class="control-wrapper">
                        <label for="password">Password</label>
                        <div>
                            <input id="password" class="form-
    control" name="password" type="password" minlength="8"
    aria-label="Type your password." required>
                            <br>
                            <input id="password-toggle"
    type="checkbox"><label for="password-toggle" class="label-
    horizontal">Show password</label>
                        </div>
                        <span id="password-error" class="error
    error-message"></span>
                    </div>
                    <button id="reset-password-button"
    class="btn btn-form" type="submit">Reset Password</button>
                    <span id="form-error" class="error error-
    message form-error-message"></span>
```

```
                    <span id="form-message" class="form-
    message"></span>
                    <input type="hidden" id="username"
    name="username" value="<?php echo $username ?>">
                    <input type="hidden" id="vercode"
    name="vercode" value="<?php echo $ver_code ?>">
                    <input type="hidden" id="user-verb"
    name="user-verb" value="reset-password">
                    <input type="hidden" id="token" name="token"
    value="<?php echo $_SESSION['token']; ?>">
                </div>
            </form>
<?php
    endif;
        include_once 'common/sidebar.php';
        include_once 'common/bottom.php';
?>
```

The `submit` event handler sends the form data to `user_handler.php`, which uses the hidden `user-verb` value of `reset-password` to route the Ajax request to the `User` object's `resetPassword()` method:

```
public function resetPassword() {

    // Store the default status
    $server_results['status'] = 'success';

    // Get the form data
    $username = $_POST['username'];
    $ver_code = $_POST['vercode'];
    $password = $_POST['password'];

    // Sanitize the username and verification code, just to
  be safe
    $username = filter_var($username, FILTER_SANITIZE_EMAIL);
    $ver_code = filter_var($ver_code, FILTER_SANITIZE_STRING);

    // Verify the user:
    // First, prepare the SQL SELECT statement
    $sql = "SELECT *
            FROM users
            WHERE username=?
            AND verification_code=?
            AND verified=0";
```

```
  $stmt = $this->_mysqli->prepare($sql);
  $stmt->bind_param("ss", $username, $ver_code);
  $stmt->execute();
  $result = $stmt->get_result();
  $row = $result->fetch_all(MYSQLI_ASSOC);

  // If a row is returned, it means the user is verified so
the password can be reset
  if ($result->num_rows > 0 AND $this->_mysqli->errno === 0) {

      // Was the password sent?
      if(empty($password)) {
          $server_results['status'] = 'error';
          $server_results['control'] = 'password';
          $server_results['message'] = 'That\'s weird: the
password is missing. Please try again.';
      } else {

          // Sanitize it
          $password = filter_var($password, FILTER_SANITIZE_
STRING);

          // Is the password still valid?
          if (!$password) {
              $server_results['status'] = 'error';
              $server_results['control'] = 'password';
              $server_results['message'] = 'Sorry, but the
password you used was invalid. Please try again.';
          }
          // Is the password long enough?
          elseif (strlen($password) < 8 ) {
              $server_results['status'] = 'error';
              $server_results['control'] = 'password';
              $server_results['message'] = 'Sorry, but the
password must be at least 8 characters long. Please try
again.';
          } else {

              // If all's well, hash the password
              $password = password_hash($password, PASSWORD_
DEFAULT);

              // Set the distance unit session variable
              $distance_unit = $row[0]['distance_unit'];
```

```
                $_SESSION['distance_unit'] = $distance_unit;
            }
        }
    } else {
        $server_results['status'] = 'error';
        $server_results['control'] = 'form';
        $server_results['message'] = 'Oh, man, a database error
occurred! Please try again.';
    }

    // If we're still good, it's time to reset the password and
reverify the user
    if($server_results['status'] === 'success') {

        // Get the user's ID
        $row = $result->fetch_all(MYSQLI_ASSOC);
        $user_id = $row[0]['user_id'];

        // Set the user's password and verified flag in the
database
        $sql = "UPDATE users
                SET password=?, verified=1
                WHERE username=?";

        $stmt = $this->_mysqli->prepare($sql);
        $stmt->bind_param("ss", $password, $username);
        $stmt->execute();
        $result = $stmt->get_result();

        // Was there an error?
        if ($this->_mysqli->errno === 0) {

            // if not, sign in the user
            $_SESSION['username'] = $username;

            // Get the user's log ID
            $sql = "SELECT *
                    FROM logs
                    WHERE user_id=?";
            $stmt = $this->_mysqli->prepare($sql);
            $stmt->bind_param("i", $user_id);
            $stmt->execute();
            $result = $stmt->get_result();
```

```
            // Set the log_id session variable
            $row = $result->fetch_all(MYSQLI_ASSOC);
            $log_id = $row[0]['log_id'];
            $_SESSION['log_id'] = $log_id;

        } else {
            $server_results['status'] = 'error';
            $server_results['control'] = 'form';
            $server_results['message'] = 'Yikes. A database
    error occurred. Please try again.';
        }
    }
    // Create and then return the JSON data
    $JSON_data = json_encode($server_results, JSON_HEX_APOS |
    JSON_HEX_QUOT);
    return $JSON_data;
}
```

This code is very similar to `verifyUser()`, which I discuss earlier.

Deleting a User

The final user task the app needs to handle is deleting a user's account. This is accomplished by clicking the Delete Your Account link in the Your Account page (`your_account.php`). This displays the `delete_account.php` page, shown in Figure 4-6.

DELETE YOUR FOOTPOWER! ACCOUNT?

Whoa, are you sure you want to do this? You'll lose all your data!

Password

Show password

YEP, I'M SURE

FIGURE 4-6: The FootPower! Delete Your Account form.

Here's the `delete_account.php` page code:

```
<?php
    include_once '../private/common/initialization.php';
    $page_title = 'Delete Your FootPower! Account?';
    include_once 'common/top.php';

    // Is the user signed in?
    if(isset($_SESSION['username'])):
?>
            <p>
                Whoa, are you sure you want to do this? You'll
  lose all your data!
            </p>
            <form id="user-delete-form">
                <div class="form-wrapper">
                    <div class="control-wrapper">
                        <label for="password">Password</label>
                        <div>
                            <input id="password" class="form-
  control" name="password" type="password" minlength="8"
  aria-label="Type your password." required>
                            <br>
                            <input id="password-toggle"
  type="checkbox"><label for="password-toggle" class="label-
  horizontal">Show password</label>
                        </div>
                        <span id="password-error" class="error
  error-message"></span>
                    </div>
                    <button id="delete-user-button" class="btn
  btn-form" type="submit">Yep, I'm Sure</button>
                    <span id="form-error" class="error error-
  message form-error-message"></span>
                    <span id="form-message" class="form-
  message"></span>
                    <input type="hidden" id="username"
  name="username" value="<?php echo $_SESSION['username'] ?>">
                    <input type="hidden" id="user-verb"
  name="user-verb" value="delete-user">
                    <input type="hidden" id="token" name="token"
  value="<?php echo $_SESSION['token']; ?>">
                </div>
            </form>
```

```
<?php
    else:
?>
        <!-- Display the sign-in page -->
        <meta http-equiv="refresh" content="0;sign_in.php">
<?php
    endif;
    include_once 'common/sidebar.php';
    include_once 'common/bottom.php';
?>
```

When the user clicks the Yep, I'm Sure button, the form's `submit` event handler sends the form data to the `user_handler.php` script, which uses the hidden `user-verb` value of `delete-user` to route the Ajax request to the `User` object's `deleteUser()` method:

```
public function deleteUser() {

    // Store the default status
    $server_results['status'] = 'success';

    // Get the username and password
    $username = $_POST['username'];
    $password = $_POST['password'];

    // Sanitize the username, just to be safe
    $username = filter_var($username, FILTER_SANITIZE_EMAIL);

    // Make sure the username exists in the database
    $sql = "SELECT *
            FROM users
            WHERE username=?
            LIMIT 1";
    $stmt = $this->_mysqli->prepare($sql);
    $stmt->bind_param("s", $username);
    $stmt->execute();
    $result = $stmt->get_result();
    // Get the user's ID
    $row = $result->fetch_all(MYSQLI_ASSOC);
    $user_id = $row[0]['user_id'];

    // If the username doesn't exist, num_rows will be 0
    if ($result->num_rows === 0) {
```

```
      $server_results['status'] = 'error';
      $server_results['control'] = 'form';
      $server_results['message'] = 'Sorry, but we can\'t find
your account. Please try again.';
  } else {

      // Now check the password
      // Was the password sent?
      if(empty($_POST['password'])) {
          $server_results['status'] = 'error';
          $server_results['control'] = 'password';
          $server_results['message'] = 'That\'s weird: the
password is missing. Please try again.';
      } else {

          // Sanitize it
          $password = filter_var($password, FILTER_SANITIZE_
STRING);

          // Is the password still valid?
          if (!$password) {
              $server_results['status'] = 'error';
              $server_results['control'] = 'password';
              $server_results['message'] = 'Sorry, but the
password you used was invalid. Please try again.';
          } else {

              // Confirm the password
              if(!password_verify($password, $row[0]
['password'])) {
                  $server_results['status'] = 'error';
                  $server_results['control'] = 'password';
                  $server_results['message'] = 'Sorry, but the
password you used was incorrect. Please try again.';
              } else {

                  // Delete the user
                  $sql = "DELETE
                          FROM users
                          WHERE username=?
                          LIMIT 1";
                  $stmt = $this->_mysqli->prepare($sql);
                  $stmt->bind_param("s", $username);
```

```
            $stmt->execute();
            $result = $stmt->get_result();

            // Was there an error?
            if ($this->_mysqli->errno !== 0) {
                $server_results['status'] = 'error';
                $server_results['control'] = 'form';
                $server_results['message'] = 'MySQLi
error #: ' . $this->_mysqli->errno . ': ' . $this->_mysqli-
>error;
            } else {

                 // Get the user's log ID
                $sql = "SELECT *
                        FROM logs
                        WHERE user_id=?
                        LIMIT 1";
                $stmt = $this->_mysqli->prepare($sql);
                $stmt->bind_param("i", $user_id);
                $stmt->execute();
                $result = $stmt->get_result();
                $row = $result->fetch_all(MYSQLI_ASSOC);
                $log_id = $row[0]['log_id'];

                // Delete the user's activities
                $sql = "DELETE
                        FROM activities
                        WHERE log_id=?";
                $stmt = $this->_mysqli->prepare($sql);
                $stmt->bind_param("i", $log_id);
                $stmt->execute();
                $result = $stmt->get_result();

                // Was there an error?
                if ($this->_mysqli->errno !== 0) {
                    $server_results['status'] = 'error';
                    $server_results['control'] = 'form';
                    $server_results['message'] = 'MySQLi
error #: ' . $this->_mysqli->errno . ': ' . $this->_mysqli-
>error;
                } else {
                    // Delete the user's master data
record (log)
```

```
                                $sql = "DELETE
                                        FROM logs
                                        WHERE log_id=?
                                        LIMIT 1";
                                $stmt = $this->_mysqli-
    >prepare($sql);
                                $stmt->bind_param("i", $log_id);
                                $stmt->execute();
                                $result = $stmt->get_result();

                                // Was there an error?
                                if ($this->_mysqli->errno !== 0) {
                                    $server_results['status'] =
    'error';
                                    $server_results['control'] =
    'form';
                                    $server_results['message'] =
    'MySQLi error #: ' . $this->_mysqli->errno . ': ' . $this->_
    mysqli->error;

                                } else {
                                    // Free up all the session
    variables
                                    session_unset();
                                }
                            }
                        }
                    }
                }
            }
        }
        // Create and then return the JSON data
        $JSON_data = json_encode($server_results, JSON_HEX_APOS |
    JSON_HEX_QUOT);
        return $JSON_data;
    }
```

After performing the usual data validation and sanitization, the code runs three prepared SQL `DELETE` statements to delete the user from the `users` table, delete the user's data from the `activities` table, and delete the user's log from the `logs` table.

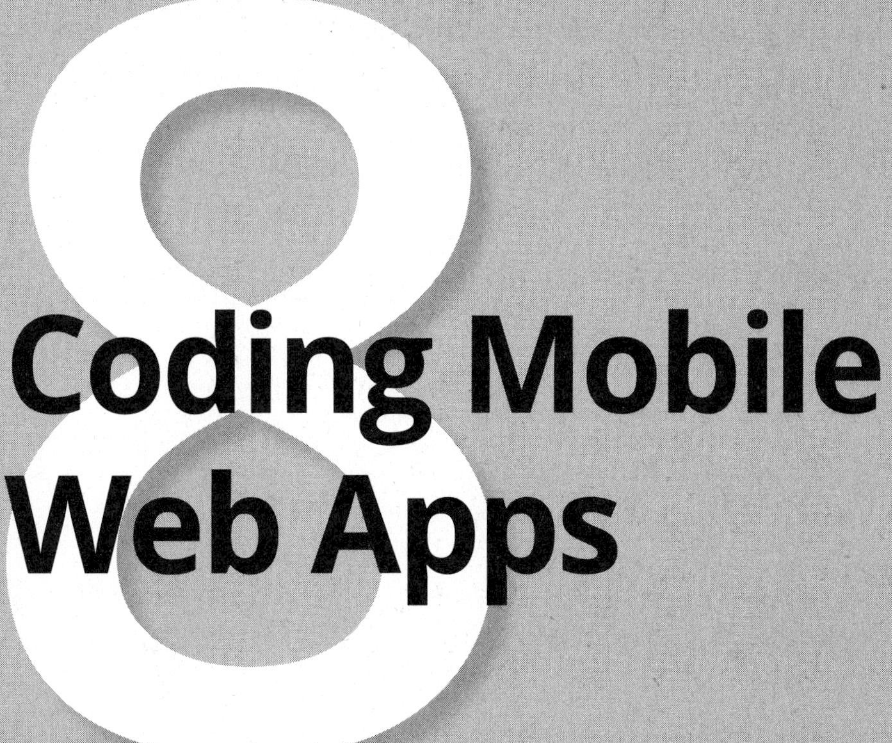

8 Coding Mobile Web Apps

Contents at a Glance

IN THIS CHAPTER

» Learning about mobile-first web development

» Understanding the main principles of coding a mobile-first site

» Getting started with jQuery Mobile

» Delivering images responsively to mobile users

» Storing user data in the web browser instead of on the server

Chapter 1

Exploring Mobile-First Web Development

Don't be afraid to start small. Some of the biggest successes in mobile today came from small experiments and teams of passionate web designers and developers. You don't need to know everything about mobile — just take what you do know and go.

— LUKE WROBLEWSKI

If you've been hanging around the web for a while, you probably remember the days when you'd surf to a site using a small screen such as a smartphone or similar portable device, and instead of seeing the regular version of the site, you'd see the "mobile" version. In rare cases, this alternate version would be optimized for mobile viewing and navigation, but more likely it was just a poor facsimile of the regular site with a few font changes and all the interesting and useful features removed.

Seen from the web developer's viewpoint, the poor quality of those mobile sites isn't all that surprising. After all, who wants to build and maintain two versions of the same site? Fortunately, the days of requiring an entirely different site to support mobile users are long gone. Yes, using responsive web design enables you to create a single site that looks and works great on everything from a wall-mounted display to a handheld device. But in modern web development, there's a strong case to be made that all web pages should be built from the ground up as though they were going to be displayed only on mobile devices. In this chapter, you explore the principles and techniques behind this mobile-first approach to web development.

What Is Mobile-First Web Development?

As I discuss in Book 7, Chapter 1, when you develop a web page to look good and work well on a desktop-sized screen, there are a number of responsive tricks you can employ to make that same code look good and work well on a mobile device screen:

- » You can use percentages for horizontal measurements.
- » You can use relative units such as `em` and `rem` for vertical measurement and font sizes.
- » You can use media queries to remove elements when the screen width falls below a specified threshold.

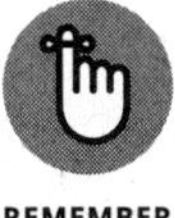

That third technique — the one where you remove stuff that doesn't fit on a smaller screen — is known in the web coding trade as *regressive enhancement (RE)*. RE has ruled the web development world for many years, but lately there's been a backlash against it. Here's why:

- » RE relegates mobile screens to second-class web citizens.
- » RE leads to undisciplined development because coders and designers inevitably stuff a desktop-sized screen with content, widgets, and all the web bells and whistles.

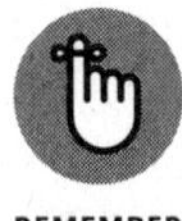

What's the solution? You've probably guessed it by now: *progressive enhancement*, which means starting with content that fits on a base screen width and then adding components as the screen gets bigger. When that original content represents what's essential about your page, and when that base screen width is optimized for mobile devices — especially today's most popular smartphones — then you've got yourself a *mobile-first* approach to web development.

Learning the Principles of Mobile-First Development

Let me be honest right off the top: Mobile-first web development is daunting because if you're used to having the giant canvas of a desktop screen to play with, starting instead with a screen that's a mere 320- or 400-pixels across can feel a tad claustrophobic. However, I can assure you that it only seems that way because of the natural tendency to wonder how you're possibly going to shoehorn your massive page into such a tiny space. Mobile-first thinking takes the opposite approach by ignoring (at least at the beginning) large screens and, instead, focusing on what works best for mobile screens which, after all, represent the majority of your page visitors. Thinking the mobile-first way isn't hard: It just means keeping a few key design principle in mind.

Mobile first means content first

One of the biggest advantages of taking a mobile-first approach to web development is that it forces you to prioritize. That is, a mobile-first design means that you include in the initial layout only those page elements that are essential to the user's experience of the page. This essential-stuff-only idea is partly a response to having a smaller screen size in which to display that stuff, but it's also a necessity for many mobile users who are surfing with sluggish Internet connections and limited data plans. It's your job — no, scratch that, it's your duty as a conscientious web developer — to make sure that those users aren't served anything superfluous, frivolous, or in any other way nonessential.

That's all well and good, I hear you thinking, but define "superfluous" and "frivolous." Good point. The problem, of course, is that one web developer's trivial appetizer is another's essential meat and potatoes. Only you can decide between what's inconsequential and what's vital, depending on your page goals and your potential audience.

So the first step towards a mobile-first design is to decide what's most important in the following content categories:

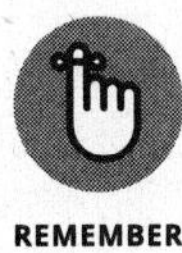

REMEMBER

» **Text:** Decide what words are essential to get your page's message across. Usability expert Steve Krug tells web designers to "Get rid of half the words on each page, then get rid of half of what's left." For a mobile-first page, you might need to halve the words once again. Be ruthless. Does the user really need to see that message from the CEO or your "About Us" text? Probably not.

- **Images:** Decide what images are essential for the user, or whether any images are needed at all. The problem with images is that, although everyone likes a bit of eye candy, that sweetness comes at the cost of screen real estate and bandwidth. If you really do need to include an image or two in your mobile-first page, then at least serve up smaller images to your mobile visitors. To learn how to do that, see "Delivering images responsively," later in this chapter.
- **Navigation:** All users need to be able to navigate your site, but the recent trend is to create gigantic menus that include links to every section and page on the site. Decide which of those links are truly important for navigation and just include those in your mobile-first layout.
- **Widgets:** Modern web pages are festooned with widgets for social media, content scrollers, photo lightboxes, automatic video playback, and, of course, advertising. Mobile users want to see content first, so consider ditching the widgets altogether. If there's a widget you really want to include, and you're sure it won't put an excessive burden on either the page's load time or the user's bandwidth, push the widget to the bottom of the page.

Pick a testing width that makes sense for your site

REMEMBER

For most websites, testing a mobile-first layout should begin with the smallest devices, which these days means smartphones with screens that are 320 pixels wide. However, you don't necessarily have to begin your testing with a width as small as 320px. If you have access to your site analytics, they should tell you what devices your visitors use. If you find that all or most of your mobile users are on devices that are at least 400 pixels wide, then that's the initial width you should test for your mobile-first layout.

Get your content to scale with the device

For your mobile-first approach to be successful, it's paramount that you configure each page on your site to scale horizontally with the width of the device screen. You do that by adding the following `<meta>` tag to the `head` section of each page:

```
<meta name="viewport" content="width=device-width, initial-
  scale=1.0">
```

This instructs the web browser to do two things:

- Set the initial width of the page content to the width of the device screen.
- Set the initial zoom level of the page to 1.0, which means the page is neither zoomed in nor zoomed out.

Build your CSS the mobile-first way

When you're ready to start coding the CSS for your page, understand that the style definitions and rules that you write will be your page defaults — that is, these are the styles the browser will display on all devices, unless you've defined one or more media queries to override these defaults. (I talk more about mobile-first media queries shortly.) You shouldn't have to write any special rules as long as you follow a few basic tenets of responsive web design:

REMEMBER

- Use the relative units `%` or `vw` for horizontal measures such as width and padding.
- Use the relative units `rem` or `em` for vertical measures and font sizes.
- Make all your images responsive.
- Use flexbox for the page layout, and be sure to apply `flex-wrap: wrap` to any flexbox container.

It's also important to make sure that your mobile-first layout renders the content just as you want it to appear on the mobile screen. This means avoiding any tricks such as using the flexbox `order` property to mess around with the order of the page elements.

Finally, and perhaps most importantly, be sure to hide any unnecessary content by styling that content with `display: none`.

In the end, your mobile-first CSS should be the very model of simplicity and economy.

Pick a "non-mobile" breakpoint that makes sense for your content

Your mobile-first CSS code probably includes several elements that you've hidden with `display: none`. I assume you want to show those elements eventually (otherwise, you'd have deleted them altogether), so you need to decide when you want them shown. Specifically, you need to decide what the minimum screen width is that will show your content successfully.

Notice I didn't say that you should decide when to show your hidden content based on the width of a target device. For example, many developers consider a screen to be "wide enough" when it's at least as wide as an iPad screen in portrait mode, which is 768 pixels. Fair enough, but will future iPads use this width? In fact, the current iPad Pro is 1,024 pixels wide in portrait mode.

TIP

Devices change constantly and it's a fool's game to try and keep up with them. Forget all of that. Instead, decide what minimum width is best for your page when the hidden content is made visible. How can you do that? Here's one easy way:

1. **Load your page into the Chrome web browser.**
2. **Display Chrome's developer tools.**

   Press either Ctrl+Shift+I (Windows) or ⌘+Shift+I (Mac).
3. **Use your mouse to adjust the size of the browser window:**
   - If the developer tools are below or undocked from the browser viewport, drag the right or left edge of the browser window.
   - If the developer tools are docked to the right or left of the browser viewport, drag the vertical bar that separates the developer tools from the viewport.
4. **Read the current viewport dimensions, which Chrome displays in the upper right corner of the viewport.**

   The dimensions appear as width x height, in pixels, as pointed out in Figure 1-1.
5. **Narrow the window to your mobile-first testing width (such as 320px).**
6. **Increase the width and, as you do, watch how your layout changes.**

   In particular, watch for the width where the content first looks the way you want it to appear in larger screens. Make a note of that width.

REMEMBER

The width where your full content looks good is the basis for a CSS media query breakpoint that you'll use to display the elements that were hidden in the mobile-first layout. For example, say that your mobile-first layout hides the `aside` element and that you found that your full content looks right at a width of 742px. You then can set up the following media query (using 750px for a round number):

```
@media (min-width: 750px) {
    aside {
        display: block;
    }
}
```

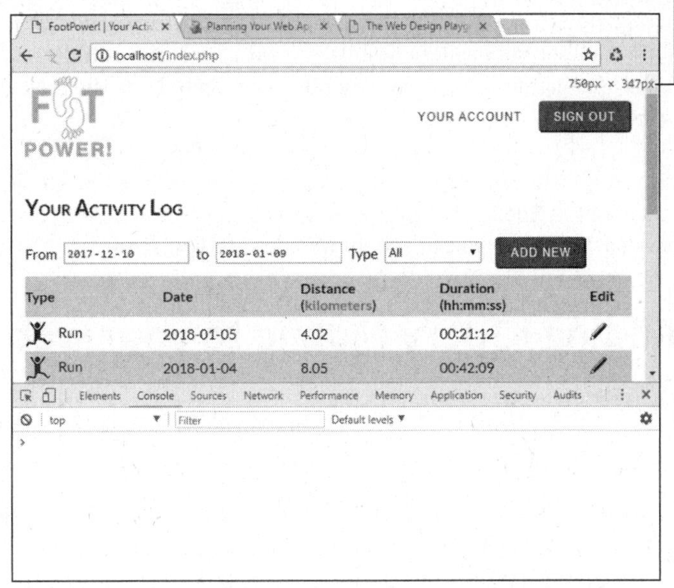

FIGURE 1-1: With Chrome's developer tools displayed, as you change the width of the browser window, Chrome displays the current viewport width and height.

This media query tells the browser that when the screen width is `750px` or more, display the `aside` element.

Going Mobile Faster with jQuery Mobile

I talk quite a bit about jQuery in Book 4, and it's safe to say that jQuery makes web development faster, easier, and even more pleasurable. I also introduce jQuery UI in Book 4, Chapter 3, and I show that it's an easy way to incorporate sophisticated components such as dialog boxes and tabs into your web projects. Now I'm going to talk briefly about yet another jQuery library: jQuery Mobile, which offers widgets optimized for mobile web apps.

What is jQuery Mobile?

Most folks nowadays have a mobile device of some description, which means that most of us are used to doing our digital duties using mobile interfaces. These interfaces include standard mobile elements such as fixed headers and footers, navigation bars, list views, tabs, switches that turn on and off, and hidden menus invoked by a "hamburger" icon.

Coding elements such as these is possible, but it would be a ton of work. Fortunately, you can skip all of that because the hardcore geeks at jQuery Mobile have done it all for you. jQuery Mobile is a set of mobile-optimized widgets that make it easy for you to design your mobile web app to have the look and feel of a native mobile app.

Best of all, the jQuery Mobile components work just like the jQuery UI widgets I talk about in Book 4, Chapter 3, so you already know how to use them. Now all you have to do is incorporate jQuery Mobile into your app.

Adding jQuery Mobile to your web app

jQuery Mobile consists of two files:

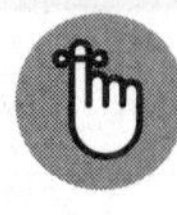

REMEMBER

- A JavaScript (`.js`) file that you add to your page by using a `<script>` tag with a reference to the external script file.
- A CSS (`.css`) file that you add to your page by using a `<link rel="stylesheet">` tag with a reference to the external CSS file.

How do you get these files? You have three ways to go about it:

REMEMBER

- **Download the files and use the default jQuery Mobile styles.** In this case, surf to `jquerymobile.com/download` and click the ZIP File link. The file you get will have a name like `jquery.mobile-1.`*`x`*`.`*`y`*`.zip`, where *x* and *y* denote the current version. Decompress the ZIP file and then copy the `jquery.mobile-1.`*`x`*`.`*`y`*`.min.js` and `jquery.mobile-1.`*`x`*`.`*`y`*`.min.css` files to your mobile web app's JavaScript and CSS folders. Then set up your `<link>` and `<script>` tags to reference the files:

  ```
  <link rel="stylesheet" href="/css/jquery.mobile-1.x.y.min.
    css">
  <script src="/js/jquery.mobile-1.x.y.min.js"></script>
  ```

  (Remember to replace *x* and *y* with the actual version numbers of your downloaded file.)
- **Use custom jQuery Mobile styles.** In this case, surf to `themeroller.jquerymobile.com` and use the ThemeRoller app to set your custom colors, fonts, and other styles. Click the Download Theme ZIP File button, type a theme name, and then click Download ZIP. Decompress the downloaded ZIP file, copy the CSS file from the Themes folder, and then add it to your mobile web app's CSS folder. Then set up your `<link>` tag to reference the file:

  ```
  <link rel="stylesheet" href="/css/custom.min.css">
  ```

Replace *custom* with the custom theme name you provided. Note that this only gives you the CSS for jQuery Mobile. You still need to download the jQuery Mobile JavaScript file, as I describe previously.

- **Link to a remote version of the file.** Several content delivery networks (CDNs) store the jQuery Mobile files and let you link to them. Here are the tags to use for Google's CDN:

```
<link rel="stylesheet" href="https://ajax.googleapis.com/
  ajax/libs/jquerymobile/1.x.y/jquery.mobile.css">
<script src="https://ajax.googleapis.com/ajax/libs/
  jquerymobile/1.x.y/jquery.mobile.min.js"></script>
```

Again, in both cases, be sure to replace *x* and *y* with the actual version numbers of the latest version of jQuery Mobile.

I hold off talking about specific jQuery Mobile widgets until Book 8, Chapter 2, where I build a mobile web app using a number of jQuery Mobile components.

WARNING

You also need to add jQuery to your page, as I describe in Book 4, Chapter 1. However, as I write this, jQuery Mobile is only compatible with version 2 of jQuery, so be sure to link to that version, not version 3.

Working with Images in a Mobile App

When planning a mobile web app, you always need to consider the impact of images, both on your design and on your users.

Making images responsive

On the design side, you need to ensure that your images scale responsively, depending on the screen width or height. For example, if the user's screen is 1,024 pixels wide, an image that's 800 pixels wide will fit no problem, but that same image will overflow a 400-pixel-wide screen. As I mention in Book 7, Chapter 1, you create responsive images with the following CSS rule:

```
image {
    max-width: 100%;
    height: auto;
}
```

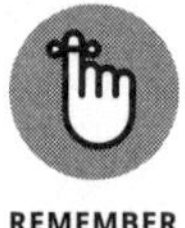

REMEMBER

Here, *image* is a selector that references the image or images you want to be responsive. Setting `max-width: 100%` enables the image width to scale smaller or larger as the screen (or the image's container) changes size, but also mandates that the image can't scale larger than its original width. Setting `height: auto` cajoles the browser into maintaining the image's original aspect ratio by calculating the height automatically based on the image's current width.

TIP

Occasionally, you'll want the image height to be responsive instead of its width. To do that, you use the following variation on the preceding rule:

```
image {
    max-height: 100%;
    width: auto;
}
```

Delivering images responsively

On the user side, delivering images that are far larger than the screen size can be a major problem. Sure, you can make the images responsive, but you're still sending a massive file down the tubes, which won't be appreciated by those mobile surfers using slow connections with limited data plans.

Instead, you need to deliver to the user a version of the image file that's appropriately sized for the device screen. For example, you might deliver the full-size image to desktop users, a medium-sized version to tablet folk, and a small-sized version to smartphone users. That sounds like a complex bit of business, but HTML5 lets you handle everything from the comfort of the `<img>` tag. The secret? The `sizes` and `srcset` attributes.

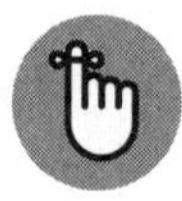

REMEMBER

The `sizes` attribute is a collection of *expression-width* pairs:

- » The *expression* part specifies a screen feature, such as a minimum or maximum width, surrounded by parentheses.
- » The *width* part specifies how wide you want the image displayed on screens that match the expression.

For example, to specify that on screens up to 600 pixels wide you want an image displayed with a width of `90vw`, you'd use the following expression-width pair:

```
(max-width: 600px) 90vw
```

A typical `sizes` attribute is a collection of expression-width pairs, separated by commas. Here's the general syntax to use:

```
sizes="(expression1) width1,
       (expression2) width2,
       etc.,
       widthN"
```

Notice that the last item doesn't specify an expression. This tells the web browser that the specified width applies to any screen that doesn't match any of the expressions.

Here's an example:

```
sizes="(max-width: 600px) 90vw,
       (max-width: 1000px) 60vw,
       30vw"
```

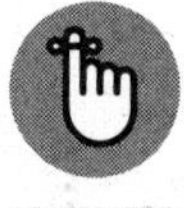

REMEMBER

The `srcset` attribute is a comma-separated list of image file locations, each followed by the image width and letter `w`. Here's the general syntax:

```
srcset="location1 width1w,
        location2 width2w,
        etc.">
```

This gives the browser a choice of image sizes, and it picks the best one based on the current device screen dimensions and the preferred widths you specify in the `sizes` attribute. Here's a full example, and Figure 1-2 shows how the browser serves up different images for different screen sizes:

```
<img src="/images/img-small.jpg"
     sizes="(max-width: 600px) 90vw,
            (max-width: 1000px) 60vw,
            30vw"
     srcset="/images/img-small.png 450w,
             /images/img-medium.png 900w,
             /images/img-large.png 1350w">
```

WARNING

The `sizes` and `srcset` attributes don't always work the way you might expect. For example, if the browser finds that, say, the large version of the image is already stored in its cache, then it will usually decide that it's faster and easier on the bandwidth to just grab the image from the cache and scale it, instead of going back to the server to download a more appropriately sized file for the current screen.

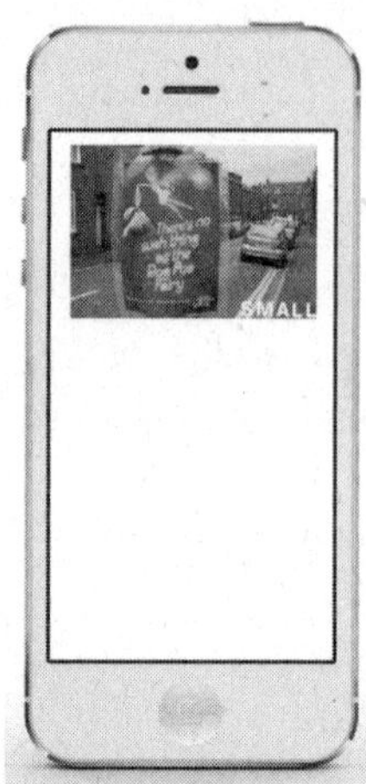

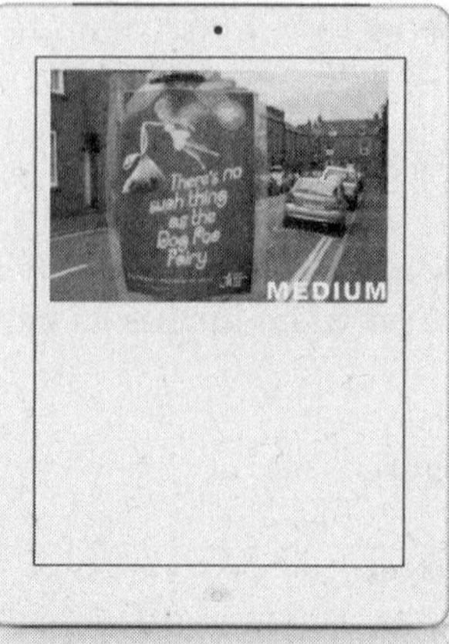

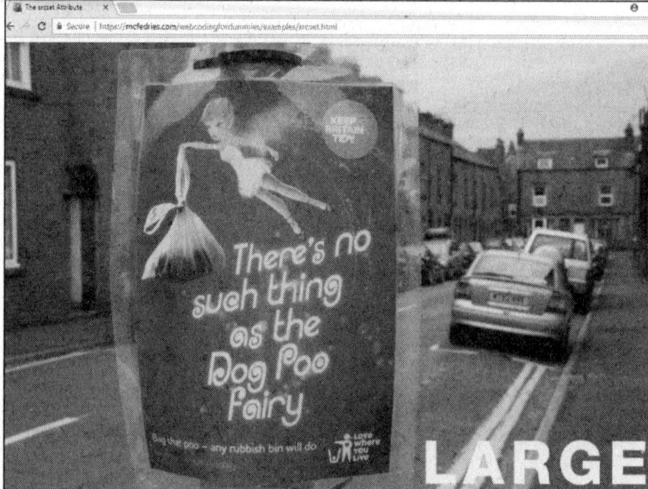

FIGURE 1-2: With the `<img>` tag's `sizes` and `srcset` attributes on the job, the browser serves up different versions of the image for different screen sizes.

Storing User Data in the Browser

I spend big chunks of this book talking about using MySQL to store data on the server, using PHP to access that data, and using JavaScript/jQuery Ajax calls to transfer data between the browser and the server. It's a robust and time-tested technique, but no sane person would describe it as trivial.

What's a web developer to do, then, when she wants to save just a few small or temporary tidbits of data for the current user? For example, perhaps her mobile web app enables each user to set custom background and text colors. That's just two pieces of data, so setting up the MySQL-PHP-Ajax edifice to store that data would be like building the Taj Mahal to store a few towels.

Fortunately, our developer doesn't have to embark on a major construction job to save small amounts of data for each user. Instead, she can take advantage of a technology called *web storage* that enables her to store data for each user right in that person's web browser.

Understanding web storage

Web storage is possible via an HTML5 technology called the Web Storage API (application programming interface), which defines two properties of the `window` object:

- `localStorage`: A storage space created within the web browser for your domain (meaning that only your local code can access this storage). Data within this storage can't be larger than 5MB. This data resides permanently in the browser until you delete it.
- `sessionStorage`: The same as `localStorage`, except that the data persists only for the current browser session. That is, the data is erased when the user closes the browser window.

It's also possible for users to delete web storage data by using their browser's command for removing website data. If your mobile web app really needs its user data to be permanent (or, at least, completely under your control), then you need to store it on the server.

Both `localStorage` and `sessionStorage` do double-duty as objects that implement several methods that your code can use to add, retrieve, and delete user data. Each data item is stored as a key-value pair.

Adding data to storage

You add data to web storage using the `setItem()` method:

```
localStorage.setItem(key, value)
sessionStorage.setItem(key, value)
```

- *key*: A string that specifies the key for the web storage item.
- *value*: The value associated with the web storage key. The value can be a string, number, Boolean, or object. Note, however, that web storage can only store strings, so any value you specify will be converted to a string when it's stored.

Here's an example:

```
localStorage.setItem('bgcolor', '#ba55d3');
```

It's common to store a collection of related key-value pairs as a JSON string. For example, suppose you collect your data into a JavaScript object:

```
var userData = {
    bgcolor: "#ba55d3'",
    fgcolor: "#f8f8f8",
    subscriber: true,
    level: 3
}
```

Before you can add such an object to web storage, you have to *stringify* it — that is, turn it into a JSON string — using the `JSON.stringify()` method:

```
localStorage.setItem('user-settings', JSON.stringify(userData));
```

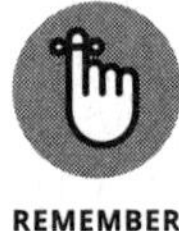

REMEMBER

When you store user data using web storage, that data is only available to the user in the same web browser running on the same device. For example, if you save data for a user running, say, Safari on an iPhone, when he returns to your site using, say, Chrome on a desktop computer, that data will not be available to him. Therefore, a good reason for going to the trouble to store user data on the server is that this makes the data available no matter what browser or device the user brings to your site.

Getting data from web storage

To retrieve an item from web storage, use the `getItem()` method:

```
localStorage.getItem(key)
sessionStorage.getItem(key)
```

» *key:* A string that specifies the key for the storage item

Here's an example:

```
var userBG = localStorage.getItem('bgcolor');
```

If you stored a JavaScript object as a JSON string, use `JSON.parse()` to restore the object:

```
var userData = JSON.parse(localStorage.getItem('user-
  settings'));
```

Removing data from web storage

If you no longer require data in web storage, use the `removeItem()` method to delete it:

```
localStorage.removeItem(key)
sessionStorage.removeItem(key)
```

» *key:* A string that specifies the key for the storage item

Here's an example:

```
localStorage.removeItem('bgcolor');
```

If you want to start fresh and delete everything from web storage, use the `clear()` method:

```
localStorage.clear();
sessionStorage.clear();
```

IN THIS CHAPTER

- » Building a mobile web app from the ground up
- » Putting a few jQuery Mobile widgets through their paces
- » Setting up the app's structure with HTML
- » Defining the look of the app with CSS
- » Making the app do something useful with JavaScript and jQuery

Chapter 2 Building a Mobile Web App

Learning the art of programming, like most other disciplines, consists of first learning the rules and then learning when to break them.

— JOSHUA BLOCH

In this chapter, I show you how to build an app that's designed for the mobile web. In particular, my goal here is to build an app that satisfies three of the most common criteria in mobile web app development. For starters, the app must work well first and foremost on a smartphone. That is, it must be a mobile-first design, as I describe in Book 8, Chapter 1. Second, the app must look at least a little like the so-called native apps that are available in the App Store for iOS and Google Play for Android. Although the code will live on the web, this isn't a website we're building, it's a web app, so it should look applike. Our new friend jQuery Mobile, which I introduce in Book 8, Chapter 1, will help with that. Finally, the app should be self-contained, meaning that it doesn't require a back end either to get the data it requires or to save any data that the user creates.

All of this might sound limiting, but constraints are the essence of creativity and can be liberating in the sense that they focus your attention on a smaller subset of what's possible. You'll be amazed at the incredible things you can build on even the smallest web development canvas. The screens you're coding for might be small, but that doesn't mean your ambitions can't be big.

Building the Button Builder App

The example I demonstrate in this chapter is called Button Builder, and it's a mobile web app that generates the CSS code for a button. That might strike you a tad trivial at first blush, but creating beautiful and unique buttons isn't easy. For example, here's some typical button code:

```
.btn {
    background-color: hsl(0, 68%, 30%);
    background-image: linear-gradient(to bottom, hsl(0, 68%,
  50%) 0%, hsl(0, 68%, 30%) 100%);
    border-color: hsl(0, 0%, 0%);
    border-radius: 10px;
    border-style: solid;
    border-width: 3px;
    color: hsl(0, 0%, 100%);
    font-family: Verdana, sans-serif;
    font-size: 1.25rem;
    font-style: normal;
    font-variant: normal;
    font-weight: normal;
    letter-spacing: 1.5px;
    padding-bottom: 10px;
    padding-left: 20px;
    padding-right: 20px;
    padding-top: 7px;
}
.btn:hover {
    background-color: hsl(0, 68%, 30%);
    background-image: linear-gradient(to bottom, hsl(0, 68%,
  30%) 0%, hsl(0, 68%, 50%) 100%);
}
```

There are no less than 19 CSS declarations here, and getting them to work in harmony to create a pleasing button is no easy task. The app I'm going to build makes button production a snap by offering controls such as text boxes, sliders, and color pickers to change a button's properties and display the results — and the underlying CSS code — in real time.

Getting Some Help from the Web

The Button Builder app has two features that require some attention from the start:

- **Color pickers:** I need color pickers for the button's text, background, and border colors. Unfortunately, as I write this, the standard HTML5 color picker (that is, an `<input>` tag with `type="color"`) doesn't work in iOS, so I need an alternative. My favorite third-party color picker is Spectrum, written by Brian Grinstead. It's simple, small, and works perfectly in all browsers. You can download it from `http://bgrins.github.io/spectrum`, and then include the files `spectrum.css` and `spectrum.js` in your project.
- **Copy to clipboard:** Button Builder will have a Copy the Button CSS command, which copies the CSS code to the device clipboard, enabling you to then paste the code into a text editor, an email message, or wherever you need it. One of the most popular tools for enabling this copying feature is Clipboard.js. You can either download it from `https://clipboardjs.com` and then include the file `clipboard.min.js` in your project, or you can use one of the content delivery networks (CDNs) that are linked from the Clipboard.js page.

Building the App: HTML

Building a Mobile Web App

The Button Builder app, like most mobile web apps, consists of just a single page: `index.html`. In the next few sections, I go through the process of building the HTML for this page.

Setting up the home page skeleton

To get started, set up the skeleton for the page. Here's the top part of the page:

```
<!DOCTYPE html>
<html lang="en">
<head>
    <meta charset="utf-8">
    <meta name="viewport" content="width=device-width,
  initial-scale=1.0">
    <title>Button Builder</title>
```

```
  <!-- External CSS Files -->
  <link
href="https://fonts.googleapis.com/css?family=Source+
Sans+Pro:400,700|Source+Code+Pro|" rel="stylesheet">
  <link
href="https://ajax.googleapis.com/ajax/libs/
jquerymobile/1.4.5/jquery.mobile.css" rel="stylesheet">
  <link href="css/spectrum.css" rel="stylesheet">
  <link href="css/styles.css" rel="stylesheet">

  <!-- External JavaScript Files -->
  <script
src="https://ajax.googleapis.com/ajax/libs/jquery/2.2.4/
jquery.min.js"></script>
  <script
src="https://ajax.googleapis.com/ajax/libs/jquerymobile/1.4.5/
jquery.mobile.min.js"></script>
  <script src="js/spectrum.js"></script>
  <script src="js/clipboard.min.js"></script>
  <script src="js/code.js"></script>

  <!-- Custom CSS for the button will appear here -->
  <style id="button-css" type="text/css">
  </style>

  <script>

      $(document).ready(function() {

      });
  </script>
</head>
```

There are four main sections to note here:

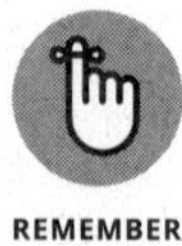

REMEMBER

- The external CSS files include a couple of Google fonts (Source Sans Pro and Source Code Pro), the jQuery Mobile CSS, the Spectrum CSS, and the app's CSS (`styles.css`).
- The external JavaScript files include the jQuery and jQuery Mobile libraries, the code for Spectrum and Clipboard.js, and the app's JavaScript (`code.js`).

- The `<style>` tag is where the app writes the custom CSS for the button. Note that this tag gets overwritten by the app, so if you want to store any CSS in a `<style>` tag, you need to create a separate `style` element.
- The `<script>` tag includes jQuery's standard `ready` event handler, which is where the app initialization and event handlers will reside.

Here's the rest of `index.html`:

```
<body>
    <main role="main" data-role="page" class="ui-responsive-
  panel">
        <header data-role="header" data-position="fixed">
        </header>
        <article role="contentinfo" class="ui-content">
        </article>
        <aside id="menu-panel" role="complementary" data-
  role="panel" data-display="overlay" data-theme="a">
        </aside>
    </main>
</body>
</html>
```

Within the `<body>` tag, there are four elements you should note:

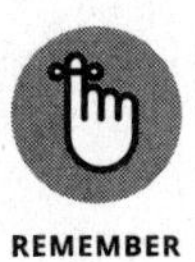

REMEMBER

- `main`: Holds all the HTML for the app. Note, in particular, that it has the attribute value `data-role="page"`. The `data-role` attribute is used by jQuery Mobile to specify what type of widget to apply to an HTML element. A Page widget is the main container for a jQuery Mobile app. The class `ui-responsive-panel` sets up the page as a responsive panel, meaning it accommodates any screen size and includes a "hamburger" button that, when tapped or clicked, reveals a menu of options.
- `header`: Defines a header at the top of the screen. In Button Builder, the header will hold the app title, the menu button, and the button preview. Adding `data-position="fixed"` configures the header to stay on screen even when the user scrolls vertically.
- `article`: Holds the app's content. For Button Builder, this will be a series of jQuery Mobile Collapsible widgets that hold the controls that enable the user to build a custom button.
- `aside`: Holds the app's menu commands. It's a jQuery Mobile Panel widget that appears when the user taps or clicks the menu button in the header. Setting `data-display` to `overlay` means the menu slides in on top of the main panel. Other display modes you could try are `push` and `reveal`.

Configuring the header

Here's the HTML for the app's `header` element:

```
<header data-role="header" data-position="fixed">
    <h1>Button Builder</h1>
    <a href="#menu-panel" data-icon="bars" data-iconpos="left"
  style="height: 3rem; background-color: #e8e8e8; border: none;
  box-shadow: none;"></a>
    <div id="button-preview" class="control-row button-preview-
  wrapper">
        <label for="built-button">Preview:</label>
        <div id="built-button" class="btn">Button</div>
    </div>
</header>
```

There are three elements to note:

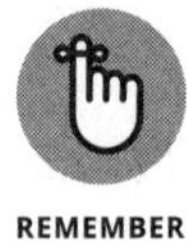

REMEMBER

- `h1`: Defines the app title.
- a: Defines the button that the user clicks to display the menu. The `href` attribute links to the ID (`menu-panel`) of the aside that contains the menu commands. The `data-icon` attribute adds a built-in jQuery Mobile icon: In this case, `bars` is the three horizontal lines that have come to be known as the *hamburger* icon.
- `div`: Holds the text `Preview:` and a nested `div` that the app uses to apply the custom CSS, which is applied to the `btn` class.

Figure 2-1 shows the app header.

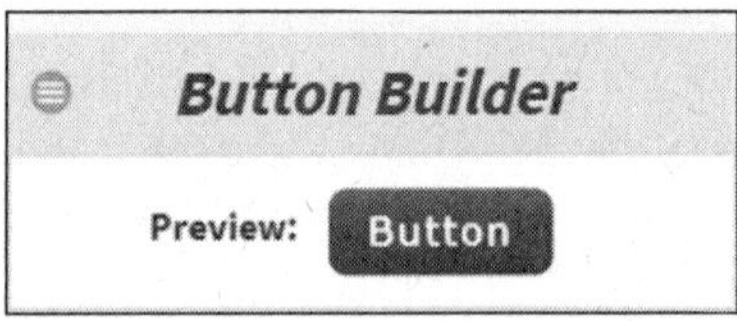

FIGURE 2-1: The Button Builder header showing the app title, menu icon, and a preview of the custom button.

TIP

To eyeball the complete list of jQuery Mobile icons, see `http://api.jquerymobile.com/icons`.

Creating the app menu

Here's the HTML for the app's menu:

```
<aside id="menu-panel" role="complementary" data-role="panel"
    data-display="overlay" data-theme="a">
      <ul data-role="listview">
          <li data-icon="delete"><a href="#" data-
    rel="close">Close menu</a></li>
              <li data-icon="check"><a id="save-button"
    href="#" data-rel="close">Save Your Button</a></li>
              <li data-icon="action"><a id="copy-button"
    href="#" data-rel="close">Copy the Button CSS</a></li>
              <li data-icon="recycle"><a id="reset-button"
    href="#" data-rel="close">Reset the Button CSS</a></li>
      </ul>
</aside>
```

Note, in particular, the nested `<ul>` tag, which is configured as a jQuery Mobile ListView widget. This displays each `li` element as an item in a vertical list, as shown in Figure 2-2, which shows the menu that appears when the user clicks or taps the menu icon.

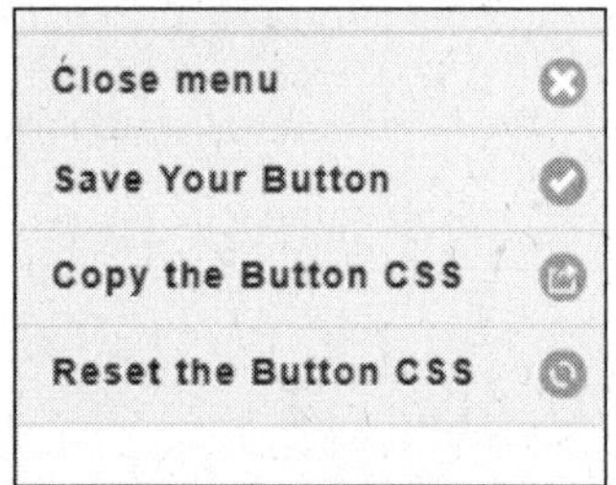

FIGURE 2-2: The Button Builder menu.

Adding the app's controls

Now it's time to populate the app with the actual controls for manipulating the button to get the look you want. The app divides the controls into four sections:

- **Text Styles:** Customizes the button text, especially the typography
- **Box Styles:** Customizes the button's box model, especially the padding and border

- **Color Styles:** Customizes the button's text, background, and border colors
- **CSS Code:** Displays the custom CSS created by the preceding controls

Each of these sections is a jQuery Mobile Collapsible widget, which is a useful mobile web app tool because it enables you to place a large amount of content onto a page, but hides that content behind section headings. When the user taps or clicks a heading, the content is revealed.

Here's the skeleton code that creates these Collapsible widgets:

```
<div id="text-settings-collapsible" data-role="collapsible"
  data-inset="false">
    <h2>Text Styles</h2>
    <section>
    </section>
</div>

<!-- Box Settings -->
<div id="box-settings-collapsible" data-role="collapsible"
  data-inset="false">
    <h2>Box Styles</h2>
    <section>
    </section>
</div>

<!-- Color Settings -->
<div id="color-settings-collapsible" data-role="collapsible"
  data-inset="false">
    <h2>Color Styles</h2>
    <section>
    </section>
</div>

<!-- CSS Code -->
<div id="css-code-collapsible" data-role="collapsible" data-
  inset="false">
    <h2>CSS Code</h2>
    <section id="css-code" class="css-code">
    </section>
</div>
```

Some notes:

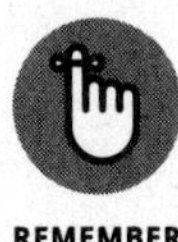

REMEMBER

- Each `div` element is given a `data-role` value of `collapsible`, which tells jQuery Mobile to configure the `div` as a Collapsible widget. These widgets normally have margins around them, but adding `data-inset="false"` tells jQuery Mobile to do without those margins.
- Each `<h2>` tag defines the text that appears in the header of each Collapsible widget.
- The `section` elements are where the app's controls will appear. The exception here is the `css-code` section, which the app itself populates with the generated CSS for the custom button.

Figure 2-3 shows the app with the Collapsible widgets added.

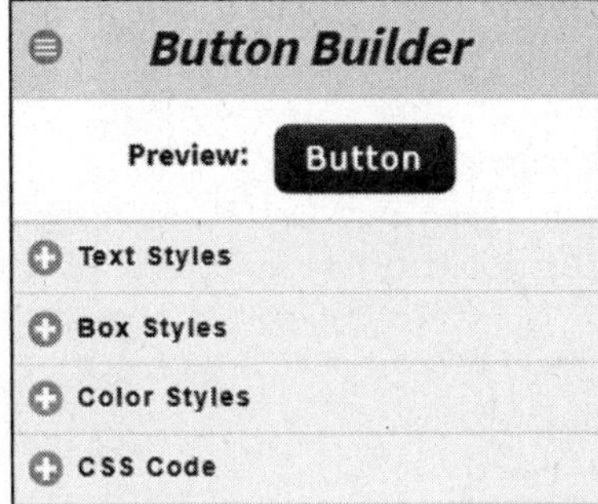

FIGURE 2-3: Button Builder with the Collapsible widget sections added.

Adding the text controls

Here's the HTML I used for the Text Styles section:

```
<h2>Text Styles</h2>
<section>
    <div class="control-row">
        <label for="button-text">Button text:</label>
        <input id="button-text" type="text" value="Button"
  aria-label="Enter the button text">
    </div>
    <div class="control-row">
        <label for="font-family">Font family:</label>
        <select id="font-family" data-role="selectmenu" aria-
  label="Select a font family">
```

Building a Mobile Web App

```
            <option value="Arial, sans-serif">Arial</option>
            <option value="Tahoma, sans-serif">Tahoma</option>
            <option value="'Trebuchet MS', sans-serif">Trebuchet
MS</option>
            <option value="Verdana, sans-serif">Verdana</option>
            <option value="Georgia, serif">Georgia</option>
            <option value="Palatino, serif">Palatino</option>
            <option value="'Times New Roman', serif">Times New
Roman</option>
            <option value="'Courier New', monospace">Courier
New</option>
        </select>
  </div>
  <div class="control-row">
        <label for="font-size">Font size (rem):</label>
        <input id="font-size" type="range" min="0.5" max="3"
step=".05" data-unit="rem" aria-label="Select a font size in
rems">
  </div>
  <div class="control-row">
        <label for="letter-spacing">Letter spacing (px):</label>
        <input id="letter-spacing" type="range" min="0" max="6"
step=".05" data-unit="px" aria-label="Select the letter
spacing in pixels">
  </div>
  <div class="control-row">
        <label for="font-weight">Bold:</label>
        <select id="font-weight" data-role="flipswitch" aria-
label="Toggle bold on and off">
            <option value="normal">Off</option>
            <option value="bold">On</option>
        </select>
  </div>
  <div class="control-row">
        <label for="font-style">Italic:</label>
        <select id="font-style" data-role="flipswitch" aria-
label="Toggle italics on and off">
            <option value="normal">Off</option>
            <option value="italic">On</option>
        </select>
  </div>
  <div class="control-row">
```

```
        <label for="font-variant">Small caps:</label>
        <select id="font-variant" data-role="flipswitch" aria-
    label="Toggle small caps on and off">
            <option value="normal">Off</option>
            <option value="small-caps">On</option>
        </select>
    </div>
</section>
```

There are seven controls here:

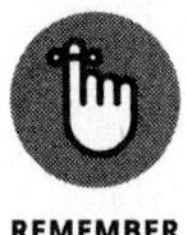

- **Button text:** The text that appears on the button face.
- **Font family:** The typeface for the button text (CSS property: `font-family`). This `select` element is given a `data-role` value of `selectmenu`, which turns it into a jQuery Mobile SelectMenu widget.
- **Font size:** The type size, measured in rems (CSS property: `font-size`). When you give an `input` element a `type` value of `range`, jQuery Mobile automatically enhances the input with a Slider widget, which enables the user to drag the slider to set the input value.
- **Letter spacing:** The space between the button text letters, measured in pixels (CSS property: `letter-spacing`).
- **Bold:** Toggles bold on and off (CSS property: `font-weight`). The `data-role` value of `flipswitch` turns this `select` into a jQuery Mobile FlipSwitch widget, which enables the user to choose between two values by tapping to "flip" the switch. The standard values are `On` and `Off`, but you can use the `option` elements' `value` attributes to set custom values (`normal` and `bold`, in this case).
- **Italic:** Toggles italics on and off (CSS property: `font-style`).
- **Small caps:** Toggles small caps on and off (CSS property: `font-variant`).

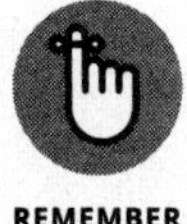

Note here that most of the controls use `id` values that are the same as the associated CSS property. For example, the `id` value of the Font Size control is `font-size`. As I describe a bit later, this makes it easy for the app's code to know which CSS property to generate for each control.

When the user taps Text Styles, the controls shown in Figure 2-4 appear.

Building a Mobile Web App

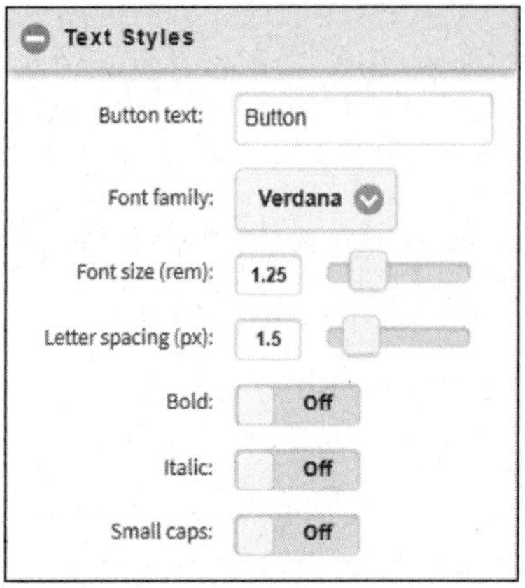

FIGURE 2-4: The controls in Button Builder's Text Styles section.

Adding the box controls

Check out the HTML code for the Box Styles section:

```
<h2>Box Styles</h2>
<section>
    <div class="control-row">
        <label for="padding-top">Padding top (px):</label>
        <input id="padding-top" type="range" min="0" max="60"
  step="1" data-unit="px"aria-label="Enter the top padding">
    </div>
    <div class="control-row">
        <label for="padding-right">Padding right (px):</label>
        <input id="padding-right" type="range" min="0" max="60"
  step="1" data-unit="px"aria-label="Enter the right padding">
    </div>
    <div class="control-row">
        <label for="padding-bottom">Padding bottom (px):</label>
        <input id="padding-bottom" type="range" min="0" max="60"
  step="1" data-unit="px"aria-label="Enter the bottom padding">
    </div>
    <div class="control-row">
        <label for="padding-left">Padding left (px):</label>
        <input id="padding-left" type="range" min="0" max="60"
  step="1" data-unit="px"aria-label="Enter the left padding">
    </div>
    <div class="control-row">
        <label for="border-radius">Border radius (px):</label>
        <input id="border-radius" type="range" min="0" max="25"
  step="1" data-unit="px"aria-label="Enter the border radius">
    </div>
```

```
    <div class="control-row">
        <label for="border-width">Border width (px):</label>
        <input id="border-width" type="range" min="0" max="10"
  step="1" data-unit="px" aria-label="Enter the border width">
    </div>
    <div class="control-row">
        <label for="border-style">Border style:</label>
        <select id="border-style" data-role="selectmenu" aria-
  label="Select a border style">
            <option value="solid">solid</option>
            <option value="dashed">dashed</option>
            <option value="dotted">dotted</option>
            <option value="double">double</option>
        </select>
    </div>
</section>
```

The first four controls set the padding values, in pixels (CSS properties: `padding-top`, `padding-right`, `padding-bottom`, and `padding-left`). The next two controls set the border radius, in pixels (CSS property: `border-radius`), and the border width, in pixels (CSS property: `border-width`). The Border Style `select` element sets the border style (CSS property: `border-style`).

Figure 2-5 shows the Box Styles section.

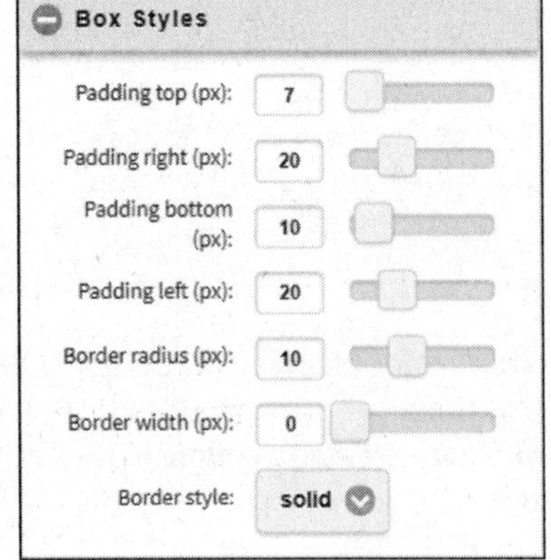

FIGURE 2-5: The controls in Button Builder's Box Styles section.

Adding the color controls

Here's the HTML code that populates Button Builder's Color Styles section:

```
<h2>Color Styles</h2>
<section>
    <div class="control-row">
        <label for="color">Text color:</label>
        <input id="color" type="text" aria-label="Select a text
  color">
    </div>
    <div class="control-row">
        <label for="background-color">Background color:</label>
        <input id="background-color" type="text" aria-
  label="Select a background color">
    </div>
    <div class="control-row">
        <label for="border-color">Border color:</label>
        <input id="border-color" type="text" aria-label="Select
  a border color">
    </div>
    <div class="control-row">
        <label for="gradient">Gradient:</label>
        <input id="gradient" type="checkbox" data-
  role="flipswitch" aria-label="Toggle the background gradient
  on or off" checked>
    </div>
    <div class="control-row">
        <label for="hover">Hover effect:</label>
        <input id="hover" type="checkbox" data-role="flipswitch"
  aria-label="Toggle the hover effect on or off" checked>
    </div>
</section>
```

This section uses three Spectrum color pickers: Text Color (CSS property: `text-color`), Background Color (CSS property: `background-color`), and Border Color (CSS property: `border-color`). There are also a couple of jQuery Mobile FlipSwitch widgets that toggle two effects:

- **Gradient:** When On, applies a gradient effect to the button's background color (CSS property: `background-image`)
- **Hover effect:** When On, adds the `.btn-hover` class to the CSS, which swaps the gradient colors when the user hovers the pointer over the button

USING HUE, SATURATION, AND LUMINANCE TO SPECIFY CSS COLORS

TECHNICAL STUFF

In the Button Builder app, I define most of the colors using the *HSL* method, which uses the following three components:

- **Hue:** Specifies a position, in degrees, on the color wheel. Acceptable values are between 0 and 359, where lower numbers indicate a position near the red end of the spectrum (with red equal to 0 degrees), and higher numbers move through the yellow, green, blue, and violet parts of the spectrum. Hue is pretty much equivalent to the term *color*.
- **Saturation:** Sets a given hue's purity, expressed as a percentage. 100% means that the hue is a pure color, whereas lower numbers indicate that more gray is mixed with the hue until, at 0%, the color becomes part of the grayscale.
- **Luminance:** Sets the hue's brightness, as a percentage. Lower percentages are darker (with 0% producing black), and higher numbers are brighter (with 100% creating white).

To apply the HSL method in CSS, use the `hsl()` function as the value of a color property (such as `text-color` or `background-color`):

```
hsl(hue, saturation, luminance)
```

- *`hue`*: Specifies the hue with a value between 0 and 359.
- *`saturation`*: Specifies the saturation with a value between 0% and 100%.
- *`luminance`*: Specifies the luminance with a value between 0% and 100%.

I used HSL in Button Builder because it helps to simplify both the gradient and hover effects:

- For the gradient, I set the bottom color to be the same as the background color, and then I defined the top color to be the background color with the luminance reduced by 20 percentage points (from 50% to 30%):

```
background-color: hsl(0, 68%, 30%);
background-image: linear-gradient(to bottom, hsl(0, 68%, 50%)
   0%, hsl(0, 68%, 30%) 100%);
```

- For the hover, I reversed the top and bottom colors in the gradient:

```
background-color: hsl(0, 68%, 30%);
background-image: linear-gradient(to bottom, hsl(0, 68%, 30%)
   0%, hsl(0, 68%, 50%) 100%);
```

Building a Mobile Web App

Figure 2-6 shows the controls in the Color Styles section.

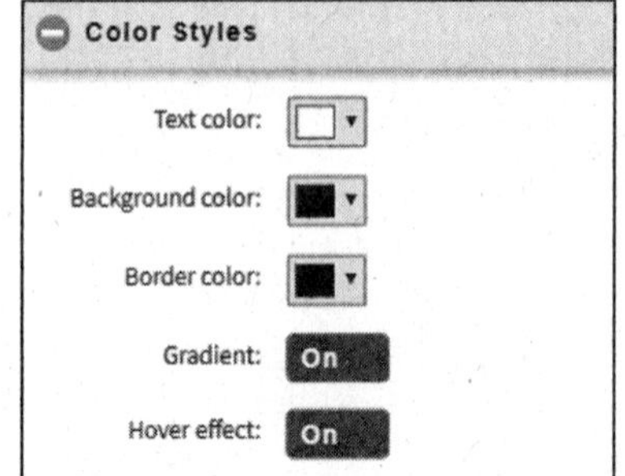

FIGURE 2-6: The controls in Button Builder's Color Styles section.

Building the App: CSS

Most of the heavy lifting for the Button Builder CSS is handled by jQuery Mobile, so the custom CSS mostly involves either app-specific rules or tweaks to the jQuery Mobile styles.

I begin with a standard CSS reset:

```
* {
    box-sizing: border-box;
}
body{
    margin: 0 auto;
    padding: 0;
    font-weight: normal;
    font-style: normal;
    font-size: 100%;
}
```

From there, I set up a few rules for some of the page elements:

```
html,
body {
    font-family: 'Source Sans Pro', Verdana, sans-serif;
    overflow-x: hidden;
}
```

```
main {
    padding-top: 0 !important;
}
h1, h2 {
    font-family: 'Source Sans Pro', Verdana, sans-serif;
    font-weight: bold;
}
label {
    font-family: 'Source Sans Pro', Verdana, sans-serif;
}
a {
    letter-spacing: 1.5px;
}
```

This is mostly typography, but I set `overflow-x: hidden` on the `html` and `body` elements to prevent horizontal scrolling on narrow devices.

Next I style a few app classes:

```
.button-preview-wrapper {
    border-top: 2px solid #ddd;
    padding: 1rem 0;
    background-color: #fff;
}
.button-preview-wrapper label {
    font-size: 1.25rem;
    font-weight: bold;
}
.control-row {
    display: flex;
    align-items: center;
}
.control-row label {
    width: 40%;
    margin-right: 1rem;
    text-align: right;
}
.css-code {
    font-family: 'Source Code Pro', 'Courier New', monospace;
    white-space: pre;
    overflow-x: auto;
}
```

These classes style the button preview `div`, the rows used to display each control, and the appearance of the CSS code.

From there I add a few tweaks to the jQuery Mobile classes:

```
.ui-header .ui-title {
    margin: 0;
    padding: .5rem 0;
    color: hsl(217, 66%, 32%);
    font-size: 2rem;
    font-style: italic;
    overflow: visible;
}
.ui-input, ui-input-text {
    width: 100%;
}
.ui-flipswitch .ui-btn.ui-flipswitch-on {
    text-indent: -3.6em;
}
.ui-flipswitch .ui-flipswitch-off {
    margin-top: -2rem;
    text-indent: 3em;
}
.ui-slider-track {
    width: 125%;
    touch-action: none
}
```

This is mostly just fiddling with properties to get things looking good. However, note the `text-indent` and `margin-top` values applied to the `ui-flipswitch` class. These are necessary to get the FlipSwitch widget to display the text values properly. You might have to fiddle with these in your own code.

Finally, because this is a mobile-first app, I added a media query to handle screens with widths greater than or equal to 800px:

```
@media (min-width: 800px) {
    .ui-mobile-viewport,
    .ui-header,
    .ui-content
     {
        width: 800px !important;
        margin: 0 auto !important;
    }
}
```

All this code does is set the width of the app's three main jQuery Mobile areas to 800px and center them within the viewport with `margin: 0 auto`.

Building the App: JavaScript and jQuery

With the app's HTML structure in place and the CSS styles making everything look respectable, it's time to wire everything together with JavaScript and jQuery.

A mobile web app that uses internal data will often need to perform four tasks using that data:

REMEMBER

- Initialize the data.
- Use the data to set the value of each of the app's controls.
- Get the values from the app's controls and store them in the app's data structure.
- Generate the app's output from the data.

The specifics of these tasks are covered in the next four sections.

Setting up the app data structures

Like many mobile web apps, Button Builder doesn't require data from a server. Instead, it uses its own internal data structures to store four chunks of button-related data:

- The button text
- Whether the button has a gradient (`true` or `false`)
- Whether the button uses a hover effect (`true` or `false`)
- The button's CSS property-value pairs

I use two JavaScript objects to store the data: one that holds the default button data and one that holds the custom button data generated by the user. Here's the code that defines the default button data:

```
var defaultButton = {};
defaultButton.text = 'Button';
defaultButton.gradient = true;
```

```
defaultButton.hover = true;
defaultButton.styles = {};
defaultButton.styles['background-color'] = 'hsl(0, 68%, 30%)';
defaultButton.styles['background-image'] = 'linear-gradient(to
   bottom, hsl(0, 68%, 50%) 0%, hsl(0, 68%, 30%) 100%)';
defaultButton.styles['border-color'] = 'hsl(0, 0%, 0%)';
defaultButton.styles['border-radius'] = '10px';
defaultButton.styles['border-style'] = 'solid';
defaultButton.styles['border-width'] = '0px';
defaultButton.styles['color'] = 'hsl(0, 0%, 100%)';
defaultButton.styles['font-family'] = 'Verdana, sans-serif';
defaultButton.styles['font-size'] = '1.25rem';
defaultButton.styles['font-style'] = 'normal';
defaultButton.styles['font-variant'] = 'normal';
defaultButton.styles['font-weight'] = 'normal';
defaultButton.styles['letter-spacing'] = '1.5px';
defaultButton.styles['padding-bottom'] = '10px';
defaultButton.styles['padding-left'] = '20px';
defaultButton.styles['padding-right'] = '20px';
defaultButton.styles['padding-top'] = '7px';
```

Notice that the object's `styles` property is itself an object.

For the custom button, the app declares the following:

```
var customButton = {};
customButton.styles = {};
```

Setting the app's control values

You could initialize the app's controls by adding `value` attributes where appropriate, but it's almost always better to set up a default data object and then use that object to populate the controls via code. That way, if you decide to change the defaults, you need only edit the object's values. Also, if your app offers a "reset" feature, as does Button Builder, then you can also use the default data to perform the reset.

Here's the function that sets the Button Builder's control values:

```
function setButtonValues(button) {

    // Set the Button Text value
    $('input[id=button-text]').val(button.text);
    $('input[id=button-text]').textinput('refresh', true);
```

```
  // Set the Gradient value
  if (button.gradient) {
      $('input[id=gradient]').prop('checked', true);
  } else {
      $('input[id=gradient]').prop('checked', false);
  }
  $('input[id=gradient]').flipswitch('refresh', true);

  // Set the Hover value
  if (button.hover) {
      $('input[id=hover]').prop('checked', true);
  } else {
      $('input[id=hover]').prop('checked', false);
  }
  $('input[id=hover]').flipswitch('refresh', true);

  // Loop through the styles
  for (var propertyName in button.styles) {

      // Skip the background-image property, which doesn't
have a setting
      if (propertyName !== 'background-image') {

          // Set the control ID from the property name
          var propertyID = '#' + propertyName;

          // Get the current property value
          var propertyValue = button.styles[propertyName];

          // Is it a color property?
          if (propertyName.includes('color')) {

              // If so, apply the color to the color picker
              $(propertyID).spectrum('set', propertyValue);
          }
          // Otherwise, is the property associated with a
<select> tag?
          else if ($(propertyID)[0].tagName === 'SELECT') {

              // If so, is it a SelectMenu widget?
              if ($(propertyID).attr('data-role') ===
'selectmenu') {
                  // If so, set the SelectMenu's selected
option
```

Building a Mobile Web App

```
                  $('select[id=' + propertyName + '] >
option[value="' + propertyValue + '"]').attr('selected', true);
                  $('select[id=' + propertyName + ']').
selectmenu('refresh', true);
              } else {

                  // Otherwise, set the FlipSwitch's selected
option
                  $('select[id=' + propertyName + '] >
option[value="' + propertyValue + '"]').attr('selected', true);
                  $('select[id=' + propertyName + ']').
flipswitch('refresh', true);
              }
          } else {

              // For all other inputs, first remove the unit
(rem or px)
              propertyValue = propertyValue.replace(/rem|
px/, '');

              // Set the control's value
              $('input[id=' + propertyName + ']').
val(propertyValue);
              $('input[id=' + propertyName + ']').
textinput('refresh', true);
          }
      }
  }
}
```

This function takes a button object — which will either be `defaultButton` or `customButton` — as a parameter. The function begins by setting the values for the Button Text box and the Gradient and Hover switches. Notice that jQuery Mobile requires that I invoke a `refresh` event on a changed control. For example:

```
$('input[id=button-text]').textinput('refresh', true);
```

From there, the code loops through the object's `styles` sub-object, setting and then refreshing the controls depending on the control type.

Getting the app's control values

Before a mobile web app can generate any output, it needs to gather all the current values of the app's controls and then store them in the app data structure. Here's the Button Builder code that does this:

```
function getButtonValues() {

    // Reference all the controls (that is, all the <input> and
    <select> tags)
    var $controls = $('article').find('input, select');

    // Loop through all the controls
    $controls.each(function() {

        // In most cases, the ID of each setting is also the CSS
    property name
        var cssProperty = $(this).attr('id');

        // Use a switch() to handle the exceptions
        switch (cssProperty) {

            // Write the button text
            case 'button-text':

                // Get the user's button text
                var newButtonText  = $(this).val();

                // Apply the text to the button
                $('.btn').text(newButtonText);

                // Store the button text
                customButton.text = newButtonText;

                break;

            // Apply a gradient to the button background
            case 'gradient':

                // Is the Gradient Flipswitch widget set to On?
                if($('#gradient').prop('checked')) {

                    // Turn on the button's gradient flag
                    customButton.gradient = true;
                } else {
```

Building a Mobile Web App

```
            // Turn off the button's gradient flag
            customButton.gradient = false;
        }

        // Build the gradient CSS
        buildGradient(customButton);

        break;

    // Apply a hover effect to the button background
    case 'hover':

        // Is the Hover Flipswitch widget set to On?
        if($('#hover').prop('checked')) {

            // Turn on the button's hover flag
            customButton.hover = true;
        } else {

            // Turn off the button's hover flag
            customButton.hover = false;
        }

        // Build the hover CSS
        buildHover(customButton);

        break;

    // For everything else, store the property-value
    // pair in the customButton.styles object
    default:

        // First, check for a unit associated with the
property
        var unit = $(this).attr('data-unit');

        // Does the unit exist?
        if(unit !== null) {

            // If so, add it to the property value
            if(cssProperty === 'box-shadow') {
                customButton.styles[cssProperty] =
$(this).val() + unit + ' 3px 3px #666';
            } else {
```

```
                        customButton.styles[cssProperty] =
  $(this).val() + unit;
                    }
                } else {

                    // Otherwise, just store the property value
                    customButton.styles[cssProperty] = $(this).
  val();
                }
            }
        });
}
```

This function first sets up a jQuery reference to all the controls — that is, all the `<input>` and `<select>` tags. The code loops through these controls, getting the associated CSS property name from the control's `id` value, then using a `switch()` statement to handle the exceptions: the button text and the gradient and hover flags. The `default` case handles the actual CSS property-value pairs, and these are stored in the `customButton.styles` object.

Writing the custom CSS code

Here's the function that generates Button Builder's custom CSS code:

```
function generateButtonCode(button) {

    // Set the button text
    $('.btn').text(button.text);

    // Build the gradient code
    buildGradient(button);

    // Build the hover code
    buildHover(button);

    // Sort the styles by property name
    var alphaStyles = {};
    Object.keys(button.styles).sort().forEach(function
  (propertyName) {
        alphaStyles[propertyName] = button.styles[propertyName];
    });

    // Build the CSS string
    var strCSS = "\n.btn {\n";
```

```
    for (var propertyName in alphaStyles) {
        strCSS += TAB + propertyName + ": " +
  alphaStyles[propertyName] + ";\n";
    }
    strCSS += "}\n";
    strCSS += hoverStyles;

    // Add the code to the CSS Code section
    $('#css-code').text(strCSS);

    // Build the <style> tag
    var strStyleTag = '<style id="button-css" type="text/css">'
  + strCSS + '</style>';

    // Replace the current <style> tag with the new one
    $('#button-css').replaceWith(strStyleTag);

    // Adjust the <article> padding so that it clears the new
  header size
    $('article').css('padding-top', $('header').height() + 2);
}
```

This function takes a button object as a parameter, then generates the new button and CSS, as follows:

- The button text is updated.
- The new gradient effect is generated by calling the `buildGradient()` function (not shown), which creates and stores the `background-image` property-value pair.
- The new hover effect is generated by calling the `buildHover()` function (not shown), which creates the `.btn:hover` CSS rule.
- The button's `styles` object is sorted alphabetically by property name.
- The CSS rule for the `.btn` class is generated and then added to the CSS Code section of the app.
- The `.btn` and `.btn:hover` rules are embedded in a `<style>` tag, which is then used to replace the existing `<style id="button-css">` tag. Doing this refreshes the preview button with the new CSS rules.
- The `<article>` tag's `padding-top` property is adjusted to the `header` element's height, plus 2px, to ensure that as the preview button grows or shrinks (say, because of font size changes), the `header` and `article` remain in the same relative position to each other.

Running the code

How does the code for setting the control values, getting the control values, and generating the CSS code get called? This happens in `index.html`, as part of the jQuery `ready` event handler. The first time you run the app (and each subsequent time if no custom button has been saved), the initial button is generated by calling the following two functions using the `defaultButton` object as a parameter:

```
setButtonValues(defaultButton);
generateButtonCode(defaultButton);
```

To handle control changes, the app uses the following event handler:

```
$('input, select').on('blur change input keyup contextmenu',
  function(e) {

    // Prevent the default whatever
    e.preventDefault();

    // Get all the custom button values
    getButtonValues();

    // Write the CSS code
    generateButtonCode(customButton);
});
```

This handler listens for several event types on the `input` and `select` elements. If invoked, the handler prevents the default action, then runs the `getButtonValues()` and `generateButtonCode()` functions.

Saving the custom CSS

When the user taps or clicks Button Builder's Save Your Button command, the following event handler leaps into action:

```
$('#save-button').click(function() {

    // Get the button's control values
    getButtonValues();

    // Save them
    localStorage.setItem('button-builder-data', JSON.
  stringify(customButton));
});
```

This handler calls getButtonValues() to populate the customButton object, and it then uses the setItem() function to store a JSON stringified version of the object in localStorage.

You now need to update the app's ready event handler to check for a saved button:

```
var buttonData = localStorage.getItem('button-builder-data');

// Did we get anything back from localStorage?
if (buttonData) {

    // If so, objectify it and store it in our global
   customButton object
    customButton = JSON.parse(buttonData);

    // Apply the button's styles
    setButtonValues(customButton);
    generateButtonCode(customButton);
} else {

    // If not, build the button using the default CSS values
    setButtonValues(defaultButton);
    generateButtonCode(defaultButton);
}
```

First, the app checks for a saved button. If a saved button exists, the app gets the saved data, stores it as a JavaScript object in the customButton variable, and then calls setButtonValues() and generateButtonCode() to apply the saved button CSS. Otherwise, the default button code is used.

Copying the custom CSS

To handle Button Builder's Copy the Button CSS command, the ready event's callback function includes the following Clipboard.js code:

```
var buttonCSSClipboard = new Clipboard('#copy-button', {
    text: function(trigger) {
    var textToCopy = $('#css-code').text();
    return textToCopy;
    }
});
```

This binds a new `Clipboard` object to the Copy the Button CSS command (which has an `id` value of `copy-button`). When this command is tapped or clicked, Clipboard.js grabs the text from the CSS Code section and copies it to the device clipboard.

Resetting the CSS to the default

To handle Button Builder's Reset the Button CSS command, the `ready` event's callback function includes the following handler code:

```
$('#reset-button').click(function() {

    // Rebuild the button using the default CSS values
    setButtonValues(defaultButton);
    generateButtonCode(defaultButton);
});
```

This code resets the button's default CSS by invoking both the `setButtonValues()` and `generateButtonCode()` functions using the `defaultButton` object as the parameter.

Building a Mobile Web App

Index

Symbols

A

C

D

E

F

G

H

I

K

L

M

N

O

P

Q

R

S

T

U

V

W

X

Y

Z

About the Author

Paul McFedries is the president of Logophilia Limited, a technical writing company, and has worked with computers large and small since 1975. While now primarily a writer, Paul has worked as a programmer, consultant, database developer, and website developer. Paul has written more than 90 books that have sold over four million copies worldwide. Paul is also the proprietor of Word Spy (`wordspy.com`), a website that has been tracking recently coined words and phrases since 1995. Paul invites everyone to drop by his personal website at `mcfedries.com`, or to follow him on Twitter (@paulmcf and @wordspy).

Author's Acknowledgments

If we're ever at the same cocktail party and you overhear me saying something like "I wrote a book," I hereby give you permission to wag your finger at me and say "Tsk, tsk." Why the scolding? Because although I did write this book's text and take its screenshots, those represent only a part of what constitutes a "book." The rest of it is brought to you by the dedication and professionalism of Wiley's editing, graphics, and production teams, who toiled long and hard to turn my text and images into an actual book.

I offer my heartfelt thanks to everyone at Wiley who made this book possible, but I'd like to extend some special thank-yous to the folks I worked with directly: Executive Editor Steve Hayes, Project Manager Maureen Tullis, Project/Copy Editor Scott Tullis, and Technical Editor Matthew Fecher. I'd also like to give a big shout-out to my agent, Carole Jelen, for helping to make this project possible.

Dedication

Since this book will be published just before Mother's Day, it seems only right to dedicate it to my late mother, who spent nearly 90 years on this Earth bringing love to her family and friends and a light-up-the-room smile to everyone she met. She was more of a crossword solver than a web coder, but I know she'd appreciate having this book dedicated to her memory because she was always proud of her "wee son." Mum, you are missed.

Publisher's Acknowledgments

Executive Editor: Steve Hayes
Development/Copy Editor: Scott Tullis
Technical Editor: Matthew Fecher
Editorial Assistant: Matthew Lowe
Production Editor: Tamilmani Varadharaj
Project Manager: Maureen Tullis
Cover Image: © DrHitch/Shutterstock